Genetics of
Livestock Population

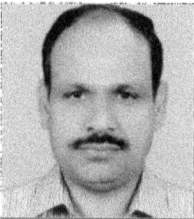

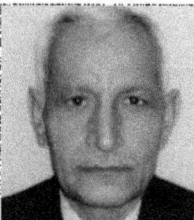

The Authors

Dr. Arun Kumar Tomar is B.Sc. (Ag.) and M.Sc. (Ag.) in A.H. and Dairying from J.V.College, Baraut, Bagpat (U.P.) and Ph.D. (Animal Breeding) from CCS, HAU, Hisar. He has worked in the capacity of Scientist (AGB) at C.S.W.R.I. Avikanagar (Rajasthan), Senior Scientist and Principal Scientist (AGB) at Project Directorate on Cattle, Meerut (U.P.). He is presently working as Head, Division of Animal Genetics and Breeding, Central Sheep and Wool Research Institute, Avikanagar, via Jaipur, Rajasthan. He has published some books and booklets and many research papers and has experience of editorial work in the capacity of Assistant Editor of Research Journal.

Professor Sukhvir Singh Tomar is B.Sc. (Ag.) and M.Sc. (Ag.) in A.H. and Dairying from J.V.College, Baraut, Bagpat (U.P.) and Ph.D. (A.G.B.) from N.D.R.I., Karnal. He started his career as Lecturer, J.V. College, Baraut (Meerut) and then at P.A.U, Hisar campus. Later on, he joined I.C.A.R. as Scientist (AGB) at C.S.W.R.I. and worked as Senior Scientist and Principal Scientist (AGB) at N.D.R.I., Karnal. He is now retired Principal Scientist (AGB) from N.D.R.I.,Karnal (I.C.A.R.) having 40 years of research experience making significant contribution in the area of Animal Breeding Research and teaching experience to M.Sc. and Ph.D. classes. He has published about 300 research articles and 3 text books on population genetics and animal breeding. He has long experience of about 28 years as Editor of Research Journal and guided a number of M.Sc. and Ph.D. students. He is still actively engaged in research and publication work.

The authors have published already a book on Animal Genetics and Breeding written as per syllabus of B.V.Sc. and A.H. and B.Sc. (Ag.) of Indian Agricultural Universities. The book has covered both the theory and practical problems.

Genetics of Livestock Population

Dr. Arun Kumar Tomar
M.Sc. (Ag.), Ph.D., A.R.S.
Head, Division of Animal Genetics and Breeding
Central Sheep and Wool Research Institute,
Avikanagar, via Jaipur
Rajasthan – 304 501

and

Prof. Sukhvir Singh Tomar
M.Sc. (Ag.), Ph.D., A.R.S.
Former Principal Scientist (AGB),
National Dairy Research Institute, Karnal

2015
Daya Publishing House®
A Division of
Astral International Pvt. Ltd.
New Delhi – 110 002

Cataloging in Publication Data--DK
Courtesy: D.K. Agencies (P) Ltd. <docinfo@dkagencies.com>

Tomar, Arun Kumar, author.
Genetics of livestock population / Dr. Arun Kumar Tomar, M.Sc. (Ag.), Ph.D., A.R.S. and Prof. Sukhvir Singh Tomar, M.Sc. (Ag.), Ph.D., A.R.S.

    pages   cm

ISBN 9789351306634 (International Edition)

1. Livestock--Genetics. 2. Animal population genetics. I. Tomar, Sukhvir Singh, author. II. Title.

DDC 636.0821   23

Published by   : **Daya Publishing House®**
                        A Division of
                        Astral International Pvt. Ltd.
                        – ISO 9001:2008 Certified Company –
                        4760-61/23, Ansari Road, Darya Ganj
                        New Delhi-110 002
                        Ph. 011-43549197, 23278134
                        E-mail: info@astralint.com
                        Website: www.astralint.com

Laser Typesetting   : **Classic Computer Services**, Delhi - 110 035

Printed at   : **Thomson Press India Limited**

PRINTED IN INDIA

Preface

The domestication has resulted to the evolutionary process of migration and selection together with the effect of small size of population and mating systems, and consequently has changed and shaped the genetic structure of animal population of domestic species. The study of the effect of evolutionary forces, population size and mating systems on the genetic variation in a population over space and time (generations) is the subject matter of population genetics. The genetic variation is studied in terms of population parameters which are character specific. These are the gene and genotype frequencies of different genetic systems of single locus with two alleles or multiple alleles present on autosomes or on sex chromosomes and two or more loci for qualitative characters, and the mean, variance and covariance for quantitative characters governed by polygenes together with partitioning of the phenotypic value and variance in to components corresponding to genetic and environmental factors using the biometrical techniques.

The population genetics was introduced at Post Graduate level almost with the commencement of SAU's in 1970's in the country. The subject matter of population genetics has been covered in different volumes of interest published abroad as well as in this country. However, the entire subject matter has not been covered in a single volume and that too as per syllabus of Post Graduate programme taught in Agricultural Universities in India. Therefore, it was felt the need of the day to compile the entire subject matter of population genetics from different published sources covering the theoretical and practical aspects and present in a simple and illustrative language in a single volume to meet the requirement.

The entire subject matter in this book has been covered in 3 parts comprising 27 chapters. The first part of 13 chapters has been devoted to the genetic structure of population in equilibrium state for different genetic systems and the changes occurred under the influence of evolutionary forces, population size and mating systems for qualitative characters. The second part comprises 10 chapters covering the partitioning of phenotypic value, variance and covariance of quantitative characters into different components attributed to additive and non-additive genetic effects. The last part of 4 chapters of the book deal with the biometrical techniques *viz.* univariate, bivariate and multivariate analysis and path analysis.

Hope this book will be of immense use to the post graduate students, teachers and those appearing in different All India Competitive Examinations like NET, SRF, and ARS conducted by ASRB (ICAR) as well as by UGC and UPSC. The subject matter has been presented in single volume in a more meaningful and desired manner and simple language with numerical examples. We do not claim any originality as the subject matter has been collected and compiled from various published sources of population genetics on both volumes of qualitative and quantitative inheritance. The authors are highly thankful to these sources.

The authors are highly thankful to Dr. R.M. Acharya, Dr. A.L. Chaudhary, and Dr. S.B. Basu for their valuable guidance, kind cooperation and help in one or the other way. Thanks are also due to Smt. Shakuntla Tomar, Dr. Ajay Kumar Tomar, Dr. Amit Kumar Tomar and other family members of the authors for their consistent encouragement and kind cooperation.

Further, we welcome the readers to point out the mistakes that are likely to be and to give suggestions for further improvement of the book.

Dr. Arun Kumar Tomar
Prof. Sukhvir Singh Tomar

Contents

Part I
Qualitative Inheritance

Chapter 1

Population Genetics

The study of genetic make up of a population is the subject matter of *Population genetics*. The genetic structure of a population is described for its equilibrium state under random mating assuming the population size to be so large that the sampling variation does not occur. The population genetics is an extension of Mendelian genetics with a difference that unit of study is the population. It is thus important to know the meaning of population before the details of genetic structure of population and then to know the importance of Population Genetics.

1.1 Concept and Definition of Population

In general, a population is a set of observations (measurements) on each individual of a group of animals, plants or any object. The observation or measurement of some quantitative property like body weight, milk yield, etc. are recorded on all individuals.

Biologically, a population refers to a group of living individuals of a species living and functioning together as a unit at a place and time.

Genetically, a population has a different concept in that the population is defined as a group of interbreeding individuals. As a result of interbreeding there is gene exchange among the individuals of the population and hence they contribute to the gene pool of the progeny generation. The gene exchange is thus the main and important factor to define a population. Therefore, a population does not accommodate the organisms reproducing asexually and by selfing because they do not share the common gene pool.

Dobzhansky (1951) thus defined a population as a reproducing group of sexual and cross fertilized individuals sharing a common gene pool.

A population geneticist considers the population as the *"Mendelian Population"* which is defined as a *group of interbreeding individuals developed over both space and time* sharing a common pool of genes, from which meaningful samples can be drawn and within which the characteristics under study follow the Mendelian rules of inheritance.

Now, it would be better to know about the gene pool and the individual. The *gene pool* is taken as the sum total of genes in a population. In other words, the gene pool includes collectively all the genetic information distributed among all the individuals of a population. The individual is a unit of population which by forming the group constitutes the population.

1.2 Limits of Population

Considering the interbreeding among the individuals of a population, a species as a whole represents Mendelian population, provided the breeding is actually or potentially occurring among all the individuals of the species, particularly considering the stages in evolutionary divergence. Therefore, a species is the largest population when all the members of that species interbred among themselves and hence share a common gene pool. Therefore, in population genetics, a *species is considered as the upper limit of population.* The groups larger than a species like sub genera and genera can not form a Mendelian population because interbreeding with another species is rare and the mating, though possible, result in sub fertile or sterile offspring,

The interbreeding among all the individuals of a species is not possible for certain reasons and hence the entire species can not be considered as a population. Therefore, a population is considered at lower level (limit). *The lower (limit of a population may be a subspecies, breed, strains within breed (e.g.* H.F., British Friesian, Canadian Friesian, Dutch Friesian), *lines within strain* (mostly in case of *poultry breeding*) *and herds* within which mating is occurring. Therefore, a population includes all animals within a large group or geographical area. It may refer to all members of a species or breed within a defined area. However, the animals of a temporary gathering, such us the animals brought in animal shows and auctions, do not constitute a Mendelian population, for the reason that such animals do not interbred.

1.3 Size of Population

It is not possible to examine all individuals of a population to know their genetic characteristics for the reason that population is normally very large. Therefore, a small group is taken under study as a measure of the characteristics of the larger population. This small group is called the sample.

The numbers of individuals constituting a population decide the size of the population. Therefore, an individual is the unit of population. The number of individuals in a population should be large enough so that the sampling variation is as small as to be negligible. Thus a population should not be affected by the sampling variation. Such a population which is not affected by the sampling variation is knows as large population and consists the number of individuals in hundreds or even in thousands rather than in tens.

The total number of individuals forming the population is important. The differential reproductive success of different individuals molds the genetic structure of a population in coming time. The counting of the number of individuals in a population is done for three purposes:

☆ To assure the existence of population,

☆ To determine the gene frequencies, and

☆ To estimate the role of chance factor played in the transmission of genes.

The numbers of Individuals of a population (species) inhabiting in a given locality (space) have the following characteristics:-

(i) The number of individuals in a local population is not constant all the time but show temporal fluctuations. They vary in numbers during different times (seasons/years) like insects,

(ii) The numbers of individuals in a population remain constant in the long run inspite of temporal changes,

(iii) The probability of extinction of a population in the long run can not be ruled out. This means that a population of species may extinct any time, For example, the Dinosaur were the dominant animals over earth at one time but now they have become extinct completely. Likewise, the American Bison have nearly extinct. Thus there is no guarantee of continued existence of a species.

1.4 Nature of Population

All the individuals of a population should be interbred among themselves so as they share the common gene pool. This assumption can be met when all the individuals of a population reside in the same locality or there is gene flow among themselves through migration of individuals or through exchange of semen.

The second assumption is that population is expected to consist the individuals of the same age group with discrete and non-overlapping generations. However, such ideal population exists only for annual/seasonal plants and insects, This second assumption is not met by the real population of farm animals and human beings, because they constitute the overlapping generations (parents and progeny are living together) and have individuals of all ages *viz.* new born, growing stock, mature/adult stock in reproductive age, and in old age unable to reproduce.

The population interacts with environment. A population is described in terms of its setting both in space and time in which it exists. The biology of a population differs from that of the cells and individuals mainly in respect of changes in number and in genetic structure along change in space and time.

1.5 Types of Population

The populations are of different types depending upon the subdivision, migratory movements, mating system followed etc.

(1) Subordinate Mendelian Population

The members of a species are not distributed homogeneously over space but they are clustered and subdivided into groups herding or flocking together due to geographical isolation (territorial limit, isolation by distance), environmental factors or social behaviour (preferential mating). Thus the individuals of a species become subdivided into various groups for a number of reasons. These groups are called as the subordinate Mendelian populations which are sub species, races/breeds/ varieties, ecotypes or local breeding groups – (herds, flocks, lines). These are local interbreeding groups and called as *local population or demes* which are fundamental units of population genetics, usually referred to as population.

(2) Closed Population or Isolates

The individuals of a population should belong to the same generation so as they may bred with one another. Therefore, the migration is excluded and the generations should not overlap. Such a population is called closed population and sometime as "isolates" or cercle (Henry, 1969) which satisfies these two conditions. Thus the word "isolate" is used for a population which is cut off from other population both in space and time. The species which behave in this manner are the many species of insects and annual plants. In human population the idea of generation is only meaningful for a family but has no meaning in the population as a whole because there is migration and overlapping of generations.

(3) Idealized verses Real Population

A population in which opposite sex gametes have equal chances of uniting with each other regardless of their relationship is called an idealized population. In other words, *an idealized population is one which produces progeny with all possible relationships between uniting gametes including selfing*. The selfing or self fertilization takes place in monoceious plants and in hermaphroditic animals such as certain marine forms (frog) that may shed sex cells (eggs and sperms) into sea for fertilization to take place. In this situation the opposite sex gametes have equal chances of uniting with each other irrespective of relationship among donors of the gametes. Therefore, such a population structure is called *"idealized"*.

Simplified Conditions for Idealized Population

The selfing can not take place in most animal populations and in many plant species. In such species the conditions for the idealized populations are simplified as under:

(i) *Population structure*: (a) An initially large random mating population (base population) becomes subdivided into a large number of sub-populations (lines) as a result of geographical or ecological conditions or under controlled breeding programme. All the lines or sub-populations constitute the whole population and each line is considered a small population in which gene frequencies are subject to the dispersive process. (b) Numbers of breeding individuals are same for all lines of all generations. (c) The generations are distinct and do not overlap.

(*ii*) *Mating Systems*: The mating is random within each line, including self fertilization and restricted to members of the same line. Thus lines are isolated having no gene flow (migration) from one line to another.

(*iii*) There is no selection at any stage.

(*iv*) The mutation is not considered.

Real Population

The conditions specified for the idealized population are not met in real populations. The populations of domestic animals and humans differ from the ideal population in the sense that generations are not distinct but overlap, migration takes place, selection occurs, mating is not restricted to any specified line, few males are used, etc. Such populations are called the real populations.

Small Population

The contribution of all the breeding individuals is equal to a gamete pool which form zygotes by random union of gametes. However, all the zygotes formed do not become breeding individuals in the next generation due to their limited and random survival. This results in sampling of genes transmitted by the gametes and unequal contribution of the parents to the next generation depending upon the chances of survival of their progeny. Thus, sampling is the only single event which reduces the large number of gametes to a small number of breeding progeny. The chances of survival of zygotes/progeny may take place at several stages but the sampling through chance survival should be random at each stage to derive the theoretical consequences based on the final number of breeding progeny. Keeping the population size constant from generation to generation, the average number of progeny per parent reaching breeding age is one or two per mated pair of parents.

(4) Panmictic Population

A population with random mating (panmixis, Weinberg~ 1908) is generally called the panmictic population. The random mating (panmixis) means the mating irrespective of the genotype, when any individual of one sex is equally likely to mate with any individual of the opposite sex. A population mating at random (without following any rule) is called as random mating population. The random mating population is called as the panmictic population under the following conditions.

(*i*) Equal viability and fertility of all individuals so that the contribution of all individuals to the next generation is equal.

(*ii*) The sex ratio is equal.

(*iii*) Both maternal and paternal parents contribute equally to the progeny, except for sex linked characters.

The random mating is usually taken as *panmixis*. However, such a random mating does not exist in real populations. There are disturbances in random mating due to differential fertility, sex ratio and mortality in the population. However, random mating holds true in so many real populations.

1.6 Individual vs Population – Dissimilarities

1. Genetic Make Up

The individual is a special and temporary collection of genes formed by uniting two gametes from preceding generation. In a diploid bisexual individual there are two alleles of a gene and a particular allele at a locus will be either present, absent, or both alleles may exist. The individual produces two gametes which was a sample of genes in the parent. An individual is characterized by its genotype and each individual has only one type of genotype *viz.* either homozygous or heterozygous. Depending upon the life and fertility of the individual the contribution of different individuals is different to next generation.

The population is a permanent collection of genes. The population is constituted with N individuals and is a sample of 2N gametes. The population will have all the alleles of a gene at a locus and the allele frequencies may take any value ranging from zero to one. Thus, all possible genotypes are present and all types of possible gametes for a locus are produced in a population. A population is characterized by gene frequencies and genotype frequencies. Any two populations may have same gene frequencies but they may differ in genotypic frequencies.

2. Change in Genetic Make Up

An individual has its fixed genetic make up over space throughout its life, except rare mutations.

A population may be in genetic equilibrium state or its genetic structure may be changed over time (generations) and space due to some forces like mutation, migration, selection, mating systems, and size of population. This change may be sudden or gradual from generation to generation.

3. Succession of Generations

There is no replacement of an individual itself. All the individuals of a population die sooner or later. The population is replaced through generations by birth and death of individuals in a continuous process. In all higher animals, there is an overlapping of generations due to gradual replacement of generation, one generation connecting the next.

4. Single vs Cluster of Measurements

An individual is described by a single measurement for each character *viz.* weight of an individual, height of an individual, milk production of a cow. On the contrary, a population is described by listing the weight, height, milk production of each individual of the population. However, such a description of all the individuals of a population is tedious, laborious and time consuming process. Therefore, a short cut and convenient method is used, to describe a population, by estimating some statistical measures- like measures of central tendency (mean) and measures of dispersion of a character based on all the individuals of a population (amount of variation from the mean within a population). The variation has no meaning for a single measurement of an individual.

5. Life Span

An individual has certain duration of its life with a definite date of its birth and death and hence an individual has limited life (mortal). The population is practically immortal, with no definite date of beginning except in few cases like origin of a plant species or variety by hybridization and likewise new breeds of animals originating at a particular time. However, the process of changing a population into another population requires many generations. Thus, the population has continuity in time.

6. Integration and Area Occupied

An individual can only be present in one place only at a time and its physical boundary is definite. Individual organism is highly organized unit bounded by skin and integrated by communication systems of nerves and hormones. The individuals in a colony are completely dependent upon one another. Individuals constantly enter or leave as migrants but cannot be merged into one another.

On the contrary, the population is spread over a limited or wide area with indefinite boundaries, and composing local sub populations each differing only a little from its neighbour hood sub-population. This makes a population to be continuous in space. Thus, population has no tangible or sharp boundaries except those confined in laboratories, no obvious communication system, and most population show almost no organization, but they behave independently of one another. Local populations shift their positions with time and may be merged into one another.

7. Tolerance Range

A population is much larger than individual in tolerance. The individual can live and reproduce only within a certain limits of physical factors in its environment, called as the "tolerance range". However, the tolerance limits vary to certain extent for different individuals which make the tolerance larger for a population than of any individual. However, neither an individual nor any population can exist beyond tolerance range. The conditions deciding the tolerance range may be climate, topography, the effect of geological parent material on soils, direct effect of other kinds of organisms such as parasites, predators, or direct interference by competitors.

1.7 Techniques to Detect Genetic Variation

The population genetics covers to determine the extent of genetic variation in a population together with covering the origin, maintenance and evolutionary importance of genetic variation.

The genetic variation, first of all exists in the form of two or more alleles (multiple alleles) of a gene at a locus. This can be revealed or detected by a number of methods. The following techniques are used to reveal and detect the genetic variation.

1. Response to Selection

Organisms develop resistance to certain agents like pesticides as a result of natural selection. The poison become ineffective to control pests as a result of arise of a mutant allele which render the poison relatively harmless.

The visible genetic variation in polygenic traits is widespread but the phenotypic differences in these traits can not be traced to the effect of particular gene. The best way to detect the genetic variation in a polygenic trait is to measure the genetic gain (improvement in progeny generation due to selection) and breeding of genetically superior parents. Thus the genetic gain is an evidence of the genetic variation.

2. Inbreeding Effects

Some types of hidden genetic variation can he studied by the inbreeding effects. The inbreeding increases the proportion of homozygous genotype at the expense of heterozygous genotype. This results for the rare recessive alleles to become homozygous. Most of the recessive homozygous genotypes lead to severe physical or mental disability or death of the individual. The inbreeding is thus used to detect the lethal genes which affect viability as well as other characters. Therefore, much of the genetic variation revealed by inbreeding is harmful. The effect of inbreeding for polygenic trait can be observed from the inbreeding depression.

The mating of unrelated individuals (outbreeding) has its effect opposite to that of inbreeding. The homozygosity is reduced and heterozygosity is increased. The increase in heterozygosity for polygenic traits is reflected from hybrid vigour or heterosis which is opposite in sign but equal in amount to the inbreeding depression.

3. Electrophoresis

The electrophoresis is the widely used method to reveal the genetic variation in enzymes and other proteins. This method is used to detect mutation that result in differences in electrophoretic mobility of the corresponding enzyme. An amino acid substitution in an enzyme of an individual leads to a difference in the overall ionic charge of the molecule and the electrophoretic mobility of the enzyme is altered. Thus the enzyme moves at a different rate. The rate of movement of enzyme of the same size and shape is determined largely by the ratio of the number of positively charged amino acids (mainly lysine, arginine and histidine) to the number of negatively charged amino acids (mainly the aspartic acid and glutamic acid). The enzymes with different electrophoretic mobility as a result of allelic differences at a single locus are called as *allozymes*. The allozymes are thus the various electrophoretic forms of a protein that can occur. The allozyme variation in a population is an indication of genetic variation. This type of genetic variation is very common. The electrophoresis has shown the extensive allozyme variation in almost all natural population of bacteria, plants, mice, Drosophila and man. It has been observed that the proportion of polymorphic genes ranged between 15 and 40 percent and a typical individual is heterozygous at between 4 and 14 percent of its genes in various species. These allozyme variations are hidden genetic variations which can be detected by means of protein electrophoresis, though conventional electrophoresis fails to detect many amino acid substitutions. The sequential electrophoresis (running a sequence of gels at different pH values) is more powerful because the proteins that may not be separated at one pH may be separated at another pH.

4. DNA Sequences

Polymorphism occurs in DNA sequences. The hidden genetic variation occurs at the level of DNA sequence and can be detected by direct DNA sequencing of cloned genes from different individuals. The polymorphism in DNA sequences can be detected by the use of restriction enzymes that cut the DNA molecules at sites of particular nucleotide sequences (called the restriction sites of the enzyme). The DNA fragments can be separated by electrophoresis like enzymes but their identification needs special procedures like *Southern blot procedure* given by Southern (1975). The key element in this procedure is the use of a probe DNA molecule containing the nucleotide sequence of interest, which is obtained from a gene that has been cloned into, for example, bacterial cells. The polymorphisms resulting in the presence or absence of restriction sites (cleavage sites for restriction enzymes) or in the occurrence of insertions or deletions of DNA sequences can be identified because they change the length of characteristic restriction fragments. The polymorphisms in restriction fragments are *"restriction fragment length polymorphisms"* abbreviated as RFLPs. The RFLPs require only cloned DNA fragments to be revealed and distributed throughout the genome of virtually all organisms.

The allozyme and DNA polymorphism are very useful in population genetics as genetic markers for mapping the genome, to interpret the ancestral history of populations or in assessing genetic relationship among subpopulations of a species, to know the types of mating systems, and as potential genetic markers linked in the chromosome with genes that cause inherited disease (*genetic markers of disease*).

1.8 Implication of Genetic Variation

Majority of the progeny do not differ from the mean value of their parents for quantitative traits. However, recombination of genes during transmission results into a characteristic distribution of progeny from same parents for metric traits such that some are superior while others are either inferior or equal to their parents.

The gene interactions affect the phenotype of the progeny in a way that they are near to the group average than their parents. This is due to the fact that interaction variation is not transmitted as such but new gene combinations are formed and only a portion of the superiority of best parents is transmitted in the progeny.

Regarding the gene mutations these are mostly recessives, harmful and lethal or semi lethal. They produce harmful traits or abnormalities in the population. Likewise, the chromosomal aberrations mostly create abnormal traits like breeding troubles. However, the chromosomal aberrations have been exploited beneficially and new varieties and species of plants have been evolved.

1.9 Significance of Genetic Variation

The existence of genetic variation is of immense significance. This is well evidenced from the followings:

1. Identity of Individual

Without variation all the local population of a species and all the individuals of a population would have been identical. This would have become impossible to identify the different individuals and thus the individuals would have lost their identity. For example, every person has its own identity having distinguished characteristics and appearance/features for which he is recognized very easily in a large crowd of people and anywhere in the world. This has solved a number of problems and disputes among people.

2. Social Importance

The variation creates and brings beauty. Different individuals of a species have their different features to the extent of continuous gradations and they appear and have different look in their physical features. This creates attraction and affection to which the word beauty was given.

3. Economic Importance

The conservation of genetic variation in a population is of great economic importance because the genetic improvement in performance traits of plants and farm animals depends upon the amount of genetic variability. The genetic variation has helped the plant breeders to develop new varieties of plants and the animal breeder to develop new breeds 'or races of farm animals. The different varieties and breeds perform differently under different environmental conditions and there is differential ecological preference of different genotypes. This enables to grow different plant varieties and rear different breeds of domestic animals according to the environmental conditions prevailing in the area. Moreover, different varieties and breeds are used to serve different purposes.

4. Biological or Evolutionary Significance

The variations give rise to the new species to come up. The variations are essential for the survival and existence of any population or species which depends on change and not by maintaining the *status quo.* This is because it requires the variability for adoption in a changing environment. Thus without variation the possibility of adaptation to new environment, which leads to evolution through natural selection favouring some variant genotypes, would have been eliminated. Thus, the variation has allowed the present evolutionary stage. The theoretical basis of Darwinian' evolution is the existence of genetic variability among individuals of a species. The evolutionary processes of second level operate on genetic variation to change a species genetic makeup over time as per changing environment.

1.10 Population Genetics

The *population genetics* is the integral part of the Mendelian Genetics in the sense that the concepts of Mendelian genetics are extended from the individual mating to the mating in the population. Thus, the Mendelian genetics is extended to the population level. The science of genetics studied at the population level to study the genes in a population covering the genetic structure of a population over time and space is thus known as 'population genetics'. Therefore, *population genetics is the study of genetic structure (genetic variation) of a population and changes that occur from generation to generation.*

The population genetics is centered round the characterization of genetic variation in the population and hence the population genetics is the study of genetic variation of population. In a population, the genes interact with size of population, systems of mating and evolutionary forces (selection, migration and mutation) to lead fixation of desirable genes as well as to eliminate undesirable ones. Therefore, *population genetics is fundamentally concerned with the study of the amount of genetic variation within a population along with the effect of forces that change and shape the genetic variation of the population over space and time.*

Population Genetics versus Quantitative Genetics

The population genetics is trait specific. Some traits are governed by major genes showing discontinuous variation dividing the individuals of a population into distinct types/groups with no connection by intermediates. This implies that there are clear cut differences between two or more groups of individuals. Such differences are known as qualitative differences and the characters showing these differences are called as qualitative characters. Such differences are caused by major genes at one or two loci. As a gene difference at a single locus gives rise to a detectable difference in a character, the Mendelian ratios corresponding to the genotype at a locus are observed among the individuals of a population to show the mechanism of inheritance of the character. It is of interest to know the proportion or frequency of different genotypes in a population as well as the proportion or frequency of individual genes at a locus (allele frequencies) and secondly to know the changes in the gene and genotype frequencies over time (from generation to generation) under the influence of certain forces. The study of the description of genetic properties of population with reference to genes causing easily identifiable qualitative differences in a character is often called as *population genetics.*

The main aim of animal breeder is to make improvement in useful (economic) traits which are governed by many pairs of genes (polygenes) showing continuous variation. The Mendelian ratios are not shown by these characters due to continuous differences forming a continuous graded series from one extreme to the other and hence the individuals can not be placed into different groups. Such characters are measured in quantitative or metric units and hence the differences shown by such characters are known as quantitative differences. Therefore, the methods of Mendelian analysis can not be applied to study the inheritance pattern of these characters. It is also not possible to study the individual polygenes affecting the economic traits because these genes have their minor, small and unappreciable effects and further their effects are modified by the variation in environment to express the character. The presence of such minor genes (polygenes), the magnitude of their effect and the potentiality for change in genetic structure for these genes can be demonstrated by using special statistical methods. Thus, statistical methods are used to study Mendelism at population level for quantitative traits to know the genetic structure of a population. This covers the *quantitative analysis of population's genetic potential.* The population genetics thus also study the hereditary phenomenon of quantitative characters based on Mendelism at a population level using statistical methods. The population genetics dealing with inheritance pattern of quantitative characters is called as the *"Quantitative genetics"* or *"Biometrical genetics"*. The quantitative genetics is thus more statistical as it involves the application of statistical methods to study the inheritance pattern of quantitative traits in a population. Thus, the quantitative genetics is a part of population genetics limiting to the study of inheritance of quantitative characters.

Levels of Population Genetics

The population genetics is studied at the following three levels-

    (i) *Theoretical population genetics:* This is concerned with the characterization of genetic variation in population. This deals with the mathematical models taking care of the process of heredity and evolution in the analysis of characters (qualitative and quantitative) which needs statistical approach. Thus, it is mainly mathematical and statistical in nature and hence called as *statistical genetics.*

    (ii) *Experimental population genetics:* The breeding experiments are conducted at population level to study the properties of genes and to test the validity of theoretical aspects (principles) of population genetics *viz.* type of gene action, pleiotropism, linkage, selection theory, G-E interaction, inbreeding depression and hybrid vigour.

    (iii) *Applied population genetics:* The important aspect is the application of the principles of population genetics to plant and animal improvement. The genetic variation in a population is exploited by formulating and executing the breeding plans which includes the selection of genetically superior individuals and the ways they should be mated (mating systems) for improvement of future generation.

1.11 Importance of the Study of Population Genetics

The knowledge of population genetics is very essential for a number of reasons: The genes are self-reproducing, thousands in numbers in each individual, organized into larger units (chromosomes) and function by interacting among themselves as well as with the prevailing environment to produce the individual's phenotype for various characteristics like growth, production, reproduction etc. The analysis of these characters of individual organism is very important to know the nature and function of genes *viz.* as a unit of segregation, recombination, mutation etc. These aspects of genes organization and their functions are very much vital to understand about the heredity. However, the study of primary gene products and their interaction cannot answer many aspects of heredity only by studying individuals alone in terms of gene organization and functions.

The evolutionary significance of natural genetic variation and the role of quantitative aspects to develop breeding method cannot be recognized simply by examining the detailed physiological and biochemical properties of genes and genotypes. The genetic variations in a population are the basic material upon which the evolutionary forces operate to change a species make up over time and space. It is thus of evolutionary significance to know how the total genotype was evolved, maintain its balance and change over time. The genotype changes over generations and the effect of a new genotype on individual's adaptability (effect of gene on fitness) can be observed from the analysis of a population. The adaptation is the ability of an organism to exploit an environment for successful living and this ability of an individual is actually the response of the population rather than of individual. This is because the tolerance, which is an adaptive trait, is the result of selection in a variable environment and is not suddenly new for a single individual but it is a function of the entire population's adjustment to the environment. The new individuals having genotype for better adaptability (having tolerance power) survive in a new environment and acquaint themselves over many generations. The better adopted individuals under variable conditions survive and reproduce to produce next generation and built up a population well adapted to that environment. It is thus most important and essential to study and describe a population in terms of the different types of genotypes (individuals) existing in a population, to what extent they are uniform or variable, and the way of utilizing (exploiting) the genetic variability by the population to be adopted.

1.12 Applications of Population Genetics

The knowledge of population genetics is very useful for the genetic improvement of any species. The use (application) of this science of genetics can be viewed as under.

1. Population Genetics and Evolution

The population genetics is fundamental to the study of evolutionary process. The population genetics covers the effects of the evolutionary forces on the genetic structure of population overtime. The different evolutionary forces are the random drift, migration, mutation and selection.

2. Population Genetics and Livestock Improvement

The variability exists in a population which decides the adaptability of a population to new (changed) environment over time. A population with greater genetic variability is capable to adopt the new (changed) environment or vice versa. The study of population genetics is of immense use to know that how much of the genetic variation in a species would be for expected change in environment so that a suitable breeding plan can be devised for creating and maintaining genetic variation sufficient to meet the changes in environment.

The genetic variation is of fundamental significance for evolution and in the application of genetics to animal breeding and plant breeding by affording material for selection. The population genetics deals with the study of genetic variation in a population and the forces which govern the changes in genetic structure of a population. The aim of an animal breeder is to improve the performance of domestic animals in desired direction by exploiting the genetic variation through selection and mating systems that form the breeding plan. The right decision of a proper breeding plan is very important to produce desirable phenotypes.

The theory of population genetics consists to know the consequence of Mendelian inheritance in population and to simultaneous segregation of polygenes together with covering the change in genetic variation under the influence of various factors such as mating types, population size, mutation, migration and selection. An animal breeder exploits the genetic variation by the application of these factors to improve the performance of domestic animals in desired direction. The study of population genetics is helpful to know that which force may quickly fix the desirable genes in the population and may eliminate the undesirable genes from the population.

In *small size population* the genetic structure is changed. The populations of domestic animals are of small size. Therefore, the gene frequencies are subjected to random fluctuations due to sampling of gametes in small population. This random change of gene frequency is the dispersive process which has the effects of random drift of gene frequencies, differentiation between sub populations, uniformity within subpopulation due to increase in homozygosity with consequent decrease in heterozygosity.

The *mating system* (inbreeding) does not change the gene frequency but changes the genotype frequencies. The inbreeding leads to an increase in homozygosity and a consequent decrease in heterozygosity. The recessive alleles in homozygous state are harmful causing either death of the individual or affect the viability and fertility or lower down the value of the trait. The animal breeder may use this information to eliminate the recessive genes from the population by producing homozygous individuals through inbreeding system of mating. The inbreed animals can be produced and the high producing animals can be selected through recurrent selection and reciprocal recurrent selection for bringing genetic improvement.

The *mutation* is a rare phenomenon and being random in direction is beyond the control of animal breeder.

The effect of *migration* on the change of gene frequency depends upon the rate of migration and the difference in gene frequency between migrants and native population. An animal breeder may use this knowledge for bringing genetic improvement by introducing new and better genes in the native population.

The change of gene frequency by *selection* depends on the selection coefficient. The *selection* in favour or against any gene can be done by selective elimination of one or the other genotype that carry the undesirable gene causing the reduction in the value of the trait. The number of generations required to bring a desired change in gene frequency can be estimated. The change in phenotypic mean by selecting genetically superior stock can be predicted from the knowledge of population genetics for metric characters. The genetics of metric characters more specifically known as quantitative genetics deals with the study of variation in the trait together with partitioning the variation into its components attributed to genetic and environmental causes. The partitioning of variation is important to provide the information about the relative importance of heredity and environment to influence a metric trait.

The genetic variance (V_G) is the only component of total phenotypic variance (V_p) which is transmitted to the progeny which implies that the genetically determined superiority of the individual is transmitted to its progeny. The amount of genetic variance provides the estimation of the degree of genetic determination (H^2) to which a trait is determined by genes as $H^2 = V_G/V_P$. However, out of the total genetic variance, only the additive genetic variance (V_A) arisen from additive gene effects is fixed and shown by the progeny of the individual. The amount of V_A is expressed in terms of heritability as $h^2 = V_A/V_P$. The estimation of additive genetic variance as h^2 is important to predict the breeding value of an animal and hence in identifying the genetically superior animals: $B.V. = h^2 P$.

The amount of V_A estimates the fraction of parent's superiority to be passed on (transmitted) to its progeny and responsive to selection. Therefore, h^2 is used to predict the response to selection (genetic improvement by selection) as: $\Delta G = h^2 S$

The selection is effective only when the amount of additive genetic variation is high. The selection based on non-additive genetic variance is not effective. Thus, the knowledge of the amount of additive genetic variance is helpful to formulate the breeding plan for bringing genetic improvement.

3. Medical Science

The population genetics has its applications in medical science. There are individual/family differences in susceptibility/resistance to disease, the effectiveness of the medicine and the mode of action of drugs. This means that individuals of different genotypes respond differently to different drugs/medicines. The chance of evolution to drug immunity among pathogens can be minimized by proper application of population genetics.-

4. Genetic Counselling

The population genetics has an important role in genetic counselling.

Chapter 2
Genetic Structure of Population

The genetic structure or constitution of a population is given by the population parameters for one or more traits for a given period of time and secondly, the changes that occurred over space and time. These population parameters are character specific which means different for qualitative and quantitative characters, for the reason of the number of gene loci affecting these characters. The population parameters for any trait are given for a group of individuals (population), in genetic equilibrium state, in general. Such a population is a large random mating population with Hardy-Weinberg equilibrium genotype frequencies in which no special breeding method (selection, mating system) is applied and hence there is no change in the genetic structure of the population over time.

2.1 Genetic Structure of Qualitative Trait

The population parameters used to describe the genetic structure of a population for a qualitative trait are the *array of genotypes* for a character and the *gene distribution* (*array of genes*).

The *genotypic array* (known as the genotypic structure of a population) is given by specifying the numbers of genotypes and the frequency of each genotype, for a trait in the population. Any combination of two alleles (in a diploid bisexual individual) in a pair or a series of multiple alleles at one or more loci affecting a character is called the *genotype*. The *genotype frequency* is the percentage or proportion of individuals having a particular genotype, formed by a pair or series of alleles at one or more loci affecting a character, among the total individuals in a population. The genotype frequency is represented as P_{ii} for homozygous genotypes and as p_{ij} for the heterozygous genotypes, where i indicate the ith allele at a locus.

The *array of genes* (known as genic structure) is given by specifying the number of loci affecting a trait, the number of alleles present at a locus (two or more *viz.* multiple alleles) affecting the character and the frequencies of different alleles at each locus in a population. The *gene frequency* or more specifically and more correctly, the **allele frequency** is defined as the proportion of a given allele in a pair of alleles or in a series of multiple alleles at a locus to the total number of alleles at that locus in the population. The gene frequency is represented as p_i

The genetic structure of a population thus includes the study of gene and genotype frequencies and secondly the prediction of these frequencies in progeny generation, presuming the mechanism of heredity applied to Mendelian genetics.

The different genetic systems are single locus with two alleles, with multiple alleles, sex-linked genes and two loci case. The genetic structure of population for different genetic systems controlling the traits has been given here dealing with the H.W. principles.

2.2 Genetic Structure – Single Locus Two Alleles

The two alleles at a locus on autosomes may be same (identical) or different in structure and function (A_1 and A_2). These two alleles are represented as A_{ij}. An individual is called as homozygous that carries identical alleles at the locus (A_{ii}). The individual is called heterozygous that carries different alleles at a locus (A_{ij}). The frequencies of two alleles (A_1 and A_2) are represented as p and q, respectively.

In case of diploid population of N individuals, the two alleles in an individual may be present in either combination (genotypes) as A_1A_1, A_1A_2 and A_2A_2 These gene combinations in an individual are called as genotypes represented as D, H and R, and their respective frequencies are denoted as p^2, $2pq$ and q^2.

Now considering N total individuals in a population, there will be N_{11} individuals with A_1A_1 gene combination (genotype), N_{12} individuals with A_1A_2 genotype and N_{22} individuals with A_2A_2 genotype, so that the genotype frequencies of three genotypes will be as:

Genotypes	No. of Individuals	Genotype Frequencies
A_1A_1	N_{11}	$\dfrac{N_{11}}{N} = D = P_{11} = p^2$
A_1A_2	N_{12}	$\dfrac{N_{12}}{N} = H = 2P_{12} = 2pq$
A_2A_2	N_{22}	$\dfrac{N_{22}}{N} = R = P_{22} = q^2$
Total	N	1.0

2.3 Genetic Structure – Single Locus Multiple Alleles

The multiple alleles are represented as $A_1, A_2,....,A_i, A_j, A_k$ with their respective frequencies as p, q,...., r, s, t. As only two alleles are present in an individual at a locus, the different alleles of multiple series will be present at that locus in different individuals. The homozygote having identical alleles at a locus is represented to have A_iA_i genotype with its frequency as P_{ii} whereas the heterozygote having different alleles at the locus is represented as A_iA_j with frequency as P_{ij}.

The frequency of an allele (p_i) will be obtained as:

$$P_i = P_{i1} + P_{i2} + ... + P_{ik} = \Sigma P_{ij,}$$

Provided all the genotypes are identifiable as in case of no dominance or co-dominance. Therefore, the frequency of an allele is obtained by adding the frequency of the homozygote for that allele to half of the frequency of all the heterozygote having that allele.

The representation of different alleles at a locus along with their frequencies is known as the genic structure of a population.

Considering 3 alleles at a locus in an equilibrium population, the frequencies of 3 alleles and 6 genotypes with their frequencies can be represented as:

Alleles and their frequencies			Genotypes and their frequencies					
A_1	A_2	A_3	A_1A_1	A_2A_2	A_3A_3	A_1A_2	A_1A_3	A_2A_3
p	q	r	p^2	q^2	r^2	2pq	2pr	2qr

The sum of gene frequencies of all the multiple alleles must equal to unity and hence p + q + r = 1.0. The sum of all the genotype frequencies must also be equal to unity and hence $p^2 + q^2 + r^2 + 2pq + 2pr + 2qr = 1.0$. The homozygotes are equal to the sum of the squared allelic frequencies $(p^2 + q^2 + r^2)$ while the heterozygote are equal to the twice of the product of each pair of frequencies *viz.* 2 (pq + pr + qr).

The possible genotypes with multiple alleles at a locus are more in number compared to that of two allelic genetic systems. Taking k as the number of multiple alleles at a locus, the number of homozygote (A_iA_i), heterozygote (A_iA_j) and total genotypes produced will be as under:

No. of total genotypes	=	*No. of homozygote*	+	*No. of heterozygote*
k (k + 1)/2	=	k	+	k (k – 1)/2

The number of total phenotypes depends on the dominance between multiple alleles and they are lesser than the number of genotypes if dominance of alleles exists.

2.4 Genetic Structure – Sex-Linked Genes

The genes present on sex chromosomes are called as sex linked genes. The two sex chromosomes are different in size and shape in the two sexes. One of the two sexes has two X chromosome (XX) which are equal in size and shape, and hence homologous. This sex is called as homogametic sex producing two similar gametes. It is the females in mammals and Drosophila. The other sex has one X chromosome and one Y chromosome, represented as XY which are not equal in size and shape, for which the two chromosomes (X and Y) are not homologous to each other and hence the individual is called heterogametic (hemizygous) which is male in mammals and Drosophila. The situation is reverse in birds.

The X chromosome is longer than Y chromosome. The X chromosome is genetically active (have genes) whereas the Y chromosome is known as genetically inert having no gene, though some genes have been found to be present on Y chromosome.

The heterogametic sex (males in mammals) is haploid for X chromosome and has zygotic frequencies equal to the allelic frequencies. Thus, the heterogametic sex has only two genotypes (X^A Y and X^a Y) and each individual has only one gene (either A or a) instead of two. Thus, the gene frequency is equal to the genotype frequency. The frequency of recessive genotype in heterogametic sex estimates directly the frequency of recessive allele.

The homogametic sex (females in mammals) is diploid for two X chromosomes (XX) and hence will have three genotypes like autosomal gene. The three genotypes with two alleles (A and a) can be represented as: $X^A X^A$, $X^A X^a$ and $X^a X^a$.

Considering single locus with two alleles (A and a) the genotypes and their frequencies of two sexes can be written as:

	Males (XY)		Females (XX)		
Genotypes	X^A Y	X^a Y	$X^A X^A$	$X^A X^a$	$X^a X^a$
Frequencies	p	q	p^2	2pq	q^2

2.5 Genetic Structure for Two Loci

Each individual has a large number of gene loci, possibly thousands. Some characters are controlled by two or more loci. The number of possible genotype for more loci are increased with the number of loci affecting a character and becomes equal to 3^n with two alleles at each locus where **n** is the number of loci. Therefore, the number of possible genotypes with two alleles at each of 1, 2, 3, 4, 5, 6 loci would be 3, 9, 27, 81, 243, 729, respectively. Thus, a complete description of any population for all loci is not possible in terms of genotypic array. The genotypic array, gene array and gametic array for two loci case have been given in chapter 6.

2.6 Relation between Genic and Genotypic Structure

The genic structure of a population can be estimated from the genotypic structure. The frequency of an allele is estimated as: $p_i = p_{ii} + \frac{1}{2} p_{ij}$

On the contrary, the genotypic structure of a population cannot be estimated from the genic structure of the population, unless the population is large and random mating. In a large random mating population, both genic and genotypic structures remain constant from one generation to the next and show the following relation:

$$(p + q)^2 \qquad = \qquad p^2 + 2pq + q^2 \qquad = \quad D + H + R$$

$$\text{(Sum of gene freq.)}^2 \quad = \quad \text{genotype frequencies.}$$

Thus, the genotypic structure of a large random mating population can be predicted from the knowledge of the genic structure or vice versa. The relationship between gene frequencies and genotype frequencies has a great significance in many calculations.

2.7 Difference between Gene Frequency and Genotype Frequency

These differ with respect to the followings-

1. **The *genotype frequency*** represents the proportion of individuals having a particular genotype at a particular locus or loci affecting a character among the total individuals of a population. **The gene frequency** represents the proportion of a particular allele in a pair of alleles or in a series of multiple alleles at a locus among the total number of alleles of that locus in the population.

2. The *gene frequency* is represented as p_i whereas the genotype frequency is represented as P_{ii} for homozygous genotypes and as P_{ij} for the heterozygous genotypes, where i indicates the ith allele at a locus. The condition is that each individual is diploid and

   $p + q = D + H + R = 1.0$

   where, $p = D + \frac{1}{2} H$ and $q = R + \frac{1}{2} H$

3. The frequencies of different alleles and different genotypes at a locus are the sources of genetic differences within the population whereas different frequencies of genes and genotypes in different populations are the sources of genetic variation between the populations.

4. The two concepts of gene frequencies and genotype frequencies are two different ways to characterize a population genetically. In a population they are dependent on each other. The gene frequency in a population depends on the genotype frequencies in the present generation whereas in the subsequent generation the genotype frequencies depend on the gene frequencies of the parent generation.

5. The gene frequencies and genotype frequencies may be different in different populations. However, it is also true that the gene frequencies may be same in different populations but with different genotype frequencies.

6. The gene frequencies are estimated from genotype frequencies but the genotype frequencies cannot be estimated from gene frequencies if the population is not in genetic equilibrium. The frequency of an allele is the square root of the frequency of its homozygous genotype carrying that allele if the population is in genetic equilibrium.

2.8 Importance of Gene Frequency

The gene frequency has its importance as given below:

1. These are the genes that are transmitted from one generation to the next. The genotypes are not transmitted as such but they are broken in gametes during cell division (meiosis) in sex cells as a requirement of genetic transmission.

2. The gene is a stable entity but the genotypes are not stable in next generation. Therefore, it is necessary and better to describe the genetic structure of a population by the genes present in the population and their frequencies at one or more loci (genic structure).

3. It is easy to give the genic structure of a population compared to the genotypic structure. For example, it is not possible to specify all the possible genotypes for all the loci affecting a character whereas the genic structure can be given by specifying the number of loci with the frequencies of alleles present on those loci. Suppose 10 loci are under consideration for which a population has to be described genetically. This can be done to specify 10 gene loci with the frequencies of different alleles at each of 10 loci, but it is not possible to specify the total number of genotypes possible for these 10 loci.

4. The method of gene frequency analysis is useful in testing the genetic hypothesis for traits for which the mating is random.

5. Evolutionary importance: The phenotypic change over time indicates the evolution and is accompanied by a genetic change which in turn depends upon the genetic variability in terms of the gene frequency. A population with large genetic variation is more flexible to adapt itself to the changing environment. Therefore, the capacity of a population to adapt itself in changing environment depends upon the genetic variability (genetic structure) of the population.

A comparison of samples, taken from different local populations or from one population at different times (generations), for the gene frequencies is made. The significant differences in gene frequencies between samples over space and time reveal the micro evolutionary changes in space and time. Therefore, the estimation of gene frequency has its evolutionary importance.

2.9 Genetic Structure for Quantitative Traits

The gene array and genotype array for the gene loci affecting any metric trait can not be estimated. This is because these are polygenic traits. Therefore, some other population parameters are used to describe the genetic structure of a population for metric trait. These are as under:

(i) The Mean of the Trait

The population mean indicates the mean genotypic value of the population for a trait. The group means are used to estimate the effect of a certain factor *viz.* the effect of genetic and environmental factors. The genetic factors are those which influence the phenotypic value of a character via genes effect *viz.* the effect of sire (family), line, strain and breed whereas the environmental factors are all those other than genes effect, which affect the phenotypic value. Each genetic and environmental factor has a number of levels of the effect *viz.* number of breeds, number of strains, number of sires within a breed, number of seasons in a year, number of years for entire period of study, number of feeding levels, number of age groups, etc. The means are estimated for different levels of a factor, known as group means. The magnitude of an effect of a certain factor is reflected in the form of the different means of the different levels of an effect (group means). These group means are compared to know the effects of these genetic and environmental factors. Now, the important point to consider is to know whether the means of different levels of an effect (group means) differ in real sense due to the causing factor or the differences in group means have arisen just by chance. This is tested by partitioning the variance in a character arisen due to the different levels of the causing factor.

(ii) The Variance in the Trait

The variability in a character is caused by different levels of certain causing factor and it is measured by the variance. The variance, caused in a character due to causing factor, is used to test the reality of an effect of a certain factor. This is known as significance of difference, in statistical term. This is done by partitioning the variance into different causal factors causing the differences in a character. The partitioning means the analysis and thus the analysis of variance means the partitioning of variance. The analysis of variance is done to partition the total variance into causing factors *viz.* genetic variance and environmental variance (variation due to breed, sire, season, year, age, etc.) and the significance of the proportionate contribution of a particular factor is tested by F-test developed by Fisher. The genetic variance is further partitioned into additive genetic variance, dominance variance and interaction variance to describe the genetic structure of a population.

(iii) The Covariance among Relatives and among Traits as well

The covariance among relatives is estimated as a measure of resemblance among relatives and to estimate the different components of genetic variance (additive, dominance and interaction variance). The covariance among traits is estimated to know the association between them and to know the extent of genetic cause of correlation among characters.

The mean, variance and covariance for a metric trait are the population parameters whose genetic basis explains the properties of genes controlling a trait so as to specify the genetic architecture (structure) of a population for any metric trait. The main *properties of genes* are the manner in which the genes produce their effects for expression of phenotypic value of a trait, like additive effect, the degree of dominance at a locus, combined effect of genes at different loci (epistasis), pleiotropic gene action, the linkage relationship among genes involved, effect of genes on fitness (fitness of genotype), and finally their interaction with the environment.

Change in Population

The change in population is the second aspect to describe a population. The change may be evolutionary or historical. The history of breeds/plants varieties/races in humans cover the historical description for a short period of time while evolutionary change includes the change extending over long period of time. When the genetic structure does not change over time from generation to generation but remain constant over generations, it is said to be at equilibrium (or genetic equilibrium) or equilibrium gene frequencies and equilibrium genotypic frequencies.

A number of **biological factors** determine the *maintenance* or *change* in the genetic equilibrium. These forces may be grouped as: the *breeding behaviour* (breeding systems *viz.* inbreeding and out breeding), the *genetic* factors (mutation), the *environmental factors* (selection and migration) which act on individuals of a population affecting their survival and fertility, and the *population size*. The study of the effect of these factors on change in genetic structure of a population is the subject matter of population genetic.

Chapter 3
Genetic Equilibrium – Single Locus Two Alleles

The equilibrium is a state of no change and hence a constant state. The genetic equilibrium is thus concerned with the constant state of the genetic structure of population. Yule (1902), Castle (1903) and Pearson (1904) reported the genetic equilibrium for the special case of equal gene frequencies ($p = q = 0.5$) at a locus with two alleles. W.E. Castle (1903) of USA was actually the founder of genetic equilibrium principle. He worked on the genetic equilibrium for a case of equal gene frequencies at a locus based on the inheritance of coat colour in mice. He supported Mendelism and rejected Galtonian basis of blending inheritance by illustrating the law of purity of gametes. Karls Pearson (1904) though rejected Mendelism but generalized the principle of segregation and showed that the F_2 ratio of ¼ AA: ½ Aa: ¼ aa is maintained with random mating in a large population.

3.1 Genetic Equilibrium

The *genetic equilibrium* means no change in genetic structure of population (gene and genotype frequencies) from one generation to the next. In a genetic equilibrium population, there is a relationship between the gene frequencies and the genotype frequencies. According to the relationship between the two, the genotype frequencies are equal to the square of the sum of gene frequencies and hence this is also called as *square law*. This is as under:

$$(p + q)^2 = p^2 + 2pq + q^2 \qquad\qquad 3.1$$

in such a way that $p + q = 1.0$ and $p^2 + 2pq + q^2 = 1.0$

This relationship is the *test of genetic equilibrium.* A population with above relationship between gene frequencies and genotype frequencies is said to be in genetic equilibrium. The genetic equilibrium is observed under many possible conditions. The first equilibrium condition is the random mating for different genetic systems *viz.* single locus for two alleles and multiple alleles (autosomes), single locus for sex linked genes, and two or more loci case.

3.2 Hardy-Weinberg Law

Hardy, G.H. (1908) of England (Mathematician of Cambridge University) and W. Weinberg (1908) of Germany (Physician) reported independently that the principle of genetic equilibrium in a large random mating population can be applied for any value of gene frequencies. They also described the genetic equilibrium under certain conditions. Therefore, this law of genetic equilibrium under random mating is known as the Hardy-Weinberg law or H.W. principle.

The *HW law states* that in a large random mating population the genetic structure (gene and genotype frequencies) remains constant from generation to generation in the absence of evolutionary forces (mutation, migration and selection).

Random mating is the simplest form of mating behavior in which no principle for mating is followed and hence any individual of one sex has equal chance to mate with any individual of the opposite sex. Thus, no restriction is imposed on mating. The main genetic consequence of random mating in a large population is that the genetic structure of population remains constant from generation to generation. No change in genetic structure (*genetic equilibrium*) is the consequence of random mating in a large population and hence it is also called as *"random mating principle"*.

The H.W. Equilibrium is an extension of Mendel's laws of inheritance, describes the consequence of random mating in a large population, and gives the expected relationship between the gene frequencies and the genotype frequencies in the population. H.W. Law is really a corollary of Mendel's law of segregation. The significance of H.W. equilibrium was appreciated and popularized through the "Genetics and the origin of species" (Dobzhansky, 1937).

The necessary **conditions, to hold true the H.W. law,** are the large population, random mating among parents and absence of evolutionary forces (migration, mutation and selection). The H.W. Equilibrium is disturbed leading to the change in the genetic properties of a population if the population is of small size, mating is non-random (inbreeding and out breeding) and any of the evolutionary forces (migration, mutation and selection) is working. Therefore, in a population which is not in H.W. Equilibrium any of the above conditions may be operating for not holding true the H.W. Equilibrium.

3.3 Equilibrium Proportions – Single Locus Two Alleles

When H.W. law holds true in a population, the genotype frequencies among progeny are obtained by the square of the sum of gene frequencies among parents as:

Square of sum of gene frequencies = Genotype frequencies

(among parents) (among progeny)

$(p + q)^2 = p^2 + 2pq + q^2$

such that $p + q = 1.0$ and $p^2 + 2pq + q^2 = 1.0$

The *homozygote* are equal to the sum of the squared gene frequencies (p^2+q^2) whereas the *heterozygote* are equal to twice of the product of frequencies of two allele *viz.* 2pq. The number of phenotypes depends on the dominance effect of alleles.

3.4 Proof of H.W. Law – Single locus two alleles:

The random mating in a large population leads to H.W. genotype frequencies in the absence of evolutionary forces. The random mating can be considered in either of two ways. The first is the random union of gametes and second is the random mating among individuals (genotypes). However, the genetic consequences of both the ways are equal in the sense that both ways lead to H.W. genotype frequencies. This can be shown by two ways as under

(i) Random Union of Gametes

A gamete produced by an individual for one locus is equivalent to one gene. The frequencies of two gametes produced by an individual are thus equal to the allele frequencies. The A_1 gamete will carry A_1 allele while A_2 gametes will carry A_2 allele. The frequency of A_1 gametes is taken as p and frequency of A_2 gametes as q among parents. The genotypes and their frequencies, the gametes produced and their frequencies are considered as:

Genotypes (Parents)	Frequencies of Genotypes	Gametes Produced by Parents	Frequencies of Gametes (Genes)
A_1A_1	$p^2 = D$	A_1	p
A_1A_2	$2pq = H$		
A_2A_2	$q^2 = R$	A_2	q

The arithmetic of probability of uniting two gametes of opposite sex is used to predict the zygotic (genotype) frequencies in the progeny. The probability that a zygote of a particular genotype will be formed is the joint probability of random union of two gametes. The probability that a male gamete carrying either A_1 or A_2 gene will unite with the female gamete carrying either A_1 or A_2 gene to from a zygote are independent of each other and hence these are two independent events. Thus, the zygote (genotype) frequencies are the product of the frequencies of the gametes. For example, if A_1 male gamete with its frequency p unites with the female gamete carrying A_1 gene with frequency p, then the zygotic frequency of A_1A_1 zygote will he $p \times q = p^2$ and when A_1 gamete with its frequency p unites with A_2 gamete with its frequency q, then the zygotic frequency will be $p \times q = p\ q$. Therefore, the genotype frequencies among the progeny produced by random union of gametes can be determined by multiplying the frequencies of the two uniting gametes. This has been illustrated with equal gene frequencies in two sexes:

Table 3.1: Random Union of Gametes

Genotypes			Male Parent	
		A_1A_1	A_1A_2	A_2A_2
		Gametes	$A_1(p)$	$A_2(q)$
	A_1A_1 — A_1 (p)		A_1A_1 (p^2)	A_1A_2 (pq)
Female parent	A_1A_2 — A_2 (q)		A_1A_2 (pq)	A_2A_2 (q^2)
	A_2A_2			

The total results in the progeny (the genotypes produced among progeny generation and their frequencies) as a consequence of random union of gametes among parents will be as under-

$$p^2 (A_1A_1): 2pq (A_1A_2): q^2 (A_2A_2)$$

The third step assumes equal survivability of all the zygotes till identified as genotypes. This results the same genotype frequencies among adults as were among zygotes. Lastly, these genotype frequencies among the progeny generation will give the following gene frequencies:

Freq of A_1 allele $= p^2 + \frac{1}{2}(2pq) = p^2 + p q = p (p + q) = p$

Freq. of A_2 allele $= q^2 + \frac{1}{2}(2pq) = q^2 + p q = q (q + p) = q$

This has proved the H.W. law because the gene frequencies in the progeny generation are the same as were in the parent generation and that the genotype frequencies in the progeny depend on the gene frequencies among the parents irrespective of the genotype frequencies. Thus when the mating is random the gene frequencies do not change from one generation to the next and the genotype frequencies among progeny are the square of the sum of gene frequencies among parents as per equation 3.1.

(ii) Random Mating of Genotypes

This procedure has two steps:

(a) Mating Types and their Frequencies

With complete random mating among the three genotypes taking their equal frequencies in two sexes, the mating frequencies of different genotypes will be obtained by multiplying together the frequencies of the 3 genotypes as shown in Table 3.2.

There are nine types of mating with some mating types being equivalent by ignoring the sex of the parent and thus these nine types are reduced to six types for the reason that DH = HD, DR = RD and HR = RH. This is because the mating of A_1A_1 male with A_1A_2 female (DH) will give equivalent result to the mating of A_1A_1 female with A_1A_2 male (HD). Thus DH = HD and similarly DR = RD and HR = RH.

Table 3.2: Mating Types and their Frequencies with Random Mating

			Genotypes and their Frequency in Female Parent		
	Genotypes	Frequencies	D	H	R
Genotypes,	A_1A_1	D	D^2	DH	DR
their freq. in male parent	A_1A_2	H	HD	H^2	RH
	A_2A_2	R	RD	RH	R^2

(b) Genotypes and their Frequencies among Progeny

The above six mating types will produce the genotypes of offspring. Among the total progeny produced the frequency of different genotypes in the progeny can be obtained. The A_1A_1 will produce only A_1 gametes and hence the $A_1A_1 \times A_1A_1$ mating will produce only A_1A_1 progeny. The frequency of A_1A_1 genotype among parent is D and hence in the total progeny the A_1A_1 genotype will be in the frequency of D^2 from $A_1A_1 \times A_1A_1$, mating. Likewise, the mating of homozygous parents with A_2A_2 genotype ($A_2A_2 \times A_2A_2$) will produce only A_2A_2 progeny with a frequency of R^2 among total progeny. Similarly, the mating of parents homozygous for different alleles (*e.g.* $A_1A_1 \times A_2A_2$) will produce only the heterozygous progeny of A_1A_2 genotype with a frequency of 2 DR in the total progeny.

The mating of heterozygous with heterozygous parent (heterozygous mating of $A_1A_2 \times A_1A_2$) will produce three genotypes in a ratio of 1:2:1 according to the Mendelian ratios. Thus ¼ of the total progeny from this mating will be of A_1A_1 genotype, ½ of A_1A_2 genotype and ¼ of A_2A_2 genotype.

The mating of heterozygous parent (A_1A_2) with homozygous parent for A_1 allele (A_1A_1) will produce progeny of two genotypes, A_1A_1 and A_1A_2 in equal frequency (DH). Similarly, the mating of heterozygous parent (A_1A_2) with another homozygous parent for A_2 allele (A_2A_2) will produce progeny of two genotypes (A_2A_2 and A_1A_2) in equal frequency (HR). The total results explained above have been shown in a tabular form below:

Table 3.3: Genotypes and their Frequencies among Progeny

Mating among Parents		Genotypes and their Frequency in Progeny		
Types	Freq.	A_1A_1	A_1A_2	A_2A_2
$A_1A_1 \times A_1A_1$	D^2	D^2	—	—
$A_2A_2 \times A_2A_2$	R^2		—	R^2
$A_1A_1 \times A_2A_2$	2DR	—	2DR	—
$A_1A_2 \times A_1A_2$	H^2	¼ H^2	½ H^2	¼ H^2
$A_1A_2 \times A_1A_1$	2DH	DH	DH	—
$A_1A_2 \times A_2A_2$	2HR	—	HR	HR

The frequency of each genotype in the total progeny can be obtained by adding the frequencies of progeny of different genotypes produced by each type of mating as under-

Frequency of A_1A_1 genotype: $= D^2 + DH + \frac{1}{4}H^2 = (D + \frac{1}{2}H)^2$

$\qquad\qquad\qquad\qquad\qquad = p^2 \qquad\qquad\qquad$ since $D + \frac{1}{2}H = p$

Frequency of A_1A_2 genotype: $= DH + 2DR + \frac{1}{2}H^2 + HR$

$\qquad\qquad\qquad\qquad\qquad = 2\,(\frac{1}{2}DH + DR + \frac{1}{4}H^2 + \frac{1}{2}HR)$

$\qquad\qquad\qquad\qquad\qquad = 2\,[D\,(\frac{1}{2}H + R) + \frac{1}{2}H\,(\frac{1}{2}H + R)]$

$\qquad\qquad\qquad\qquad\qquad = 2\,(\frac{1}{2}H + R)\,(D + \frac{1}{2}H)$

$\qquad\qquad\qquad\qquad\qquad = 2pq \qquad$ since $\frac{1}{2}H + R = q$ and $\frac{1}{2}H + D = p$

Frequency of A_2A_2 genotype: $= R^2 + HR + \frac{1}{4}H^2 = (R + \frac{1}{2}H)^2$

$\qquad\qquad\qquad\qquad\qquad = q^2$

The frequencies of the three genotypes so obtained are the H.W. equilibrium frequencies. This proves that H.W. E. frequencies are approached by one generation of random mating, irrespective of the genotype frequencies in the parent generation.

The important point about the two ways of random mating (random union of gametes and random mating of individuals) is that they have equivalent genetic consequences. The total result of random mating between individuals and the subsequent random union of gametes produced by the mates is equivalent to complete random union of all the gametes produced by population. The use of the principle of random union of gametes is simple particularly when dealing with multiple alleles, sex linked genes and two or more loci case because the complete enumeration of all possible mating frequencies become tedious. The genetic composition of any generation can be determined by the principle of random union of gametes very easily by finding the total gamete output of the parent generation and uniting the gametes at random.

3.5 Approach to Equilibrium – Single Locus Two Alleles

The rate of approach to equilibrium depends upon whether the gene frequencies in the population are equal or different in the two sexes.

(1) Equal Gene Frequencies in Two Sexes

If a population is not in equilibrium, it will attain equilibrium in next generation if the random mating is followed and the gene frequencies are equal in two sexes. For example, take the gene frequencies as $p = 0.2$ and $q = 0.8$ in both the sexes of a population. With these gene frequencies, the three genotypes may be in any proportion (frequencies) in the population as given under:

$\qquad$ (0.10, 0.20, 0.70); $\qquad$ (0.18, 0.04, 0.78); $\qquad$ (0.0, 0.4, 0.6);

$\qquad$ (0.20, 0.00, 0.80); $\qquad$ (0.05, 0.30, 0.65); $\qquad$ etc.

Now, if each of these populations are allowed to mate randomly, they will all reach the genetic equilibrium in next generation having the genotype frequencies as,

0.04, 0.32, 0.64 following the square law: $(p + q)^2 = p^2 + 2pq + q^2$. This has been shown in solved example 3.1. The genetic equilibrium will be maintained in successive generations till random mating will be allowed. Thus, the equilibrium condition is immediately established under random mating of one generation.

(2) Unequal Gene Frequencies in Two Sexes

When the gene frequencies are not equal in the two sexes, it requires two generations of random mating to approach genetic equilibrium. The initial gene frequencies may be different in the two sexes particularly when most of the migrants are of one sex (like crossbreeding zebu cows with bulls of European breeds). In such cases, the H.W. frequencies for an autosomal locus are attained in two generations of random mating. The gene frequencies in the first generation of random mating become equal in both sexes which are the average of the frequencies in the parents of two sexes. The genotype frequencies in the second generation of random mating attain equilibrium. This has been verified by an example 3.2.

It may be concluded that if genotype frequencies confirm to the H.W. law or the square law, then mating among parents was probably at random and other conditions of H.W. equilibrium were probably met. However, such a conclusion should not be based on a single generation.

3.6 Properties of Equilibrium Population

A population for single locus with two alleles has the following properties:

1. Relationship between Gene Frequencies and Genotype Frequencies

The gene frequencies and genotype frequencies has a relationship between them. The genotypic frequencies are determined by the square of the sum of the gene frequencies so that $(p + q)^2 = p2 + 2 pq + q^2$. Accordingly a change in gene frequency will lead to a change in genotype frequencies.

2. Proportion of Heterozygote

The proportion of heterozygote is as under —

(i) Under two allelic systems for a locus, the proportion of heterozygote (H) is 2pq. The value of H is maximum when p = q 0.5 and it (H = 2pq) can never exceed more than 0.50 for the diploid population in equilibrium.

(ii) The value of H decreases when the p and q move away from the point of equality (when p and q are away from 0.5). The H moves from maximum to an intermediate frequency, and the point of change is when H = D or R (2pq = p^2 or q^2) and when $p = \dfrac{2}{3}$ then H =D or when $q = \dfrac{2}{3}$ then H = R. Beyond this value of p (p = $\dfrac{2}{3}$) the p^2 > 2pq> q^2. The value of heterozygote may be greater than D or R but never greater than the sum of the two homozygote (H is never greater than D + R).

(*iii*) When an allele is very rare, it occurs almost exclusively in the heterozygous condition. This most often happens with a recessive defect which has very low frequency in the population. This means that when the allele become less frequent, the heterozygote carry a much greater proportion of that allele than carried by the homozygote. Thus as q approaches to zero, the H compared to R approaches infinity.

(*iv*) When the frequency of one allele is more than twice of the other, the proportion of heterozygote is intermediate between the two homozygote.

Thus, if $p > 2q$ then $p^2 > 2pq$ and $2pq > 4q^2 > q^2$. Thus $p^2 > 2pq > q^2$

(*v*) Test of equilibrium: The proportion of H is twice the square root of the product of the two homozygous proportions.

Thus, $H = 2\sqrt{DR}$ 3.2

or $H^2 = 4\,DR$ because $H^2 = (2pq)^2 == 4p^2q^2 = 4\,DR$.

This relationship between the proportion of heterozygote and two homozygotes holds true irrespective of the gene frequencies in the population. Thus, this can be used as a test of equilibrium. This condition of $H = 2\sqrt{DR}$ should be observed to confirm the square law.

3. Frequency of Mating

There is a general theorem for equilibrium populations which is applicable not only with random mating but also with inbreed-ing. The general theorem states that in any equilibrium population, the mating between heterozygote ($A_1A_2 \times A_1A_2$) are twice as frequent as those between the two different homozygote ($A_1A_1 \times A_2A_2$). Thus $2(A_1A_1 \times A_2A_2) = A_1A_2 \times A_1A_2$ for equilibrium. This relation is independent of gene frequencies or amount of inbreed-ing. This fact of equilibrium was first noted by Fisher (1918) and then Haldane and Moshinsky (1939). The frequency of mating between heterozygote is $4\,p^2q^2$. This is twice than the mating between the two different homozygotes ($A_1A_1 \times A_2A_2$ plus $A_2A_2 \times A_1A_1 = 2\,p^2q^2$).

The reason is given as: Out of the 6 types of mating in the population, 4 types ($A_1A_1 \times A_1A_1$, $A_2A_2 \times A_2A_2$, $A_1A_1 \times A_1A_2$, $A_1A_2 \times A_2A_2$) produce offspring of the same genotypic proportions as their parents. Whereas, in $A_1A_1 \times A_2A_2$ mating the two homozygous parents are replaced by heterozygote in the next generation but in $A_1A_2 \times A_1A_2$ mating (mating between heterozygote) only half of the offspring regain the homozygous condition. Therefore, the heterozygous mating ($A_1A_2 \times A_1A_2$) must be twice as frequent as $A_1A_1 \times A_2A_2$ including reciprocals. In other words, in homozygous mating ($A_1A_1 \times A_2A_2$), the homozygote are replaced by offspring heterozygote while in mating between heterozygote ($A_1A_2 \times A_1A_2$) only half of the offspring are homozygote. Therefore, the frequency of heterozygote mating must be twice than of mating between two homozygote $[(A_1A_1 \times A_2A_2) + (A_2A_2 \times A_1A_1)]$ at equilibrium.

The relative proportion of A_2A_2 offspring, produced by the three parental mating which produce A_2A_2 offspring ($A_1A_2 \times A_1A_2$, $A_1A_2 \times A_2A_2$, and $A_2A_2 \times A_2A_2$), are in the same proportions as the genotype frequencies expected from the square law.

Parent Mating	A_2A_2 Genotype among all offspring	Relative Frequencies of A_2A_2
$A_1A_2 \times A_1A_2$	$p^2 q^2$	$\dfrac{p^2 q^2}{q^2} = p^2$
$A_1A_2 \times A_2A_2$	$2 p^2 q^3$	$\dfrac{2p^2 q3}{q^2} = 2pq$
$A_2A_2 \times A_2A_2$	q^4	$\dfrac{q^4}{q^2} = q^2$
Total	q^2	1.0

4. Equilateral Triangle Property

The equilateral triangle can be used to represent any equilibrium population by a point (P) inside the triangle. The point P inside the triangle is chosen such that all the 3 perpendiculars from this point P to the 3 sides of the triangle are equal to D, H, R. The characteristic feature of the equilateral triangle is that the sum of the 3 perpendicular distances to the sides is equal-to the altitude of the triangle. Therefore, the altitude (height) of the triangle is taken as unity because $D + H + R = 1.0$. For convenience, the perpendicular distance from P to the base is taken equal to the proportion of heterozygote (H) and the perpendicular distances from P to the two sides of the triangle are taken equal to D and R. The point P representing the equilibrium population will fall on the parabola satisfying the equation $4DR = H^2$. Thus any equilibrium population corresponds to a point on the parabola but if the point P does not fall on the parabola, then the population is not in equilibrium. Further if a perpendicular is drawn from P to the base of the triangle, then the two segments of the base are proportional to the gene frequencies.

3.7 Estimation of Gene Frequencies – Two Allelic Systems

This depends on the type of gene action *i.e.* dominance-recessive relation between alleles.

1. Co-dominance System

There are two methods to estimate gene frequencies:

(i) Gene Counting Method

Each individual has two alleles at each locus and so there are a total of 2N genes at a locus in the population of N diploid individuals. Each A_1A_1 individual will have 2 A_1 alleles, each A_1A_2 individual will have one A_1 allele and one A_2 allele, and each A_2A_2 individual will have 2 A_2 alleles. The procedure of estimating gene frequencies is as under:

Genotypes	No. of Individuals	Total No. of Genes
A_1A_1	N_{11}	$2\,N_{11}$
A_1A_2	N_{12}	$2\,N_{12}$
A_2A_2	N_{22}	$2\,N_{22}$
Total	N	2 N

$$\text{Frequency of } A_1 \text{ allele (p)} = \frac{(2N_{11} + N_{12})}{2N} = \frac{\text{Total } A_1 \text{ alleles}}{\text{Total alleles}}$$

$$\text{Frequency of } A_2 \text{ allele (q)} = \frac{(2N_{22} + N_{12})}{2N} = \frac{\text{Total } A_2 \text{ alleles}}{\text{Total alleles}}$$

(ii) Genotype Frequency Method

The A_1A_1 genotype contains all the A_1 alleles, A_2A_2 has all the A_2 alleles while A_1A_2 genotype has one half of the A_1 alleles and another half the A_2 alleles. The Mendelian segregation partitions the two alleles of heterozygote into the two gamete pools. Thus, the frequency of an allele equals to the sum of the frequency of homozygous genotype plus half of the heterozygous genotype. Therefore, the frequency of A_1 allele (p) and A_2 allele (q) are estimated as:

$p_{(A1)} = D + \frac{1}{2}H$ and

$q_{(A2)} = R + \frac{1}{2}H$

As an example to illustrate the numerical estimation of gene frequencies from genotype frequencies, the case of MN blood group of 1000 British people may be cited here from example 3.3.

2. Dominance System

The gene frequencies for the two alleles with dominance can only be estimated in a population with H.W.E. genotype frequencies. The dominance at a locus does not change the equilibrium genotype frequencies because equilibrium is a function of the gene frequencies and not of the type of gene action.

Assuming that the population is in H.W.E., the gene frequency of recessive allele is estimated as the square root of the genotype frequency of the recessive homozygote. This is because the frequency of recessive homozygote (R) is taken as q^2 and the frequency of recessive allele is q.

Therefore, $q = \sqrt{R} = \sqrt{q^2}$ and $p = 1 - q$

The *coat colour* in Aberdeen-Angus cattle has only two phenotypes *viz.* black and red. The red colour is recessive and hence the red cattle are homozygous recessive. Another example is *dropsy in calf* of Ayrshire breed of cattle caused by a recessive autosomal gene.

3.8 Sex Influenced Traits

The genes controlling the sex influenced characters are present on autosomes. The dominance-recessive relationship of the alleles is reverse in two sexes for these traits which results the heterozygous genotype to produce different phenotype in two sexes. The allelic interaction is such that one allele is dominant in one sex but recessive in opposite sex. This changed or opposing dominance is due to the presence of different sex hormones in two sexes. The examples of such characters are presence of horns in some breeds of sheep, mahogany and white colour in Ayrshire breed of cattle, pattern baldness, short length of index (second) finger, white forelock, ichthyosis (skin abnormality) in human, beard in goat. The genes controlling these characters show dominance in males but recessive in females.

The procedure to estimate the gene frequency of these genes is like that of autosomal alleles which show dominance. Therefore, $q = \sqrt{R}$.

3.9 Application of H.W. Law

This law is useful in following ways:

1. *Maintenance or change in genetic structure*: This law suggests that the genetic structure of a population can be conserved under random mating. Therefore, random mating is advocated if the population has optimum fitness. However, the animal breeder remains interested to change the genetic structure in a desired direction and level. The knowledge of this law is useful for bringing a change in genetic structure by violating one or more conditions under which the H.W. law holds true. The most important and practical force is the selection for bringing genetic change.

2. *Estimation of genotypic frequencies:* Provided the population is large, the mating is random and no evolutionary force is operating, the genotypic frequencies in progeny generation can be estimated from gene frequencies in parent generation by using the square law as: $(p + q)^2 = p^2 + 2pq + q^2$

3. *Estimation of gene frequencies*: When there is dominance relation between alleles, the estimation of gene frequencies is not possible either by gene counting or from genotypic frequencies. Under this situation, the frequency of recessive allele may be estimated as square root of frequency of recessive homozygote as $q = \sqrt{q^2}$

4. *Test of genetic equilibrium*: The genotypic frequencies observed in a population should be in agreement to that expected genotypic frequencies based on the square law of the relation of gene and genotypic frequencies. This is the test of genetic equilibrium. A significant deviation between observed and expected genotypic frequencies indicates that the population is not in genetic equilibrium and hence one or more of the assumptions of holding true the H.W. law is not satisfied. The chi-square test is applied to test the significance of deviation as-

$$\chi^2 = \frac{(A - p^2N)}{p^2N} + \frac{(B - pqN)^2}{2pqN} + \frac{(C - q^2N)^2}{q^2N}$$

$$= \left[\frac{A^2}{p^2N} + \frac{B^2}{2pqN} + \frac{C^2}{q^2N} \right] - N$$

where, A, B and C are the observed numbers of three genotypes

N = A + B + C It is tested at one degree of freedom.

5. *To establish Mendelian hypothesis i.e. mode of inheritance*: The H.W. law can be used to establish a genetic theory about the mode of inheritance of a trait. Some of the examples are as under:

(i) Wright (1917) established the evidence of genetic basis of coat colour in Short horn breed of cattle being controlled by a single locus with two co-dominant alleles rather than two loci hypothesis proposed earlier. He compared the observed frequencies of progeny genotypes with the expected frequencies based on square law for 2 loci and single locus.

(ii) Bernstein (1925) established the genetic basis of A, B, O blood antigens as three alleles of a single locus rather than two loci hypothesis proposed in 1911. He found that the observed frequency data was not in agreement with that expected on two loci with dominance.

(iii) Neel (1950) established the monofactorial basis of thalassemia major and minor which was earlier thought to be the result of interaction of two dominant factors.

(iv) Establishment of hypothesis for the genetic determination of a character controlled by major genes requires the analysis of family data for two generations or for a single generation (sib pairs), particularly when there is dominance so as the heterozygotes are distinguished from dominant homozygotes by conducting genetic analysis or by biochemical and immunological techniques.

Snyder (1932) collected family data on the ability to taste the synthetic substance *phenylthiocarbamide* (PTC) and studied the inheritance of human ability to taste PTC. He found that the ability to taste PTC is dominant (TT, Tt) over lack of ability to taste the substance by people (tt).

The observed ratios of recessive progeny produced from the mating of D x D, D x R, and R x R parents are compared with the expected ratios for recessive progeny from these mating (Snyder's ratios). Three types of mating, their frequencies, the frequencies of dominant (D) and recessive (R) progenies under random mating if dominance is present are shown below:

Table 3.4: Snyder Ratios

Types of Mating	Mating Frequencies Dominant	Frequency of Recessive	Progeny Recessive	Ratio of
D x D	$(1 - q^2)(1 - q^2)$ $= p^2(1 + q)^2$	$p^2(1 + 2q)$	p^2q^2	$\dfrac{q^2}{(1+q)^2} = S_2$
D x R	$2(1 - q^2)q^2$ $= 2pq^2(1 + q)$	$2pq^2$	$2pq^3$	$\dfrac{q}{(1+q)} = S_1$
R x R	$(q^2)(q^2) = q^4$	0	q^4	

Snyder (1932) worked out two ratios as:

Expected recessive progeny from D x R (dominant x recessive) mating,

$$S_1 = \frac{R}{D+R}$$

$$= \frac{2pq^3}{\left[2pq^2 + 2pq^3\right]}$$

$$= \frac{q}{(1+q)} \text{ and}$$

Expected recessive progeny from D x D (dominant x dominant) mating,

$$S_2 = \frac{R}{D+R}$$

$$= \frac{p^2q^2}{\left[p^2(1+2q)+p^2q^2\right]}$$

$$= \frac{q^2}{(1+q)^2}$$

The, S_1 and S_2 are called as *Snyder's ratios or population ratios*. The S_1 and S_2 are expected ratios based on square law, for single locus two allelic systems with dominance, and obtained from the value of q. The value of q is estimated from observed sample data (number of parents and progenies) as:

Mating Types (Parents)	Numbers of Mating	Number of Progeny		
		Dominant	Recessive	Total
D x D	N_{01}	N_{11}	N_{21}	N_{31}
D x R	N_{02}	N_{12}	N_{22}	N_{32}
R x R	N_{03}	N_{13}	N_{23}	N_{33}
Total	N_{04}	N_{14}	N_{24}	N_{34}

$$q^2 = \frac{[\text{No. of recessive parents + rec. progeny}]}{[\text{Total parents + totalprogeny}]} = \frac{[(2N_{03} + N_{02}) + N_{24}]}{[2N_{04} + N_{34}]}$$

$$q = \sqrt{q^2}$$

The observed ratios of recessive progenies out of total progenies from D x D mating (S_2) and from D x R mating (S_1) are worked out from sample data. The observed and expected ratios are compared as:

Expected ratio based on HWL   Observed ratios (sample data)

$$S_2 = \frac{q^2}{(1+q)^2} \qquad\qquad\qquad\qquad \frac{N_{21}}{N_{31}}$$

$$S_1 = \frac{q}{(1+q)} \qquad\qquad\qquad\qquad \frac{N_{22}}{N_{32}}$$

An agreement between observed and expected ratios is tested provided the hypothesis for single locus autosomal gene holds good. A close agreement indicates that the trait is controlled by single autosomal locus with two alleles having dominance.

The Snyder's ratios have a relationship that $S_2 = S_1^2$. Secondly, these Snyder's ratios differ from Mendelian ratios. The Mendelian ratios are constant for all traits and all populations but the population ratios (S_1 and S_2) differ from trait to trait in the same population and from population to population for the same trait.

6. Square law and *mating system*: A close fit between the observed and expected frequency data indicates the random mating whereas the deficiency of heterozygotic frequency is an indication of inbreeding, in general.

7. *Estimate the micro-evolutionary changes*: The micro evolutionary changes can be known by comparing the gene and genotype frequencies of different samples from two localities to know the change over space or from one population at different times (generations) to know the changes over time. Significant deviation between populations over space and over time for a population indicate the micro-evolutionary changes in space and time.

Solved Examples and Exercises

Example 3.1

The genotypic frequencies for 3 genotypes in a population were recorded to be as 0.0, 0.4 and 0.6. Estimate the frequencies of two alleles, apply test of genetic equilibrium and show the approach to genetic equilibrium under random mating.

Solution

(i) The frequencies of two alleles can be estimated from genotypic frequencies as:

Frequency of A_1 allele (p) = ½ (0.4) = 0.2

Frequency of A_2 allele (q) = ½ (0.4) + 0.6 = 0.8

(ii) Test of genetic equilibrium:

The genotypic frequencies as per square law will be as:

$(p + q)^2 = p^2 + 2pq + q^2$

$(0.2 + 0.8)^2 = 0.04 + 0.32 + 0.64$

Thus, the genotype frequencies in parental generation were not in genetic equilibrium because they were not in accordance with the gene frequencies.

(iii) Approach to equilibrium: The genotype frequencies in the progeny generation, produced by random union of gametes of parental population, which was not in equilibrium, become as:

$p^2_{(A1A1)} = 0.04$; $2pq (A_1A_2) = 0.32$; $q^2 (A_2A_2) = 0.64$.

These genotype frequencies are in genetic equilibrium because these can be determined by the square of gene frequencies in the parent generation as shown above. Thus, the population (which was not in equilibrium but had equal gene frequencies in the two sexes) attains an equilibrium structure of the genotype proportion in the first generation of random mating.

Example 3.2

The gene frequencies in two sexes were found unequal as under -

Gene frequencies in males p $_{m(A1)}$ = 0.4, q $_{m(A2)}$ = 0.6;

Gene frequencies in females p $_{f(A1)}$ = 0.8, q $_{f(A2)}$ = 0.2

Where, the subscripts *m* and *f* indicate the male and female sex.

Show the approach to genetic equilibrium of this population under random mating.

Solution

The population will attain the genetic equilibrium in two generations of random mating. This can be verified by random union of gametes. The new gene frequencies in the first generation will be the average of the respective gene frequencies among the parents and hence

$p_1 = \frac{1}{2}(0.4 + 0.8) = 0.6$ and $q_1 = \frac{1}{2}(0.6 + 0.2) = 0.4$

It is interesting to note that the genotype frequencies in the progeny of first generation do not follow the square law because these are not in accordance of the gene frequencies in the parents. Thus the progeny of first generation are not in HW Equilibrium.

Second generation of random mating:- In the next generation (G_2) the genotype frequencies can be determined from the gene frequencies in G_1. Thus the genotype frequencies in second generation (G_2) will be as:

$(p_1 + q_1)^2 = p_1^2 + 2p_1q_1 + q_1^2$ and hence,

$(0.6 + \mathbf{0.4})^2 = 0.36 + 0.48 + 0.16$

Now this second generation (G_2) is in H.W. equilibrium and will remain in equilibrium under the assumption of H.W. law.

Example 3.3

The *MN blood group* in man is controlled by two alleles at one locus showing no dominance. These two alleles are designated as M and N; having co-dominance relation between them, producing molecules (substance) on the surface of RBC of the individuals. The genetic structure for this locus of MN blood group in a sample of 1000 British (Race and Sanger, 1975) is given as under:

Phenotypes (Blood Groups)	M	MN	N	Total
Genotypes				
No. of individuals	298	489	213	1000
Per cent individuals	29.8	48.9	21.3	100.0
Proportion of individuals	0.298	0.489	0.213	1.0
(genotype frequencies)	$P_{11} = D$	$(2P_{12}) = H$	$(P_{22}) = R$	

Solution

Total numbers of genes (2N) were 2x 1000 = 2000.

Number of M alleles were (2 x 298) + 489 = 1085

Frequency of M allele (p) = $\dfrac{1085}{2000}$ = 0.5425.

Number of N alleles out of total 2000 alleles were (2 x 213) + 489 = 915

Frequency of N allele (q) = $\dfrac{915}{2000}$ = 0.4575.

Example 3.4

The frequency of dropsy calves is about 1 in 300 births. Find out the frequencies of two alleles showing dominance relation and proportion of heterozygous.

Solution

$$R = q^2 = \frac{1}{300} = 0.0033 \text{ and so}$$

$$q = \sqrt{\frac{1}{300}} = \sqrt{0.0033} = 0.057$$

The frequency of dominant allele (p) will be $1-q = 1-0.057 = 0.943$

Exercises

3.5. Find the proportions of 3 genotypes in next generation produced by random mating in case of the following populations- 0.25, 0.0, 0.75; 0.20, 0.40, 0.40; 0.15, 0.25, 0.60

3.6. From the composition of the following population. Check whether these are in genetic equilibrium. Estimate the equilibrium proportions for those which are not in equilibrium:

0.20, 0.32, 0.48; 0.30, 0.25, 0.35; 35, 15, 5; 0.50, 0.50, 0; 0.9, 0.10, 0.81; 27, 36, 12

3.7. Verify the following relations, taking $p + q = 1$:

(i) $p^2q + pq^2 = pq = q-q^2$

(ii) $p^2-q^2 = p-q$

(iii) $p+2q = 1+2q = 1+q = 2-p$

(iv) $(1-2q)^2 = (1-2p)^2$ (v) $1-2q = p-q = 2p-1$

(vi) $2q-p = 1-2p = q-p$

(vii) $p(1+q) = 1-q^2 = p(2-p)$

3.8. A character is controlled by single locus with no dominance among alleles. The genotypic frequencies in the population observed were 0.24 AA, 0.52 Aa and 0.24 aa in one population while these were 0.27 AA, 0.20 Aa and 0.53 in second population. Examine whether these population are in HWE state and find out the genotypic frequencies in next generation assuming random mating.

3.9. Calculate gene frequency of A and a gene in a population having 500 AA, 600 Aa and 950 aa individuals. What is the expected number of each genotype if the population is in HWE state? If the frequency of allele **a** is 0.45, estimate the expected number of individuals of three genotypes in a random mating population of 500 size.

3.10. What is the frequency of heterozygote (Aa) in a random mating population (i) if the frequency of recessive phenotype aa is 0.09 and (ii) when the frequency of all dominants is 0.19?

3.11. Consider three genotypes (PP, Pp and pp) in a random mating population of cattle in which the individuals with genotypes PP and Pp were polled but with genotype pp were non-polled. It was found that 36 out of 100 cattle were non-polled. Calculate the relative frequencies of (i) two alleles, (ii) 3 genotypes and (iii) two phenotypes.

3.12. In a random mating population, it was found that one-fourth of the normal individuals were carrier for a defect controlled by single locus two alleles. Find out the frequency of recessive allele.

(Hint: The frequency of recessive, normal and carrier individuals among normal individuals is q^2, $1-q^2$ and $2pq/1-q^2$, respectively. Thus equate $2pq/1-q^2 = ¼$ and find the answer).

3.13. Consider that black coat colour in cattle is dominant over red colour. Find out the gene frequency of black and red alleles and the number of heterozygous individuals if there were 72 red animals in a sample of 450 animals.

Chapter 4
Genetic Equilibrium – Multiple Alleles

Presence of more than two alleles at a locus in the population is common. These alleles are called as multiple alleles. The presence of additional allele at a locus does not introduce any difficulty to follow the square law. The consequences of random mating in a large population are same as for two alleles at a locus. Weinberg (1909) showed that H.W. law is also applicable to the case of multiple alleles. The zygotes are formed proportionately by random mating of two sexes having equal allelic frequencies according to the square of sum of gene frequencies.

4.1 Equilibrium Proportions – Multiple Alleles

The genotype frequencies for multiple alleles in a large random mating population are obtained from expansion of square of a multinomial. For example, consider 3 alleles (A_1, A_2 and A3) at locus A with their frequencies as p, q, r, respectively such that p + q + r = 1.0. In this case there will be 6 genotypes with their proportions as under:

Alleles and their Frequencies				Genotypes and their Frequencies					
A_1	A_2	A_3		A_1A_1	A_2A_2	A_3A_3	A_1A_2	A_1A_3	A_2A_3
$(P + q + r)^2$			=	p^2 +	q^2 +	r^2 +	2pq +	2pr +	2 qr

The sum of allelic frequencies must be equal to unity and hence p + q + r = 1.0. Likewise, the sum of the genotype frequencies must also be equal to unity and hence $p^2 + q^2 + r^2 + 2pq + 2pr + 2qr = 1.0$. The homozygote are equal to the sum of the squared frequencies $(p^2 + q^2 + r^2)$ while the heterozygote are equal to the twice of the product of each pair of frequencies *viz.* $2 (pq + pr + qr)$. In general, the genotypes in an equilibrium population can be represented as:

$$(\Sigma p_i A_i)^2 = \Sigma p_i (A_i A_i)^2 + 2 \Sigma (A_i A_j)$$

$$= \text{Homozygote} + \text{Heterozygote}$$

Taking K as the number of alleles at a locus, the number of homozygotes, heterozygotes and total genotypes produced will be as under :

No. of genotypes = No. of homozygotes + No. of heterozygotes

$$\frac{K(K+1)}{2} = K + \frac{K(K-1)}{2}$$

The number of phenotypes depends on the interaction of multiple alleles (dominance). The numbers of phenotypes are lesser than the number of genotype if dominance among alleles is involved.

4.2 Proof of H.W. Law – Single Locus Multiple Alleles

The H.W. equilibrium frequencies of genotypes can be proved by the same two methods as done in case of two allelic system *i.e.* random union of gametes and random mating of genotypes.

The random mating of genotypes procedure becomes cumbersome, labourious and time consuming due to more number of combinations of 6 genotypes (with 3 alleles at a locus). There will be 36 combinations of mating with 6 genotypes, out of which 15 combinations will be similar and therefore there will be only 21 different types of mating among 6 genotypes.

The random union of gamete method is used to test the equilibrium condition as was done for two allelic systems.

4.3 Approach to Equilibrium – Multiple Alleles

(i) **Equal gene frequencies in two sexes:** A population which is not in genetic equilibrium state will approach equilibrium after one generation of random mating provided there are equal gene frequencies in two sexes, as in case of two alleles.

(ii) **Unequal gene frequencies in two sexes:** When the gene frequencies are not equal in two sexes, it requires 2 generations of random mating to reach the equilibrium state. In the first generation of random mating, the gene frequencies become equal in the two sexes which will be equal to the average of the gene frequencies in parents. In the second generation (produced by random mating) the genotypic frequencies attain equilibrium state.

The approach to equilibrium state for multiple alleles having their unequal frequencies can be illustrated by taking 3 alleles at a locus as:

Gene frequencies in male sex $p_{m(A1)} = 0.3$, $q_{m(A2)} = 0.5$ and $r_{m(A3)} = 0.2$

Gene frequencies in female sex $p_{f(A1)} = 0.4$, $q_{f(A2)} = 0.3$ and $r_{f(A3)} = 0.3$

Gene frequencies in G_1 generation after one generation of random mating will be:

$$P_{1(A1)} = 0.35, q_{1(A2)} = 0.4 \text{ and } r_{1(A3)} = 0.25.$$

These new gene frequencies in G_1 generation under random mating are equal to the average of the respective gene frequencies among the parents but these are not in accordance to the square law and hence G_1 generation is not in HWE. But in next generation (G_2), produced after random mating, the genotype frequencies can be determined from the gene frequencies in G_1 generation. The genotype frequencies in G_2 generation will be as under:

$$(p_1 + q_1 + r_1)^2 = p_2^2 + q_2^2 + r_2^2 + 2 p^2 q^2 + 2 p^2 r^2 + 2 q^2 r^2$$

$$(0.35 + 0.40 + 0.25)^2 = 0.122 + 0.16 + 0.062 + 2 (0.14 + 0.087 + 0.10)$$

The above values can be verified from random mating among two sexes of G_1 generation. The genotypic frequencies in G_2 generation are in HWE and will remain in equilibrium in future generations under the conditions of H.W. law. Thus, if the gene frequencies in a population are not equal in the two sexes for multiple alleles, it will require two generations of random mating to attain HWE.

4.4 Properties of Genetic Equilibrium – Multiple Alleles

1. There exists a relationship between gene frequencies and genotype frequencies

$$(p + q + r)^2 = p^2 + q^2 + r^2 + 2pq + 2pr + 2qr$$

2. The heterozygotes for multiple alleles have the proportion as:

   (i) The heterozygote may exceed to 0.50 which is maximum for two alleles. The frequencies of heterozygote are maximum when the frequencies of multiple alleles are equal. Thus, if there are k alleles at a locus, the frequencies of all the multiple alleles should be equal to $1/k$ to make the proportion of heterozygote maximum.

   (ii) The relationship of the number of multiple alleles to heterozygosity is that the maximum heterozygosity for k alleles will equal to $(k-1)/k$. It can be observed that the heterozygosity increase with increase in number of alleles, approaching a limit nearly 100 per cent with their frequencies being equal. The total heterozygosity decreases for unequal gene frequencies.

   The total number of genotypes $= k (k + 1)/2$, out of which the number of homozygote are equal to number of multiple alleles at a locus (k) and the number of heterozygotes $= k (k -1)/2$ with maximum frequency of heterozygote $= (k-1)/k$.

4.5 Estimation of Gene Frequencies – Multiple Alleles

The gene frequencies are estimated considering the type of allelic interaction among multiple alleles *viz.* absence or presence of dominance and mixture of dominance and co-dominance.

1. Absence of Dominance (Co-dominance)

The number of different alleles are counted and divided by the total number of genes in the population at that locus. Considering 3 alleles at a locus (A_1, A_2 and A_3), there will be 6 genotypes (A_1A_1, A_2A_2, A_3A_3, A_1A_2, A_1A_3 and A_2A_3) and 6 corresponding phenotypes. The frequency of A_1 allele can be estimated as a proportion of total number of A_1 alleles to that of total number of alleles (2N) in the population. Thus, the frequencies of three alleles will be estimated as-

$$P_{(A1)} = \frac{(2A_1A_1 + A_1A_2 + A_1A_3)}{2N}$$

$$q_{(A2)} = \frac{(2A_2A_2 + A_1A_2 + A_2A_3)}{2N}$$

$$r_{(A3)} = \frac{(2A_3A_3 + A_1A_3 + A_2A_3)}{2N}$$

The allele frequencies can also be estimated from the genotypic frequencies. For example, with 3 alleles at a locus, the frequency of A_1 allele will be estimated as-

$$P_{(A1)} = f\,A_1A_1 + \tfrac{1}{2}(f\,A_1A_2 + f\,A_1A_3),$$

where, f stands for the frequency of the genotype.

Example

There exists hemoglobin polymorphism in human controlled by 3 alleles at a locus represented by A (normal hemoglobin), S (sickle cell hemoglobin), and C (mild anemia). The hemoglobin S is produced when the amino acid, glutamic acid present in normal hemoglobin at 6 [th] place is replaced by amino acid valine, and causes RBC to sickle under reduced oxygen tension resulting in hemolytic anemia which is fatal before the age of 20. The hemoglobin C (Hb^C) produced at the same position (residue 6 of β chain) causes mild anemia with hemolysis. The 6 possible genotypes produced for hemoglobin are AA, SS, CC, AS, AC, SC and all these 6 genotypes produce 6 phenotypes due the co-dominance among the 3 alleles.

2. Dominance System

The number of phenotypes equals the number of alleles. The genotypes of some heterozygote show dominance which results in some of the heterozygote and homozygote to become indistinguishable. This makes difficult the estimation of gene frequencies. In such case, random mating is assumed. In case of complete dominance between 3 or more alleles in succession, the gene frequency can be estimated with the most recessive allele by taking its frequency as square root of the recessive genotype frequency.

Let the 3 alleles at a locus be designated as A, a′ and a with dominance hierarchy as A > a′ > a, and representing their corresponding frequencies as p, q, r. This condition of dominance hierarchy produces only 3 phenotypes from 6 genotypes.

(i) The genotypes AA, Aa' and Aa with their respective genotypic frequencies of p^2, $2pq$, $2pr$ are grouped in first phenotypic class, denoting the observed number of individuals of this phenotypic class by the letter a and its proportion as $\dfrac{a}{N}$.

(ii) The genotypes a'a' and a'a with their respective genotypic frequencies of q^2 and $2pr$ are grouped in second phenotypic class, denoting the observed number of individuals of this class by the letter b and its proportion as $\dfrac{b}{N}$.

(iii) The remainder sixth genotype (aa) with its genotypic frequency of r^2 is the third phenotypic class, denoting the observed number of individuals of this third class by the letter c or a. and its proportion as $\dfrac{c}{N}$ which is the frequency of most recessive genotype (r^2).

The proportion of three phenotypic classes will be as under:

$$\text{Proportion of phenotype I} \quad = \frac{(AA + Aa' + Aa)}{N} = \frac{a}{N}$$

$$= p^2 + 2pq + 2pr$$

$$\text{Proportion of phenotype II} \quad = \frac{(a'a' + a'a)}{N} = \frac{b}{N}$$

$$= q^2 + 2qr$$

$$\text{Proportion of phenotype III} \quad = \frac{aa}{N} = \frac{c}{N}$$

$$= r^2$$

(i) The frequency of most recessive allele (a) represented by r is estimated as:

$$r = \sqrt{r^2} \text{ or } r = \sqrt{\frac{c}{N}}$$

(ii) The frequency of second recessive allele (a') in hierarchy represented by q is estimated as-

$$q = \sqrt{\frac{b}{N} + \frac{c}{N}} - \sqrt{\frac{c}{N}} \quad \text{(Wiener and others)}$$

$$= 1 - \sqrt{\frac{b}{N} + \frac{c}{N}} \quad \text{(Bernstein, 1925)}$$

(iii) The frequency of most dominant allele (A) is estimated by difference as:
$p = 1 - (q + r)$.

Examples

(1) Coat colour of rabbit is controlled by three alleles at a single autosomal locus with dominance hierarchy as: $C > c^h > c$ occurring with the frequencies as p. q and r, respectively. The allele c produces albino rabbits, c^h produces Himalayan colour rabbit (white body with pigmented ears, nose, tip of feet and tail) and C produces agouti (full colour).

(2) Land snail (Copaca memoralis in Europe) is the most common polymorphic for shell color and banding patterns. The colour pattern is governed by 3 alleles at a locus showing dominance hierarchy as Brown > pink > yellow and thus yellow colour is the most recessive. The 3 alleles can be represented as B, P, Y, respectively for the 3 colours with frequencies as p, q and r, respectively. The phenotypes of 3 colours in land snail are represented as:

Phenotypes	Brown	Pink	Yellow
Frequencies	$p^2 + 2pq + 2pr$	$q^2 + 2qr$	r^2

3. Mixture of Dominant and Co-dominant Allele

The alleles A and B are co-dominant to each other but both are dominant over the third allele O. The procedure to estimate the allelic frequencies is the same as that for the alleles showing dominance. The best example is the *ABO blood group system in man* controlled by three alleles (A, B and O).

Bernstein (1930) explained that the allele A produces antigen A, B allele produces antigen B while the allele O does not produce any antigen. The three alleles follow the ordinary Mendelian inheritance that the alleles A and B are co-dominant to each other but both are dominant over the allele O. The frequencies of three alleles A, B and O are taken, respectively, as p. q and r. This produces six genotypes but only four phenotypes known as blood groups. The phenotypes, genotypes and their frequencies are as under:

Phenotypes (Blood Groups)	Genotypes	Genotype Frequencies	Serum Agglutinin
A	AA, AO	$p^2 + 2pr$	Anti-B
B	BB, BO	$q^2 + 2qr$	Anti-A
AB	AB	$2pq$	None
O	OO	r^2	Anti-A and Anti-B

The genotype frequencies are obtained from the expansion of gene frequencies as:

$$(p + q + r)^2 = p^2 + q^2 + r^2 + 2pq + 2pr + 2qr$$

This can be obtained from random union of gametes.

Estimation of Allelic Frequencies for Multiple Alleles

(i) Freq. of most recessive allele, $r = \sqrt{r^2}$

= $\sqrt{}$genotypic freq. of blood group O

(ii) Frequencies of co-dominant alleles are estimated from combined frequencies of either of the co-dominant allele (p or q) with most recessive allele (r) as:

(a) Freq. of one co-domonant allele (p) is estimated as:

$(p + r)^2 = p^2 + 2pr + r^2$ combined frequency of blood group A and O

Thus, $(p + r) = \sqrt{(A + O)}$ and hence

$p = (p + r) - r$

$= \sqrt{(A + O)} - \sqrt{O}$ = frequency of A allele.

(b) Similarly, frequency of other codominant allele (q) is estimated as:

$(q + r)^2 = q^2 + 2pq + r^2$ combined frequency of blood group B and O

Thus, $(q + r) = \sqrt{(B + O)}$ and hence

$q = (q + r) - r$

$= \sqrt{(B + O)} - \sqrt{O}$ = frequency of allele B

Alternately, the frequency of codominant allele can be estimated by difference as:

$p = 1 - (q + r) = 1 - \sqrt{(B + O)}$ and

$q = 1 - (p + r) = 1 - \sqrt{(A + O)}$

Where, A, B, and O are the frequencies of blood groups.

Solved Examples and Exercises

Example 4.1

The following data on hemoglobin polymorphism controlled by multiple alleles showing co-dominance in American Negros was given by Levingstone (1967) as:

Hb Types	AA	AS	AC	SS	SC	CC	Total
Numbers	2501	213	64	14	4	4	2800
Frequencies	0.8932	0.0776	0.0229	0.0059	0.0014	0.0014	100.0

Solution

The gene frequencies can be estimated by gene counting method as well as from the frequencies of genotypes containing that particular allele. The allelic frequencies so estimated were found as:

Hb A = 0.9427; Hb S = 0.0437; Hb C = 0.0136

Example 4.2

The following data on shell colour polymorphism of land snail were recorded. Estimate the frequencies of 3 alleles, showing dominance relationship.

Phenotypes	Brown	Pink	Yellow	Total
Observed No.	173	443	115	731

Solution

The allelic frequencies of 3 alleles producing shell colour can be estimated as under:

Frequency of most recessive allele (r_y) $= \sqrt{r^2} = \sqrt{\dfrac{115}{731}} = 0.3966$

Frequency of pink gene (q) $= \sqrt{\left[\dfrac{443+115}{731}\right]} - \sqrt{\dfrac{115}{731}}$

$= 0.8737 - 0.3966 = 0.4771$

Frequency of brown gene (p) $= 1 - (q + r)$

$= 1 - (0.4771 + 0.3966) = 0.1263$

Example 4.3

ABO blood group in human follow the dominance relation as A = B > O. Find out the allelic frequencies in a population having 29 AB, 371 B, 54 A and 436 O blood groups.

Solution

Frequency of most recessive allele O (r)

$= \sqrt{\text{genotype frequency of blood group O}} = \sqrt{r^2}$

$= \sqrt{\dfrac{436}{890}} = \sqrt{0.4898} = 0.699$

Frequency of A allele (p) $= \sqrt{\dfrac{(54+436)}{890}} - \sqrt{\dfrac{436}{890}}$

$= \sqrt{\dfrac{490}{890}} - 0.4898 = \sqrt{0.551} - 0.4898$

$= \sqrt{0.061} = 0.246$

Frequency of B allele (q) $= 1 - p - r = 1 - \sqrt{A + O}$

$= 1 - 0.246 - 0.699 = 0.052$

4.4. The followings are the allelic frequencies at a locus with 3 alleles: $A_1 = 0.3$, $A_2 = 0.5$ and $A_3 = ?$ Calculate the frequency of A_3 allele and write down all the possible genotypes at this locus with their frequencies.

4.5. The *RBC acid phosphatase enzyme* controlled by three alleles (A, B, and C) at a locus with co-dominance among all of them have been recorded in a sample of 500 people with the following results

Genotype	AA	BB	CC	AB	AC	BC
Frequency	0.09	0.35	0.0	0.48	0.03	0.05

Estimate the frequency of three alleles. Explain why there was no CC individual in the sample.

4.6. The three alleles at a locus (A, S and C) control the *Hb variation in humans* showing co-dominance among all the three alleles. Calculate the frequencies of three alleles from the data. Find out the percentage of heterozygote and predict the genetic structure of next generation assuming random mating.

Genotype	AA	AS	AC	SS	SC	CC
Numbers	719	199	114	2	5	3

4.7. Taking the order of dominance as agouti (full colour) > Himalayan >albino colour allele in rabbit, estimate the frequencies of 3 alleles in a sample having 570 agouti, 140 himalayan and 20 albino rabbits and in another sample of 500 rabbits having 25 per cent agouti, 50 per cent Himalayan and rest albino in a random mating population.

4.8. A survey of 600 people conducted on ABO blood group system revealed that there were 37 people having blood group A and rest had the group O. Find out the allelic frequencies assuming random mating.

Chapter 5
Genetic Equilibrium – Sex Linked Genes

The homogametic sex (XX, female in case of mammals and Drosophila) having two sex linked alleles at each locus transmits one gene to all of the progeny of both the sexes (sons and daughters). The heterogametic sex (XY, males in case of mammals and Drosophila) having only one sex linked gene at each locus on X chromosome transmits its genes to sons only. Thus, the female offspring receive one X chromosome from their mother and other X chromosome from their father, and both the parent have equal genetic contribution to its female offspring. On the contrary, the male offspring receive X chromosome from their mother and Y chromosome from their father, thus male parent does not contribute any sex linked gene to it male offspring. The genetic contribution of male parent is thus not equal to its offspring of two sexes.

5.1 Equilibrium Proportion – Sex Linked Genes

When mating frequencies are determined randomly and the allelic frequencies are equal in two sexes, it can be shown that the population remains at equilibrium. The frequencies of six types of mating and the expected progeny at equilibrium for X – linked alleles are shown as in Tables 5.1.

Table 5.1

(i) Mating Frequencies

Males	Females		
	p^2 (A1 A1)	$2\ pq$ (A1 A2)	q^2 (A2 A2)
P (A1Y)	p^3	$2\ p^2q$	pq^2
q (A2Y)	p^2q	$2\ pq^2$	q^3

(ii) Expected Progeny Produced at Equilibrium

Mating Types	Frequency of Mating	Progeny Produced				
		Females			Males	
		A_1A_1	A_1A_2	A_2A_2	A_1Y	A_2Y
$A_1 A_1 \times A_1 Y$	p^3	p^2	...	...	p^3...	
$A_1 A_2 \times A_1 Y$	$2\ p^2q$	p^2q	p^2q	...	p^2q	p^2q
$A_2 A_2 \times A_1 Y$	pq^2	...	pq^2	...	...	$p\ q^2$
$A_1 A_1 \times A_2 Y$	p^2q	...	p^2q	...	p^2q	...
$A_1 A_2 \times A_2 Y$	$2\ pq^2$	...	pq^2	pq^2	pq^2	pq^2
$A_2 A_2 \times A_2 Y$	q^3	...	...	q^3	...	q^3

These are the same frequencies in both the sexes as were in the parent population. Therefore, the gene and genotype frequencies for sex-linked genes remain constant from generation to generation under the conditions of H.W. law.

5.2 Approach to Equilibrium – Sex Linked Genes

(i) Equal Gene Frequencies

If sex-linked alleles are at equilibrium in the population, it is expected that allelic frequencies should be equal inn the two sexes. Conversely, if the allelic frequencies for sex linked genes are equal in the two sexes, the population is in equilibrium. If the allelic frequencies for autosomal genes are not equal in the two sexes, they become equal in the first generations under random mating and they are equal to the average of the two parent's gene frequencies and attain genetic equilibrium after two generations of random mating.

(ii) Unequal Gene Frequencies

The situation is complicated for sex-linked genes and follow an oscillating (zig zag) approach to equilibrium. The complication is due to the two facts that the gene frequencies among male progeny are determined by those of their mothers ($p_m = p'_f$) and secondly the average gene frequency in the two sexes (p) is not simply half the sum of the parental gene frequencies but is the average weighted by the dosage of the X chromosomes (2 X in female + 1 X in males divided by three).Thus, p = 1/3 (2p_f + p_m). This p is constant and is the ultimate equilibrium value of gene frequency after several generations of random mating.

The initial population with different gene frequencies in the two sexes will be as under:

	Males (XY)		Females (XX)		
Genotype	A_1Y	A_2Y	A_1A_1	A_1A_2	A_1A_2
Frequency	p	q	r	2s	t

such that p + q = r + 2s + t = 1 among females and   p + q = 1 among males

The principle of random mating between individuals equivalent to random union of gametes is used to estimate the genotypic frequencies of next generation. The females produce two types of gametes *viz.* A_1 (r + s) and A_2 (s + t). The proportion of A_1 female gametes is r + s and the proportion of A_2 female gametes produced is s + t. When they unite with Y gamete of males, they produce male offspring in those proportions. When the female gametes unite with X gamete of males, they produce female offspring in the following proportion.

Table 5.2: Female Progeny of different Genotypes Produced with Expected Proportions

		Female Gametes and their Frequencies	
		A_1 (r + s)	A_2 (s + t)
Male Gametes	A_1 (p)	$A_1 A_1$ = p (r+s)	$A_1 A_2$ = p (s + t)
and their freq.	A_2 (q)	$A_1 A_2$ = q (r + s)	$A_2 A_2$ = q (s + t)

The total female progeny will be produced in the ratio of p (r + s) with $A_1 A_1$ genotypes, p (s + t) + q (r + s) with $A_1 A_2$ genotypes and q (s + t) with $A_2 A_2$ genotypes. Therefore, the next generation of two sexes will be produced in the following proportions:

Male progeny: r + s with A_1Y genotype and s + t with A_2Y genotypes

Female progeny: p (r + s) $A_1 A_1$: p (s + t) + q (r + s) $A_1 A_2$: q (s + t) $A_2 A_2$

The approach to equilibrium for sex-linked genes with random mating for unequal gene frequencies in the two sexes follow an oscillating (zig zag) approach to equilibrium and it has been illustrated with the help of example 5.1.

5.3 Properties of Equilibrium Population

The values in the table are an illustration of the approach to equilibrium in an oscillating manner. The following properties of sex linked genes showing relation between any generations to the next are evident:

(i) *Gene frequency in males* (p_m): This depends on the gene frequency of their mothers because the males get their X-linked alleles only from their mothers. Therefore, the gene frequency among the males in any generation is the same as was in the females of the preceding generation. Thus,
$$p_m = p'_f$$

(ii) *Gene frequency in females* (p_f): This is the mean of the gene frequencies of their both parents, ands hence equal to the average gene frequency of two sexes in preceding generation. This is because the females get X-linked alleles equally from both parents. Thus, $\qquad p_f = \frac{1}{2}(p'_m + p'_f)$

(iii) *Difference in gene frequency between two sexes* (d): The difference is halved in each generation of random mating but with opposite sign.

$$
\begin{aligned}
d \quad &= p_f - p_m \\
&= \frac{1}{2}(p'_m + p'_f) - p'_f \qquad \text{in terms of previous generation} \\
&= \frac{1}{2}p'_m - 1/2\,p'_f \\
&= -\frac{1}{2}\,d'
\end{aligned}
$$

Where, d indicates the difference,

prime (') indicates the preceding generation.

The negative sign tends to oscillate the gene frequency in the two sexes. The oscillation of gene frequency means that if p_f is greater than p_m in one generation. then p_m will he greater than the p_f in the next generation. The decrease in difference of gene frequency in two sexes to the extent of half in each generation leads to the gene frequencies in the two sexes to become equal and the population is said to approach in equilibrium state. Thus the gene frequencies among males and females are equal in an equilibrium population.

(iv) *Average gene frequency in the whole population of two sexes* (p): This is given as:

$$\overline{P} \quad = \frac{1}{3}\,P_m + \frac{2}{3}\,P_f$$

$$= \frac{1}{3}\,(P_m + 2\,P_f)$$

$$= \frac{1}{3}\,(p'_m + 2\,p'_f)$$

= Equilibrium gene frequency = Constant

The equilibrium value of gene frequency (p) is approached in both sexes and this can be calculated from any generation.

The genes remain shuttling from one sex to the other and this shuttling of genes does not affect the relative frequencies of two alleles among the total number of X chromosomes. After a number of generations of random mating, the gene frequency in both the sexes approaches equality with no difference in gene frequency between two sexes (d = 0) and p is equilibrium value common to the two sexes.

(v) *Deviation of gene frequency from equilibrium value*: This can he obtained for any generation by putting the equation of p as follows -

$$P_m - \overline{P} = -2(p_f - p)$$

This can be obtained from $\overline{p} = \dfrac{1}{3}(P_m + 2p_f)$

$3\overline{p} = 2p_f + P_m$ by cross multiplication and rearranging

$$P_m + 2p_f = 2\overline{p} + \overline{p}$$

$$P_m - \overline{p} = -2p_f + 2\overline{p}$$

$$= -2(p_f - \overline{p})$$

This shows that in any generation, the deviation of p_m from equilibrium values is twice as great as that of the deviation of p_f from equilibrium value but on the other side of the equilibrium value. The deviation of gene frequency from equilibrium value in either sex is halved in each generation of random mating with opposite sign.

The above equations can also be used to estimate alternately the followings_

(i) Gene frequencies in either sex (p_m and p_f):

$$P_m \quad = 3\overline{p} - 2p_f$$

$$= 1.5\,\overline{p} - \tfrac{1}{2}p'_m = \tfrac{1}{2}(3\overline{p} - p'_m)$$

$$p_f = 1.5\,\overline{p} - \tfrac{1}{2}p'_f = \tfrac{1}{2}(3\overline{p} - p'_f)$$

(ii) Gene frequency in either sex of any generation: It is the average of the gene frequencies of two preceding generations of the same sex. Therefore,

$$P_m = \tfrac{1}{2}(p'_m + p''_m)$$

$$p_f = \tfrac{1}{2}(p'_f + p''_f)$$

(iii) Average gene frequency: The equilibrium value (p) which is also the average gene frequency, can also be expressed in terms of the difference in gene frequency (d) between two sexes as:

$$\overline{P} \quad = \dfrac{1}{3}P_m + \dfrac{2}{3}P_f$$

$$= P_f - \dfrac{1}{3}d$$

$$= P_m + \dfrac{2}{3}d \text{ where, } d = p_f - P_m$$

Thus $\overline{p}$ is one-third the distance from p_f and two-third the distance from P_m.

5.4 Estimation of Sex-Linked Allelic Frequencies

When the gene frequencies are equal in the two sexes, they can be estimated in females as for the autosomal genes whereas in males the genotypic frequencies are the direct estimate of gene frequencies. However, there is usually a difference in gene frequencies between the two sexes. When the allelic frequencies are not equal in two sexes, the frequencies of X-linked alleles in both sexes as a whole (p) are estimated differently for two situations *viz.* when there is no dominance and when there is dominance between alleles.

(1) No Dominance: Co-dominance

Where there is no dominance, the heterozygous females can be recognized phenotypically and so there are 3 phenotypic classes. The gene frequencies in two sexes can be estimated either by gene counting or by genotypic frequencies. However, the allelic frequency in the whole population of two sexes (q) is estimated as:

$$q = \frac{(2C + B + C_y)}{(2N_f + N_m)}$$

$$= \frac{(2R_f + H_f + R_m)}{(2N_f + N_m)}$$

$$p = 1 - q = \frac{(2A + B + A_y)}{(2N_f + N_m)}$$

$$= \frac{(2D_f + H_f + D_m)}{(2N_f + N_m)}$$

where, N_f = no. of total females = A + B + C

                 N_m = no. of total males = Ay + Cy

                 A, B, C = no. of homozygous dominant (D_f), heterozygous (H_f), and homozygous recessive (R_f) females, respectively

                 Ay, Cy = no. of dominant and recessive males, respectively.

                 Coat colour in cat is controlled by sex linked codominant alleles.

(2) Dominance

In this situation, there will be 4 phenotypic classes (two in each sex). The expected numbers in the four classes will be:

D_m = Dominant males = Ay

R_m = Recessive males = Cy

D_f = Dominant females

R_f = Recessive females

$$q_m = \frac{R_m}{N_m}$$

$$q_f = \sqrt{\frac{R_f}{N_f}}$$

$$q = -Ay + \sqrt{\left\{ \frac{\left[(Ay)^2 + 4(2N_f + N_m)(2C + Cy) \right]}{2(2N_f + N_m)} \right\}}$$

Examples

Colour blindness in man, hemophilia (excessive bleeding) in man, white eye in Drosophila, are the traits governed by sex linked recessive genes.

The allelic frequencies for sex linked loci are not equal in the two sexes due to a number of causes and hence the unequal gene frequencies in two sexes indicate one of the following causes:

1. Non random mating system which may arise due to selective differences in mating success.

2. Sex limited or sex influenced differences in effective selective forces.

3. More than one locus is affecting the trait.

When the allelic frequencies are unequal in the two sexes, it indicates that the population is not in equilibrium. When the sex linked alleles are at equilibrium in the population, it is expected that the gene frequencies are equal in the two sexes.

5.5 Characteristic Features of Sex Linked Traits

1. Sex Linked Recessive Traits

A trait governed by sex linked recessive gene expresses itself in the following way:

(i) Considering the zygotic expectations, it is clear that the incidence of sex linked recessive trait is more in males (q_f) than in females (q). The proportion of male recessive to female recessive is 1: q if the recessive gene is more. Taking the proportion 1 in male, the proportion in female will be $q^2/q = q$. The red-green colour-blindness in humans is due to sex linked recessive (colour blind) gene. The frequency of colour blindness is more in men than in women.

Rare recessive genes: For q being very small, the q^2 would be so small that there would be hardly any homozygous recessive females at all and the recessive gene of the females will remain hidden in the heterozygous condition.

Hemophilia is a sex linked recessive trait and it is extremely rare in women for two reasons- one is the low frequency of the recessive gene for hemophilia and other is that homozygous females are nonviable.

(ii) The other feature of the recessive sex linked traits is that they appear to "*skip a generation*". In case of hemophilia, one of the conditions (number of offspring of the various possible types of marriages) for the H.W. law does not hold true. The inheritance of a recessive sex linked trait (colour blindness) is shown below:

G_0 $X^X X^X$ x $X^C Y$

       Normal female   ↓   Colour blind Male

G_1 $X^X X^C$ $X^X Y$

       Carrier female   Normal male

       (Normal)   ↓

G_2 $X^X X^X$ $X^X X^C$ $X^X Y$ $X^C Y$

       Normal   Carrier   Normal   Colour blind

       female   female   Male   Male

             (Normal)

The reciprocal crossing produces different results for the sex linked genes. When the sex linked recessive gene is present in male parent, the trait (recessive) disappears in the F_1 progeny, but reappears in males of F_2 progeny. This type of cross is called *criss cross* or skip type of inheritance. The skip generation inheritance occurs when the female is hómozygous. Thus, the recessive trait does not appear in males of two consecutive generations: But when the female is heterozygous the recessive trait appears in father as well as in sons.

The results of reciprocal crossing for sex linked recessive trait (colour blindness in human) arc given below:

G_0 $X^C X^C$ x $X^X Y$

       Colour blind   ↓   Normal

G_1 $X^X X^C$ $X^C Y$

       Normal (Carrier)   ↓   Colour blind

G_2 $X^C X^C : X^X X^C$: $X^C Y : X^X Y$

       Colour blind   Normal   Colour blind   Normal

         female   Female   male   male

2. Sex Linked Dominant Traits

The trait controlled by a dominant sex linked gene has the following type of inheritance:

(i) All the carrier females will express the trait. The female dominants are always more numerous than the male dominants. Thus the dominant trait is present mostly in females than in males. The ratio of female dominant to male dominant will be $p^2 + 2pq/p = 1 + q: 1$. If p is very rare, the ratio is approximately 2: 1. Thus, the frequency of carrier female plus dominant female is about twice the frequency of affected males in the population.

(ii) The inheritance pattern of dominant sex linked trait is quite different from that of recessive sex linked trait. The mating of affected male (AY) and a normal female ($X^X X^X$) produces the female progeny of' $X^X X^C$ genotype which are all affected but will produce the male progeny of $X^X Y$ genotype which is normal. The reciprocal [normal male ($X^X Y$) and an affected female ($X^X X^C$)] produces all the affected progeny if the female was $X^X X^X$ but half the affected progeny if it was of $X^X X^C$ genotype, irrespective of their sex. Therefore, there is no "skipping" of generation for dominant sex-linked traits as with recessive sex linked traits. *Ocular albinism* in man is controlled by partially dominant gene. It can be concluded that if the female parent does not express the trait, it is not expressed in the male progeny from mother. The trait is expressed in all female progeny of a male which expresses the trait.

(iii) The third feature is that the females do not express the trait unless the recessive trait occurs in the paternal parent.

3. Y-linked Genes

The genes present on Y chromosome in the male are very rare and hence the Y chromosome is often called as genetically inert or inactive. The traits governed by the Y-linked genes have a very simple pattern of inheritance. All the male offspring expresses the trait of the father whereas none of the female progeny expresses the trait. The inheritance is controlled by Y linked gene is called *haulandric inheritance*.

Solved Examples and Exercises

Example 5.1

Coat colour in cat is due to a co-dominant sex-linked gene. All the three genotypes are recognizable in females, the heterozygous have tortoise shell or calico, and the two homozygotes have black and yellow coat colour. A female population with yellow colour is mated at random with black males. The gene frequencies and genotype frequencies in the two sexes, average gene frequency in both the sexes and difference in gene frequency between two sexes over several generations can he estimated as under

Solution

The females are homozgyous for yellow colour and hence the frequency of yellow gene in female population is $p_f = 1.0$. The males are of black colour and hence the frequency of yellow gene in male population is zero ($p_m = o$). The frequency of yellow and black genes and the genotypic frequencies in two sexes, the average gene frequency in both sexes combined and the difference in gene frequency for yellow gene between two sexes in successive generations will take the values as shown in table below.

Approach to Equilibrium for Sex-linked Gene

Generation	Males				Females				
	p_m	q_m	Gene Freq.		Genotype Frequencies			$\bar{p}$	d
	Yellow	Black	p_f	q_f	Yellow	Tortoise	Black		
0	0	1	1	0	1	0	0	0.666	1
1	1	0	0.5	0.5	0	1	0	0.666	– 0.5
2	0.5	0.5	0.75	0.25	0.5	0.5	0	0.666	– 0.25
3	0.75	0.25	0.625	0.375	0.375	0.5	0.125	0.666	– 0.125
4	0.625	0.375	0.687	0.312	0.437	0.43	0.097	0.666	– 0.0625
5	0.687	0.312	0.656	0.344	0.43	0.45	0.12	0.666	– 0.0312
6	0.656	0.344	0.672	0.328	0.45	0.44	0.11	0.666	– 0.0156
7	0.672	0.328	0.664	0.336	0.44	0.45	0.11	0.666	– 0.0078
.									
.									
∞	0.666	0.333	0.666	0.333	0.44	0.45	0.11	0.666	0.00

$p_m = p'_f ; \ q_m = q'_f ; \ p_f = \frac{1}{2}(p'_m + p'_f);$ $\qquad q_f = \frac{1}{2}(q'_m + q'_f)$

$\bar{p} = 1/3 (p_m + 2 p_f); \qquad d = p_f - p_m$

Example 5.2

The following data were recorded for the presence of the antigen in human which is controlled by a sex linked locus with dominance relation between two alleles at the locus.

Sex	Dominant Phenotype	Recessive Phenotype	Total
Males	25	56	81
Females	90	61	151

(i) Estimate the frequency of two alleles in males, females and whole population.

(ii) Estimate the expected numbers of all the four phenotypic classes under random mating and apply χ^2 test for goodness of fit.

Hint

(i) $q_m = \dfrac{C_y}{N_m} = \dfrac{56}{81} = 0.69$

$q_f = \sqrt{\dfrac{C}{N_f}} = \sqrt{\dfrac{61}{151}} = 0.63$

(ii) Use q to estimate the expected number of 4 phenotypic classes. The degree of freedom will be $1 = 3 - 1$ (estimate of p) $- 1$ (estimation of expected no of males).

5.3 The white eye of Drosophila is due to a sex linked recessive allele and red eye (wild type) to its dominant allele. It was observed that there were 60 males and 20 females with white eye in a sample of 260 males and 380 females. Calculate the frequency of white gene using all the data (q). Ans: q = 0.19

5.4 Colour blindness in human is a sex linked recessive trait. It was observed that 30 men were colour blind in a sample of 750 men.

  (i) What is the freq. of two alleles?

  (ii) Find out the proportion of women expected to be colour blind, carrier and normal.

  (iii) Find out the proportion of marriage in which both husband and wife are expected to be colour blind.

Hint: (i) $q_m = \dfrac{30}{750} = 0.04$

  (ii) $q_f = q_m = 0.04$ under H.W.E.

  (iii) Proportion of marriage $= q_m\, q^2_f = 1$ in 16000

5.5 The frequency of females showing the sex linked recessive trait was 19.36 per cent. Find out the percentage of males that would he expected to show this trait.

Hint: Percentage of males $= \sqrt{q^2_f}$

5.6. The percentage of female dominants for sex linked trait was observed to be 60.64. Find out the recessive males.

5.7. With a frequency of dominant sex linked gene as 0.003, find out the percentage of dominant females. Also estimate the ratio of the female dominant to that of the males.

5.8. Estimate the changes occurred under random mating in a population for a sex linked gene having the genetic structure for males as 0.4 A and 0.6 a while for females as 0.3 AA, 0.5 Aa and 0.02 aa.

5.9. The freq. of rare recessive allele was observed to be equal in two sexes as q = 0.07 with gentoypic distribution as:

Males 0.93 A + 0.07 a and Females 0.90 AA + 0.06 Aa + 0.04 aa

  (i) Find out the genotypic distribution at equilibrium and the number of generations required to approach equilibrium.

  (ii) Find out the proportion of women carrier and the women expressing the trait.

Hint: (i) The population with equal gene frequencies in two sexes will approach genetic equilibrium in one generation of random mating with genotypic frequencies as:

Male: 0.90 A + 0.07 a; Females: 0.8649 AA + 0.1302 Aa + 0.0049 aa

(ii) Proportion of women carrier for recessive allele = 2pq and the proportion of women expressing the trait = q2.

5.10. The polymorphism of X-linked phospho-glucomutase gene in Drosophila persimilis with two alleles (Pgm^A and Pgm^B) has been studied with their gene frequencies as 0.3 arid 0.7. Estimate the expected genotypic frequencies in the two sexes under random mating.

Hint: Among males: $Pgm^A = 0.3$ and $Pgm^B = 0.7$;

Among females: $Pgm^{AA} = (0.3)^2 = 0.09$, $Pgm^{AB} = 2(0.3)(0.7) = 0.42$, $Pgm^{BB} = (0.7)^2 = 0.49$

5.11. The reduced ability of blood to clot when exposed (excessive bleeding) called as hemophilia is a genetically controlled disease governed by a sex linked gene with two alleles. In a gene pool of certain population one percent gametes have hemophilic allele. What is the expected frequency of hemophilia in males and females?

Hint: Expected freq. of hemophilia males = q, Exp. freq. of hemophilia females = q2

where, q = 1/100 = 0.01.

5.12. Coat colour in cat is controlled by a sex-linked locus with co-dominant alleles (C^B and C^Y). A cat population yielded the following data.

	Black	Tortoise	Yellow	Total
Males	510	—	50	560
Females	280	60	10	350

Find out the allelic frequencies in two sexes and a combined estimate

Hint: Use the method of gene counting.

$q_m = 0.09$, $q_f = 0.11$ and $q = 0.10$

$$q = \frac{(2C + B + Cy)}{2N_f + N_m}$$

Chapter 6
Genetic Equilibrium – Two Pairs of Genes

The principle of random mating can he extended to two or more loci whether they are independently assorting (present on different homologous chromosomes or present far apart on the same pair of chromosome) or they are linked (present nearer on the same pair of chromosome).The random mating leads to genetic equilibrium for both loci considered jointly. Logically it seems that when two loci reach equilibrium separately, they should also he in equilibrium considered jointly. But this is not true.

6.1 Genetic Structure for Two Loci

Consider two pairs of genes each with two alleles. The first is A-a pair at locus A and second is B-b at locus B. The frequencies of two alleles **A** and **a** at locus A are represented as **p** and **q,** and the frequencies of the two alleles, **B** and **b** at locus B as **u** and **v**. Considering these two loci jointly, there will he 9 genotypes in a population. These 9 genotypes can be arranged in a systematic pattern by a zygotic matrix of 3 x 3 size and can be represented by Z as under:

Genotype Arrays

		Total							*Total*
	AABB	AABb	AAbb	AA		Z_{11}	Z_{12}	Z_{13}	$Z_{1.}$
	AaBB	AaBb	Aabb	Aa	and	Z_{21}	Z_{22}	Z_{23}	$Z_{2.}$
	aaBB	aaBb	aabb	aa		Z_{31}	Z_{32}	Z_{33}	$Z_{3.}$
Total	BB	Bb	bb			$Z_{.1}$	$Z_{.2}$	$Z_{.3}$	

The sum of all the 9 genotypes is unity. The sums of row totals of zygotic matrix give the genotypes for locus A (AA, Aa, aa) while the sums of column totals give the genotype for locus B (BB, Bb, bb).

Gamete Arrays

The 9 genotypes for two loci produce 4 types of gametes which are AB. Ab, aB and ab. These 4 types of gametes can be arranged in a pattern similar to the zygotic matrix and can be represented by gamete matrix (g) of 2 x 2 size as:

$$\begin{vmatrix} AB & Ab \\ aB & ab \end{vmatrix} \quad \text{and} \quad g = \begin{vmatrix} g_{11} & g_{12} \\ g_{21} & g_{22} \end{vmatrix}$$

The sum of all the 4 gametes is unity. The sums of two rows of gamete matrix give the gene frequencies of A-a pair and the sums of the two columns give the gene frequencies of B-b pair.

The **types of gametes** produced by different genotypes (gamete output) assuming Mendelian independent segregation of alleles for two loci are as:

(i) *Double homozygous genotype*: These have been arranged at the 4 corners of the zygotic matrix Z. They each produce only one kind of gamete. The genotype AABB produces only AB gametes. AAbb genotype produces only Ab gamete, aaBB produces only aB gamete and aabb genotype produces only ab type gamete.

(ii) *Single homozygote or single heterozygote*: These have been arranged in the middle of first and third rows and in the middle of first and third columns of the zygotic matrix. They all produce two types of gametes in equal proportion whether the two loci are linked or independent

AABb genotypes produce 50 per cent AB and 50 per cent Ab gametes.

AaBB genotypes produce 50 per cent AB and 50 per cent aB gametes,

Aabb genotypes produce 50 per cent Ab and 50 per cent ab gametes.

aaBb genotypes produce 50 per cent aB and 50 per cent ab gametes,

(iii) *Double heterozygous genotype (AaBb)*: This has been arranged in the middle of the zygotic matrix. It will produce 4 kinds of gametes *viz*. AB, Ab. aB and ab. The proportion of these 4 gametes depends on the linkage between two loci. When the two loci are independent the proportion of 4 gametes is equal but when they are linked the proportion of four gametes produced depends upon the strength of linkage (r, which denotes recombination fraction).

6.2 Frequencies of the Genotypes, Gametes and Genes

The population at equilibrium will produce four types of gametes with their frequencies as:

$$g = \begin{vmatrix} AB & Ab \\ aB & ab \end{vmatrix} = \begin{vmatrix} pu & pv \\ qu & qv \end{vmatrix} = \begin{vmatrix} w & x \\ y & z \end{vmatrix}$$

The random union of these four types of gametes will produce the progeny generation having 9 types of genotypes.

(i) Genotypic Arrays with their Frequencies

These can be obtained in three ways as under:

(a) Squaring the gamete output:

$$\begin{vmatrix} AB & Ab & aB & ab \\ pu + qv + qu + qv \end{vmatrix}^2 = \begin{vmatrix} AABB & 2AABb & AAbb \\ 2AaBB & 4AaBb & 2Aabb \\ aaBB & 2aaBb & aabb \end{vmatrix}$$

Totals

$$= \begin{vmatrix} p^2u^2 & 2p^2uv & p^2v^2 \\ 2pqu^2 & 4pqv^2 & 2pqv^2 \\ q^2u^2 & 2q^2uv & q^2v^2 \end{vmatrix} \begin{matrix} p^2 \\ 2pq \\ q^2 \end{matrix}$$

Totals $\quad u^2 \quad 2\ uv \quad v^2$

(b) Product of genotypes frequencies of two loci: The sums of the three rows totals give the genotype frequencies for the three genotypes produced for A locus while the sums of the three columns totals give the genotype frequencies for the three genotypes produced for B locus. Therefore, the zygotic arrays of 9 genotypes in an equilibrium population can also be obtained from the product of the row by column totals of genotypes as:

$(p^2 + 2pq + q^2)\ (u^2 + 2uv + v^2)$,

(c) From product of the squares of the gene frequencies of two loci as:

$(p + q)^2\ (u + v)^2$.

(ii) Gamete Frequencies

These can be estimated from the genotypic frequencies in a population at equilibrium as under -

f (AB)	= AABB + ½ (2AABb +2 AaBB) + ¼ (4 Aa Bb)	
	= p²u² + ½ (2 p²uv + 2 pq u²) + ¼ (4 pq uv)	
	= pu (pu + pv + qu + qv)	
	= pu	Since pu + pv + qu + qv = 1.0
f (Ab)	= AAbb + ½ (2 AABb) + 2 Aa bb + ¼ (4 Aa Bb)	
	= p² v² + p² uv + pq v² + pq uv	
	= pv (pv +pu + qv + qu)	

$$= pv$$

f(aB) $= aaBB + \frac{1}{2}(2AaBB + 2\ aa\ Bb) + \frac{1}{4}(4\ Aa\ Bb)$

$= q^2u^2 + pq\ u^2 + q^2\ uv + pq\ uv$

$= qu\ (qu + pu + qv + pv)$

$= qu$

f(ab) $= aabb + \frac{1}{2}(2\ Aabb + 2\ aa\ Bb) + \frac{1}{4}(4\ Aa\ Bb)$

$= q^2v^2 + pq\ v^2 + q^2\ uv + pq\ uv$

$= qv$

(iii) Gamete and Gene Frequencies for the Alleles at Two Loci

This can be estimated from the gamete set and from genotypic frequencies.

(a) Gamete Arrays and Frequencies of Gametes and Genes

$$
\begin{array}{ccccccc}
& & & & & \text{Total} & \\
g & = & \begin{vmatrix} AB & Ab \\ aB & ab \end{vmatrix} & = & \begin{vmatrix} pu & pv \\ qu & qv \end{vmatrix} & \begin{array}{c} p \\ q \end{array} & = & \begin{vmatrix} w & x \\ y & z \end{vmatrix}
\end{array}
$$

$$
\begin{array}{ccc}
\text{Total} & u & v
\end{array}
$$

The sum of the four gamete frequencies is unity. The sums of two rows of gamete matrix (g) are equal to the gene frequencies of the A-a pair while the sums of the two columns of gamete matrix give the gene frequencies of the B-b pair.

$$p = f(AB) + f(Ab) = pu + pv = w + x$$
$$q = f(aB) + f(ab) = qu + qv = y + z$$
$$u = f(AB) + f(aB) = pu + qu = w + y$$
$$v = f(Ab) + f(ab) = pv + qv = x + z$$

(b) Genotypic Set and Gene Frequencies

The gene frequencies from the genotypic frequencies are estimated directly as:

$$p = Z_{1.} + \frac{1}{2} Z_{2.}$$
$$q = Z_{3.} + \frac{1}{2} Z_{2.}$$
$$u = Z_{.1} + \frac{1}{2} Z_{.2}$$
$$v = Z_{.3} + \frac{1}{2} Z_{.2}$$

where, $Z_{i.}$ indicates the sum of the ith row of the zygotic matrix,

$Z_{.i}$ indicates the sum of the jth column of zygotic matrix.

6.3 H.W. Equilibrium for Two Loci

The genotypes for two loci jointly and their frequencies in a population at equilibrium under random mating can be represented by Z matrix.

Totals

$$Z \;=\; \begin{vmatrix} AABB & 2AABb & AAbb \\ 2AaBB & 4AaBb & 2Aabb \\ AaBB & 2aaBb & aabb \end{vmatrix} \;=\; \begin{vmatrix} p^2u^2 & 2p^2uv & p^2v^2 \\ 2pqu^2 & 4pqv^2 & 2pqv^2 \\ q^2u^2 & 2q^2uv & q^2v^2 \end{vmatrix} \begin{matrix} p^2 \\ 2pq \\ q^2 \end{matrix}$$

Totals $\qquad u^2 \qquad 2\,uv \qquad v^2$

This population, being in equilibrium for two loci jointly must also be necessarily in equilibrium for two pairs of genes taken separately. This is because the row totals of Z matrix give the genotypic frequencies for the alleles segregating at locus A (p^2, 2 pq, q^2), while the column totals give the genotypic frequencies for the alleles segregating at locus B (u^2, 2 uv, v^2)

It can be verified either from random mating of genotypes or from the random union of gametes that this population for two loci represented by Z matrix is in equilibrium under random mating

There will be $(9 \times 10)/2 = 42$ different mating possible. The procedure of random mating of genotypes to test an equilibrium population is longer and hence the alternate equivalent method of random union of gametes to produce the progeny generation can be used. This method requires finding out the gamete frequencies. The gamete frequencies can be estimated from the zygotic (genotype) frequencies as illustrated earlier. The gamete output of Z matrix is as under:

$$g \;=\; \begin{vmatrix} AB & Ab \\ aB & ab \end{vmatrix} \;=\; \begin{vmatrix} pu & pv \\ qu & qv \end{vmatrix}$$

The random union of this gamete output will produce the genotypes of the progeny generation with their frequencies as:

$$Z_1 \;=\; \begin{vmatrix} AB & Ab & aB & ab \\ pu + pv + qu + qv \end{vmatrix}^2 \;=\; \begin{vmatrix} p^2u^2 & 2p^2uv & p^2v^2 \\ 2pqu^2 & 4pquv & 2pqv^2 \\ q^2u^2 & 2q^2uv & q^2v^2 \end{vmatrix}$$

The Z_1 is the same as the Z. Therefore, the population represented by Z is in equilibrium. The genotypic array in subsequent generation is the square of the gamete array of preceding generation under random mating: Thus genotypic array with random mating is obtained from gamete array as:

$$\left[w_{(AB)} + x_{(Ab)} + y_{(aB)} + z_{(ab)} \right]^2 \;=\; \begin{vmatrix} w^2 & 2wx & x^2 \\ 2wy & 2(wz + xy) & 2xz \\ y^2 & 2yz & z^2 \end{vmatrix}$$

6.4 Linkage Equilibrium

In an equilibrium population for two loci jointly, the frequency of a gamete (carrying any particular combination of alleles) should be equal to the product of the frequencies of the alleles present in that gamete *viz.*

f (AB) = pu, f (Ab) = pv,

f (aB) = qu, and f (ab) = qv.

This means that the gametic frequency should depend on gene frequencies. In matrix from, this should be as under:

$$
g \;=\; \begin{vmatrix} AB & Ab \\ aB & ab \end{vmatrix} \;=\; \begin{vmatrix} pu & pv \\ qu & qv \end{vmatrix} \;=\; \begin{vmatrix} w & x \\ y & z \end{vmatrix}
$$

In other words, in an equilibrium population, the gametes should contain the random association (combination) of alleles for two gene pairs. The genes in this condition are said to be in a state of equilibrium or *linkage equilibrium* or gamete equilibrium.

The random association between two alleles each for the two gene pairs showing the expected gamete frequencies (when the alleles are in linkage equilibrium) can be shown as under:

Table 6.1: Linkage Equilibrium (Random Association) for Genes of Two Loci

		Alleles and their Freq. at B Locus	
		B(u)	*b(v)*
Alleles and their	A (p)	AB (pu) = w	Ab (pv) = x
freq. at A locus	a(q)	aB (qu) = y	ab (qv) = z
		Such that p + q = 1 and u + v = 1.	

The combinations of A's and B's in the square above indicate the gametes and not the genotypes.

In an equilibrium population for two loci jointly, the gamete frequencies should have the following relation:

f (AB). f (ab) = f (Ab). f (aB)

pu.qv = pv qu.

or wz = xy

Thus, pu. qv – pv. qv = 0 or wz – xy = 0

Therefore, there should be no difference in the production of the gametes of coupling phase and of repulsion phase in an equilibrium population.

6.5 Linkage Disequilibrium

When the gametes do not contain the random association of alleles of two gene pairs and hence the gamete frequencies do not depend on gene frequencies, two loci are not in equilibrium jointly. In this condition the production of gametes in the coupling state and the repulsion state are not equal and hence pu. qv – pv.qu ≠0. This condition is known as *linkage disequilibrium*.

Thus the linkage disequilibrium is represented and measured by the differ-ence in products of the gametes of coupling phase and of the repulsion phase. This difference or the linkage disequilibrium is denoted by D and is a measure of the magnitude of the departure from equilibrium state. The D is thus regarded as index of the divergence of a population from equilibrium, Therefore, the quantity D is defined as

D = pu. qv – pv. qu

$\quad$ = wz – xy

The gamete frequencies have the following relationship in terms of gene frequencies and D:

w = pu + D;x = pv – D;

y = qu – D; z = qv + D

To understand the above relationship, consider first w. Take that the two loci are independent. In case of independence between the two loci, the probability of a gamete AB should be equal to the product of the probability of drawing A allele from gene pool and the probability of drawing B allele from gene pool. Therefore, when two loci are independent, then w must be equal to pu. Similarly, x will equal to pv, y will be qu and z will be equal to qv. Taking these values of gamete frequencies and putting these values in the above equations, it can he seen that D is zero. This confirms that when loci are independent, then D is zero.

When the loci are not independent, but linked, then D is not zero. Thus, the extent to which the gamete frequencies differ from their values which would have been if the loci were independent is indicated and measured by the parameter D. This amount of D is referred to as the *'linkage disequilibriun coefficient'*. When D is zero and hence when w = pu, etc. the condition is said as linkage equilibrium or gamete equilibrium. However, the value of D is not concerned with linkage at all and hence the term equilibrium applies to independent as well as linked loci.

Causes of Linkage Disequilibrium

The linkage disequilibrium between loci can arise irrespective of linkage between loci. Thus linkage disequilibrium may occur for the two loci which are either linked or independent (segregating independently). The disequilibrium can arise as a number of factors, like, breeding of two populations with different gene frequencies, chance event in small population (sub divisions of population into divergent subgroups), selection favouring some combinations of alleles over others, differential inbreeding (the inbreeding may increase the frequencies of certain phenotypes).

6.6 Approach to Equilibrium

A population in linkage disequilibrium reached to linkage equilibrium for nine genotypes under random mating and in the absence of evolutionary forces. However, the equilibrium is not attained in one generation of random mating but the approach to equilibrium is gradual with very slow rate compared to the approach of H.W. frequencies for single locus.

The gene frequencies in a population with random mating remain in constant from generation to generation, But there is change in gamete frequencies under random mating till they become equal to the product of gene frequencies for two foci jointly. The proportion of those gametes present in excess amount in initial population is reduced in progeny generation while the proportion of those gametes that are deficient increase in proportion by random union of gametes. This process results in reducing the difference in the product of gamete frequencies of coupling and repulsion phase gametes (D) in the progeny generation compared to the parent generation. The difference vanishes completely (D is reduced to zero) after a number of generations with random mating and the population reaches in linkage equilibrium.

6.6.1 Factors Affecting Rate of Approach to Equilibrium

The change in gamete frequencies towards the linkage equilibrium depends upon the combined effects of the recombination fraction (r) which indicates the strength of linkage and the relative frequencies of four types of gametes produced by double heterozygous genotype which in term depends upon the origin of double heterozygous individuals from coupling phase or repulsion phase.

The rate with which the difference (amount of disequilibrium, D) is reduced in each generation of random mating can be estimated by finding out the gamete frequencies in progeny generation. This is the change in the gamete proportion of progeny generation compared to parent generation with random mating.

(i) Recombination Fraction

The change in gamete frequencies from generation to generation under random mating towards linkage equilibrium depends upon the extent to which the recombination occurs between the two loci. The recombination fraction is denoted by r and this (r) measures the strength of linkage. The values of r vary from 0 to ½. The value 0 and close to 0 indicates that recombination between the two loci does not occur and hence there is strong linkage. Thus, r = 0 means strong linkage. On the other hand, when r is near to ½ it indicates loose linkage and when r = ½ it then indicates that the two loci are independent (unlinked) and hence the segregation at meiosis is independent between the two loci. Thus r = ½ means no linkage.

(ii) Gamete Output of Double Heterozygous Individual

The effect of recombination can only be detected from the double heterozygous genotypes. The linkage does not affect the gámete output of genotypes that are either double homozygous (homozygous for both loci _viz._ AABB, AAbb, aaBB, and aabb or the single homozygous for one or other gene pair _viz._ AABb, Aa BB, Aa bb, aaBb which are called as single homozygotes or single heterozy-gotes. For example aaBb genotype produces 50 per cent aB gametes and 50 per cent ab gametes whether the loci are linked or independent. Likewise the genotypes homozygous for both loci (double homozygote) produce only one kind of gamete _viz._ AA BB genotype produces only AB type gametes. The linkage affects the gamete output of only double heterozygous genotype (Aa Bb). The rate of approach to linkage equilibrium depends upon the relative frequencies of 4 types of gametes produced by double heterozygous individuals.

Coupling or Repulsion Phase Double Heterozygote

The double heterozygous individual produce 4 types of gametes (AB, Ab, aB and ab) out of which two gametes are parental type and other two are recombinant types not present among parents. Which of the two are parental and which are recombinant type gametes depends upon the fact whether the double heterozygote are from coupling phase or from repulsion phase.

The linkage modifies the gamete output of double heterozygote (relative frequency of 4 types of gametes) depending upon whether the double heterozy-gote are in the coupling or repulsion phase.

(a) Gamete Output from Coupling Phase Double Heterozygote

The double heterozygote individual in coupling phase (AB/ab) will produce 4 types of gametes in the following frequencies:

Gametes	Types	Frequency of Gametes		
		General	Linkage $(r = 0)$	No Linkage $(r = ½)$
AB	Parental	$(1-r)/2$	½	¼
ab	"	"	½	¼
Ab	Recombinant	$r/2$	0	¼
aB	"	"	0	¼

(b) Gamete Output from Repulsion Phase Double Heterozygote

The double heterozygous individual in repulsion phase (Ab/aB) will produce the 4 types of gametes with the following frequencies-

Gametes	Types	Frequency of Gametes		
		General	Linkage $(r = 0)$	No Linkage $(r = ½)$
AB	Parental	$(1-r)/2$	0	¼
ab	"	"	0	¼
Ab	Recombinant	$r/2$	½	¼
aB	"	"	½	¼

Thus r is very important to determine the amount of disequilibrium (D). The rate of approach to linkage equilibrium depends upon the recombination fraction (r,) because this determines the relative frequencies of parental and recombinant type gametes.

6.6.2 Estimation of the Amount of Linkage Disequilibrium (D)

The D can be estimated from the frequency of any of the 4 gametes produced in progeny generation. For example, the AB gamete will be produced by AABB genotype to the extent of 100 per cent ,by AABb genotype to the extent of 50 per cent, by Aa BB genotype also to the extent of 50 per cent of the total gametes, while the double heterozygous genotype (Aa Bb) will produce the AR gametes in two ways $viz.$ the chromosome may undergo crossing over with a probability of r out of which half of the total gametes will be of aB type and another half will be of Ab type whereas the chromosome which might fail to undergo crossing between two loci with a probability of $1-r$ will produce AB and ab gametes each with a probability of ½ (1-r). Therefore, the total gamete output of AB gamete in progeny generation will be estimated as:

f (AB) = AABB + ½ (2AABb + 2AaBB) + ½ r (2AaBb) + ½ (1- r) (2AaBb).

w_1 (AB) = w^2 + ½ (2wx + 2wy) + ½ r(2xy) + ½(1- r) (2wz)

$$\text{Recomb.} \qquad \text{Parental}$$

$$= w^2 + \tfrac{1}{2}\,(2wx + 2wy) + \tfrac{1}{2}\,(2wz) - \tfrac{1}{2}\,r\,(2wz) + \tfrac{1}{2}\,r\,(2xy)$$

$$= w\,(w + x + y + z) - r\,(wz - xy)$$

$$= w - rD_0 \qquad \text{Since } wz - xy = D_0$$

Similarly, the frequency of other 3 types of gametes can be estimated. The frequencies of Ab gametes (x_1), aB gametes (y_1) and ab gametes (z_1) will be as:

$f(x_1) = x + rD_0$

$f(y_1) = y + rD_0$

$f(z_1) = z - rD_0$

The value of D in progeny generation (D_1) will be obtained as:

$$
\begin{aligned}
D_1 \;&= w_1 z_1 - x_1 y_1 \\
&= (w - rD_0)\,(z - rD_0) - (x + rD_0)\,(y + rD_0) \\
&= wz - wrD_0 - zrD_0 + r^2 D^2{}_0 - xy - xrD_0 - yrD_0 - r^2 D^2{}_0 \\
&= wz - xy - rD_0\,(w + x + y + z) \\
&= D_0 - rD_0 \qquad\qquad \text{Since, } w + x + y + z = 1 \text{ and } wz - xy = D_0 \\
&= (1- r)\,D_0
\end{aligned}
$$

Thus, $D_0 = (1- r)\,D_{n-1} = (1-r)^n D$

The value $(1- r)\,D_0$ indicates the rate of decrease in linkage disequilibrium caused by recombination between loci and this is also the rate of attaining the linkage equilibrium. Thus the rate with which the linkage equilibrium is approached depends upon r (strength of linkage).

I. Independent Loci

The value of r is ½ for independent loci (no linkage) which indicates that the recombination fraction is 50 per cent. Thus 50 per cent gametes are recombinant types and another 50 per cent gametes are of parental types from double heterozygous individuals when the two loci are segregating independently. Therefore, the production of 4 types of gametes is in equal proportion (1/4) from the double heterozygous individuals. Thus, the rate of decay of linkage disequilibrium per generation for independent loci is 50 per cent or half of' that in preceding generation because the value of $r = 0.5$ (proportion of recombinant gametes produced) and hence

$$D_1 = (1-r) D_0$$
$$= (1-0.5) D_0 = 0.5 D_0$$

The $r = 0.5$ is the maximum value of r when loci are independent.

The gametic output in progeny generation under random mating becomes as:

$$f(AB)_1 = f(AB) - \tfrac{1}{2} D$$
$$f(Ab)_1 = f(Ab) + \tfrac{1}{2} D$$
$$f(aB)_1 = f(aB) + \tfrac{1}{2} D$$
$$f(ab)_1 = f(ab) - \tfrac{1}{2} D$$

The change in gamete production is in such a way that the quantity $D = wz - xy$ is reduced by one-half in each generation of random mating. Therefore, after n generation of random mating,

$$D_n = \tfrac{1}{2} D_{n-1}$$
$$= (\tfrac{1}{2})^n D_0 \text{ as n approaches infinity.}$$

When the population reached in equilibrium, $wz = xy$.

This means that $f(AB).f(ab) = f(Ab).f(aB)$ and the gamete frequencies will be

$$w = pu = (w + x)(w + y)$$
$$= w - D_0, \text{ etc.}$$

This makes the gamete output as:

$$d = \begin{vmatrix} w - D_0 & x + D_0 \\ y + D_0 & z - D_0 \end{vmatrix} = 0$$

The gamete frequencies in the initial population differ from the gamete frequencies in equilibrium population by the amount D. The D is the index of the divergence of an initial population from equilibrium. The maximum value of D is 1/4 and halved in each generation with random mating. Thus, the approach to equilibrium is very rapid.

In a large random mating population (equilibrium population), the D is expected to be zero and hence no association between particular alleles at the two loci. The lack of independence can be expressed by taking the difference between the observed value of any gamete frequency and the corresponding row by column product (expected value) *e.g.* taking the frequency of double dominant gamete (AB)) as pu, the value of D will be:

D $\quad$ = pu.qv – pv.qu

D (AB) $\quad$ = observed freq. of AB – expected freq. of AB

$\qquad$ = pu – (pu + pv) (pu + qu)

$\qquad$ = pu – $p_A u_B$

$\qquad$ = f (AB) – f (A). f (B)

The non zero value of D indicate lack of independence or linkage disequilibrium. A non zero value of D may also be in the absence of linkage between loci. An excess or deficiency of a particular gamete combination may occur whether the loci concerned are linked or independent.

Some Cases of Reaching in Equilibrium in One Generation of Random Mating

(i) An arbitrary population whose gamete output is such that D = 0 and hence (wz – xy = 0) may not necessarily be in equilibrium with respect to its genotypic proportions but the equilibrium is attained in one generation of random mating.

(ii) The first generation of crossbreds produced by mating of two purebreds are composed entirely of double heterozygous individuals (F, produced by AABB x aabb or AAbb x aa BB). The p u = ½ in this case. The equilibrium is attained in one generation of random mating of F_1 with F_1 and the genotype frequencies in F_2 population are symmetrical with respect to both diagonals. Thus the F_2 population derived from an original cross between two pure lines is always in equilibrium condition. Subsequent generations produced by random mating will remain the same with respect to genotype frequencies.

II. Linked Loci

The value of r is less than 0.5 for linked loci. This means that the proportion of recombinant gametes (produced by crossing over in the double heterozygote) are less than 50 per cent while the proportion of parental type gametes is more than 50 per cent for linked loci. The value of *r* is decreased with the increase in the strength of linkage between loci. Therefore, the proportion of recombinant type gametes produced by double heterozygous individuals is reduced and consequently the production of parental type gametes is in higher proportion. Therefore, the value of D is higher in case of linked loci and hence the rate of approach to equilibrium is slower when the intensity of linkage is higher. The value of (1- r), the parental type gamete proportion, is greater than 0.5 and hence the quantity D is reduced at a slower rate per generation. I however, the limiting value of D is also zero because $D_n = (1- r) D_{n-1} = (1- r)^n D = 0$ as the numbers of generations (n) goes on infinity.

When equilibrium is reached, D = 0 and hence wz = xy or (pu.qv = pv. qu) similar to the case of independent loci. This means that the coupling zygotes (AB/ab) and the repulsion zygotes (Ab/aB) are equal in proportion of the 2pquv in an equilibrium population. Further the final gamete proportions in an equilibrium population are also the same in case of linked loci as those for independent loci *viz.* w = pu = pu – D, etc.

6.7 Detection (Evidence) of Linkage

In a random mating equilibrium population the genotype frequencies for two pairs of linked genes are identical to those of independent genes. That is to say that the genotype frequencies are determined by gene frequencies. Therefore, an examination of genotypic or phenotypic frequencies in an equilibrium population can not be used to detect the linkage between loci. This is the main problem to detect linkage in random mating population. Therefore, if there is a correlation between two traits in a population under random mating it is not correct to conclude that the correlation between two traits is due to linked genes. The correlation in such a population between two traits may be due to other factors like, pleiotropy, maternal or common environmental effects, differential inbreeding, subdivision of population in divergent groups, bias in sampling, physiological effects of development of traits etc.

The linkage can only be revealed in the segregation ratios among progenies whose at least one parent is heterozygous for both pairs of genes. This is because the linkage affects the gamete output of only double heterozygous individuals and not the gamete output of any other genotype.

When both positive and negative correlations for two traits are observed in about equal numbers of sib ship it is then a strong evidence of linkage, though in the total population there is no correlation between the two traits. This is because that the double heterozygous individuals, produced by coupling phase and repulsion phase gametes, are about equal in the general population under random mating.

6.8 Differential Gametic Array and Differential Recombination Fraction in Two Sexes

The disequilibrium in the gamete frequencies caused by these two situations are transient and cancelled out in one generation of random mating. Neither of the two situations changes the results appreciably.

6.9 Constancy in Gene Frequency

The gene frequency within a locus remains constant under random mating from generation to generation. This can be illustrated as under:

The genotypic array at equilibrium is obtained by random union of gametes as:

(w AB + x Ab + y aB + z ab)

or (pu + pv + qu + qv)

The frequency of allele A is given by p and hence denoting the two generations by the subscripts 1 for progeny generation and 0 for parent generation, the frequency of A gene in progeny generation will be the same as in parent generation-

$$P_1 \quad = w_1 + x_1$$
$$= (w_0 - rD) - (x_0 + rD)$$
$$= w_0 + x_0$$
$$= P_0$$

Thus there is no change in gene frequency with random mating from one generation to the next.

The change only occurs in the gamete frequencies and consequently in the genotypic frequencies during the process of approaching the equilibrium from disequilibrium.

At equilibrium the gamete frequency become equal to the product of frequencies of alleles contained in the gamete. The gamete frequency is equal to the corresponding row by column product. For example,

$$f(AB) \quad = (w + x)(w + y) \qquad \text{Row by column product}$$
$$= w^2 + wy + wx + wz \ (\text{Taking } xy = wz)$$
$$= w(w + y' + x + z)$$
$$= w \qquad\qquad (\text{Since } w + x + y + z = 1.0)$$

or $f(AB) \quad = pu$
$$= (pu + pv)(pu + qu) \ \text{From row by column product}$$
$$= p^2u^2 + pqu^2 + p^2uv + pquv$$
$$= pu(pu + qu + pv + qv)$$
$$= pu \qquad (\text{Since } pu + qu + pv + pv = 1.0)$$

6.10 No. of Generations Required

The number of generations required to reduce the linkage disequilibrium from initial value (D_0) to a certain value (D_n) can be estimated. The proportion r required to be reduced to its initial value is represented by $\dfrac{1}{k} = \dfrac{D_n}{D_0}$. Therefore,

$$\frac{D_n}{D_0} = \frac{1}{k}$$

$$\frac{D_0(1 - r)^n}{D_0} = \frac{1}{k}$$

$$(1 - r)^n = \frac{1}{k}$$

$$n = \frac{\log\left(\frac{1}{k}\right)}{\log(1-r)}$$

6.11 Estimaton of Gene Frequencies with Dominance

When the two loci are in linkage equilibrium and have complete dominance but without epistasis between two loci, the gene frequencies can be estimated from the phenotypic frequencies. Consider that the allele A is dominant over the allele a at locus A and the allele B is dominant over its allele b at locus B. There will be only four phenotypic classes in the following proportions:

	B-	Bb	Total Freq.
A-	$(1\text{-}q^2)\,(1\text{-}v^2)$	$(1\text{-}q^2)\,v^2$	$1\text{-}q^2$
Aa	$q^2\,(1\text{-}v^2)$	q^2v^2	q^2
Total	$1\text{-}v^2$	v^2	1.0

The product of the double-dominant (AABB) and double recessive (aabb) phenotype is equal to the product of the two single dominants in a condition of linkage equilibrium.

The gene frequencies can be calculated by proceeding first to estimate the frequency of recessive allele from row and column totals. The frequency of recessive allele *a* can be estimated from the sum of second row (q^2) as:

$f(aa) = q^2$

$$q = \sqrt{q^2} = \sqrt{[(aa\ B\text{-}) + (aa\ \ bb)]}$$

$p = 1\text{-}q$

Similarly the frequency of recessive allele b at B locus can be estimated from sum of second columns (v^2) as

$f(bb) = v^2$

$$v = \sqrt{v^2} = \sqrt{[(A\text{-}bb) + (aa\ bb)]}$$

6.12 Application of Two Loci Case

1. Type of mating being followed: The knowledge of the linkage disequilibrium helps to know to some extent the history of population. When a population is in linkage disequilibrium with high value of D, it then gives an indication that random mating is not being followed in the population for long while the value of D very close to zero gives an evidence of the random mating practice in the population.

2. Causes of genetic correlation: When a strong genetic association exists between two traits in a random mating population for many generations, it then helps to assign the cause of genetic correlation. The linkage between two loci can not be the cause of genetic correlation in an equilibrium population for two loci but it may be more probably due to pleiotropic gene action or it indicates the possibility of intermixture of two breeds.

3. Mating plan of intercrossing to be followed: The existence of linkage in a crossbred population indicates that the desired combination of genes will be compared to the genes segregating independently. Therefore, this suggests that free intercrossing should be allowed for few generations so as the crossing over takes place to form desirable combination of genes. Such a mating scheme of free intercrossing should be a pre-requisite of selection and to develop new line or breed.

Exercises

6.1. The following genotypic frequencies occur in a certain population for two loci, A and B, each with two alleles represented by Z:

$$Z = \begin{matrix} 0.09 & 0.18 & 0.09 \\ 0.12 & 0.24 & 0.12 \\ 0.04 & 0.08 & 0,04 \end{matrix}$$

Find out the gamete and allelic frequencies and check the equilibrium?

6.2. In a random mating population consider the two loci A and B with two alleles at each locus. Write down the complete array of genotypes along with expected frequencies when the gene frequencies are as under-

$A_1 = 0.3, A_2 = 0.7, B_1 = 0.5, B_2 = 0.5$

6.3. Consider one population entirely of double heterozygote, second population having equal proportion of four double homozygotes and third one having equal proportions of four single homozygotes.

  (i) Estimate the gamete output of each of them

  (ii) Find out the constitution of their next generation on random mating within each population?

  (iii) What will be the constitution of hybrid population produced by crossing second and third population?

Hint: (i) $p = u = 0.5$

  (ii) Equilibrium will be established in one generation for first population

6.4 The two loci each with two alleles are segregating and their gamete frequencies are as:

$$\begin{vmatrix} W & X \\ Y & Z \end{vmatrix} = \begin{vmatrix} 0.35 & 0.35 \\ 0.25 & 0.05 \end{vmatrix}$$

(i) Find out the frequencies of nine genotypes of the initial population mating at random?

(ii) Test if the population is in linkage equilibrium. Find out the value of D if the population is not in linkage equilibrium.

6.5 The two loci (MN and Ss) have been reported to be located closely on the same chromosome with a recombination fraction of $r = 0.01$. Estimate the types and frequencies of the gametes to be produced by MS Ns and Ms NS individuals.

Hint: Find out the parental types and recombinant types of gametes and then their frequencies as $\dfrac{(q-r)}{2}$ and $\dfrac{r}{2}$ respectively for the two individuals separately?

6.6. The linkage disequilibrium is taken as $D = wz - xy$ with the gamete frequencies of four types of gametes as w, x, y, z (AB, Ab, aB and ab) with r as the recombination fraction, Find out the equilibrium value of D and estimate the amount of equilibrium to be approached.

6.7 The genotypes for two loci MN and Ss blood groups are found in H.W. proportions separately with the gene frequencies as

$P_M = 0.5425$ (p_1); $q_N = 0.4575$ (p_2);

$P_S = 0.308$ (q_1); $q_s = 0.692$ (q_2)

Among 1000 people following results were obtained for gamete types, their frequencies and observed numbers:

MS $(p_1q_1) = 474$, Ms $(p_1q_2) = 611$,

NS $(p_2q_1) = 142$, Ns $(p_2q_2) = 773$

(i) Test whether the two loci are in linkage equilibrium?

(ii) If not find out the amount of linkage disequilibrium

Hint: (i) Find out the expected numbers of four types of gametes as p_1q_1 $2N$ and apply chi-square test with 1 degree of freedom [4-1-1 for estimating $p_1 - 1$ for estimating q_1] ?

(ii) The amount of linkage disequilibrium can be obtained by estimating the gamete frequencies (p_1q_1) from observed numbers as a ratio of observed number to the total number of genes in the population *viz.* for MS gametes $(p_1q_1) = 474/2N = 474/2000 = 0.2370$. Now $D = p_1q_1 \, p_2 \, q_2 - p_1q_2 \, p_2 \, q_1$ from the estimated gamete frequencies and

$D_{min} = p_1 \, q_2$ or $- p_2 \, q_2$ (which ever is larger)

$D_{max} = p_1 \, q_2$ or $p_2 \, q_1$ (which ever is smaller)

Amount of linkage equilibrium (per cent) = D/D by putting the value of D max which ever in smaller. $= 0.07/0.4 = 0.50 = 50$ per cent of its theoretical maximum in this problem.

6.8. The recombination fraction (r) is 0.20 in a population which is not in linkage equilibrium for two linked loci. Estimate how many generations will be required for the population to reach half equilibrium.

Hint: $\dfrac{D_n}{D_0} = \dfrac{1}{2}$, $n = \dfrac{\log\left(\dfrac{1}{2}\right)}{\log(1-r)} = \dfrac{0.67}{0.223} = 3$

Chapter 7
Factors Affecting Gene Frequency: Systematic Processes (Mutation and Migration)

The random mating in a large population results in a genotype distribution according to the frequencies of genes (square law) and hence maintains the genetic equilibrium in a population. The H.W. law states about the conditions necessary to maintain the genetic equilibrium. The population in which these conditions are met is called the ideal or idealized population. The *ideal population* is one which produces progeny with all possible relationships between uniting gametes, including self fertilization. Therefore, in idealized population, the opposite sex gametes have equal chance of uniting in all possible combinations and the genetic equilibrium is maintained because no disturbing force comes in action to upset the genetic equilibrium. The specified conditions for ideal population are large population size, random mating (mating with all possible combinations including selfing), absence of evolutionary forces of selection, migration and mutation, and the distinct generations without overlapping.

The populations of farm animals are not ideal and hence the genetic equilibrium is disturbed. First of all, the farm animals are bisexual and hence selfing can not take place. Secondly, the *real population* of farm animals also differs from idealized population because the population size is small, the migration takes place, the selection is occurring, mating is restricted, mutation may takes place though very rare and the generations are not distinct but overlap.

It is thus obvious that most of the conditions for ideal population to maintain the genetic equilibrium are not fulfilled. Therefore, the genetic equilibrium is not observed in population of farm animals and the change in genetic structure of population is likely to occur in all practical situations. The genetic properties of a population are affected during transmission of genes from one generation to the next, if any of the conditions of idealized population or H.W. law is violated. The change can be brought to favourable direction and magnitude after having the knowledge of the genetic effects of the breeding policy which mainly covers the selective breeding and migration. Therefore, it is most essential for a breeder to know the effects of different forces leading to the change in genetic structure of population.

7.1 Forces Changing Genetic Structure

The genetic structure from one generation to the next is under the control of some biological forces. These forces act on individuals mainly by affecting their survival and reproduction and hence determine the relative genotype frequencies of a population. The forces capable to change the genetic structure of a population can be classified by several criteria given as under-

1. First Criterion of Classification

Natural Vs. artificial factors: Both nature and human activities disturb the existing genetic equilibrium. One or the other force come into operation in changing the genetic structure either through man's activities or through the role of nature, as explained under-

(i) Man's Activities to Change the Genetic Structure

The breeders are interested to change the existing genetic structure of his animal's population in a desired direction to exploit the existing genetic variability to make his animals more productive and more useful. The aim of animal breeder to produce better performing animals is achieved in a number of ways which are as under-

Firstly, the animal breeder selects the better productive animals and eliminates the low productive and inferior ones. This is called the *artificial selection.*

Secondly, the selected animals are mated following certain criteria of mating rather than allowing random mating in the herd. Thus, the *mating is preferential (non-random or* assortative mating or *selective breeding)* and this is done for certain valid reasons *viz.* to avoid inbreeding, to combine the best characters of different breeds, to get advantage of hybrid vigour etc. Thus, the random mating is not allowed but it is based on choice under certain natural and artificial conditions (livestock breeding at organized farms).

Thirdly, the breeders are compelled to keep their animals in relatively *small herds/flocks* for a number of reasons *viz.* breeding space, capital required etc. This results in *small population size* which upsets the genetic equilibrium. The small population affects the genetic structure of population for two reasons. First is that the inbreeding is inevitable in small size. Second is that the possibility of producing the expected genotype frequencies is low in small population due to sampling effect (lesser number of animals). According to the probability higher numbers of events make the expectation more close to reality. Thus, smaller number of animals in the herd results in the occurrence of errors in sampling due to chance events. This leads to differentiation of gene frequencies in local populations resulting from sampling and is known as *random drift.*

The *fourth activity* of breeders is the trade breeding under which the animals are sold or transferred to another breeder's herd and thus *migration* of animals occurs. Moreover, the advances in animal breeding due to artificial insemination and frozen semen technology have made possible the transportation of semen from one herd to another herd located far apart within or outside the country. This has thus further increased the possibility of gene flow (*migration*) from one corner to other corner of the country or the world.

(ii) Role of Nature to Change Genetic Structure

The factors which are under the control of nature to upset the genetic equilibrium are the *mutation* (change in genetic structure of a gene) and the *natural selection.* The gene mutation occurs due to many factors and changes the genetic material (mutation and chromosomal aberrations). The natural selection operates through differential fertility and viability. The fertility and survivability of individuals results in non-random mating and selective breeding.

2. Second Criterion

Factors involved at individual and population level: The first is the change at gene level (mutation). The second is the change at population level by gene flow (migration), selection, small population size, and by a change in mating system from random mating to preferential mating (non-random mating).

3. Third Criterion

Type of change involved: The genetic change may be brought in genotype distribution without affecting the gene frequencies or the change may occur in gene frequencies which accompanied change in genotype frequencies. The *first category of force* is the *non-random mating* (genetic assortative mating) which leads to a change only in genotype frequencies without affecting the gene frequencies. The genotype frequencies are changed because of a different combination of genes. The change persists for as long as the mating is nonrandom and the switch to random mating brings the population to its original genetic structure. This is because the gene frequencies are not changed under assortative mating and hence switching to random mating the genotype frequencies in progeny generation are determined by the gene frequencies of the parent generation.

The *second category of forces* brings a change in gene frequencies between generations and consequently result a change in genotype frequencies. These forces include *gene mutation, gene flow (migration), selection, small population size* and disassortative mating. The genetic change brought by the forces of second category is permanent even after switching to random mating. This is because these forces involve the change in gene frequencies.

4. Fourth Criterion

Amount and direction of change: On this basis, all the forces are divided into two groups. The first group is the deterministic or *systematic forces* which are also called as the vectorial process. The *systematic forces* tend to change the gene frequencies predictable both in amount and direction, and consequently the genotypic frequencies are changed. These are *mutation, migration and selection.*

The second category is the stochastic process or random or *dispersive process.* This process arises in *small population* from the effect of sampling. The change brought by dispersive process is predictable only in amount but not in direction.

7.2 Mutation and Change of Gene Frequency

The mutant allele has an effect different to that of the normal allele. Thus, mutation provides new genetic material on which the different forces can operate. The effect of mutation to cause genetic change depends upon the recurrence of mutation (single mutation or recurrent mutation) and the balancing effect of reverse mutation.

1. Single Mutation (Non-Recurrent) and its Fate

A newly mutant gene arisen in an individual may increase or decrease in its frequency or may be lost from the population by chance elimination in the progeny generation. The frequency of the mutated gene (q) when it occurs just once as a single mutational event is extremely low and it is equal to $1/(2N)$. However, it has an equal chance of survival or being lost. The probability of extinction of a single mutant gene is 0.3679 in the first generation. The probability that it should be lost in second generation after its occurrence is 0.5315 and the probability of being loss of new mutant gene goes on increasing in subsequent generations if the gene is neutral (neither beneficial non harmful) to the individual carrying it. The great majority of single mutant alleles are lost within a few generations after they arise and only a few ones become established in the population. This is because the loss of a new single mutant gene is an irreversible process. Thus, a unique mutation has no effect on the change of population without its selective advantage. The fate of a new single mutation depends on population size, selective advantage, and the distribution of progenies in families in which the mutant gene is arisen.

2. Recurrent Mutation

When each mutational event recurred regularly it is called as recurred mutation. This result to an increase in the frequency of the mutant allele in a large population and thus the mutant allele can not be lost by sampling but they are established in the population. The frequency of this mutant allele depends on the rate of mutation per generation which varies for different loci but seems to be reasonably constant for a particular locus from generation to generation under constant environmental conditions.

Considering, the original gene A which mutates to its alternate form **a** (**A** mutates to **a**) with a mutation rate denoted by **u** per generation (**u** is the proportion of all **A** genes that mutate to *a* between one generation and next) and the frequency of **A** in one generation as *p*, then the frequency of **a** gene (mutant gene) in the next generation will be equal to **u p**. This makes the frequency of **A** gene in the next generation as $p - up$ because the change of gene frequency is $-up$. The frequency of allele a in the next generation is increased by the amount up. At any generation (t) the frequency of mutant gene (q) may be obtained as:

$$q_t \quad = q_{t-1} + u\, p_{t-1}$$

$$q_t \quad = q_{t-1} + u\,(1 - q_{t-1}) \quad \text{By putting } p_{t-1} = 1 - q_{t-1}$$

$$= q_{t-1} + u - u\, q_{t-1}$$

$$= u + (1-u)\, q_{t-1}$$

and $q_{t+1} = u + (1-u)\, q_t$

where, **up**$_{t-1}$ is the proportion of **A** allele mutated to a in the population of **t** generation,

q_{t-1} is the frequency of allele **a** in previous generation (**t-1**).

This can be taken as the sequence equation of the q_i series. The repeated substitution of the values of q_{t-1} and q_{t-2} expresses the general terms as:

$$q_t = u + (1 - u)\,[u + (1 - u)\, q_{t-22}]$$

$$= u + (1-u)\,u + (1-u)^2 q_{t-2}$$

This produces a geometric series in which the last term with q_0 refers to the initial generation:

$$q_t = u + (1-u)\,u + (1-u)^2 u + (1-u)^3 u + . + (1-u)^t q_0$$

The sum of t terms in this geometric series is $(1-u)^t$. Therefore,

$$q_t \quad = 1 - (1-u)^t + (1-u)^t q_0$$

$$= 1 - (1-u)^t (1 - q_0)$$

$$(1-u)^t \quad = \frac{(1 - q_1)}{(1 - q_0)}$$

$$= \frac{p_t}{p_0}$$

$$t \log(1-u) \; = \log\left(\frac{p_t}{p_0}\right)$$

$$t \quad = \frac{\log\left(\dfrac{p_t}{p_0}\right)}{\log(1-u)}$$

This will help to estimate the gene frequency after a given number of generations or to estimate the number of generations required to change the gene frequency to a given level, if q_0 and **u** are known. The number of generations required (t) is inversely proportional to the mutation rate (u).

Secondly, if the recurrent mutation from **A** to **a** in one generation is not opposed, all the A genes in the population will be **a** after a number of generations. The amount of change in **q** per generation (Δq) is:

$$\Delta q = q_{t+1} - q_t = u + (1-u)\, q_t - q_t$$

$$= u\,(1 - q_t)$$

The amount of increase in allele **a** per generation is larger in the beginning when the frequency of **q** is small than when allele **a** in the population is abundant.

3. Reverse Mutation

The gene mutates in both directions which means that all the alleles mutate. The mutation of **A** gene into **a** allele is termed as _forward mutation_ and when _a_ mutates into **A,** it is called as _backward_ or _reverse mutation._ It has been indicated that when forward mutation (A to a) is slow, reverse mutation (a to A) is usually slow. Therefore, when an allele is rare the detection of mutation to other alleles is difficult because of low rate of mutation. The forward and backward mutations are important when the frequency of an allele is abundant.

7.3 Mutation Equilibrium

Taking Δq as the increment in **a** allele, _u_ = mutation rate per generation from **A** to **a,** and **v** = reverse mutation rate from **a** to A, then the gain in **a** = **up** and loss in **a** = _v q_. This means that after one generation there is a gain of **a** genes equal to _u p_ as a result of mutation (A to _a_) and loss in **a** genes equals to _v q_. The net amount of change in the frequency of **a** gene per generation (Δq) is:

$$\Delta q = \text{gain} - \text{loss}$$

$$= up - vq$$

Thus the relative magnitude of gain or loss per generation will decide the increase or decrease of q. If the forward and backward mutation rates are equal then q will become zero. This will lead no change in q in next generations and thus an equilibrium condition will be reached.

Thus, $\Delta q = 0$ which makes u p = v q, when population is at equilibrium.

and v q $= u\,(1\text{-}q)$

         $= u\text{-}u\,q$

u $= v\,q + u\,q$

         $= q\,(v + u)$

Thus, the _gene frequencies at equilibrium_ are as under:

$$q = \frac{u}{u+v} \quad \text{and}$$

$$p = \frac{v}{u+v}$$

It has been observed that the reverse mutation (**a** to A) is less frequent than forward mutation (A to a). Thus, the **mutation rate** *from wild type mutant* is more than mutation from mutant to the wild type. This resulted in to mutants as the more common form whereas the wild type as rare form. However, this condition is not observed in natural populations due to the effects of selection. The approach to mutational equilibrium is thus very slow.

Regarding equilibrium state of q, it is important to note that:

☆ The rate of forward and backward mutation (u and v) are constant which makes the q stable

☆ The value of $\hat{q}$ at equilibrium is independent of initial gene frequencies in the population but determined entirely by the relative amount of **u** and **v.**

☆ The value of **q** is decreased in subsequent generation if **q** is higher than the value of $\hat{q}$ at equilibrium and the decrease continues till the value of **q** at equilibrium is reached and the vice versa is also true. As a result if the value of q deviates from q value at equilibrium due to some reason, it comes back to equilibrium slowly as soon as the causal factor ceases to operate.

☆ The rate of approaching the q value to equilibrium is low and depends on the extent of deviation of the actual q from its equilibrium value. Thus if the actual q deviates from $\hat{q}$ at equilibrium, the change per generation (Δ q) will be:

$$q \quad = u\,p - v\,q$$
$$= u\,(1 - q) - v\,q$$
$$= u - u\,q - v\,q$$
$$= (u + v)\,\hat{q} - (u + v)\,q \text{ since } u = (u + v)\,q$$
$$= - (u + v)\,(q\text{-}\hat{q})$$

The number of generations required to bring a specific change in gene frequency can be estimated from the above expressions of Δ q by treating it a differential equation by replacing Δ q by dq/dt where t represents the generations required:

$$t \;=\; \log_{e} \frac{\dfrac{\left(q_0 - \hat{q}\right)}{\left(q_t - \hat{q}\right)}}{\left(u + v\right)}$$

7.4 Migration and Change of Gene Frequency

The migration means the transfer or movement of animals from one herd (sub population) to another. The animals are migrated through purchase or under exchange system in trade breeding by transferring the animals to another breeder's herd. The sires of improved breeds are imported from other countries for genetic improvement of other breeds. The technique of AI and frozen semen has made possible the transfer of semen from one herd to another inside or outside the country and has made faster the process of gene flow or gene migration without migration of the animals. Therefore, the genes of improved breed (s) migrate by transferring or importing the sire as such or their semen to be used in an inferior herd under the crossbreeding programme or upgrading the local, the non- descript animals. Thus, there is gene flow or gene migration through migration of animals or their semen.

The individuals leaving the population are called as *emigrants* but after joining other population are called *immigrants* or *migrants.* Thus the individuals which enter a population are called immigrants or migrants. The individuals of the population to which the migrants join are called the native animals or the native population. The migrants take part in reproduction of the native population. Thus the migrants genetically unit the native one and make a link to cause all members of a species to share a common pool of genes. The migration is closely related to mating systems because migrants take part into the breeding structure of a population.

The migration may occur in several ways *viz.* one way migration, mutual or reverse migration, fusion of sub populations etc. The effects of all the three types of migration on genetic structure of population have been discussed separately.

7.4.1. One-way Migration

When migration occurs from one population to another without any amount of migration in the reverse direction, it is called as the one-way migration.

Single Versus Recurrent Migration

The single and recurrent migration has their different effects. As a result of single migration of animals, genetic structure of population is changed but a new genetic equilibrium is attained after random mating on the basis of new genetic structure. In case of recurrent migration (when local sires are completely replaced by extraneous ones) the mixed population eventually turned like that of migrants resulting the ousting of the existing genes of native population. The recurrent (continuous) migration is like that of upgrading through continuous back crossing of crossbred progeny with sires of improved breed. This leads the genes of the improved breeds to be fixed in the progeny generations and the frequency of the alleles introduced become $(2^t-1)/2^t$ after t generation. The genes from migrants become numerous gradually and thereby reducing the frequency of the existing genes of native population. Thus migration brings about change in gene frequencies and so creates differences in genotypic relationship. This results in a marked reduction in the frequency of occurrence of original genotypes and appearance of new genotypes due to combination of the original and new genes if the migrants belong to other breed.

Consider two populations before migration. Some individuals migrate from one population (population 2, migrants) to join the other population (population 1, which is native population) and form a mixed population:

Population 1 (Native)	Population 2 (Migrants)

Freq. of A = p_n Freq of A = p_m

Freq. of a = q_n Freq. of a = q_m

Mixed population (Native + Migrants)

[Migrants (m), p_m and q_m]

[Native (1- m), p_n and q_n]

The migration is similar to mating system *viz.* crossbreeding, out crossing and grading up. The genetic effect of migration can be described considering the rate of migration (**m**) and the gene frequencies (**q**) in the two populations as:

$$\mathbf{m} = \text{Migration rate} = \text{proportion of migrants} = \frac{n_2}{n_1 + n_2}$$

where, n_1 are the number of individuals in the native population,

               n_2 are the number of migrants, respectively.

               1 – m = Proportion of native individuals in the mixed population,

               q_m = gene frequency among migrants

               q_n = gene frequency among natives.

               q_1 = gene frequency in mixed population

               q_t = gene frequency in tth generation of recurrent migration

Among humans, the migration rate depends upon a number of factors *viz.* sex, marital status, socio-economic status, population density, education, business etc.

The gene in the mixed population after migration will come from native (host) population with a probability of (1-m) q_n and from the migrants with a probability of m q_m. Therefore, the *gene frequency after migration* (q_1) will be:

$q_1 = m\, q_m + (1\text{-}m)\, q_n$

     $= m\, q_m + q_n - m\, q_n$

     $= q_n + m\, (q_m - q_n),$

     $= q_n - m\, (q_n - q_m)$ 7.1

This can be expressed in terms of the proportion of natives (1- m). This is done by adding and substracting q_m in the above equation of q_1. On solving, the value of q_1 will be as

$q_1 = q_m + (1\text{-}m)\, (q_n - q_m)$ 7.2

The gene frequency with recurrent migration for a number of *t* generations (q_t) will be as:

$q_t = q_m + (1\text{-}m)^t (q_n - q_m)$ 7.3

The *rate of change in gene frequency* in one generation (Δq) can be estimated from the difference in gene frequency in natives before and after migration as

$$\Delta q = q_1 - q_n$$
$$= q_n + m(q_m - q_n) - q_n$$
$$= m(q_m - q_n) \qquad\qquad\qquad .... 7.4$$

It can be noted that the change in gene frequency (Δq) depends on the migration rate (m) and the difference in gene frequency of all natives and migrants ($q_m - q_n$). The change is proportional to both these factors.

The *difference in gene frequency* between two populations is reduced after migration. The reduction in difference of gene frequency can be obtained as:

$$q_1 - q_m = [q_n + m(q_m - q_n)] - q_m$$
$$= q_n - q_m - m(q_n - q_m)$$
$$= 1(q_n - q_m) - m(q_n - q_m)$$
$$= (1-m)(q_n - q_m) \qquad\qquad .... 7.5$$

Thus, the difference in gene frequency between two populations after migration depends upon the initial difference in gene frequency between two populations and the proportion of natives. The difference is reduced with increase in migration rate. Therefore, further migration will reduce the difference in gene frequency between two populations. It means that the two populations tend to become alike genetically or homogeneous in gene frequencies with continuous migration. The frequency of gene present in the migrants is continuously increased with continuous migration. Therefore, in a crossbreeding programme with continuous use of sires of improved breed on the crossbred female progeny or in an upgrading programme of mating non descript female with sires of improved breed will increase the frequency of genes of improved breed leading to fixation of the allele after a number of generations. The frequency of alleles introduced becomes $(2^t - 1)/2^t$ after t generations if the gene frequency is zero in the native or non-descript population. In this situation of crossbreeding and upgrading, the migration rate is *0.5* because the sires of improved breed contribute half of the total genes of the next progeny generation.

The amount of genetic migration (m) can be estimated from the allele frequency data as:

$$m = \frac{\Delta q}{(q_m - q)} \qquad\qquad .... \text{from equation 7.4}$$

$$= \frac{(q_1 - q_n)}{(q_m - q_n)}$$

The migration rate (m) per generation after a number of t generations of continuous migration can be estimated using the equation of q_t from equation 4.3 as:

$$q_t = q_m + (1-m)^t (q_n - q_m) \qquad\qquad .... \text{from equation 7.3}$$

$$(1-m)^t = \left[\frac{(q_t - q_m)}{(q_n - q_m)}\right] \qquad \text{...............7.6 (a)}$$

$$(1-m) = \left[\frac{(q_t - q_m)}{(q_n - q_m)}\right]^{\frac{1}{t}} \qquad \text{...............7.6 (b)}$$

$$m = 1 - (1 - m)$$

7.4.2. Reverse or Mutual Migration

The migration is also practiced for another purpose when the individuals of two or more populations are reciprocally exchanged under associated herd improvement programme. The interchange of individuals between sub populations is called as reverse migration.

To estimate the effect of reverse or mutual migration the migration rate (m) from and to both the populations is taken equal as well as both these populations are assumed to be large enough to ignore the effect of random drift. In this case, the frequency of gene among the migrants is taken equal to the average gene frequency in the two populations ($\bar{q}$). Therefore, substituting the value of $\bar{q}$ in place of q_m in the estimation equation of (q_1) obtained in case of one-way migration (eq. 7.1). The gene frequency after migration can be estimated as:

$$q_1 = m\,\bar{q} + (1 - m)\,q_0$$

$$= q_0 - m\,(q_0 - \bar{q})$$

$$\Delta q = q_1 - q_0 = m\,(\bar{q} - q_0)$$

where, q_0 is the initial gene frequency in a particular group.

The gene frequency after t generation will be

$$q_t = m\,\bar{q} + q_{t-1}\,(1 - m)$$

$$= \bar{q} + (1 - m)^t\,(q_0 - \bar{q}) \qquad \text{...............equivalent to eq. 7.3}$$

The example of reverse or mutual migration is the associated herd progeny testing programme under which the animals are exchanged between two or more herds. The migration rate is fixed for all generations to estimate the change in gene frequency over time (generations). The gene frequency is increased in herd (s) having initial gene frequency lower than average gene frequency of all herds ($\bar{q}$) while the gene frequency is reduced towards q in those herds having initial gene frequency higher than $\bar{q}$. The magnitude of convergence in t generation ($q_t - \bar{q}$, measured as Δq_t) towards equilibrium gene frequency can be estimated as:

$$q_t - \bar{q} = (1-m)^t\,(q_0 - \bar{q}) \qquad \text{...............equivalent to eq. 7.5}$$

The average gene frequency in two or more subpopulation ($\bar{q}$) remains same in all the generations ignoring the random genetic drift, mutation and selection.

The possibility of reverse migration is more among the neighbouring herds or subpopulations. The change in gene frequency is less because the neighbouring sub populations have lesser differences in their gene frequency due to frequent interchange of animals. Therefore, with frequent exchange of animals between any sub populations, the gene frequencies become nearly equal in such populations.

7.4.3. Fusion of Subpopulations–Isolate Breaking

As a result of migration, the isolated subpopulations are fused (mixed) together which is known as isolate breaking. The subdivision of a population into small lines produces a deficiency of heterozygote and a corresponding increase of the frequency of homozygote (See next chapter of small population). The fusion of two subpopulations into one population has an effect on the genotype frequencies. This effect is reverse to that of the subdivision of a population. The fusion of populations reduces the frequency of homozygote and a consequent increase in the frequencies of heterozygote. This effect of isolate breaking (Fusion of subpopulations into one population) is a part of *Wahlund's principle*.

The Wahlund's principle of isolate breaking which results in to lesser frequency of homozygotes in fused population after random mating can be expressed in two ways *viz.* fixation index (pqF) and variance of gene frequency among subpopulations ($\sigma^2 q$).

(i) Fixation Index

The *Wahlund's effect of isolate breaking* (reduction in the frequency of homozygote in fused population after random mating) in terms of *fixation index*. This can be observed considering the frequency of allele **a** as q_1 and q_2 in two populations with their average as $\bar{q}$. The average frequency of aa homozygote of two subpopulations should be mean of the square of recessive gene frequency $\left(q^2\right)$ which is greater than square of average gene frequency $\left(\bar{q}\right)^2$ before fusion. As the subdivision has inbreeding like effect, the frequency of homozygote is increased in subdivided population. The average frequency of aa homozygote in all the subpopulations is $\bar{q}^2\,(1-F) + \bar{q}\,F = \bar{q}^2 + \overline{pq}\,F$. The F is called as the fixation index denoted as F_{ST} (inbreeding coefficient in subpopulation relative to total population). The frequency of aa homozygote after fusion and one generation of random mating will be q^2 which is lesser than their average frequency before fusion by the amount equal to $\overline{pq}\,F$ as shown –

<table>
<tr><td>Before fusion</td><td>After fusion</td></tr>
<tr><td>$[\,\bar{q}^2\,(1-F) + \bar{q}\,F] - \left(\bar{q}\right)^2$</td><td>$\bar{q}\,F - \left(\bar{q}\right)^2 F$</td></tr>
<tr><td></td><td>$= \bar{q}\,F\,(1-\bar{q}) = \overline{pq}\,F$</td></tr>
</table>

(ii) Variance of Gene Frequency

Secondly, the *Wahlund's principle of isolate breaking* (reduction in the frequency of homozygote in fused population after random mating) can also be expressed in terms of *variance of gene frequency* among subpopulations. The variance measures the degree of dispersion of a set of numbers from the mean or how closely the individual numbers cluster around the mean. Mathematically, the variance is calculated as the mean of the squared values minus the square of mean ($\sigma^2_q = \overline{q^2} - \overline{q}^2$.). This can be shown as:

Population	1	2	Mixed
Freq. of allele **a**	q_1	q_2	q
Freq. of genotype **aa**	$(q_1)^2$	$(q_2)^2$	q^2
Av. freq. of allele **a** $(\overline{q}) = \frac{1}{2}(q_1 + q_2)$			
Av. freq. of genotype aa $(\overline{q^2}) = \frac{1}{2}[(q_1)^2 + (q_2)^2] = $ Mean of squares			

The frequency of recessive homozygote (aa) before fusion is the mean of squares of gene frequency $\left(\overline{q^2}\right)$ whereas after fusion is the square of the mean gene frequency $(\overline{q})^2$. Therefore, the difference in the frequency of recessive homozygote before and after fusion is the variance in allele frequency among sub populations which indicates the reduction in the frequency of recessive homozygote due to fusion:

Variance of gene freq. = Freq. of **aa** before fusion – Freq. of **aa** after fusion

$$\left(\sigma^2\right) \qquad = [\text{Mean square, } \overline{q^2}] - [\text{Square of the mean, } (\overline{q})^2]$$

The mathematical illustration of Whalund's principle of isolate breeding (fusion of subpoplation into one population) on the reduction in the frequency of homozygotes in pooled population after random mating has been shown in example 7.1.

Utility of Wahlund's Principle

In human populations, there are a number of harmful recessive genes at high frequency in certain population *viz.* sickle-cell anemia in Negros (q= 0.05 to 0.1), Tay-Sachs disease (q=0.013) which is degenerative disorder of brain among Ashkenazi Jews, albinism in Southwest American Indians (q= 0.077), antitrypsin deficiency (q = 0.024) and cystic fibrosis (q= 0.022) in Caucasians. The frequency of children born with genetic defects resulting from these recessive genes in homozygous condition can be reduced by migration in the population in which they are relatively high.

The variance is large when the individual values deviate more from the mean. Similar is the case for the variance of gene frequency among sub populations. When sub populations have higher variation in allele frequencies, the variance in allele frequency among sub populations will be more and if the allele frequencies are equal in all sub-populations the variance in allele frequency among subpopulations will be zero.

7.5 Relation between σ^2_q and F

The frequency of recessive homozygote after fusion of two populations (isolate breaking) is reduced equal to variance of gene frequency ($\sigma^2 q$) among subpopulations and is also equal to pqF as well. ***Therefore, $\sigma^2 q = pqF$ and thus $F = \sigma^2 q/pq = F_{ST}$.*** The F_{ST} is fixation index due to subdivision or reduction in heterozygosity of a subpopulation due to random drift. The F_{ST} is the average inbreeding of subpopulation in relation to total population. This relation is useful to estimate F from allele frequency data as shown below:

Sub Populations		$\sigma^2 q = \overline{q_i^2} - \left(\overline{q_i}\right)^2$		F
q_1	q_2	$= \frac{1}{2}(q_1^2 + q_2^2) - [\frac{1}{2}(q_1 + q_2)]^2$		$= \sigma^2 q/\overline{pq}$
0.5	0.5	0.25	0	0
0.6	0.4	0.25	0.01	0.04
0.7	0.3	0.25	0.04	0.16
0.8	0.2	0.25	0.09	0.36
0.9	0.1	0.25	0.16	0.64
1.0	0.0	0.25	0.25	1.00

where, $\overline{q_i^2}$ = Mean of square (before fusion)

$\left(\overline{q_i}\right)^2$ = Square of mean (after fusion)

The magnitude of $\sigma^2 q$ depends on the deviation of q among subpopulations from the average value of $\overline{q}$ in all subpopulations. The $\sigma^2 q$ affects the magnitude of F. Both $\sigma^2 q$ and F increase linearly with the increase in differences in q among subpopulations.

7.6 Effect of Migration on σ^2_q and F

The continuous migrations make the gene frequencies of the various groups more nearly alike and render the total population more homogeneous. The deviation of q in any group from its average value in all the groups $(\overline{q})$ is $(q_i - \overline{q})$. This deviation is reduced in the next generation after migration as:

$$(q_1 - \overline{q}) \quad = [q_i - m(q_i - \overline{q}) - \overline{q} \quad \text{Since } q_i = m\overline{q} + (1-m)\,\overline{q}_i = q_i - m(q_i - \overline{q})$$

$$= q_i - \overline{q} - m(q - \overline{q})$$

$$= (q_i - \overline{q})(1 - m) \qquad \text{................ equivalent to eq. 7.5}$$

Now taking $\sigma^2 q$ as the variance of q among subgroups in one generation, this variance in next generation will be reduced to:

$$\sigma^2 q = (1-m)^2 (q_i - \overline{q})^2$$

$$= (1-m)^2 \sigma^2 q \qquad \text{considering that q remains constant.}$$

The variance of gene frequency ($\sigma^2 q$) is a measure of the heterozygosity or genetic differentiation of the total population divided into groups. Therefore, decrease in $\sigma^2 q$ implies that the sub populations, among which migration takes place, become more uniform. Now $F = \sigma^2 q / \overline{pq}$ and hence with the decrease in variance the F relative to the total population will also decrease due to migration. However, the change in q of any sub group is limited to $\overline{q}$.

7.7 Migration Limits Genetic Divergence among Sub-Populations

The subdivision of a population into many small groups of size N with random mating within each group leads to a loss of heterozygosity at the rate of $1/(2N)$ per generation with ultimate fate of small group to reach complete homozygosis. In such small group the F increases. The subdivision of a population into small groups leads to genetic differentiation among subpopulations. Considering F as the value in one generation, it will increase to $\dfrac{1}{(2N)} + \left[1 - \dfrac{1}{2N} \right]$ in the next generation under complete random union of gametes. Now if migration takes place between small groups, it will not only prevent the small groups to attain complete homozygosis but will bring the gene frequencies in small groups nearer to the q (average value of total population) and hence it will prevent significant genetic divergence among subpopulations resulted from random genetic drift. Consequently the variance of gene frequencies among groups ($\sigma^2 q$) reduces to $(1-m)^2 \sigma^2 q$ in the next generation as illustrated above. Reduction in $\sigma^2 q$ reduces the F also in the same proportion because $\sigma^2 q = \overline{pq}$ F or F = $\sigma^2 q / \overline{pq}$. The F is thus decreased with the increase in number of migrants.

The effect of the number of migrants on F is as:

When $N_m = 0$, F = 1.0

$N_{(m)} = 0.25$ (one migrant every fourth generation), F = 0.50

$N_{(m)} = 0.50$ (one migrant every second generation), F = 0.33

$N_{(m)} = 1$ (one migrant each generation), F = 0.20

$N_{(m)} = 2$ (Two migrants each generation), F = 0.11.

It is thus very much obvious that migration is a potent force which acts against genetic divergence that arises due to random genetic drift among subgroups.

7.8 Joint Effect of Migration and Mutation

A large population under random mating remains in genetic equilibrium in the absence of evolutionary forces. The effects of different evolutionary process on the change of gene frequency have been discussed in preceding chapters. However, if different evolutionary processes operate for long enough, the population will eventually reach a state of equilibrium depending upon the balance of a single process (mutation in both directions with equal rate, selection favouring heterozygote) or due to the joint effect of two or more forces working in opposite direction. The gene frequency at equilibrium is determined by equating the change of gene frequency under two processes. The change of gene frequency at equilibrium due to one process should be equal to the change brought by second process. Thus, the balance between two processes (the relative magnitude of their effects) decides the equilibrium point.

The genetic equilibrium attained under selection (when selection favours heterozygote) and mutation has been discussed along with the effect these forces, separately on change of genetic structure of population.

These two forces (Migration and mutation) jointly have similar effect on the gene frequencies. The migration affects the gene frequencies of the local subgroups in a similar way as do the mutation for the population gene frequencies.

Under migration, $\Delta q = -m(q - \bar{q})$

$$= m\bar{q}(1-q) - m\bar{p}q$$

Under Mutation, $\Delta q = -(u+v)(q - \bar{q})$

$$= u(1-q) - vq$$

The joint effect of migration and mutation will change the gene frequency (Δq) as:

$\Delta q \qquad = -m(q - \bar{q}) - (u+v)(q - \bar{q})$

$$= -(m+u+v)(q - \bar{q})$$

Or from $\Delta q \quad = m\bar{q}(1-q) - mq\bar{p} - u(1-q) - vq$

$$= (m\bar{q} + u)(1-q) - (m\bar{p} + v)q$$

The constant $m\bar{q}$ may be substituted for **u** (forward mutation rate), while $m\bar{p} = m(1 - \bar{q})$ can be taken for v (reverse mutation rate), and proportion of migration (m) can be taken as equal to the sum of the two mutation (u + v).

Also $\Delta q = 2up - 2vq$ in terms of mutation after substituting the constant

$$mq = u \text{ and } m\bar{p} = v$$

$$= -2m(q - \bar{q}) \quad \text{in terms of migration after substitution of } u + v = m.$$

The equilibrium gene frequency ($\hat{q}$) can be obtained by setting $\Delta q = 0$ under the joint effect of migration and mutation.

$\Delta q \qquad = up - vq \qquad\qquad$ under mutation

$\Delta q \qquad = -m(q - \bar{q}) \qquad\qquad$ under migration

and hence $\Delta q \quad = up - vq - m(q - \bar{q}) \qquad$ under joint effect

$$= u(1-q) - vq - mq + m\bar{q}$$

$$= u - uq - vq - mq + m\bar{q}$$

$$= u - q(u + v + m) + m\bar{q}$$

$$= -(u + v + m)q + u + m\bar{q}$$

Therefore, $\hat{q} \quad = \dfrac{(u + m\bar{q})}{(u + v + m)}$

7.9 Significance of Migration

The genetic change in the population is quite obvious in case of migration. Consequent to migration, new alleles are introduced which *create new genetic variation* like mutation, equalize the genetic differences between sub population and continuous migration reduces the chance of fixation of alleles. The migration holds the subpopulations close together genetically reducing the genetic divergence and hence it is a sort of *genetic glue (gelatine)*. It has its homogenizing effect on the genetic structure of subpopulations. On the other hand, the species become differentiated genetically in the absence of migration, as in case of self fertilizing plants, asexual reproducing organisms and closed populations. The migration between two populations located distantly is practiced to introduce, from other population, the genes that are rare or absent in one population (native or non-descript). This purpose is achieved by one- way migration. The main effect of isolate breaking is to decrease the overall frequency of homozygote. This information can be utilized to reduce the frequency of genetic defects arise from homozygous recessive genes that are harmful.

Solved Examples and Exerecises

Example 7.1

Mathematical illustration of Whalund's principle of Isolate breaking (Reduction of frequency of homozygous)

Genotypes

Sub Population	Allele Frequency		Genotypic Frequencies		
	p	q	p^2	$2pq$	q^2
1	0.9	0.1	0.81	0.18	0.01
2	0.3	0.7	0.09	0.42	0.49
Average of two sub populations	0.6	0.4	0.45	0.30	0.25
After fusion and random mating	$(0.6+0.4)^2$		0.36	0.48	0.16
Difference in genotype frequencies			0.09	− 0.18	0.09

The average frequency of aa homozygote in two sub populations $\left(\overline{q^2}\right)$ is higher (0.25) than the frequency of homozygote (0.16) after fusion of two sub-populations and one generation of random mating $\left(\overline{q}^2\right)$.

In the above example of fusion of two sub populations in which the frequency of recessive allele was 0.1 and 0.7, the average of the variance of gene frequency (mean of squares) before fusion was 0.25 (average frequency of homozygote, $\overline{q^2}$) and the variance of the average gene frequency [square of the mean gene frequency, $\overline{q}^2$] after fusion was 0.16 which is the frequency of recessive homozygote after fusion. Thus the variance equals 0.25 − 0.16 = 0.09. Therefore, the variance between sub populations is 0.25 − 0.16 = 0.09. This indicated that the frequency of recessive homozygote has been reduced by 9 percent as a result of fusion of two sub populations.

Example 7.2

The initial gene frequencies of the two alleles (A and a) are 0.4 and 0.6. The A allele mutates to allele *a* with the mutation rate of 6 per thousand with reverse mutation rate from *a* to A as 2 per thousand. Estimate the change in gene frequency in one generation due to mutation. What will be the equilibrium gene frequency ?

Solution

$$\Delta q = up - vq \text{ where, } u = \frac{6}{1000} = 0.006$$

$$\text{and } v = \frac{2}{1000} = 0.002$$

$$p = 0.4 \text{ and } q = 0.6$$

Therefore, $\Delta q = up - vq \quad = 0.006 \times 0.4 - 0.002 \times 0.6$

$$= 0.0024 - 0.0012 = 0.0012$$

Gene frequency at equilibrium $(\hat{p}) = \dfrac{v}{u+v} = \dfrac{0.002}{[0.006+0.002]}$

$$= \frac{2}{8} = 0.25$$

and $\hat{q} = 1 - \hat{p} = 1 - 0.25 = 0.75$

Example 7.3

The allele A mutates to *a* at a rate of 1 in 1000 and the revere mutation rate of 1 in 10000. Find out the genotypic frequencies at equilibrium in a random mating population, considering equal fitness of all the three genotypes. What will be the result if the mutation rate is doubled in both the directions?

Solution

The frequency of gene **a** at equilibrium $(\hat{q}) = \dfrac{u}{u+v}$

$$= \frac{10^{-3}}{10^{-3}+10^{-4}}$$

$$= \frac{1}{\left(1+10^{-1}\right)}$$

$$= \frac{10}{11} = 0.909$$

The HW frequencies of three genotypes can be obtained.

Doubling the mutation rate will not affect the result.

Example 7.4

Consider initial gene frequency of an allele among the native population as 0.3 and among immigrants as 0.6. The migration rate was 10 per cent. What will be the frequency of gene in the mixed population?. Estimate the change in gene frequency.

Solution

Given migration rate (m) = 10 per cent = 0.1; $q_n = 0.3$; $q_m = 0.6$

Gene frequency after migration (mixed population, $q_1) = q_n - m\,(q_n - q_m)$

$$= 0.3 - [0.1(0.3\text{-}0.6)] = 0.3 + 0.03 = 0.33$$

Change in gene frequency (Δq) $= m\,(q_m - q_n) = 0.1\,(0.6\text{-}0.3) = 0.03$

or Δq $= q_1 - q_n = 0.33 - 0.30 = 0.03$

Example 7.5

The gene frequency of an allele in native population was observed as 0.4 whereas among migrants it was 0.7 and after migration the gene frequency in mixed population was 0.5. Find out the migration rate.

Solution

$$\text{Migration rate (m)} = \frac{(q_1 - q_n)}{(q_m - q_n)}$$

$$= \frac{(0.5 - 0.4)}{(0.7 - 0.4)} = \frac{0.1}{0.3} = 0.33$$

Thus, the migration rate was 33 per cent.

Example 7.6

Find out the frequency of an allele after 20 generations in two populations which have initial gene frequency as 0.2 and 0.8. Assume a fixed reverse migration rate of 10 per cent in all generations

Solution

In this case 10 per cent of the animals are interchanged between two populations, amounting $m = 0.1$, average gene frequency in two populations ($\bar{q}$) will be $0.5 = (0.2 + 0.8)/2$ and q_0 is 0.2 and 0.8 in two populations in the beginning before migration.

$$q_{20} = \bar{q} + (q_0 - \bar{q})(1 - m)^{20}.$$

First population will attain the gene frequency after **20** generation as:

$$q_{20} = 0.5 + (0.2 - 0.5)(1 - 0.1)^{20}$$
$$= 0.5 + (-0.3)(0.1216)$$
$$= 0.4635$$

Second population will have the reduced gene frequency after 20 generation to:

$$q_{20} = 0.5 + (0.8 - 0.5)(1 - 0.1)^{20}$$
$$= 0.5 + (0.3)(0.1216)$$
$$= 0.5365$$

Average gene frequency after 20 generation in the two populations

$$\bar{q}_{20} = \frac{0.4635 + 0.5365}{2}$$

$$= 0.50$$

Example 7.7

Find out the migration rate per generation taking the initial gene frequencies among two populations as 0.474 (natives) and 0.507 (migrants) while the gene frequency was 0.484 in 10th generation.

Solution

$$q_t \quad = q_m + (1-m)^t (q_n - q_m) \qquad\qquad \text{Eq. 7.3}$$

$$(1-m)^t \quad = \frac{(q_t - q_m)}{(q_n - q_m)}$$

$$(1-m) \quad = \left[\frac{(q_t - q_m)}{(q_n - q_m)} \right]^{\frac{1}{t}}$$

$$= \left[\frac{-0.023}{-0.033} \right]^{\frac{1}{10}}$$

$$= 0.9645$$

$$m \qquad = 0.0355$$

It can be concluded that in any generation about **3.5 per cent** of the alleles were introduced by genetic migration in the native population.

Example 7.8

Find out the migration rate per generation with reverse migration among two populations having average gene frequency of 0.5, and the initial gene frequency in one of the two populations as 0.2 which rose to 0.4635 alter 20 generation of reverse migration. What was the initial gene frequency in second population?

Solution

$$1-m \quad = \left[\frac{(q_t - \bar{q})}{(q_1 - \bar{q})} \right]^{\frac{1}{t}}$$

$$= \left[\frac{(0.4365 - 0.5)}{(0.2 - 0.5)} \right]^{\frac{1}{20}}$$

$$= \left[\frac{-0.0365}{-0.3} \right]^{\frac{1}{20}}$$

$$= (0.12166)^{\frac{1}{20}}$$

$$= 0.900$$

Therefore, $m = 1 - (1 - m)$

$$= 1 - 0.900$$

$m \qquad = 0.1 = 10 \text{ per cent}$

$q_2 \qquad = 2q - q_1 \text{ Since } q = \dfrac{(q_1 + q_2)}{2}$

$$= (2 \times 0.5) - 0.2$$

$$= 0.8$$

Example 7.9

How many generations will be required to increase the gene frequency from 0.2 to 0.4635 with a migration rate per generation as 10 per cent taking the gene frequency among migrants as 0.5.

Solution

The number of generations required to bring a specific change in gene frequency can be estimated as under:

$q_t = q_m + (1 - m)^t (q_n - q_m)$ Eq. 7.3

$(1 - m)^t (q_n - q_m) = q_t - q_m$

$$(1 - m)^t = \frac{(q_t - q_m)}{(q_n - q_m)}$$

$$t \log (1 - m) = \log \frac{(q_t - q_m)}{(q_n - q_m)}$$

$$t = \frac{\log \dfrac{(q_t - q_m)}{(q_n - q_m)}}{\log (1 - m)}$$

$$= \frac{\log \dfrac{(0.4365 - 0.5)}{(0.2 - 0.5)}}{\log (1 - 0.1)}$$

$$= \frac{\log \dfrac{(-0.0365)}{(-0.3)}}{\log (0.9)}$$

$$= \frac{\log 0.12166}{\log 0.9}$$

$$= \frac{-0.9148521}{-0.0457574}$$

$= 19.99$ generations

Exercises

7.10. The Tay sachs disease (degenerative disorder of brain) is controlled by autosomal gene leading to death in infancy. Find out the incidence of the disease among the offspring of the mating between two populations having the incidence as 1 in 6000 and 1 in 5000,000 births. Also find out the incidence of the disease among the offspring of hybrid population mated randomly.

Hint: $q_1 = \sqrt{1/6000}$, $q_2 = \sqrt{1/500000}$

Expected freq. of rec. among the offspring of mating between two populations
$= q_1 q_2$

Allele freq.(q) in hybrid population $= \frac{1}{2}(q_1 p_2 + q_2 p_1) + q_1 q_2$

Freq. of homozy. Rec. $= (\bar{q})^2$

7.11. Consider the black Africans as ancestral population of blacks with MN blood group $p_{0(M)} = 0.474$, in black Georgian at percent $(p_t) = 0.484$ and the white Georgian be taken as the source of migration with $\bar{p} = 0.0507$ for the white population. The blacks were migrated to Georgia from Africa about 300 years ago (t = 10 generations). Estimate the amount of migration (m).

Hint: $p_1 = p_{t-1}(1-m)\bar{p}_m$

$= \bar{p} + (p_0 - \bar{p})(1-m)^t$ in term of p_0.

Answer: m = 0.035 per generation. This means that about 3.5 per cent of the alleles of MN blood group in any generation were newly introduced by genetic migration from white in the genetic history of the black Georgian.

Chapter 8
Change of Gene Frequency: Systematic Processes (Selection)

It is common practice to speak of selection in the sense of favouring the objects. When the objects are animals, the selection implies for giving preference to certain animals in the population to reproduce than others and hence selection is the choice of individuals to produce the next generation. In genetic term, the selection is the differential propagation of genetic material to the next generation. This is the result of differential survival and reproductive ability of different individuals of a population. Some animals are capable to survive and to produce their progeny while others are not, and some others produce more numbers of their progeny than others. Therefore, there is differential survival and reproductive success among the individuals of a population. The *process of differential survival and reproduction of individuals is known as "selection".*

8.1 Forces of Selection

The survival and reproductive success are two ingredients of selection. These are influenced by a number of life-cycle components at gamete and zygotic stage which in turn are under the control of two forces *viz.* natural and artificial.

(1) Natural Selection

This involves forces of nature which decide that which animal will reproduce and leave viable progeny to continue the process. This is the *"survival of fittest"* in a given environment. The survival of the fittest is determined/measured by the survivability and the reproductive success of the individual. Therefore, survivability and the reproductive status are known as the fitness or adaptive characters. The individuals that are not fit to survive and to produce their progeny died of their genetic death without leaving any offspring. This is the natural selection. The natural selection is thus a consequence of the differences between individuals for their capacity to produce viable progeny when living together under the same environmental conditions and hence have inequality of genetic contribution to future generation. All individuals are not equally fit to compete in a particular environment and the individuals having more progeny are known as better fit and adapted.

Large populations have all the time a great store of potential genetic variability known as the *plasticity of a population.* Every individual contains thousands of gene loci forming very large numbers of gene combinations beyond calculation. Secondly, diversity of environments over space and time is very well recognized. The different genotypes of a population have differential response to this diversity of environment (variations in climate, physical features, biological interactions and other environmental exigencies). This results some genotypes to become more efficient in their living and utilizing the available resources to create their own biomass leading them to evolve new gene pools and to become adapted and fit for survival and reproduction than others. Thus the environment imposes rigid rules and restrictions on the genotypes for their successful survival and reproduction. The genetic potential for change must exist in the population for selection to achieve a response to environmental stresses. Any unselected population or a plastic population is more fit because such population shows better response to environmental necessities by changes in its gene pool in a way that gives improved chances of survival and reproduction. When environmental conditions change, the existing genotypes may no longer be fit for survival but a plastic population may be able to go through genotypic recombination is so that new and more fitting types are produced. Thus, the *adaptability is a response of the population rather than of the individual* who cannot react to the needs of the changing environment by purposefully and immediately producing beneficial mutations where and when they are needed. The hereditary variations produced by mutation are molded into varieties and species due to the action of that environment through the mechanism of natural selection. Many adaptive characters of organisms are the result of natural selection.

Sub-populations of a species live different environments. Natural selection acts differently according to the environmental conditions provided to different sub-populations. When sub-populations live in different environments, the natural selection promotes the genetic divergence among them through the effect of increasing the adaptation of each sub-population to its own environment. When the sub-populations live in similar environment the natural selection tends to prevent genetic divergence again through the effect of increasing adaptation.

Stages of Life Cycle and their Components to Affect Natural Selection

The selection may operate at any stage of the life cycle of an organism and the means of selection may vary widely for different cases. However, the survival of fittest is determined by the survivability and fertility status of the individual which are under the control of life-cycle components at gamete and zygotic stages. Some major life cycle components contributing to Darwinian fitness (differences in survival and reproductive success in terms of the total number of progeny over several generations) in sexually reproducing diploid individuals are listed as under:

Gamete Stage

1. Segregation of homologous chromosomes at meiosis for gamete formation - (Segregation distortion).
2. Gamete competition or compatibility of ova and sperm before fertilization.

Zygotic Stage

3. Embryonic growth and development
4. Maturity rate (Early or late puberty),
5. Mating ability
6. Fecundity, age-specific fertility, gamete production, care and protection of young,
7. Total progeny produced
8. Survival at different age *viz.* embryonic stage, birth to maturity and adulthood.

The factors which affect survival are:

(a) Resistance to disease, outbreak of disease

(b) Protection from danger- wild animals (predation) and natural calamities. The wild animals kill the weak, very young and old animals *e.g.* killing of sheep by wolves.

(c) Accident, hunger

(d) Competitive ability to use resources

(e) *Differential ability to cope with climate and other environmental conditions*: Difference in survival of man due to differences in skin pigmentation is an example of climate effect. Differences in skin pigmentation from light to dark or black are due to genetic variation caused by mutation of genes. In Africa, the dark skinned individuals survive in large numbers than persons with a lighter skin. On the other hand, white skin men survive in a greater proportion in Europe because they are better adapted to less intense sunlight and low temperature. But the dark skinned Eskimos are residing in the polar regions of North and this may be because their dark skin could prevent sunburn from intense light rays reflected by the snow.

Like the climatic conditions, the survival is for the particular environmental conditions where the population is living. For example, the polled conditions in cattle being governed by the dominant gene, the number of polled cattle should have been more than the horned cattle. But actually the reverse is true. This might be, because that the polled cattle were in disadvantage in an environment when they had to move among wild animals in ancient period. This affected their survival and their contemporary horned cattle which were in few numbers could survive and reproduce new population with horns.

The population growth rate is high in areas where almost all basic living facilities are available than in desert and hilly areas. This either affects the survivability or compels the individuals to migrate in better area.

(f) *Differential survival of certain genotypes*: The human blood group (A, B and O) can be cited here. The individuals with blood group A, and O are said to be in more susceptible to gastric cancer and peptic ulcer, respectively.

(g) *Lethal genes*: The mutation causes the lethal genes which are eliminated from the population due to their low survival or low fertility.

(2) Artificial Selection

The second force of selection is man made which depends upon the choice of the breeder to allow the animals to produce the next generation. This is called as artificial selection. It is under the control of breeder who decides that to which animals he wants to retain and allow becoming parents of next generation. The choice of the breeder is objective specific and hence the artificial selection has certain purposes. Some genotypes are either more attractive, productive or more efficient functionally and hence preferred by the breeder.

The process of sum total of environmental forces including the choice of man acting to decide the survival and reproduction of a particular genotype in a population is the selection. Therefore, selection is regarded as a function of survival and reproductive success.

The two forces may act simultaneously on the same trait or on different traits and their action may be antagonistic (opposite) in a way that the individuals to which the breeder wants to favour to reproduce may be less fit in certain fitness traits (*e.g.* may be reproductively less fit or may not reach the breeding age, or may not survive longer after reaching reproductive age etc.). Therefore, there is undesirable genetic correlation between natural fitness and choice of animal breeder. Thus natural selection may oppose artificial selection. This results less than expected response to artificial selection.

8.2 Fitness and Selection Coefficient

A genotype is better fit and adapted if it produces and leaves more number of offspring than others in the same environment. Therefore, the *fitness (adaptive value or selective value)* of an individual indicates its contribution of offspring to the next generation and hence is a function of the survival and reproductive success of the individual in a given environment compared to its competitors in the population The simplest form of measuring the fitness is counting the number of offspring produced and left by an individual (genotype) compared to that produced by another optimum genotype (individual) having maximum number of offspring. The *fitness of an individual is thus defined as the relative survival and reproductive success.* This relative fitness is also called as the ***Darwinian fitness*** of individual.

The fitness of different genotypes of a population is known as the ***absolute fitness*** which is converted into relative (Darwinian) fitness by assigning the value 1.0 to the absolute fitness of the genotype with largest fitness in the population. For example, the females of three genotypes at a locus (AA, Aa and aa) produces on an average 80, 80 and 64 eggs, respectively. These values are the absolute fitness. Now assigning the females with highest absolute fitness (AA and Aa) as 1.0, the relative fitness of three genotypes will be 80/80, 80/80, 64/80 or 1.0, 1.0 and 0.8, respectively. Thus, the ***relative fitness (Darwinian fitness)*** *is* assigned to the individual of each genotype within a population. These are called as the adaptive values or **selective values** denoted by W_i. Thus, W_i indicates the relative fitness (selective value) of ith genotype of a population.

Selection Coefficient

In the example above, the aa genotype had less contribution to next generation and hence the selection is operating against *aa* genotype. The *proportionate reduction in contribution of a genotype selected against compared to the contribution of the favoured genotype with highest fitness* (W = 1.0) is called as the selection coefficient denoted by **S.** The selection coefficient indicates the strength of selection. The contribution of a favoured genotype (fitness) is taken as 1.0 and that of the genotype with reduced contribution (for the genotype selected against) is taken as 1 – S. Thus, **1-S** is *fitness of the genotype* selected against relative to the other favoured genotype. Therefore, the fitness of a genotype is conversely related to the selection coefficient as:

Fitness (W) = 1-S

The S is the **selection coefficient** *and indicates the fraction of genotypes which do not reproduce and hence do not contribute to the next generation.* Thus **S** expresses the amount by which the adaptive value is reduced or S is the proportionate reduction in gamete contribution of a genotype compared to the standard genotype having its fitness as 1.0. Thus, S is used to measure the relative fitness of different genotypes as 1- S_1 = W_1, 1- S_2 = W_2, ..., etc. taking the relative fitness of the most favoured genotype as 1.0.

However, the term adaptability is used for population rather than for the individual because an individual is powerless to respond to changed environment in changing its genotype in a favourable direction. The population or species, through ages, evolves new gene pools which become adapted under new environmental conditions. It is, therefore, estimated the average fitness of a population denoted by **W**. The *average fitness of a population* $\left(\overline{W}\right)$ is taken as the mean of the selective value of different genotypes weighted by their relative frequencies. Thus

$$\overline{W} = p_i p_j w_{ij} = \Sigma f_i w_i$$

The **dominance for fitness** may differ from the dominance of gene (phenotypic effect). This is because most of the mutant alleles are completely recessive to the wild type in phenotypic effect but the heterozygote may not have fitness equal to that of the wild type homozygote. The nature of dominance for fitness is independent to the dominance effect of gene on the phenotype. This is important to study the effect of selection. The effect of selection is taken in terms of dominance of fitness than dominance of phenotype. The examples of creeper condition in fowl, coat colour in mice and other characters may be cited to make clear the difference.

The *creeper condition (short legs) in fowl* is due to a dominant gene (C) which is lethal. The normal birds are recessive (cc) while the creepers (short and deformed legs and wings) are heterozygous (Cc) and the dominant homozygote (CC) die before birth. Thus, creeper condition is due to a dominant gene but this dominant gene has its adverse effect on vitality when homozygous (recessive for fitness). The yellow *coat colour in mice* is produced by a dominant gene A^Y but this gene is recessive for lethality causing $A^Y A^Y$ homozygote to die whereas the gene *"a"* is recessive for phenotypic expression of coat colour producing albino mice but dominant for fitness. The mating of heterozygous yellow produce a ratio of 2:1 instead of 3:1 because $A^Y A^Y$ homozygote die but heterozygote yellow (A^Ya) survive. Thus yellow colour gene is dominant for coat colour but cause lethality and hence recessive for fitness. Similarly, the gene for *platinum colour in fox* is dominant but cause lethality before birth in homozygous condition. The *brachydactyly* and the *thelessemia* in man and *polydactyly* in cattle are dominant characters but cause lethality before sexual maturity.

8.3 Fisher's Fundamental Theoram of Natural Selection (Improvement of Average Fitness Due to Selection)

The fitness is a trait of greatest significance in natural selection and it is taken as the capacity to survive and reproduce in the existing environment. The average fitness $(\overline{W})$ is the sum of the individual genotype fitness time its frequency and this is set equal to 1.0, Therefore,

$$\Sigma f_i w_i = \quad \overline{W} = 1.0 \qquad\qquad 8.1$$

The essence of the theory of evolution through selection is that there exists genetic variation in fitness among the individuals of a population and some contribute more number of offspring than others in the same environment. This results a change in the genetic make up of the next generation to that of the parent generation leading to substantial changes over generations. Thus evolution depends upon the existence of genetic variation in the population. The magnitude of change depends upon the magnitude of the genetic variation. The natural selection tends to increase the frequency of those genes which increases the fitness of the individuals carrying those genes. Consequently, the fitness is increased following selection till an adaptive peak is reached. The rate of change in fitness due to selection is related to the variability in fitness of the population. Fisher (1930) described that there is a relationship between the genetic variance in fitness and the increase in the average fitness of the population that occur in one generation. He called this relationship as the *"fundamental theorem of natural selection"*. This theorem states that the increase in average fitness in one generation of natural selection in a population with non overlapping generations equals the additive genetic variance in fitness divided by the average fitness. Thus Δ W = σ^2_A/W. Most accurately the fundamental theorem is that of Wright (1931): "the *rate of increase in fitness of a population at any time is equal to its genetic variance in fitness at that time.*"

Fisher's fundamental theorem of natural selection can be demonstrated from the frequencies (f) and relative fitness (W) of various genotypes (g) in two successive generations of a population as: '

First generation:

Genotypes	g_1	g_2	g_3 .... g_n
Frequencies	f_1	f_2	f_3...f_n
Fitness	w_1	w_2 w_3. ....w_n

Average fitness $\left(\overline{W}\right)$ = $1.0 = f_1 w_1^2 + f_2 w_2^2 + f_3 w_3^2 +. f_n w_n$

Second generation:

Genotypes	g_1	g_2	g_3.....g_n
Frequencies	$f_1 w_1$	$f_2 w_2$ $f_3 w_3$ .... $f_n w_n$
Fitness	w_1	w_2 w_3 +.... w_n

Average fitness $\left(\overline{W}\right)$ = $f_1 w_1^2 + f_2 w_2^2 + f_3 w_3^2 + ... f_n w_n$

The variance in fitness equals the average of squared deviation from the mean (mean of the squares) minus square of the mean. Therefore, the genetic variance in fitness (σ^2_W) is:

$$\sigma^2_W \quad = \Sigma f_i w_i^2 - \overline{W}^2$$
$$= \Sigma f_i w_i^2 - 1.0$$
$$= \Sigma f_i w_i^2$$

The initial frequency of each genotype is changed due to selection and the new frequency equals the product of the original frequency time its corresponding fitness ($f_i w_i$) whose sum equals $\overline{W}$ or 1.0.

The new average fitness (second generation) denoted as W_2 is calculated which equals to the sum of the new frequencies times the corresponding fitness as:

$$\overline{W}_2 = \Sigma(f_i W_i)(W_i) = \Sigma f_i W_i^2$$

Since the individuals with low viability and reproductive success will be relatively less numerous after selection than before, so the average fitness of the selected population $\overline{W}_2$ will be higher than that of the preceding generation $\overline{W}_1$. Therefore, the change or increase in the average fitness ($\Delta \overline{W}$) due to selection will be as:

$$\Delta \overline{W} \quad = \text{Av. fitness in second generation} - \text{Av. fitness of first generation}$$

$$= \overline{W}_2 - \overline{W}_1$$

$$= \Sigma f_i W_i^2 - \overline{W}$$

$$= \Sigma f_i\, W_i^2 - 1.0$$

$$= \Sigma f_i\, W_i^2 = \sigma^2_w$$

$$= \text{Genetic variance in fitness}$$

Therefore, the rate of increase in fitness (ΔW) of any organism at any, time is equal to its genetic variance in fitness (σ^2_w) at that time. Thus σ^2_w, is a measure of the rate of increase in fitness.

The effect of selection is the change of gene frequencies. The frequencies of the genes associated with fitness are increased and hence the change in gene frequencies results in an improvement of the average fitness. That is to say that the improvement or gain in average fitness of a population by selection is in fact due to the changes in gene frequencies. In view of this the effect of selection can be described by two different ways of estimating either $\Delta \overline{W}$ (change in fitness) or Δq (change in gene frequency).

The use of ($\Delta \overline{W}$) or Δq depends upon the nature of the problem. The effect of selection on polygenic traits is measured by ($\Delta \overline{W}$) while Δq is used as a measure of the effect of selection for qualitative traits.

Fitness as a Quantitative Trait

The increase in mean fitness in one generation (($\Delta \overline{W}$)) due to natural selection is the response (R_w) and therefore, Fisher's theorem can be taken as

$$R_w = \sigma^2_{A(w)} / \overline{W}$$

$$= \Delta W$$

where,   R is the increase in mean fitness (ΔW)'

   $\sigma^2_{A(w)}$ is the additive genetic variance in fitness,

   $\overline{W}$ is the average fitness of the parental generation which corresponds to μ.

and $R = h^2 S$ for a quantitative trait

where, h^2 is the heritability

   S is the selection differential

   R is the response

Therefore, $R = Rw$ and so $h^2 S = \dfrac{\sigma^2_{A(w)}}{\overline{W}}$

Now, $S = \left[\dfrac{\sigma^2_{A(w)}}{\overline{W}}\right]\left(\dfrac{1}{h^2}\right)$

$\quad\; = \left[\dfrac{\sigma^2_{A(w)}}{\overline{W}}\right]\left(\dfrac{\sigma^2_P}{\sigma^2_A}\right)$

$$= \frac{\sigma p^2}{\overline{W}}$$

where, σ^2_p is the total phenotypic variance in fitness.

Intensity of selection (i) is taken as:

$$i \quad = \frac{S}{\sigma_P} = \frac{\sigma^2_P}{\overline{W}\sigma_P} \qquad \text{Since} \quad S = \frac{\sigma^2_P}{\overline{W}}$$

$$= \frac{\sigma_P}{\overline{W}}$$

Thus, for fitness, the selection differential is a ratio of the phenotypic variance of the trait to the mean value of the trait while the intensity of selection is a ratio of the phenotypic standard deviation of the trait and the mean value of the trait. However, these calculations are based on the assumption that fitness is normally distributed

what is doubtful. Crow J.F. (1966; Bioscience 16, 863-867) called the quantity $i^2 = \dfrac{\sigma^2_P}{\overline{W}^2}$

as the *index of opportunity for selection.* This indicates that how much potential genetic selection is inherited in the pattern of birth and death.

Marginal Fitness of Genotypes

The marginal fitness of the alleles **A** and **a** equals to the average fitness of all the genotypes containing that allele (A or a) weighted by their relative frequency and the number of A or a alleles they contain. For example, allele A occurs in AA and Aa genotype with relative proportions p and q. Therefore, the marginal fitness $\left(\overline{W}_1\right)$ of genotype containing **A** allele equals:

$$\overline{W}_1 = p\, w_{11} + q\, w_{12.}$$

Similarly, marginal fitness of genotype containing **a** allele $\left(\overline{W}_2\right)$ is:

$$\overline{W}_2 = p\, w_{12} + q\, w_{22.}$$

The **s** is the selection coefficient against the aa genotype and **h** indicates the degree of dominance of allele **a.** The value of **h** may be either 0, or ½ or 1.

When h = 0, the fitness of AA, Aa, aa will be 1, 1, 1 – s, respectively and **a** is recessive.

When h =1, the fitness will be 1, 1 – s and 1 – s, respectively for the three genotypes and **a** is dominant to A or say that A is favoured recessive.

When h= ½, the fitness will be respectively as 1, 1 – ½ s, 1 – s, the allele A is favoured and the alleles are additive in effects on fitness.

8.4. Change of Gene Frequency by Selection

General Case

The effect of selection depends on the intensity of selection (selection coefficient) and initial frequency of allele. The change in gene frequency per generation (Δq) is taken as the difference in gene frequency between two generations. Thus, $\Delta q = q_t - q_{t-1}$.

Steps to Estimate the Effect of Selection: General Expression

When all the genotypes are equally fit, the population remains in HWE. Therefore, the effect of selection is described by the relative fitness of each genotype. The steps involved to determine the effect of selection on gene frequencies are as:

1. Initial gene frequencies, genotype frequencies (p_{ii}, p_{ij}) and relative fitness (W_{ij}) of different genotypes are determined.

2. Gamete contribution (frequencies) of genotypes after selection ($p_i p_j W_{ij}$):- These are obtained as the products of genotypic frequencies and corresponding fitness values as $p_i p_j W_{ij}$. These are the proportion of each genotype after selection. Therefore, the ratio of AA: Aa: aa among adults is $p^2 w_{11}: 2pq\ w_{12}: q^2 w_{22}$. The ratio of A: a between the gametes of the next generations is therefore, as under:

$$= p^2 w_{11} + \tfrac{1}{2}(2pq\ w_{12}): q^2 w_{22} + \tfrac{1}{2}(2pq\ w_{12})$$
$$= (p^2 w_{11} + p\ q\ w_{12}): q^2 w_{22} + p\ q\ w_{12}$$
$$= p\ (p\ w_{11} + q\ w_{12}): q\ (q\ w_{12} + p\ w_{12})$$

3. Average Fitness $(\overline{W})$: This is the total gamete contribution of the population of different genotypes after selection and is equal to the sum of the products of genotype frequencies with their fitness as

$$\overline{W} = \Sigma\, p_i p_j\, w_{ij} = p^2 W_{11} + 2pq\ w_{12} + q^2 w_{22}$$

4. New genotypic frequencies after selection: These are the relative genotypic frequencies obtained for each genotype as the fitness of each genotype multiplied by its frequency (gamete contribution after selection, $p_i p_j W_{ij}$) divided by the average fitness of the population ($\overline{W} = \Sigma\, p_i p_j w_{ij}$). Thus,

$$\text{new genotypic frequency} = \frac{p_i p_j w_{ij}}{\overline{W}}.$$

5. Gene frequency after selection (q_1): It is obtained by dividing the gamete ratio with average fitness as: $q_1 = \dfrac{(q^2 w_{22} + pq w_{12})}{\overline{W}}$

6. Change in gene frequency (Δq):

$$\Delta q = q_1 - q_0$$
$$= pq\,[p\,(w_{12} - w_{11}) + q\,(w_{22} - w_{12})]$$
$$\Delta p = 1 - \Delta q$$

8.5. Patterns of Selection and their Effect

There are three modes of selection depending on the choice of individuals to be selected on the basis of their phenotypes. These are directional selection, disruptive selection (Bidirectional selection) and stabilizing selection.

The **directional selection** is when the genotype selected against is either homozygous recessive or the genotype may contain dominant gene (homozygous dominant or heterozygote). Thus, the selection is in one direction. The **bidirectional selection** is when selection is against the heterozygote and in favour of both types of homozygotes. Thus, the selection is in both the directions. The **stabilizing selection** is when the selection is in favour of heterozygote and against both the homozygote.

8.5.1 Directional Selection

This is also called as *one way upward selection* or linear or dynamic selection in which the individuals with extreme phenotypic values (genetically superior) are selected.   This type of selection is of great importance to the animal breeder.

(i) Selection against the Recessive Genotype

The gene A is favoured dominant: This can be taken under two situations – first is when there is partial selection against recessive and second is when there is complete elimination of recessive individuals due to lethal gene when all the recessive homozygote die prior to breeding age and also due to artificial selection against unwanted recessive in a breeding programme.

(a) Partial Selection against Recessive (Recessive with low fitness)

The dominant are favoured because of their higher fertility or lower mortality or better performance. The A allele is favoured dominant and hence h = 0. As a consequence the recessives produce only $(1-s)$ offspring where s is the coefficient of selection. The effect on population can be obtained from the table given below.

1. | Genotypes | AA | Aa | aa |
   |---|---|---|---|
   | Initial frequencies | p^2 | $2pq$ | q^2 |
   | Relative fitness | (w_{11}) | (w_{12}) | (w_{22}) |
   | (Darwinian) | 1 | 1 | 1-s |

2. | Gamete contribution | $p^2 w_{11}$ | $2pq w_{12}$ | $q^2 w_{22}$ |
   |---|---|---|---|
   | after selection | $= p^2$ | $2pq$ | $q^2(1-s)$ |

3. Average Fitness $(\overline{W}) = p^2 + 2pq + q^2(1-s) = 1 - s\,q^2$

4. New genotypic frequencies $\dfrac{p^2}{1-sq^2} ; \dfrac{2pq}{1-sq^2} ; \dfrac{q^2(1-s)}{1-sq^2}$

   (Zygotes after selection) $= \dfrac{p_i p_j w_{ij}}{W}$

5. Gene frequency after selection (q_1 or p_1)

$$P_{1\,(A)} = \frac{p^2}{1-sq^2} + \frac{pq}{1-sq^2} = \frac{p}{1-sq^2}$$

$$q_1\,(a) = \frac{pq}{1-sq^2} + \frac{q^2(1-s)}{1-sq^2} = \frac{q-sq^2}{1-sq^2}$$

6. Change in gene frequency: $\Delta q = q_1 - q = \left[\frac{q-sq^2}{1-sq^2}\right] - q$

$$= \frac{-sq^2(1-q)}{1-sq^2}$$

$$= \frac{-spq^2}{1-sq^2}$$

The frequency of recessive allele decreases by the amount per generation equal

to $\frac{-spq^2}{1-sq^2}$. When the recessive allele is at low frequency the amount of change in its

frequency per generation (Δq) will be low and equal to $-sq^2$ but appreciable when the q is at intermediate. The change will also be low if q is higher than intermediate. Therefore, selection is most effective for common traits in a population but less effective for rare traits.

(b) Complete Elimination of Recessive Genotype (Lethal Recessive)

This would apply to natural selection against a recessive lethal. In this case the fitness (w) of recessive genotype is zero (w = 1- s = 1-1= 0). This is because the selection coefficient is equal to one (S = 1). The frequency of recessive allele in the progeny generation (q_1) under partial selection against recessive phenotype is obtained as under.

$$q_1 = \frac{[q-sq^2]}{[1-sq^2]}$$

Now taking, s = 1 (complete elimination of recessives)

$$q_1 = \frac{(q-q^2)}{(1-q^2)}$$

$$= \frac{q(1-q)}{[(1+q)(1-q)]}$$

$$= \frac{q}{(1+q)}$$

Likewise, $p_1 = \frac{p}{(1-q^2)} = \frac{1}{(1+q)}$

The change in gene frequency $(\Delta q) = q_1 - q$

$$= \left[\frac{q}{(1+q)} \right] - q$$

$$= \frac{-q^2}{(1+q)}$$

There is only the heterozygote which produces the gametes having *a* gene, when the aa individuals either die or are completely infertile. In each generation the aa progeny die or fail to reproduce and therefore there is a consequent decrease in the frequency of recessive allele. The gene frequency in t generation can be predicted taking S=1 as:

$$q_1 = \frac{q}{(1+q)} = \frac{q_0}{(1+q_0)}$$

$$q_2 = \frac{q_1}{(1+q_1)} = \frac{q_0}{(1+2q_0)}$$

Likewise, $q_t = \frac{q_0}{(1+t\,q_0)}$ where, t indicates the number of generations.

From the above expression of q_t, the number of generations (t) required to effect a specific change in frequency of recessive allele can be estimated as:

$$q_t = \frac{q_0}{(1+t\,q_0)}$$

$$t\,q_0 = \left(\frac{q_0}{q_1} \right) - 1$$

$$= \frac{(q_0 - q_t)}{q_t}$$

$$t = \frac{(q_0 - q_t)}{q_t q_0}$$

$$= \left(\frac{q_0}{q_t q_0} \right) - \left(\frac{q_t}{q_t q_0} \right)$$

$$= \frac{1}{q_t} - \frac{1}{q_0}$$

Thus, t depends on the initial gene frequency and its frequency after t generations. More generations are required to reduce the abnormality if the allele is rare. Thus, the effect of selection against recessive allele is very slow.

(ii) Selection against Recessive Gene, a

(a) No Dominance

The allele A is favoured and both the alleles are additive in their effect on fitness. The allele A will be fixed by this type of selection. When there is no dominance of fitness, the heterozygote is distinguishable and has it fitness (phenotypic value) exactly intermediate between the fitness (phenotypic values) of two homozygotes. It this case of additive effects, the $h = \frac{1}{2}$. This is partial selection against incomplete recessive.

1. Genotypes   AA   Aa   aa

	AA	Aa	aa
Initial frequencies	p^2	$2pq$	q^2
Relative fitness	1	$1 - \frac{1}{2}s$	$1 - s$
2. Gamete contribution	p^2	$2pq(1 - \frac{1}{2}s)$	$q^2(1 - s)$

3. Average Fitness, $\overline{W} = $ $1 - sq$

4. Genotypic proportion $\dfrac{p^2}{(1 - sq)} : \dfrac{2pq\left(1 - \dfrac{1}{2}s\right)}{(1 - sq)} : \dfrac{q^2(1 - s)}{(1 - sq)}$

5. Gene freq. after selection

$$P_{1\,(A)} = \frac{\left[p^2 + pq\left(1 - \frac{1}{2}s\right) \right]}{(1 - sq)}$$

$$= \frac{p - \frac{1}{2}spq}{(1 - sq)}$$

$$q_1(a) = \frac{p - \frac{1}{2}spq - sq^2}{(1 - sq)}$$

6. Change in gene frequency $(\Delta q) = q_1 - q$

$$= \left[\frac{q - \frac{1}{2}spq - sq}{(1 - sq)} \right] - q$$

$$= \frac{\frac{1}{2}spq}{(1-sq)}$$

(b) Incomplete Dominance in Fitness

This is the case when the selection is against the heterozygote and recessive but the relative fitness of heterozygote is greater than the average of the homozygotes and hence greater than the fitness of recessive homozygote. Thus $W_1 > w_2 > W_3$ and it is similar to the case of no dominance. Considering the AA genotype as the favourable genotype, the relative fitness for AA, Aa, aa genotypes will be 1, 1-hs, 1-s, respectively and the average fitness (W) = 1- sq²-2pq hs. The new gene frequency will be:

$$P_1 = \frac{p(1-qhs)}{(1-2pqhs-sq^2)}$$

$$q_1 = \frac{q(1-qhs-sq)}{(1-2pqhs-sq^2)}$$

The change in gene frequency will be:

$$\Delta q = q_1 - q = \frac{-spq[q+h(p-q)]}{(1-2pqhs-sq^2)}$$

$$= \frac{-spq[q+h(p-q)]}{(1-sq)[q+h(p-q)+h]}$$

In this case, the fitness of heterozygotes (w_2) is expressed as some proportion of the selection coefficient in w_3. The heterozygote selection coefficient is taken as *hs* which is expressed as a proportion of the recessive's selection coefficient (s). Thus *h* is the fraction of selection coefficient of recessive found in heterozygote. The h is the amount to which the heterozygotes are at selective disadvantage compared to that of the recessive selection coefficient.

For example, $w_1 = 1.0$, $W_2 = 0.85$, $W_3 = 0.70$.

Thus $w_3 = 1- s = 0.70$, hence s = 0.30 and

$w_2 = 1- hs = 0.85$, hence *hs* = 0.15 and so h = 0.5.

Therefore, the heterozygotes selective disadvantage is 50 per cent of the recessives. The *hs* = 0.15 is 50 per cent of the value of *s* = 0.30.

The rate of change in gene frequency can be now compared for completely 1- ½ 2s because of the average being ½ (1+ 1- s) = ½ (2 – s) = 1 – ½s. The new gene frequency and the amount of change in gene will be obtained as for recessive allele and for incomplete dominance in fitness (the present case). Taking q = 0.9, s = 0.3 and h = 0.2 the change in (Δ q) = – 0.0268 in the present case of incomplete dominance and Δ q = – 0.0321 in case of compite recessive. Thus the rate is slightly lower in the present case of incomplete dominance than in case of complete recessive.

The incompletely recessive gene when rare is eliminated more rapidly than for complete recessive gene. When q = 0.1, the Δ q = -0.071 for depressed heterozygote (incomplete recessive) compared with Δ q = -0.0027 for the complete recessive case.

When h = 0.5,   the heterozygote is exactly intermediate between two homozygotes in fitness and hs becomes equal to 1/2s. Thus,

$$\Delta q = - \frac{-\frac{1}{2}spq}{1-sq}$$

When h = 0, Δ q = $\frac{-spq^2}{1-sq^2}$ equal to non lethal recessive with low fitness.

This type of selection will fix the A gene. When the selection is against recessives the frequency of recessive become rare and the selection against recessive is less effective in later generation. Thus more number of generations will be required for a decrease as the frequency of a recessive gene reduces.

(iii) Selection against Dominant Phenotype

There may be complete dominance or co-dominance in fitness:

(a) Complete Dominance of Fitness

This has equal meaning that selection is in favour of recessive phenotype and against A gene. When the selection is against the dominant phenotype, the fitness is equal for AA as well as for Aa genotype which will be (1- s) and the fitness for aa genotype will be equal to 1.0. Consequently the frequency of recessive allele will be increased in each generation till it becomes fixed. The change is demonstrated as follows:

1. Genotypes | AA | Aa | aa
    Initial frequencies | p^2 | 2pq | q^2
    Relative fitness | 1-s | 1-s | 1
2. Gamete contribution | $p^2(1\text{- }s)$ | 2pq (1- s) | q^2
    after selection (final frequencies)

3. Average Fitness $= \overline{W} = 1\text{- }s(1\text{- }q^2)$

4. Genotypic proportion $\dfrac{p^2(1-s)}{1-s(1-q^2)} : \dfrac{2pq(1-s)}{1-s(1-q^2)} : \dfrac{q^2}{1-s(1-q^2)}$

5. Gene freq. after selection $\quad P_{1\ (A)} \quad = \dfrac{p^2(1-s)+pq(1-s)}{1-s(1-q^2)}$

$$= \frac{p(1-s)}{1-s(1-q^2)}$$

$$q_{1\,(a)} = \frac{q-spq}{1-s(1-q^2)}$$

6. Change in gene frequency $\Delta q = q_1 - q$

$$= \frac{q-sq+sq^2}{1-s(1-q^2)} - q$$

$$= \frac{spq^2}{1-s(1-q^2)}$$

When the dominant phenotypes will be completely eliminated, there is no source for dominant gene to be transmitted in the progeny. Therefore, after one generation of complete elimination of dominant phenotype the frequency of recessive allele will become one. *It is thus more effective.* If s is small, the change in gene frequency become nearly equal but in opposite direction in two cases when the selection is against the recessive phenotype. The ultimate fate of A allele is that it will lost.

(b) No Dominance of Fitness

In this case, the value of $\Delta q = \frac{1}{2} sq (1-q)$.

8.5.2 Bidirectional Selection: Selection against Heterozygote

This is also called as *two way selection* or diversifying or centrifugal or *disruptive selection.* The individuals having extreme phenotypes on both the sides are selected and thus, the heterozygote is at selective disadvantage. This selection favours two diverse types at a time and results in two populations with better and poor performance. This selection results in little change in the phenotypic values in the next generation. This type of selection does not change the gene frequency but change the genotypic frequencies, the heterozygous genotypes are reduced. Under some circumstance the fitness of heterozygote may be less than the homozygote. In a random mating population the effect of selection against heterozygote on the change of gene frequency can be estimated as:

1. Genotypes
	AA	Aa	aa
Initial frequencies	p^2	2pq	q^2
Relative fitness	1	1-s	1

2. Gamete contribution after Selection (Final frequencies)

	AA	Aa	aa
	p^2	2pq (1-s)	q^2

3. Average Fitness = $\overline{W}$ = 1- 2pqs

4. Genotypic proportion
$$\frac{p^2}{1-2pqs} : \frac{2pq(1-s)}{1-2pqs} : \frac{q^2}{1-2pqs}$$

5. Gene freq. after selection
$$P_{1(A)} = \frac{p^2 + pq(1-s)}{1-2pqs} = \frac{p-pqs}{1-2pqs}$$

$$q_{1(a)} = \frac{q^2 + pq(1-s)}{1-2pqs} = \frac{q-pqs}{1-2pqs}$$

6. Change in gene freq. Δq
$$= q_1 - q$$
$$= \frac{pqs(q-p)}{1-2pqs}$$

The interesting point of this type of selection is that when $q = \frac{1}{2}$ the proportion of the two homozygote are equal ($p^2 = q^2 = \frac{1}{4}$) in a random mating population. Consequently there will be no change in gene frequency either the heterozygote is eliminated completely or partially and the population will be in its original genotypic frequencies in the next generation on random mating. Secondly if p# q but p>q the heterozygote will have higher proportion of the rare alleles than in the recessive homozygote. Thus selection against heterozygote will affect more to the rare alleles than the common allele and consequently the frequency of rare allele will be further decreased.

The *well known example of selection against the heterozygote* is the *Rh factor in men.* The heterozygous baby (Rh rh) from Rh negative women (*rh rh*) will have a hemolytic disease known as *"Erylhroblastosis fatalis"* which may cause death of the child. Such a case will only happen if such heterozygous baby is born to a recessive mother (rh rh, said to be rh-negative). Thus, in this case the selection is against the heterozygote born to recessive mothers rather than born to heterozygous or Rh positive mothers which will bore **normal children.**

8.5.3 Stabilizing Selection: Selection Favours the Heterozygote (Over Dominance) and Disfavours both the Homozygote

This is also called as *balanced selection* or centripetal or unifying selection. This is the case of over-dominance (heterosis). This selection is based on the superiority of heterozygote over both the homozygote. This selection does not change the mean of progeny generation and to some extent reduces the variance. This selection preserves both the alleles, so it is called as *balanced polymorphism or balanced lethal* when both the homozygotes are lethal and the only surviving genotype is the heterozygote.

The change in gene frequency due to this selection will be:

1. Genotypes	AA	Aa	aa
Initial frequencies	p^2	$2pq$	q^2
Relative fitness	$1-s_1$	1	$1-s_2$

2. Gamete contribution $\quad p^2(1-s_1) \qquad 2pq \qquad q^2(1-s_2)$
   after selection (final frequencies)

3. Average Fitness $= \overline{W} = 1 - s_1 p^2 - s_2 q^2$

4. Genotypic proportion $\dfrac{p^2(1-s_1)}{[1-s_1 p^2 - s_2 q^2]} : \dfrac{2pq}{[1-s_1 p^2 - s_2 q^2]} : \dfrac{q^2(1-s_2)}{[1-s_1 p^2 - s_2 q^2]}$

5. Gene freq. after selection $\qquad P_{1\ (A)} = \dfrac{p^2(1-s_1)+pq}{1-s_1 p^2 - s_2 q^2}$

$$= \dfrac{p-s_1 p^2}{1-s_1 p^2 - s_2 q^2}$$

$$q_{1\ (a)} = \dfrac{pq+q^2(1-s_2)}{1-s_1 p^2 - s_2 q^2}$$

$$= \dfrac{q-s_2 q^2}{1-s_1 p^2 - s_2 q^2}$$

6. Change in gene frequency $\qquad \Delta q = q_1 - q$

$$= \dfrac{pq(s_1 p - s_2 p)}{1-s_1 p^2 - s_2 q^2}$$

Equilibrium under Selection

The consequence of selection favouring heterozygotes leads to an increase in the frequency of heterozygote and a consequent decrease in frequency of both homozygotes than their initial frequencies. The gene frequencies will eventually reach a stable equilibrium value instead of being lost or increased to unity as a limit. The increase or decrease in gene frequency depends on the proportion of $s_1 p$ and $s_2 q$. When $s_1 p = s_2 q$, then there will be no change in gene frequency and an equilibrium state will reach and thus q = 0. This will happen when $s_1 p = s_2 q$ or $p\ (w_{11} - w_{12}) = q$ $(w_{12}-w_{22})$. Therefore, the gene frequency at equilibrium will be as under:

$s_1 p = s_2 q$, $\quad \dfrac{p}{q} = \dfrac{s_2}{s_1}$, $\quad \dfrac{(1-q)}{q} = \dfrac{s_2}{s_1}$

$s_1 - s_1 q = s_2 q \qquad\qquad$ and hence

$s_1 \qquad = s_2 q + s_1 q$

$\qquad\quad = q\ (s_1 + s_2)$

$\hat{q} \qquad = s_1 / (s_1 + s_2) \qquad\qquad$ and

$\hat{p} \qquad = s_2 / (s_1 + s_2)$

Therefore, the values of p and q at equilibrium are independent of their initial values in the population but entirely determined by the intensity of selection (selection coefficient) of two homozygotes. Thus, it is not only the degree of superiority which decides the gene frequencies at equilibrium but it is the relative disadvantage of one homozygote (1- s_1) compared with that of others (1- s_2). The gene frequencies at equilibrium are such that the average fitness of the population is maximum provided the fitness of genotypes are constant. When q is below its equilibrium point, it will increase in each generation and when q is greater it will decrease till equilibrium is attained. This is because when q is below its equilibrium point s2q will be less than s1p and therefore, Δ q will be positive.

When the heterozygote is superior irrespective of its degree, the gene frequencies at equilibrium are at more or less intermediate gene frequencies. The intermediate gene frequencies are expected when selection favours the heterozygote. This is one of the possible reasons for the existence of polymorphism.

The effect of birth weight on infant mortality is an example of stabilizing selection, because the new born having their extreme birth weight to either side are likely to die. The best example of *superiority of heterozygote is the sickle cell anemia.* The homozygote suffers from anemia characterized by sickle shape of erythrocyte. This disease is fatal. The hemoglobin of homozygote is of the abnormal types. On the other hand, the heterozygote does not suffer from anemia. The gene causing sickle cell is recessive for anaemia, partially dominant for haemoglobin synthesis and overdominance for fitness. The selective advantage of heterozygote has been shown to be associated with their resistance to malaria. The sickle cell homozygote ($Hb^S Hb^S$) is anemic severely having sickle of RBC but resistant to malaria while the normal homozygote ($Hb^+ Hb^+$) is not anemic have normal hemoglobin but susceptible to malaria and the heterozygote is mild anemic but resistant to malaria for which the heterozygote has advantage over both homozygotes. There is high frequency of sickle cell in the area of high incidence of malaria.

8.5.4 Other Condition of Selection

(1) Unequal Selection Intensities in Two Sexes

This is the most prevalent situation in farm animals that the selection intensities for males and females are different. Taking the selection coefficients for males and females recessive as S_1, and S_2, respectively, the proportion of recessive in the whole population in the next generation will not be equal to q^2 but it will be lower than q^2 and equal to q $[1- \frac{1}{2} (S_1 + S_2)]$.

This assumes that males and females are equal in number in a random mating population. The change in gene frequency will be of the same magnitude as if the S = $\frac{1}{2} (S_1 + S_2)$ for the recessive genotype of both sexes equally.

(2) Selection for Sex Linked Genes

The selection for sex linked genes is more effective against the sex linked recessive in both the sexes compared to the selection against the autosomal genes, for equal fitness. The selection for sex linked genes is equivalent to gamete selection in males because of their XY genetic constitution and is equivalent to zygotic selection in females because of their XX genetic constitution. The effect of selection against the recessive lethal allele has been described here.

Sex	Male		Female		
Genotype	A	a	AA	Aa	aa
Frequency	p	q	p^2	2pq	q^2
Relative fitness	1	0	1	1	0

Gene Frequency

1. Initial : p q p and q
2. After selection among survivors:

    Males   p (A) $= p$

                    q(a) $= 0$

    Females   p (A) $= \dfrac{\left(p^2 + pq\right)}{p^2 + 2pq} = \dfrac{1}{\left(1+q\right)}$

                     q (a) $= \dfrac{pq}{\left(p^2 + 2pq\right)} = \dfrac{q}{\left(1+q\right)}$

3. In next generation:

    Males   p (a) $= p'f$

                    q (a) $= q'f$

                         $= \dfrac{q}{1+q}$ because $P_m = p'_f$

    Females   p (A) $= \tfrac{1}{2}\,(P'_m + P'_f)$

                     q (a) $= \tfrac{1}{2}\,(q'_m + q'_f)$

                         $= \tfrac{1}{2}\,\dfrac{q}{1+q}$

    Overall (q) $= \dfrac{2}{3}q_f + \dfrac{1}{3}q_m$

    = Overall gene frequency (q) among survivors of both sexes.

               (Δq) $= q_{1} - q = \dfrac{2q}{3(1+q) - q}$

                         $= \dfrac{-q(1 + 3q)}{3(1+q)}$

(3) Gamete Selection: Haploid Selection

It is not essential that selection acts in the zygotic stage but it may act in the gamete stage also. It happens when one gamete has selective advantage over others in fertilization. The effect of gamete selection against recessive gamete may be obtained as:

1. Gametes   A   a

     Initial frequency   p   q

     Relative fitness   1   1-s

2. Gamete contribution after selection   p   q-sq

3. Average Fitness $= \overline{W} = 1 - sq$

4. Gene frequency after selection:

$$P_{1(A)} = \frac{p}{1-sq}$$

$$q_{1(a)} = \frac{q-sq}{1-sq}$$

$$= \frac{q(1-s)}{1-sq}$$

5. Change in gene frequency:

$$\Delta q = q_1 - q$$

$$= \frac{q-sq}{1-sq} - q$$

$$= \frac{-spq}{1-sq}$$

$$\Delta p = 1 - \Delta q$$

$$= \frac{spq}{1-sq}$$

The change in gene frequency in this case (selection against the gametes) is similar to the selection against zygotes with no dominance (selection against intermediate heterozygote and recessive homozygotes, selection against *a* gene). In other words, the rate of change in q under selection against intermediate heterozygote (no dominance) is similar to the rate of change under selection against recessive gamete for a haploid population. Thus, the recessive allele has a complete effect on fitness which means that it is additive in fitness.

8.6 Joint Effect of Selection and Migration

Every species is having a number of subpopulations isolated from each other. But due to one or the other reason there is an exchange of individuals (migration) among the isolated subpopulations. The subpopulations differ in their gene frequencies. Therefore, the migrants that join the local population have different frequency for one or more allele from the local population, and they will be naturally less adapted to local conditions (flew environment). Thus there will be some selection among the migrants, and local environment will favour only some genotypes. There is possibility of equilibrium between local selective forces and migrants.

Continued intergroup migration leads to the gene frequencies of the subgroups alike and make the total population homogeneous. Suppose **q** is the frequency of gene a in a particular group, **q** in the whole population and in the migrants also, and **m** is a fraction of population which is replaced by migrants each generation. This migration will lead to a change in gene frequency in the i th sub-population in each generation as:

$$\Delta q = -m(q - \bar{q})$$

The effect of selection (taking heterozygotes with intermediate fitness between the two homozygous types ($W_1 = 1, W_2 = 1 - s$ and $W_3 = 1 - 2s$) on gene frequency is:

$$\Delta q = \frac{-spq}{1 - 2sq} = -spq \text{ for small value of s.}$$

Now, the joint effect of migration and selection on change of gene frequency in one generation will be:

$$\Delta q \quad = \text{Change due to selection} + \text{change due to migration}$$

$$= -spq - m(q - \bar{q})$$

$$= -sq(1 - q) - m(q - \bar{q})$$

$$= -sq^2 - (m + s)q + m\bar{q}$$

At equilibrium $\Delta q = 0$. The equilibrium value of q for a group receiving m immigrants from outside in each generation with some selection (s) will be:

$$q = \frac{m + s \pm \sqrt{(m + s)^2 - 4ms\bar{q}}}{2s}$$

The relative magnitude of m and s affect the equilibrium value of a group. When selection is against recessive gene the value of s is positive whereas selection in favour of recessive gene gives the s value negative because $W_1 = 1, W_2 = 1 - s$ and $W_3 = 1 - 2s$. The value of q depends upon whether the recessive gene is deleterious or favourable to the individual carrying the gene. Depending upon the relative magnitude of m and s the value of q can be obtained as:

When m = s,   m + s = 2 s if the gene is deleterious and

m + s = 0 if the gene is favourable.

Now substituting the value of m + s = 2s or 0 in the above expression of $\hat{q}$, the q will be as: $\qquad q = \sqrt{\bar{q}}$ $\qquad\qquad$ if s is negative (favourable gene)

$$= 1 - \sqrt{(1 - \bar{q})} \text{ if s is positive (unfavourable gene)}$$

Therefore, the equilibrium value of $(\hat{q})$ will depend on selection in favour or against the gene. The $\hat{q}$ local equilibrium values of the groups will differ from each other considerably.

When m < s (s is greater than m), the direction of selection will decide the gene frequencies in local groups. The equilibrium value of q, can be obtained by putting the value of m and s in the above expression of q. However, the q value for s being much larger than m, will be

$$\hat{q} = 1 - \left(\frac{m}{s}\right)(1 - \bar{q}) \qquad \text{for favourable gene}$$

$$= (m/s)\, q \qquad \text{for unfavourable gene}$$

The equilibrium value of $\hat{q}$ will be higher for beneficial gene but lower for deleterious gene. The q value for favourable and unfavourable gene will differ more in this case than when m = s. As a result, there will be more local differentiation depending upon the amount of selection (local conditions of selection). The role of migration is to prevent fixation or loss of alleles like that of mutation.

When m is larger than s (m > s), the migration will counter balance the effect of selection and hence will reduce the tendency of selective differentiation. Therefore, the deviation in equilibrium values among local groups will not be much from the average gene frequency of the whole population $(\bar{q})$. The equilibrium values of $\hat{q}$ for favourable or unfavourable genes can be obtained by substituting the values of m, s and q in the gene expression of q given above or from the following expression of q:

$$q = \bar{q} \pm \left(\frac{s}{m}\right) \bar{q}\,(1 - \bar{q})$$

obtained by dividing the equation of $\Delta q = 0$ with m as:

$$\Delta q = \frac{-sq(1 - q) - m(q - \bar{q})}{m} = 0$$

$$= -\left(\frac{s}{m}\right)q(1 - q) - q + \bar{q} = 0$$

Thus, for favourable or unfavourable genes q = $\bar{q} \pm (s/m)\, \bar{q}\,(1 - \bar{q})$ because q would be close to $\bar{q}$. The relatively larger value of m than s will bring to the local populations more close to the average value of $\bar{q}$ in the whole population.

8.7. Joint Effect of Selection and Mutation

In almost all the populations the mutation and selection operate simulta-neously and therefore it is necessary to study their effects jointly. The deleterious genes are eliminated through selection and results a decrease in their frequency. However, the deleterious alleles persist in natural populations. This is because new deleterious alleles arise through mutation. The effect of selection and mutation are in different ways. The mutation has its greater effect in increasing the frequency of a rare mutant gene because of higher chances of mutation of the unmutated genes. On the other hand, the selection is less effective when the frequency of a gene is rare.

(1) Selection against Recessive Allele

It was observed that the change in gene frequency of recessive allele in one generation under the condition of partial selection against recessive individual is:

$$\Delta q = \frac{-sq^2(1-q)}{1-sq}$$

This becomes as $\Delta q = -sq^2(1-q)$ for s being small because the denominator for small value of s will be one. The gain or increase in frequency of recessive allele (a) due to mutation of A allele to *a* allele with mutation rate u per generation is *up* or *u (1-q)*. Thus A (p) $\longrightarrow$ (q) = u (1- q)

The selection decreases the value of q while mutation increases. The gain due to mutation is *up = u (1- q)* where as the loss due to selection is spq^2 = sq^2 (1- q). The net change in q per generation in a random mating population will be:

q   = gain – loss

q   = u (1– q) – Sq^2(1– q)

At equilibrium the gain through mutation will be equal to the loss through selection making $\Delta q = 0$.

Thus loss through selection = gain through mutation

Sq^2 (1- q) = u(1-q)

Sq^2 = u

$$q^2 = \frac{u}{S}$$

$$q = \sqrt{\frac{u}{S}}$$

This equilibrium state is stable but it is approached slowly. Therefore, the forward mutation rate from dominant to recessive (u) and selection coefficient (s) against the recessive gene decide the equilibrium frequency (q) of a mutant gene in a population. With the increase in mutation rate the frequency of recessive allele will increase but with increase in selection coefficient (reduced fitness) its frequency will decrease.

When S = 1 (lethal) for aa genotype' the equilibrium frequency becomes:

u $\quad = Sq^2$

$\quad\quad = q^2$

q $\quad = \sqrt{u}$

It can therefore be concluded that the frequency of homozygous recessive lethal at equilibrium (q^2) will be about equal to the mutation rate (frequency of new genes produced by mutation) and hence $q^2 = u$.

(2) Selection against Homozygous Dominant

This type of selection decreases the frequency of dominant (A) whereas the mutation of recessive allele (a) to dominant allele (A) increases the frequency of dominant allele (A). Thus stable equilibrium may be established by mutation of recessive allele to dominant allele. The equilibrium frequency of dominant allele (p) can be obtained from situation (i) by replacing q with p and u by v. Therefore,

$$p \quad = \sqrt{\frac{v}{S}} = \sqrt{v} \quad\quad when\ S = 1$$

A familiar example of selection against dominant gene is human brachydactyly (short finger). All the individuals with this defect are heterozygous whereas the dominant homozygous condition is lethal (S = 1).

Therefore, p = $\sqrt{v}$ approximately which is a very small quantity and hence q is nearly unity. Thus 1- p = q = 1. In this case, the frequency of dominants in the population (p^2) is equal to the mutation rate ($p^2 = v$.)

(3) Selection Against 'a' Gene when No Dominance: Partial Dominance or Incomplete Recessive

When dominance is lacking (no dominance, h =½) the reduction in gene frequency per generation is ½ spq/(1- sq) = ½ spq for small values of q; and the mutation frequency to the deleterious allele is u p. Therefore, the selection – mutation equilibrium is:

Loss through selection = Gain through mutation

½ spq $\quad = u\,p$

q $\quad\quad = \dfrac{2\,u\,p}{sp}$

$\quad\quad\quad = \dfrac{2\,u}{s}$

$\quad\quad\quad = \dfrac{u}{h\,s} \quad\quad$ where, h = 0.5

Thus, the equilibrium frequency of a deleterious recessive gene in the absence of dominance is about twice that for a deleterious dominant (p = u/s).

The equilibrium frequency mentioned above can be used to estimate the mutation rate as: u = ps = mutation rate for dominant gene, provided p and S are known. This can be obtained from the population data based on the genotypic (phenotypic) frequencies and their fitness values.

The above expressions of the equilibrium gene frequency under the joint effects of selection and mutation indicated that the equilibrium gene frequency depends on the mutation rate, coefficient of selection (deleterious effect on fitness, s) and degree of dominance. Now it is important aspect to analyze the consequences of increase in mutation rate and a change in selection intensity.

Social importance of increase in mutation rate and change of selection intensity:

The increase in mutation rate will have very small effect immediately on the change of gene frequency. The change in gene frequency in one generation will be:

Δq = Gain from mutation – Change in gene frequency due to selection

(increases rate)   (with complete dominance)

$= u_1 p$ $- Sq^2 (1- q)$

$= u_1 (1- q)$ $- Sq^2 (1-q)$

$= u_1$ $- Sq^2$ (Taking $1 - q$ as unity)

$= u_1$ $- u_0$ (Since $Sq^2 = u_0$ = initial mutation rate)

The increase in mutation rate will increase the gene frequency equal to the rate of increase in mutation rate at equilibrium.

The gene frequency will increase toward a new point of equilibrium at which Sq^2 (the proportion of genetic death) will be equal to the new mutation rate (u_1).

Therefore, if the mutation rate is doubled at equilibrium, the change (increase) in gene frequency will be very low (equal to the rate of increase in mutation) and it will also double the frequency of genetic deaths at new equilibrium. For example, if the mutation rate is 10^{-6} and if it was doubled, the change in gene frequency will be:

$\Delta q = u_1 - u_0 = 2 \times 10^{-6} - 10^{-6} = 10^{-6}$

The reverse mutation is not important because of its low rate as the mutant gene is rare and hence there are few chances for the reverse mutation. The genetic death of abnormal individuals will decrease the frequency of the defects in the population.

Therefore, it is advocated to intensify the artificial selection to cull the individuals with genetic defects in order to reduce the frequency of genetic defects in the population.

But it was mentioned that the effect of selection against a recessive gene causing genetic defect, is very slow. This is because artificial selection is already working against the genetic defects and artificial selection can be maximized to the maximum of S = 1 which will he about double of the present value of S. Therefore, the present frequency of the defects can not be reduced to more than half of their present incidence.

Haldane (1939) studied the spread of harmful autosomal recessive genes in human populations and pointed out that deleterious recessives are not at their equilibrium but are at low frequencies. This is because the frequency of homozygous individuals has been reduced due to modern civilization which has reduced the rate of inbreeding in human.

It is also important here to point out that the intensity of natural selection has been reduced at present and there is relaxation selection against the minor genetic defects due to the development of medical treatment, causing an increase in the lives of susceptible people. Consequently, there will be an increase in the frequency of genes, causing the disease, towards new equilibrium at higher values. Thus it is expected that the incidence of genetic defects which are minor of course will he increased in future and therefore, efforts will have to be made for providing medical treatment at a large scale for correcting genetic defects.

X-linked Genes

A single recessive gene in hemizygous organism (male in case of man, farm animals, Drosophila) is expressed in males and hence exposed to the full effect of selection. Thus the superiority of heterozygotes has only a slight effect on the frequency of sex linked recessive. As one third of the X chromosomes are present in males, the rate of elimination of mutant alleles in one generation is about $S/3$ if the fitness for mutant allele is 1-S compared to normal males and if the heterozygous females are not impaired greatly. At equilibrium, being balanced by mutation, the frequency of recessive allele (q) will be about $3u/S$. Thus $q = 3u/S$ and hence $u = 1/3\, qS$. According to the expectation the frequency will be higher than for autosomal dominant but much less than for complete recessives. This can be used to estimate the mutation rate. For example, the incidence of hemophilia is about 1 in 25000 births with their survival value as 0.25. (S = 0.75). Thus $u = 1/3\, qS = 1/3\ (0.00004)\ (0.75) = 0.00004 = 1$ in 25000.

Non Random Mating–Balance with Inbreeding

In highly inbred population (F = 1) there will be no heterozygote and the value of h will be irrelevant. Therefore, $P_{11} = p$, $P_{12} = 0$, and $P_{22} = q$.

The q_1 after selection will be:

$$q_1 = \frac{q - sq}{1 - sq}$$

and the amount of change will be:

$$\Delta q = q_1 - q$$

$$= \frac{q - sq}{1 - sq} - q$$

$$= -sq(1-q)$$

This amount of change due to selection will be balanced by an equal amount by new mutation from A to **a** at equilibrium. The change due to mutation is up = u (1- q).

Therefore, $\hat{q}$ = u (1- q) – [- Sq (1- q)]

or,   u(1- q) = Sq(1- q)

and $q = \dfrac{u}{S}$

8.8 Genetic Polymorphism

The different forms of many genes, if not of all, exist in a population with their intermediate frequencies (0.01 to 0.9) and they are responsible to produce different forms of the same species. The blood group genes and the genes responsible for colour varieties of many species like insects, fishes and snails etc. may be cited as examples of different forms. The existence of individuals in a population with visible differences caused by genes at intermediate frequencies is called polymorphism.

8.8.1 Definition of Polymorphism

Ford (1940) defined polymorphism as the occurrence together in the same locality of two or more discontinuous forms of a species in such proportion that rarest of them can not be maintained by recurrent mutation. The term polymorphism is extended to cover all differences whether they are easily visible or not as well as to describe the gene loci having different alleles at intermediate frequencies. A gene is said to be polymorphic if its most common allele has a frequency of less than 0.95 and a gene which is not polymorphic is said to be monomorphic. The differences have been detected by electrophoresis and other methods for the amino acid composition of proteins and this has shown that many gene loci (at least one third of loci or more) are polymorphic that code for different proteins. Thus many loci had allelic differences leading to genetic variation among normal individuals of a population.

8.8.2 Factors Responsible for Polymorphism

The different evolutionary forces play their role in saving an allele from its extinction. The widespread existence of polymorphic variation is explained in two ways. The first is the influence of *selective forces* which bring the balanced polymorphism. The deleterious genes are present in the population, though with low frequency, under mutation- selection balance and they cause the appearance of rare abnormal or mutant individuals in the population. The second way is that the mutant alleles survive by random changes of gene frequency in populations of small size. Thus, mutation and chance event in small population may cause polymorphism. However, the genes causing the appearance of rare abnormal individuals form a minor part of the genetic variation. The genetic polymorphism is caused and maintained by a number of factors given below.

1. Superiority of Heterozygotes

The selection in favour of heterozygotes (the heterozygotes being at selective advantage) the population eventually approaches stable equilibrium at intermediate gene frequency and hence both alleles remain in the population. This is known as balanced polymorphism. However, the heterozygote superiority is not a general cause of polymorphism because there are relatively few cases of superior fitness of heterozygotes.

The most striking example is the sickle cell anaemia. The heterozygotes do not suffer from anaemia while homozygotes suffer having abnormal type of haemoglobin (sickle shape RBC).

2. Frequency Dependent Selection

Many phenotypes are favoured when they are rare. Thus, the rare phenotype is at selective advantage and hence the direction of selection depends on the gene frequency producing the rare phenotype. It occurs when the fitness of a genotype depends on its frequency and on the type of other genotypes present. The allele at low frequency produces the rare phenotype and is favoured but when the same allele attains high frequency it is selected against. This process of selection in favour and against its frequency leads to a stable equilibrium gene frequency and hence a balanced polymorphism is attained. There are a number of examples of frequency dependent selection *e.g.* self sterility alleles and *apostatic* selection by wild birds. There are better chances of fertilization of an ovule with pollen grains having a rare self sterility allele due to the reason that the allele is rarely present in the stigma of other plants. Likewise, the prey with rare colouration escaped from predation.

3. Multiple Niche Polymorphism

There is *heterogeneity of environment* due to change in environment over space and time. The adaptation is environment specific. This means that different individuals adapt to different environments. One allele has selective advantage in one environment and another in a different environment. This leads to stable polymorphism at the locus. This type of polymorphism occurs when the weighted fitness of both the homozygotes in different environments is lower than that of the heterozygotes. The selection in heterogeneous environment results in a gradient of gene frequency between two localities which are maintained by selection favouring one allele in one locality and another allele in another locality. The polymorphism is maintained by the process of migration between neighbouring localities and the selection in opposite directions in two environments (localities).

4. Transient Polymorphism

There are environmental changes over time and the new alleles may enter in the population either through mutation or migration over time. The different alleles have selective advantage to different environments. There may be replacement of one allele by the other due to change in environment. It takes many generations for a gene substitution to take place. A population may thus be polymorphic during the process of gene substitution (evolution). The polymorphic genes observed at present may be in a transitional stage of the evolutionary process of gene substitution. The transitional polymorphism may persist for a long time because many generations are required for gene substitution. Therefore, it is not easy to distinguish between stable and transient polymorphism. The transient polymorphism is a very small portion of polymorphism.

5. Meiotic Drive or Gamete Selection

One allele in a series of alleles is favoured either due to meiotic drive or due to gamete selection (selection in the gamete stage) and this leads to a segregation bias. This eventually leads to a stable polymorphism when the favoured allele is deleterious in the zygotic selection and hence there is a conflict between gamete and zygotic selection. The tailless t allele in mice and segregation distorter factor (SDF) in Drosophila in homozygous condition are maintained in the population despite the selective disadvantage of these alleles.

6. Neutral Polymorphism

The neutral mutation polymorphism theory was proposed by Kimura (1983). Neutral mutation is widely recognized as a major cause of polymorphism. According to this theory the mutated genes, nearly neutral for fitness, represent some of the polymorphism. The mutated genes with a small selective advantage or disadvantage are neutral in the population and total neutrality is not required by the theory. The neutral polymorphism thus occurs when a series of alleles have nearly equal fitness and the frequencies of different types are determined largely by their mutation rate. The mutation and chance survival give rise to polymorphism taking into account the population size. Most of the mutants are lost but a few survive and replace the original allele. The mutants that survive take a very long time to spread through population and during this period they rise to polymorphism.

8.8.3 Uses of Genetic Polymorphism

1. Mating System being Followed

The study of genotypic frequencies for polymorphic loci helps to know the type of mating system being followed in the population in the past for the loci of interest. A population under random mating has certain pattern of genotype frequencies. The amount of self fertilization in monocious plants and in hermaphroditic animals and the inbreed-ing in plants as well as in animals can be estimated from the genotype frequencies. This is because the different mating systems have their different effects on the relative frequencies of the phenotypes that are formed from the alleles of a polymorphic gene.

2. Genetic Relationship among Sub populations

The sub populations share the alleles due to migration. The similarity in allelic frequencies can be used to estimate the rate of migration. The common ancestry also leads to share the alleles. The anthropological and genetic studies conducted by Watanable et.al. (1975) on the Japanese have indicated that the Ainu people of northern Japan have their facial features, hairy bodies and light skin similar to that of Caucasoids but even they are more closely related to other Mongoloid groups as evidenced by genetic polymorphism they have the D allele of (transferrin) protein and Di allele of the Dieog blood group which are both restricted to Mongoloid populations but they do not have several polymorphic alleles present in Caucasoids.

3. Ancestral History of a Group of Organisms

The ancestral history can be inferred from the existing genetic polymorphism in a species. The extreme genetic uniformity present in any species indicates that the species underwent severe reduction in population number at sometime in the past. On the other hand, the widespread genetic variability in E.coli than in Eukaryotes has disproved the prejudice that species of haploid asexual organisms must be genetically uniform.

4. Genetic Markers for Diagnosis of Disease

The genetic polymorphism is useful as genetic marker which may be linked in chromosomes with harmful genes causing the disease. This helps to determine that which members of the kinship are carriers and hence it helps in early diagnosis of individuals which are likely to be suffered. The RFLPs linked to disease genes may be used as probes to identify the recombinant DNA having defective genes which may unable to pin point the function of the defective genes and hence to help in effective treatment.

5. Evolutionary Significance of Polymorphism

The genetic polymorphism ensures the existence of genetic variability in the population. The essential requirement for evolution is the genetic variability. A population with genetic plasticity is better adapted to its immediate environment and may have genotypic recombination so as to produce new and better fitting types and perpetuate them in changing environment. Thus a genetically plastic population may mold itself according to the environment. This leads to an adaptive shift in the phenotype and as a result new species/types may arise. The new genotype either through mutation or gene combination may be produced which is better adapted phenotypically. Therefore, the production of more fit genotypes is required for continuous evolution.

Solved Examples and Exercises

Example 8.1

The *cy* allele producing curly wings in D. melanogester is lethal with fitness (w_{12}) as 0.5 relative to a value of $w_{22} = 1.0$ for ++ genotype. Estimate (i) the frequency of cy allele (p) after one generation, (ii) the change in gene frequency (Δp).

Solution

Genotypes:	cy cy	cy+	++
Frequency:	0	0.67	0.33
Fitness:	0	0.5	1.0

Frequency of cy allele $(p_0) = \frac{1}{2} (0.67) = 0.335$

Therefore, $q_0 = 1 - p_0 = 0.665$

$W = p^2 w_{11} + 2pq w_{12} + q^2 w_{22}$

$= (0.335)^2 (0) + 2(0.335) (0.665) (0.5) + (0.665)^2 (1.0)$

$= 0 + 0.223 + 0.442 = 0.665$

(i) Gene freq. after one generation $(p_1) = \dfrac{\left[p_0\left(p_0 w_{11} + q_0 w_{12}\right)\right]}{W}$

$$= \dfrac{\{0.335\left[(0.335)(0) + (0.665)(0.5)\right]\}}{0.665}$$

$$= \dfrac{\left[0.335(0 + 0.3325)\right]}{0.665} = \dfrac{0.1114}{0.665} = 0.167$$

(ii) Change in gene freq. $(\Delta p) = p_1 - p_0 = 0.167 - 0.335 = -0.168$

Example 8.2

The gene frequency of recessive allele in a population was 0.3. This population was under selection with selection coefficient against homozygous recessive (aa) as 0.4. Estimate the change in gene frequency per generation of selection.

Solution

Change in gene frequency $(\Delta q) = \dfrac{-spq^2}{1-sq^2}$

Here, $\quad q = 0.3$, hence $p = 0.7$, and $s = 0.4$

$$\Delta q = \dfrac{-spq^2}{1-sq^2}$$

$$= \dfrac{\left[-0.04 \times 0.7 \times 0.09\right]}{1 - 0.4 \times 0.09}$$

$$= \dfrac{-0.0252}{1 - 0.036} = \dfrac{-0.0252}{0.964} = -0.0262$$

Therefore, the change in q per generation will be equal to -0.0262.

Exercises

8.3. If the frequency of recessive gene in a population was 0.2, compute its frequency after 5 generation of selection against homozygous recessive.

8.4. In a cattle farm of 500 animals, the frequency of red gene is 0.6, what will be the frequency of red and white genes after the death of 60 white and 40 roan animals due to sudden outbreak of a contagious disease?.

8.5. In every 1000 calves born in a large cattle herd, 10 suffer from muscular hypertrophy and if they are totally eliminated from breeding, what will be the frequency of the gene concerned with this ailment in the fifth generation taking the generation in which selection is given effect as generation zero.

8.6. The frequency of white animals in a Shorthorn cattle population is 4 per cent. What will be its frequency after two generations of complete selection against white animals?

Chapter 9
Change of Gene Frequency: Dispersive Process (Small Population)

In large population, the gene frequencies remain constant from generation to generation, excluding the effects of migration, mutation and selection. The effects of systematic processes were studied in last two chapters considering large population.

The whole population of any species is divided into sub-populations for certain reasons *viz.* geographical or ecological reason under natural conditions or as a result of breeding plans in domestic and laboratory animals. These sub-populations are the various herds/flocks of domestic animals which are small in numbers. Thus, all the populations of domestic animals are constituted of small number of animals.

If the population size is small, the gene frequencies are subject to change, even the systematic processes are not operating. The small population is a dispersive process regarding its effect in dispersing the gene frequencies. The dispersive process differs from the systematic processes. This is because its effect is predictable only in amount but it has random effect on gene frequencies in direction which implies that the direction of change in gene frequency is not predictable, in a population of small size.

The *dispersive process* arises in **small population** from the effect of sampling. The gene frequencies are under random fluctuations as a result of the sampling of gametes in small population. The gametes carry the genes and transmit to the next generation. These gametes formed in parent generation in small population are a sample of the genes of the parent generation and do not represent the whole population. It is well known that if the sample is small, the gene frequencies between two generations are subject to change and this change is random. Thus, the small population is the dispersive process because it disperses the gene frequencies in either direction which is unpredictable.

The dispersive process in small population and its consequences can be studied in two different ways:

☆ *Sampling process* and its effect on gene frequencies in terms of sampling variance. The sampling process leads to genetic drift.

☆ *Inbreeding process* and its effect on genotypic changes.

9.1 Sampling Process

It is most important to know about the sample, the process of sampling and its effect.

9.1.1 Sampling

The herds or flocks of farm animals having less number of animals represent only a sample of individuals of the whole population. In a population of small size (sample), the total gene pool is thus divided into samples (herds/flocks) of small size. This results in random sampling from the whole population and hence subjected to sampling error because small sample deviates randomly from expectations/reality as per theory of the probability of events. The theory states that there is an increasing consistency to the actual trend (reality) with the increase in number of trails. For example, the occurrence of heads and tails of a coin by tossing come close to the expectation of 50:50 when the numbers of tossing become large but deviates from expectation when the numbers of tossing (trials) are small. Therefore, the consistency of the actual with the expectation depends on the numbers of events (trails) under observation. In case of population of domestic animals, the frequency of two or more alleles of a gene pair are like head or tail of a coin and the number of animals of population are like the numbers of tossing of a coin.

The numbers of breeding animals constitute the size of a population. In small size population, the numbers of breeding animals (parents) are small. Therefore, the allelic frequencies among parents do not represent the actual frequencies of alleles of the whole population but they deviate from the actual frequencies. These allelic frequencies among parents determine the genotypic frequencies of the progeny generation which in turn decides the gene frequency among progeny generation. Therefore, the allele frequencies in different samples of small size are expected to deviate from that of the whole population.

9.1.2 Sampling Effect

The effect of sampling can be seen by considering a single locus with two alleles (A and a) with their equal frequencies as $p = q = \frac{1}{2}$. In a large random mating population, the frequency of A allele is expected to be ½ in progeny generation. But when the population is small, a few numbers of offspring are raised from the large pool of gametes produced from parental population. The gametes are sampled in a small population and the sample is not expected to have equal number of two alleles at a locus but either of the two alleles may be transmitted in greater numbers than the other. This will lead to change the gene frequency from ½ to any other value, *viz.* if the offspring raised are 20 which are formed by the union of 40 gametes drawn at random from the large pool of gametes produced by the parent generation. Exactly equal number of *A* and *a* gametes may not be sampled out of 40 gametes but it may happen that 30 gametes may carry A allele and the rest 10 gametes may carry *a* allele. Thus, the gene frequency of A allele (p) in progeny generation will be 30/40 = 0.75 instead of 0.5. Therefore, the frequency of A allele has changed from 0.5 to 0.75 in one generation. This change in gene frequency is the sampling error whose extent depends upon the size of the population. Thus, when population size is small, the sampling error occurs leading to the gene frequencies to change or fluctuate in any direction and hence the change is random.

The contribution of all the breeding individuals to the gamete pool is equal due to random mating among the individuals of a line. A large number of gametes are produced in each line and unite together at random to form the zygote. However, all the zygotes formed do not survive to become parents due to the restriction of constant population size in all generations. The survival of zygote is random and only some of them become the breeding individuals of the next generation. As a result of random survival of the zygote, the parents do not have their uniform contribution to the progeny generation but contribute according to the probability of survival of their progeny. The number of progeny is one per parent or two per mated pair to maintain the constant population size in all the generations. The random survival of the zygotes is the stage at which the sampling error occurs and has its consequence to influence the gene frequencies. This process results in the reduction of a large number of gametes produced by parental generation to a smaller number of progeny reaching the breeding age. This reduction may occur at several stages but the final number of the breeding progeny determines the consequences of the sampling process if the sampling is random at each stage.

9.1.3. Concept and Definition of Genetic Drift

In a population of small size, the numbers of parents (breeding animals) are small in numbers and hence the gene frequencies among them do not represent the actual gene frequencies of the whole population but deviate from that of the whole population. The gametes carry a sample of genes of the parental generation of small size and hence the gene frequencies are liable (expected) to change between one generation and the next.

The change in gene frequency occurs due to sampling and hence it is a sampling error. Any change has its magnitude and direction. The magnitude of the change in gene frequency due to sampling process is predictable but its direction cannot be predicted. The direction of change in gene frequency as a result of sampling error is random which means that the change may take place in any direction. Thus, there is no trend in change of gene frequency (increase or decrease) but it may take any value in either direction in the next generation. Therefore, the gene frequency may deviate (move or drift) randomly to any direction and thus the change of gene frequency from one generation to the next is random. The random change of gene frequency in small population, resulting from the sampling process, is called the **random drift** or the **"genetic drift"**, the term coined by Wright (1931).This is also called as *random genetic drift*. The random change of gene frequency due to genetic drift is the *dispersive process as* it disperses the gene frequencies.

9.1.4. Consequence of Genetic Drift

The consequences of dispersive process (random genetic drift) to change the genetic structure of population are as under:

(i) Direction of Change is Random

The effect of genetic drift on change of gene frequency can be seen from the probability distribution of the number of alleles of a gene pair transmitted to the offspring. The base population is taken to be divided into a large number of lines and each line has N breeding individuals in each generation which are equally divided in two sexes. There are thus ½ N mating pairs of N breeding individuals having 2 N alleles at a locus. Thus, each line is a random sample of parental generation and hence the gene frequencies among N individuals of a line will deviate by chance.

The direction of change in gene frequency is random due to random genetic drift, because the gene frequency in successive generation seems to drift about in either direction. The gene frequency may increase or decrease in next generation and hence there is no trend in change of gene frequency but the change is in a erratic manner from generation to generation. The gene frequency is drifted back and forth and does not reach equilibrium.

Measure & Amount of Change

It is measured as variance of gene frequency.

The change in gene frequency in small population in one generation is inversely proportional to the population size and the magnitude of change in gene frequency is reflected in the spread of gene frequency in different subpopulations.

The gene frequencies in different lines (q_i) deviate from the gene frequency in base population (q_0) due to sampling error and will be distributed around the mean gene frequency of the base population with a variance $pq/2N$. This is the bimodal variance of sample means and indicates the deviation (change) in gene frequency among lines after one generation. The variance is the measure of the differences of gene frequency in different lines after one generation. All the lines have the same gene frequency initially represented as q_0. The variance ($pq/2N$) is the difference of the change of gene frequency ($q_1 - q_0 = \Delta q$) in one generation and expresses the magnitude of change of gene frequency due to sampling (dispersive process). Therefore, the change of gene frequency due to dispersive process can be stated in terms of the variance of change in gene frequency as:

$$\sigma^2 \, \Delta q = \frac{P_0 q_0}{2N} \qquad\qquad\qquad 9.1$$

This is the change of gene frequency in one generation, denoted by $\Delta q = (q_1 - q_0)$ and measured by the variance of gene frequency among subpopulations as $\sigma^2 q = p \, q / 2N$. The amount of change in gene frequency being inversely proportional to population size, decreases with increase in population size. Therefore, the effect of random drift is less in population of large size.

Interpretation of Variance

The variance of the change in gene frequency $\left(\sigma^2 \, \Delta q = \dfrac{P_0 q_0}{2N} \right)$ can be interpreted in different ways as:

(i) Expected change in any one line: (a) Distribution of gene frequencies of different loci of one generation and (b) Distribution of gene frequencies of a particular locus over generations.

(ii) Dispersion of gene frequencies at a locus among lines after one generation. The different lines will have different gene frequencies after one generation due to sampling effect.

The genetic drift has its cumulative effect over generations. This is because each line of the next generation starts from a different gene frequency and hence each subsequent sampling leads to a further dispersion of gene frequency. The line thus has a different gene frequency from previous generation and further affected by sampling process. This leads to the lines to spread apart in gene frequencies progressively in each successive generation and hence the lines become genetically differentiated from each other.

Cumulative effect of genetic drift: The populations of domestic animals are subdivided into local groups (herds/flocks) and are of small size for which they are subjected to genetic drift leading to genetic differentiation between them. The progressive differentiation among lines increases the variance of gene frequency among lines and the variance in *t generation* becomes as:

$$\sigma^2 \, q_{(t)} = P_0 q_0 \left[1 - \left(1 - \frac{1}{2N} \right)^t \right]$$

$$= P_0 q_0 F_t \qquad\qquad \text{Since } F_t = 1 - H_t \text{ and } H_t = \left(1 - \frac{1}{2N} \right)^t$$

The increase i n differentiation among lines is equivalent to the increase in variance of gene frequency among them. The increase in variance of gene frequency due to dispersive process depends on the size of line (N), initial gene frequency and the number of generations (t). The variance between lines increases with time (generations) finally becomes twice of the original variance and variance within line

decreases @ $\left(\dfrac{1}{2N}\right)$ per generation finally reduces to zero.

(ii) Decay of Genetic Variability within Line

A population of small size ultimately reaches complete homozygosis which is known as decay of variability or genetic decay because the line losses its capacity to change genetically. The genetic variation within line is reduced and hence there is uniformity within sub-population. The rates of loss and fixation of an allele are equal because the distribution of gene frequency is uniform. Thus, the total rate of decay is

$\left(\dfrac{1}{2N}\right)$ per generation. This means that the average heterozygosity decreases at this

rate per generation out of which 50 per cent $\left(\dfrac{1}{4N}\right)$ is the rate of fixation and the

remaining 50 per cent is the rate of loss of an allele per generation. Thus, the average homozygosity is increased equal to the loss in average heterozygosity and this increase

in homozygosity is measured in terms of F. Thus F for one generation is $\left(\dfrac{1}{2N}\right)$ and it

is the F of the progeny.

This is the loss of heterozygosity on random mating in small population and also called as the rate of "**disintegration**".

(iii) Genetic Differentiation between Lines

Random drift leads to genetic differentiation between the different lines. Different lines are developed in different geographical areas and the mating take place more often among the animals of the same locality. Thus the different lines of different areas differ in their gene frequencies.

(iv) Change in Genotypic Frequencies – Increased Homozygosity: (Wahlund Formula of Breeding Structure)

The mating is assumed to be random within each sub population (line) and hence the genotypic frequencies in any one line are in H.W. proportions determined by the gene frequencies in the previous generation of that line. Therefore, the change in gene frequencies leads to a change in genotypic frequencies.

The direction of change in genotypic frequencies is towards an increase of homozygous genotype and decrease of heterozygous genotype. The increase in frequency of homozygote in the population as a whole occurs inspite of the fact that random mating is followed in all the sub populations into which a large population is subdivided. The reason is very simple.

The gene frequencies drift apart from intermediate value towards the extreme due to random drift. The frequency of heterozygote in a random mating population

(2pq) is maximum at intermediate gene frequencies (p = q = 0.5) and heterozygosity decreases with movement of gene frequencies towards the extremes. Thus, the random drift or dispersion of gene frequencies towards the extreme as a result of subdivision of population into lines leads to a decrease in the frequency of heterozygote and an excess of homozygote compared with a large single population (in which all lines are considered together as a random mating entirely).

Thus, the *subdivision of a large population into small groups increases the frequency of homozygote and a deficiency of heterozygote*. This effect of subdivision of population results from the dispersion of gene frequencies and it is like the effect of inbreeding. This is known as *stratification principle or Wahlund's principle of subdivision of population or* Wahlund's proportions of breeding structure of population because these relationships were first noted by Wahlund (1928).

Before illustration of Wahlund's principle of subdivision of population, it is better to understand about the variance of gene frequencies.

Variance of gene frequency ($\sigma^2 q$): The difference between the average frequency of the homozygote over all the lines (q)^2 and the frequency of the homozygote in the population as a whole under random mating (q)^2 equals the variance of gene frequency ($\sigma^2 q$). This variance of gene frequency is the variance of the change of gene frequency ($\sigma^2 \Delta q$) which indicates the amount of change in gene frequency. Therefore,

$$\sigma^2 q = \left| \overline{q^2} - (\overline{q})^2 \right| = \sigma^2 \, \Delta q \qquad\qquad 9.2$$

It is known that the variance is a measure of the dispersion of a set of numbers clustered around the mean. Mathematically, the variance is estimated as the mean of the squares minus the square of the mean $\sigma^2 q = \left| \overline{q^2} - (\overline{q})^2 \right|$. Thus, the difference between the frequency of recessive homozygote after and before subdivision of a population equals to the variance in gene frequencies among lines. This represents the excess amount of homozygote in the whole population over all the lines.

In a random mating breeding unit, the frequency of homozygote of an allele in the progeny generation is equal to the square of gene frequency (q^2) in previous generation. The average frequency of homozygote in the whole population (taking all the lines together) is equal to the mean of the frequencies of homozygote for all the lines $\left(\overline{q^2} \right)$. On the other hand, without dividing the population into lines, the frequency of aa homozygote in the whole population under random mating would have been $(\overline{q})^2$, taking $\overline{q}$ as the average gene frequency of all the lines. The average gene frequency does not change due to dispersive process and hence $\overline{q} = q_0$, initial gene frequency. Mathematically, the mean of squares $\left(\overline{q^2} \right)$ is greater than square of the mean $(\overline{q})^2$. Therefore, the subdivision of a large population into small groups (small population – dispersive process) having different allelic frequencies in different lines due to random sampling produces an excess amount of homozygote and a consequent decrease of heterozygote compared to a single large population.

Wahlund's Principle

The effect of subdivision of population into small groups to increase the frequency of homozygote can be better understood with the help of a numerical example as:

Table 9.1: Allelic and Genotypic Frequencies for Three Supopulations (K=3) All of Equal Size Produced by Subdivision of Large Population

Sub Populations	Allelic Frequency		Genotypic Frequencies		
	p	q	p^2	$2pq$	q^2
1	0.9	0.1	0.81	0.18	0.01
2	0.6	0.4	0.36	0.48	0.16
3	0.3	0.7	0.09	0.42	0.49
Average $\left(\overline{q^2}\right)$ of all 3 lines	0.6	0.4	0.42	0.36	0.22

Genotype freq. in whole

population $(\overline{q})^2$ $(0.6 + 0.4)^2$ $=$ 0.36 0.48 0.16

Difference: $\sigma^2 q = \left|\overline{q^2} - (\overline{q})^2\right| =$ +0.06 −0.12 + 0.06

Now, $\sigma^2 q = 0.22 - 0.16 = 0.06$

The variance of gene frequency can be used to estimate the genotype frequencies in the whole population as a whole as under:

$$\sigma^2 q = \left|\overline{q^2} - (\overline{q})^2\right|$$

Hence, $\overline{q^2} = (\overline{q})^2 + \sigma^2 q$ 　　　　　　　　　　9.3

= Average frequency of homozygote in whole population over all lines.

Table 9.2: Genotypic Frequencies in the Total Population

Genotypes	Frequencies of Genotypes in Whole Population (Wahlund proportions)
AA	$p_0^2 + \sigma^2 q$
Aa	$2p_0 q_0 - 2\sigma^2 q$
aa	$q_0^2 + \sigma^2 q$

The Wahlund proportions are the result of the subdivision.

The p_0^2 and q_0^2 are the original frequencies of the homozygote in the base (original) population. It can be noted that these genotype frequencies in the total population (mean genotype frequencies over all lines) are not in accordance of the H.W. law and hence not according to the original or mean gene frequency. The H.W. relationship between gene frequency and genotype frequencies holds true within each line separately but not for the total population. The mating is random within each line and hence the genotype frequencies in any one line are the H.W. frequencies determined by the gene frequencies of the previous generation of the line. However, after the lines drift apart in gene frequencies they become differentiated also in genotypic frequencies. Therefore, the H.W. relationship does not hold true when all the lines are considered as a single population. The effect of subdivision of population is that heterozygote are decreased equal to the twice of the variance of gene frequency $(2\sigma^2 q)$ and each homozygous proportion is increased by the amount $\sigma^2 q$ at the expense of heterozygote. This effect of subdivision results from dispersion of gene frequencies and is similar to the effect of inbreeding. This is known as *Stratification principle* or *Wahlund proportions* of breeding structure of population (Wahlund, 1928).

The change in genotype frequencies described above was for one locus in many lines. However, this can be taken equally for many loci in one line wherein the change will be an increase of the number of homozygous loci and corresponding decrease in number of heterozygous loci. Therefore, the dispersive process leads to change of genotype frequencies and this is the genetic basis of the phenomenon of inbreeding depression. The recessive alleles that are deleterious become in homozy-gous condition and this is the genetic basis of the loss of fertility, vigour and vitality that almost always results from inbreeding and known as the inbreeding depression.

Wahlund Effect of Subdivision is Equivalent to Inbreeding Effect

The variance of gene frequency $(\sigma^2 q)$ equals $\dfrac{pq}{2N}$. This can be expressed in terms of the inbreeding coefficient as:

$$\sigma^2 q = \frac{pq}{2N}$$

$$= pq\ \Delta F \text{ Since, } \left(\frac{1}{2N}\right) = \Delta F$$

$$= \overline{pq}\ F \text{ , in terms of inbreeding coefficient.}$$

Thus, taking $\sigma^2 q = \overline{pq}\ F$, it is obvious that the Wahlund proportions of genotypes as a result of subdivision of a population into separate breeding groups are equivalent to inbred changes occurred due to inbreeding within the total population. The Wahlund's proportions are the result of the subdivision of a large population into lines. Therefore, these Wahlund proportions can be used to estimate the homozygosity as a result of subdivision as:

$$\sigma^2 q \quad = \overline{pq}\ F \text{ and hence}$$

$$F \quad = \frac{\sigma^2 q}{\overline{pq}}$$

This relationship between F and $\sigma^2 q$ was obtained by Wright (1943) comparing Wahlund's genotypic proportions with those of an equilibrium population having the inbreeding coefficient F. The F so estimated applies to the total population which means that the genotypic proportions in the total population would be equal as if certain amount of inbreeding (F) had been practiced within the whole population, though the mating were at random in the subgroups. This F represents the increase in homozygosity due to subdivision and known as the *'fixation index"*.

The data given in the Table 9.1 would indicate $F = \dfrac{0.06}{0.4 \times 0.6} = 0.25$ which is equivalent to one generation of full sib mating. Therefore, this $F = 0.25 = F_1 =$ inbreeding coefficient of the total population while the inbreeding coefficient of a group (F_G) is zero.

The fixation index is related to the population size as under-

$$F = \frac{\sigma^2 q}{\overline{pq}} = \left(\frac{\overline{pq}}{2N}\right)\left(\frac{1}{\overline{pq}}\right) \qquad \text{Since } \sigma^2 q = \frac{\overline{pq}}{2N}$$

$$= \left(\frac{1}{2N}\right)$$

The fixation index (F) can be interpreted in terms of the identity of alleles by descent. This F is indeed the probability that two alleles chosen at random from within the same subpopulation are identical by descent. This F changes (increases) generation after generation because of the cumulative effect of the random genetic drift. Therefore, in any generation t, the average value of fixation index among subpopulations is represented by F_t. The value of F_t is:

$$F_t = 1 - \left[1 - \left(\frac{1}{2N}\right)\right]^t$$

$$= 1 - Ht$$

Thus, there is an increase in fixation index due to random genetic drift (subdivison of population due to random sampling).

(v) Gene Fixation

The change in gen2e frequency in small population due to random sampling is continuous till the gene frequency lies between $\left(\dfrac{1}{2N}\right)$ and $2N - \left(\dfrac{1}{2N}\right)$ and the change is in both directions. The gene frequency may take almost any value after a number of generations of random mating irrespective of its initial value. If the gene frequency comes down to a small value due to cumulative effect of genetic drift, it may be further decreased to a still lower value or may be increased in the next generation. In fact, the gene may eventually be lost in the next generation due to random sampling. In small

population the process of random sampling is a continuous one till the population eventually becomes fixed for one of the existing alleles at a locus. Thus the genetic drift leads to each allele ultimately becoming either fixed or lost. This is the genetic drift theory which states that with or without natural selection, a gene locus with alternate alleles in a small population will become fixed for one of the existing alleles sooner or later. The fixation of one or the other allele is the final consequence of genetic drift. There is no variation in gene frequency in subsequent generations once the gene is lost ($q = 0$) or fixed ($q = 1$). The points of $q = 0$ and 1 are said the *dead points* or dead ends or points of no return when the change of gene frequency is stopped. The phenomena of' approaching the dead ends is an irreversible without mutation or crossing between breeding units. Thus, the process of genetic drift become irreversible at the dead ends,

The gene frequency in a small population thus ultimately approaches dead ends irrespective of its initial value and the population becomes homozygous for one or the other allele to having either all AA or aa individuals inspite of random mating. The gene is said to he fixed in a line on reaching a frequency of one while on reaching a frequency of zero the gene is said to be lost from the line. When an allele is fixed in a line, no other allele remains present at the locus in that line and the line is then said to be fixed. In case of loss of an allele ($q = 0$) there will be no restoration of that allele in the line, it will remain homozygous for that line.

The probability of fixation of an allele at the dead end is equal to its initial frequency. This means that when Ft reaches to I. All subpopulations eventually become fixed for one allele or the other and the proportion of subpopulations that eventually become fixed for an allele is equal to the initial frequency of that allele. This is due to the reason that the average gene frequency in all the lines remains unchanged equal to the initial gene frequency. Thus the initial gene frequency of alleles at a locus determines the proportion of total lines to become fixed for different alleles *e.g.* taking p and q as the frequencies of A_1 and A_2 alleles at a locus, the A_1 allele will be fixed in proportion p of the total lines and A_2 allele in the remaining lines equal to l-p = q. The individuals of a line that is fixed for an allele are genetically identical having identical genotype. Finally all lines and all loci in a line become fixed when the random process has gone to completion. When the lines become genetically uniform (fixed) the variance of gene frequency among lines is equal to pq.

The fixation does not start immediately but after a number of generations. There is dispersion of gene frequencies in small population due to random sampling. The parental gene frequencies spread out over a wide range in the progeny generation of different lines. The distribution of gene frequency at a locus among many lines or for different loci in any line is practically uniform as a result of the continuous process of spreading for a number of generations and the spreading out is a random process. This uniform distribution of gene frequencies is responsible for no change in mean gene frequency in all the lines from that of the initial gene frequency.

Although the change in gene frequency is more with intermediate gene frequency ($p = q = 0.5$) than when it is near 0 or 1, but the chance factor for a loss or fixation of an allele is more when p or q in near 0 or 1 than when it is intermediate because there is more danger of loss or fixation of an allele in subsequent generation when p or q is near 0 or 1. The rare alleles are mostly eliminated from the population of small size. The initial gene frequency determines the time that a population will remain segregating is 2.8 N generations when the initial gene frequency is 0.5 while the average time is 1.3 N generations when the initial gene frequency is 0.1. Thus, the population remain segregating for longer time when its size is large and when the initial gene frequency is near 0.5.

Regarding the effect of genetic drift among lines, the gene may be lost in some lines, fixed in others and may be segregating in some other lines assuming any value within the range. The fixation proceeds at a constant rate. A proportion of 1/N of the lines previously unfixed (segregating) become fixed in each generation alter the steady phase is reached. The proportions of lines to be fixed, lost or segregating are as under after Wright (1952):

Fixed: $q - 3pq\left(1 - \dfrac{1}{2N}\right)^t$

Lost: $\quad p - 3pq\left(1 - \dfrac{1}{2N}\right)^t$

Segregating: $\quad 6pq\left(1 - \dfrac{1}{2N}\right)^t$

The frequencies of fixation and loss of an allele increase from generation to generation. The fixation and loss of alleles are each proceeding at the rate of $\dfrac{1}{4N}$ per generation so as the total loss of heterozygosity is $\dfrac{1}{2N}$ in the absence of systematic forces. The loss or fixation of a gene means the loss of heterozygote.

9.2 Inbreeding Process (in Small Population)

The inbreeding in a small population can be studied under 3 situations *viz.*

☆ Idealized population, with all types of mating including selfing
☆ Real population, which deviates from idealized model.
☆ Hierarchical population structure

9.2.1 Idealized Population

Consider in an idealized population of N individuals, each producing equal number of gametes uniting at random, resulting an infinite pool of gametes when each breeding individual has equal contribution. Further assumption is that each parent is heterozygous for different pairs of genes and hence having non-identical alleles. Thus, the base population has 2 N different types of gametes, in equal numbers and the alleles at a locus being A_1, A_2, $A_{3, etc.}$ The gametes of two sexes produced by 2 N individuals are:

Individuals	1	2	3	N^{th}
Male gametes	$A_1 A_2$	$A_3 A_4$	$A_5 A_6$	A_{2N-1}, A_{2N}
Female gametes	$A_1 A_2$	$A_3 A_4$	$A_5 A_6$	A_{2N-1}, A_{2N}

Any random pair of opposite sex gametes will have $\left(\dfrac{1}{2N}\right)$ chance for carrying

identical allele and hence any gamete has a $\left(\dfrac{1}{2N}\right)$ chance of uniting with another

gamete of the same kind. The probability that a gamete should unite with a gamete

from the same individual is $\left(\dfrac{1}{2N}\right)$, having identical alleles and the probability to

unite from a different individual is $\left[1-\left(\dfrac{1}{2N}\right)\right]$, having non-identical alleles.

Therefore, $\left(\dfrac{1}{2N}\right)$ is the rate of inbreeding of the progeny (F_1). Thus, F in first generation

is $F_1 = \left(\dfrac{1}{2N}\right)$

Thus, $\dfrac{1}{2N} = \Delta F$.

The variance of change of gene frequency, in terms of rate of inbreeding is :

$$\sigma^2 \Delta q = \frac{p_0 q_0}{2N} = p_0 q_0 \Delta F$$

In the second generation, the identical homozygote will be produced from inbreeding in the first generation and from new replication of genes. The probability of newly replicated genes uniting together in the form of zygote is 1/2 N again. The

rest proportion $\left[1-\left(\dfrac{1}{2N}\right)\right]$ of zygotes carry genes that have been identical from first

generation. Thus if there has been any previous inbreeding, some part of $\left[1-\left(\dfrac{1}{2N}\right)\right]$

in the population may be identical with each other with a frequency for the parent generation as F_1. As a result, a random pair that has not become identical by the fusion of gametes in second generation but by a previous inbreeding will be identical $\left[1-\left(\dfrac{1}{2N}\right)\right]$ F_1 proportion of the time. Thus conclusively,

Probability of random pairs to be identical $=\left(\dfrac{1}{2N}\right)$

(Newly replicated genes)

Probability of remainder pairs $\left[1-\left(\dfrac{1}{2N}\right)\right]$ to be identical $=\left[1-\left(\dfrac{1}{2N}\right)\right]F_1$

(due to previous inbreeding)

Sum of these two probabilities of identical homozygote (F_2) is

$$F_2 = \left(\frac{1}{2N}\right) + \left[1-\left(\frac{1}{2N}\right)\right]F_1 \qquad\qquad \text{..................9.4}$$

Where, F_1 and F_2 represent the inbreeding coefficient of generation 1 and 2, respectively.

Thus, the inbreeding coefficient in t generation will be

$$F_t = \left(\frac{1}{2N}\right) + \left[1-\left(\frac{1}{2N}\right)\right]F_t \qquad\qquad \text{..................9.4 (b)}$$

= New inbreeding + old inbreeding

The rate of inbreeding increment is $\left(\dfrac{1}{2N}\right)$, symbolized by ΔF. This ΔF represents the fraction of non-identical genes that become newly "inbred" (identical) each generation.

Therefore, the rate of inbreeding increment (ΔF) each generation in an idealized population is $\Delta F = \left(\dfrac{1}{2N}\right)$. This indicates the rate of dispersion. This rate of homozygosity increment becomes constant after some generations.

The inbreeding increment (ΔF) measures the rate of inbreeding in the term of a proportionate increase. The $\Delta F = \left(\dfrac{1}{2N}\right)$ in an idealized population while the equation $F_t = \Delta F + (1 - \Delta F)\,F_{t-1}$ is valid for any breeding system when the inbreeding coefficient is expressed in terms of ΔF. Therefore, this measure of the rate of inbreeding provides a means of comparing the inbreeding effects of different breeding systems.

9.2.2 Real Populations

The conditions of real populations are different from that of the idealized population. In a natural or real population, the total numbers of individuals may be very large but they all may not contribute to the genetic composition of the next generation because some of them may not reach the sexual maturity, others may not be able to mate while others which mate may not leave offspring that survive to maturity in the next generation. Moreover, in populations of domestic farm animals the numbers of breeding males are frequently less than the number of breeding females. Therefore, the individuals which are not taking part in breeding or those that leave no offspring do not contribute to the genetic composition of the population and the males though lesser in number have contribution equal to that of the females which are more in number. Thus, all the individuals of the real population are not effective to influence the genetic composition of the next generation and hence the numbers of breeding individuals affecting the genetic constitution of the next generation may be less than the actual number of individuals living at a time in a real population. Therefore, the breeding structure of a real or actual population is much more complicated and differs from the ideal population in many respects.

Now the important point is that how the complicated situations of real population can be simplified and reduced to the equivalent case of ideal population for which the recurrent relations of F and H have been derived. To deal with the complicated situations of real population which deviate from the ideal population, a very useful concept of effective population number or *effective population size* was introduced by Wright (1931) to meet this requirement. The concept is based on the fact that a compromise is made to convert the actual breeding size to a number equivalent to the number of individuals in the ideal population.

Effective Population Size

In a small population, there is random drift in gene frequencies due to sampling variance (variance effect) and consequently there is an increase in homozygosity (inbreeding effect). The change in the probability of identity of genes by descent (increase in homozygosity) was shown to be related with N (population size) in small population of ideal structure. Similarly, the change in gene frequency due to random genetic drift in small population is also related to N in small population with idealized structure. Any particular situation of real population that deviates from the idealized breeding structure is expressed by converting the number of breeding individuals in a real population to the effective number of breeding individuals or the effective population size.

This effective number is defined as the number of individuals that would give rise to calculated sampling variance or the rate of inbreeding, if they bred in the manner of the idealized population. Therefore, the effective number or the effective population size (Ne) of real population is the size of an ideal population that would have the same increase in homozygosity (decrease in H) as the real population. The actual breeding size of real population is thus converted to a number equivalent to the number of individuals in the ideal population that would give rise to the increase in homozygosity equivalent to that under the condition of ideal population. This number (converted) is called the effective number of breeding individuals or the effective population size of the breeding group. This effective number gives rise to the sampling variance or homozygosity increase appropriate to the ideal population if bred to the conditions of ideal population.

The concept of effective population size (Ne) can be made clear by considering the different situations of real population that differ from ideal population. The different equations for different deviated situations will be derived to convert the actual number (N) to the effective number (Ne) so as the rate of inbreeding increment become equal in real and ideal populations.

The ΔF is related to population size in an ideal population as: $\Delta F = \left(\dfrac{1}{2N}\right)$.

The effective size is related to ΔF and hence Ne can be calculated from ΔF as

$Ne = \dfrac{1}{2} \Delta F$. Therefore, if the actual number of individuals in a real population is converted into effective number and Ne is substituted for N, the conclusions drawn for ideal population are valid for any breeding structure. The effective number (Ne) can be obtained from the actual number (N) if the breeding structure is known. The rate of inbreeding (ΔF) can be estimated, after knowing the effective population size (Ne) for any breeding structure, as:

$$\Delta F = \left(\frac{1}{2\,Ne}\right)$$
............9.5

Situation 1

No self Fertilization (exclusion of closely related mating *viz.* selfing and sib mating): The self fertilization does not take place in domestic animals and hence the two uniting gametes can not come from the same parent. The closest possible relative mating could be of sibs and parent offspring which will also be excluded. The avoidance of mating between close relatives is advantageous to keep constant the rate of inbreeding in subsequent generations as well as to keep uniform the inbreeding coefficients of individuals within generations.

Wright (1969) quantified the effect of exclusion of selfing and full-sib mating in the effective numbers as:

(i) When self fertilization is excluded:

Effective number $(Ne) = N + \frac{1}{2}$
............9.6 (a)

$$\Delta F = \left(\frac{1}{2N+1}\right)$$
............9.6 (b)

(ii) When sib-mating is excluded:

$Ne = N + 2$ and $\Delta F = \left(\dfrac{1}{2N+4}\right)$

Situation 2

Unequal numbers of two sexes: The rate of inbreeding is a function of number of breeding individuals (parents) as: $\Delta F = \left(\dfrac{1}{2N}\right)$.

It is more economical to use fewer males than females in domestic animals. Different numbers of breeding individuals of the two sexes is the most common situation in domestic animals and this reduces the real breeding size (N) to a smaller effective size (Ne). If the population size is constant over generations ($N_o = N_1 = N_2$), then each parent contributes two haploid doses of genes on the average to the next generation. If the numbers of two sexes are unequal, the lesser sex (male) will contribute more than two doses on the average while the sex greater in number (female) will contribute less. In case of unequality of the numbers of males and females, the effective number of parents (Ne), contributing gametes to the generation, will not be a simple arithmetical average or total of the parental number.

The probability for any two genes to be contributed to the next generation is $\dfrac{1}{2} \times \dfrac{1}{2} = \dfrac{1}{4}$ which means that the probability that two genes in different individuals in

t generation are both derived from a male of t-1 generation is $\dfrac{1}{4}$. The probability that

both genes have come from the same male is $\left(\dfrac{1}{4}\right)\left(\dfrac{1}{Nm}\right) = \left(\dfrac{1}{4\,Nm}\right)$. Likewise, for any

individual female to contribute two genes, the probability is $\left(\dfrac{1}{4}\right)\left(\dfrac{I}{Nf}\right) = \left(\dfrac{1}{4\,Nf}\right)$.

Therefore, the total probability that any two genes have come from the same individual regardless of sex is the sum of two probabilities. Therefore,

$$\left(\frac{1}{4\,Nm}\right) + \left(\frac{I}{4\,Nf}\right) = \frac{1}{Ne}$$

$$Ne = \left(\frac{4\,Nm\,Nf}{Nm + Nf}\right) \qquad\qquad \text{.................. 9.7 (a)}$$

$$\text{and } \Delta F = \left(\frac{1}{8\,Nm}\right) + \left(\frac{1}{8\,Nf}\right) \qquad\qquad \text{.................. 9.7 (b)}$$

The Ne depends more on the sex with small numbers (males) used for breeding.

For example, there is a herd of 500 breeding individuals out of which 10 are males and 490 are females. They mate at random. The heterozygosis in this herd of 500 breedable animals will decrease at the same rate as if there were only (4 x 490 x

10)/(490 +10) = 39 breeding individuals in the group equally divided between the two sexes. The variance of gene frequency and the amount of random drift have the same magnitude as in a group of 39 animals all of which have equal chance to reproduce. Now reducing the number of males to 5 will yield Ne as:

$$Ne = \frac{4(5)(495)}{(5+495)}$$

$$= \frac{9900}{500} = \frac{99}{5} = 20$$

Thus, Ne is reduced with the reduction in the number of fewer sex (male). The value of Δ F in two cases will be 0.012 and 0.02. The use of Al has reduced the number of sires and hence consequently increased the rate of inbreeding, reduced the genetic variabil-ity and increased in the frequency of undesirable homozygote.

Situation 3

Unequal numbers in different generations: This is also a practical situation when the breeding animals are different in subsequent generations. In this case, the mean rate of inbreeding is not constant with varying numbers of breeding individuals in subsequent generations and hence each generation has to be considered. The mean rate of inbreeding will be the mean value of 1/2N of different generations. The effective number (Ne) is the harmonic mean of the number of individuals in each generation:

$$\frac{1}{Ne} = \frac{1}{t}\left[\sum \frac{1}{N_i}\right]$$

$$= \frac{1}{t}\left[\frac{1}{N_1} + \frac{1}{N_2} + \frac{1}{N_3} + \dots + \frac{1}{N_t}\right] \quad \dots\dots\dots 9.8$$

It is thus obvious that the generation with least numbers of breeding individuals (parents) will have more effect on rate of inbreeding.

An increment in inbreeding in one generation due to smaller numbers can not be counter balanced by increasing the numbers in later generations, though increasing the number will reduce the amount of new inbreeding. The average effective number is close to the minimum number compared to the maximum number in the cycle of generations. This is because the harmonic mean as compared to the arithmetic mean is more influenced by the smallest number of the terms being averaged together.

Situation 4

Unequal gamete contribution of parents: This means the number of progeny of an individual that become parents of next generation. This is also a deviated situation in real population than in ideal population in which each parent has equal chance of contributing genes in terms of the progeny of next generation. This situation of departure from ideal population is very important practically

In real population, each parent does not contribute equally because of differences in their fertility as well as survival and the survivability among their progeny. Therefore, these differences have an effect that some parents have more gamete contribution to the next generation than others. Consequently, the effective number of parents (Ne) is reduced than actual numbers. On the contrary, if the variation in gamete contribution of parent is reduced (family size become equal) by some breeding methods, it may then comparatively increases the (Ne). In case of unequal gamete contribution of parents, the effective number (Ne) is obtained as:

$$Ne = \frac{4N}{(V_k + 2)} \qquad\qquad\qquad \text{.................9.9}$$

Where, V_k is the variance of family size (k).

Situation 5

Overlapping generations: This is also an important practical situation observed in farm animals and human beings. The overlapping generation means that individuals of different generations survive together at the same time. These individuals belong to different age groups and of different stages of their life cycle. The reproductive chances are also different due to differences in their life span which increase the variance of family size (V_k). This is because the individuals having longer life have more chances to contribute more to the next generation. The equation 6.9 can be used to obtain the Ne with some adjustment for actual number (N) because it is problematic to know the total number of individual per generation. This requires the stable age-structure. It is then requires to know the number of individuals born in a particular period of time or any convenient time interval (say one year, etc). Let this number be taken as Nc. This number (Nc) is related to total number alive at any time (N_T) as: Nc $= N_T/E$. The E is taken as the mean life span. This also requires the generation length (L). Now the total number (N) can be obtained as: N = 4 Nc L and the Ne is obtained as:

$$Ne = \frac{4Nc\,L}{(V_k + 2)} \qquad\qquad\qquad \text{.................9.10}$$

9.2.3 Hierarchical Population Structure

Each breed of domestic animals has certain distinguished specific physical features and the breeds are thus recognized on the basis of some physical traits. This is mostly the criteria of identifying the animals belonging to different breeds. Therefore, the animals of a particular breed are homozygous for certain genes, controlling physical characteristics like body colour, physical traits (horn patterns – shape and size; facial expression, etc) with negligible differences, probably due to environmental variations which are not inherited. Likewise, there may be some family traits particularly observed in human families, particularly the facial characters for which a person belonging to a certain family is recognized easily. This means that the genes controlling such characters have been fixed in different breeds and families for which they are homozygous. The homozygosity indicates that the genes at a particular locus governing such traits are identical which may be identical by state or identical by descent. Each breed of farm animals is further divided into sub-populations (herds/flocks) for a number of reasons, mentioned elsewhere and hence they are subjected to homozygosity, probably due to small population size, if not by actual inbreeding.

Structured Population

The probability of homozygosity in a subdivided population compared to that of a panmictic population may be of help to understand the population structure and the Wahlund effect. The population subdivision has the inbreeding like effect and hence it is better to measure its effect in terms of the decrease in heterozygosity like that of inbreeding effect. The homozygosity is measured by computing the coefficient of inbreeding (F) with reference to a certain group of individuals as the base population.

However, sometimes it may be of interest to know the inbreeding coefficient with reference to a different base, either less or more remote in the ancestry. A full sib mating produce an individual which is 25 percent inbred ($F_1 = 0.25$) for which the reference base is its parents which may themselves be inbred with reference to a more remote base. In doing so the total population (T) is assumed to be divided into subpopulations (S) or demes each of which is further subdivided into sub-lines which are composed of certain individuals (I). Therefore, a population has three levels of its structure and such a population is called as *structured population* with a hierarchical subdivision into lines and sub-lines as shown below:

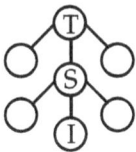

Total population (T), say one breed

Sub populations/lines (S), say different herd of a breed.

Individuals (I) in a herd (sub-line)

Figure 9.1: Showing Structured Population.

There is possibility of non random mating (inbreeding) within sub-populations. In this Figure 9.1, the letter I represents the individuals whose inbreeding coefficient is to be estimated and belongs to one of the subpopulations (S) and T is the total population representing the further-back base population.

Measures of Homozygosity

The relative homozygosity (identity between gametes) can be considered in at least three ways considering the frequencies of heterozygote as H_I, Hs and H_T among the contemporaries of I, S and T, respectively. Therefore, in this subdivided population:

H_I = *Individual heterozygosity due to inbreeding*, if followed in a subpopulation. This is interpreted as the average heterozygosity of all the genes in an individual or the probability of heterozygosity of any one gene.

H_S = *Subpopulation heterozygosity* of an individual due to random sampling in an equivalent random mating subpopulation. It is estimated from the estimated allele frequencies within subpopulations (Pt). Thus, $H_S = 2 \, p_i q_i$ for a subpopulation.

H_T = *Total heterozygosity* (H_T) of an individual due to combined effects of *subdivision and inbreeding*. It is estimated from the allele frequency in the pooled subpopulations (p_0). Thus $H_T = 2\,p_0 q_0$

Now in this subdivided population, the heterozygosity can be estimated, considering in at least three ways the relative homozygosity caused by inbreeding within sub-lines (F_{IS}), by random sampling with effects of subdivision (F_{ST}) and by the combined effects of inbreeding and subdivision (F_{IT}). These are as under:

The heterozygosity in an inbred population relative to that in a random mating population is called as the panmictic index (P). Accordingly, $P_t = H_t/H_0$ and it is the complement of the inbreeding coefficient. Therefore, the panmictic index (P_t) at generation t is:

$$P_t = 1 - F_t = \frac{H_t}{H_0} \text{ from equation 10.2 (b)}$$

This has been explained in subsequent chapter on inbreeding.

1. Homozygosity due to inbreeding effect within sub-line, measured as F_{IS}:

$$P_{IS} = \frac{H_I}{H_S}$$

          = Heterozugosity of individual (I) relative to sub-population.

          $= 1 - F_{IS}$

$$F_{IS} = 1 - \frac{H_1}{H_S} = \frac{(H_S - H_1)}{H_S}$$

          = *Homozygosity* (Inbreeding coefficient of an individual) *due to inbreeding* in its own sub-line.

Thus, F_{IS} is a measure of the increase in homozygosity due to inbreeding within sub-line. The $F_{IS} = 0$, in a random mating sub-line.

2. Homozygosity due to random sampling within subpopulation due to the effect of subdivision, measured as F_{ST}:

$$P_{ST} = \frac{H_S}{H_T}$$

          = Subpopulation Heterozygosity of individual (H_S) relative to sub-population.

          $= 1 - F_{ST}$

$$F_{ST} = 1 - P_{ST}$$

$$= 1 - \frac{H_S}{H_T} = \frac{(H_T - H_S)}{H_T}$$

          = *Homozygosity due to sub division* (Average inbreeding of the subpopulation relative to the total population),

The F_{ST} is called the *Fixation index* due to subdivision or Wahlund effect and is a measure of the increase in homozygosity of a subpopulation due to random genetic drift and hence it is a measure of the *effect of population subdivision.* This probability (F_{ST}) equals $\dfrac{\sigma^2 q}{pq}$ due to Wahlund effect, when allelic frequencies differ in different lines. This is also known as the 'fixation index" and equals $\left(\dfrac{1}{2N}\right)$. This is because $F_{ST} = \dfrac{\sigma^2 q}{pq} = \left(\dfrac{pq}{2N}\right)\left(\dfrac{1}{pq}\right) = \dfrac{1}{2N}$.

The F_{ST} is concerned with inbreeding in subpopulations (S) relative to the total population of which they are a part.

Fixation Index (F_{ST}) and Genetic Differentiations among Subpopulation: The concept of F_{ST} was developed by Wright (1978) describing the variability within and among natural populations. He interpreted the fixation index (F_{ST}) as an index of genetic divergence among subpopulations by suggesting the following guidelines

F_{ST}	$= 0$	= no genetic divergence
	$= 0$ to 0.05	= little genetic divergence
	$= 0.05$ to 0.15	= moderate genetic divergence
	$= 0.15$ to 0.25	= great genetic differentiation
	$= > 0.25$	= very great genetic differentiation
	$= 1.0$	= fixation of alternate allele in the subpopulation.

3. Homozygosity due to combined effects of inbreeding and subdivision, measured as F_{IT}:

$$P_{IT} = \frac{H_I}{H_T} = \text{Heterozygosity of individual relative to total population.}$$

$$= \frac{H_I}{H_S}\frac{H_S}{H_T}$$

$$= P_{IS} P_{ST}$$

$$1 - F_{IT} = (1 - F_{IS})(1 - F_{ST})$$

$$F_{IT} = 1 - P_{IT} = \text{Total inbreeding coefficient}$$

$$= 1 - \frac{H_I}{H_T} = \frac{(H_T - H_I)}{H_T}$$

= Inbreeding coefficient of an individual relative to the total population and hence it includes the effect of inbreeding within sub-population (F_{IS}) plus the effect of random genetic drift due to population subdivision (F_{ST}).

F_{IT} is a measure of the increase in homozygosity of an individual relative to the total population due to *inbreeding* and *subdivision*, The F_{IT} is the most inclusive measure of inbreeding as it covers both the effects of inbreeding within subpopulation (F_{IS}) and the effects of population subdivision (F_{ST}).

The F_{IS}, F_{ST} and F_{IT} are the different types of "inbreeding coefficients" but they differ with respect to reference populations. These three types of inbreeding coefficients are known as Wright's F-statistics, used to describe the structured populations and have mathematical relation among themselves. The increase in overall homozy-gosity (F_{IT}) is due to inbreeding within subpopulation (F_{IS}) combined with the effect of random sampling within subpopulations (F_{ST}) known as subdivision or the Wahlund effect.

However, the total homozygosity (F_{IT}) is not the simple sum of F_{IS} and F_{ST}. This can be illustrated by the use of panmictic index (P = I-F) which is defined in terms of heterozygosity relative to that in a panmictic population. The probability of an individual to be heterozygous relative to random mating ($1 - F_{IT}$) is the product of two probabilities of that the individual has not been produced by the random union of two genes (gametes)

(i) That are identical by descent within the subgroup measured as $1 - F_{IS}$ and

(ii) That are identical due to remote relationship measured as $1 - F_{ST}$.

Therefore, $1 - F_{IT} = (1 - F_{IS})(1 - F_{ST})$ and hence,

$$P_{IT} = P_{IS} P_{ST}$$

and $F_{IT} = F_{ST} + F_{IS}(1 - F_{ST})$.

Therefore, the overall homozygosity of an individual in the total population is for two reasons *viz.* random sampling of gametes within subpopulations (Wahlund effect) plus the portion resulting from inbreeding.

9.3 Evolutionary Significance

Species with very large number of individuals are spread over a wide area of the world. The individuals spread over the wide region are distributed in small groups. However, the distribution is not continuous and uniform and this subdivides a large species into a great number of small isolates or groups. These small groups are subjected to random sample of gene frequencies and hence have no or low genetic variability. Therefore, small populations in which all the loci have been fixed have no genetic variability and hence they are unable for genotypic reorganization it required to meet the changed environmental conditions. A purebred line fixed for all loci may be favourable under present situation but its ultimate fate is probably the extinction during the long process of evolution. Therefore, partial isolation, with some migration among sub populations, is essential to prevent complete fixation and to permit differentiation which allows more favourable conditions for evolutionary process. This helps to keep a proper and delicate balance between adaptation at present and future flexibility.

Solved Examples and Exercises

Example 9.1

Find out the inbreeding coefficient of an individuals belonging to a line after 10 generations maintaining a constant size of 10 individuals each generation under the assumption of random mating within the line,

Solution

$$F_t = 1 - \left(1 - \frac{1}{2N}\right)^t$$

$$= 1 - \left(1 - \frac{1}{20}\right)^{10}$$

$$= 1 - (0.95)^{10}$$

$$= 1 - 0.5987 = 0.4012$$

This showed that there is substantial inbreeding in small population inspite of the fact that mating is random within each line and the genotypic frequencies within the line are according to H.W. law. The inbreeding does not result from actual non random mating but due to the fact that population is of small size

Example 9.2

Calculate the inbreeding coefficients due to subdivision (F_{ST}) and due to inbreeding plus subdivision (F_{IT}) from the data given in Table 9.1, assuming that in all the three subpopulations the inbreeding has been going on at the same level and attained $F_{IS} = 0.40$ in all the lines.

Solution

$F_{IS} = 0.4$ in all the three lines due to inbreeding within the lines.

$$F_{ST} = \frac{\sigma^2 q}{pq} \text{ (Wahlund's effect due to subdivision)}$$

$$= \frac{0.06}{0.6 \times 0.4}$$

$$= 0.25$$

$$F_{IT} = F_{ST} + F_{IS}(1 - F_{ST}).$$

$$= 0.25 + 0.40\,(0.75)$$

$$= 0.55$$

The F_{IT} is the total probability of an individual being homozygous in the overall population. The F_{IT} is due to two components corresponding to the *Wahlund effect* which is subdivision effect (increase in homozygosity due to random sampling of gametes within sub-populations) and *inbreeding effect* (consanguinity or non-random mating).

Genotypic frequencies in three lines and the whole population will be as:

Subpopulations	Genotype Frequencies			
	p^2	$2pq$	q^2	F_{IS}
1	0.846	0.108	0.046	0.4
2	0.456	0.288	0.276	0.4
3	0.174	0.252	0.574	0.4
Whole population	0.492	0.216	0.298	F_{IT}

Example 9.3

A line of 10 individuals (5 pairs) is maintained for 10 generations under random mating and in eleventh generation full sib mating was allowed, Find out the inbreeding coefficient of the progeny (Fo.) from the sib pair?

Solution

$$F_{IT} = F_{ST} + F_{IS}(1 - F_{ST}).$$

(i) Now, the homozygosity due to small population (F_{ST}) will be:

$$F_{ST} = 1 - P_{ST} = \text{Wahlund effect}$$

$$= 1 - \left(1 - \frac{1}{2N}\right)^t$$

$$= 1 - \left(1 - \frac{1}{20}\right)^{10}$$

$$= 0.4012$$

(ii) The homozygosity due to inbreeding (full sib mating) will be:

$$F_{IS} = 0.25 \text{ for full sib progeny}$$

(iii) The total homozygosity (F_{IT}) will be:

$$F_{IT} = 0.4012 + 0.25 \,(0.5988)$$

$$= 0.4012 + 0.1497$$

$$= 0.5509$$

Therefore, the progeny of full sib pair mating would be expected to be homozygous at about 55 percent of their gene loci instead of 25 percent expected under constant large population size.

Example 9.4

To estimate heterozygosity and F statistics.

Levin (1978) studied the genetic variation in 43 natural subpopulations of annual phlox for two allele pgm – 2^A and pgm – 2 ^{B} for phosphogluco mutase- 2 gene (pgm-2). It was observed that pgm -2^B allele was fixed in 40 subpopulations whereas in the remaining 3 polymorphic subpopulations, the frequencies of this allele (pgm- 2^B were 0.49, 0.83. and 0.91 respectively and the observed frequency of heterozygote in these 3 polymorphic subpopulations were 0.17, 0.06, and 0.06, respectively. Based on the data, find out the different kinds of heterozygosity and F statistics.

Solution

1. *Individual heterozygosity* (H_I) : Average heterozygosity of individuals within subpopulations:

$$H_I = \frac{[(40 \times 0) + 0.17 + 0.06 + 0.06]}{43} = 0.0067$$

2. *Subpopulation heterozygostiy* (H_S): It is estimated from the estimated allele frequencies within subpopulations and the expected frequency of heterozygote under the assumption of random mating as:

$$H_S = \frac{[(40 \times 0) + 0.17 + 0.06 + 0.06]}{43} = 0.0067$$

$$= \frac{[(40 \times 0) + 2 \times 0.49 \times 0.51 + 2 \times 0.83 \times 0.17 + 2 \times 0.91 \times 0.09]}{43}$$

$$= 0.0220$$

3. *Total heterozygosity* (H_T): It is estimated from the average allele frequency in the total population (combined subpopulations) and the HW expectation of heterozygosity.

Average frequency of pgm- 2^B allele $= \dfrac{[(40 \times 0) + 0.49 + 0.83 + 0.91]}{43} = 0.9821$

H_T $= 2\, pq = 2 \times 0.9821 \times 0.019 = 0.0352$

4. *Inbreeding effect:* $F_{IS} = \dfrac{(H_S - H_I)}{H_S} = \dfrac{(0.0220 - 0.0067)}{0.022} = 0.70$

= Estimated inbreeding coefficient due to non random mating within subpopulations (inbreeding effect).

5. *Fixation index* or Wahlund effect:

$$F_{ST} = \frac{(H_T - H_S)}{H_T} = \frac{(0.0352 - 0.0220)}{0.0352} = 0.38$$

= Amount of inbreeding due to sub division

6. *Total inbreeding coefficient*:

$$F_{IT} = \frac{(H_T - H_I)}{H_T} = \frac{(0.0352 - 0.0067)}{0.0352} = 0.81$$

= Amount of inbreeding due to combined effects of non random mating within subpopulation (F_{IS}) and to random genetic drift among subpopulations (F_{ST}).

or $F_{IT} = F_{ST} + F_{IS}(1 - F_{ST})$.

$$= 0.38 + 0.70(1 - 0.38) = 0.38 + 0.043 = 0.814$$

Exercises

9.5. A mouse colony was established 30 generations back with 20 individuals in each generation from a much larger colony and the colony is ideal particularly with respect to random mating within the colony. What is the F of a mouse in the colony ?.

Hint: Total F of an individual $(F_{IT}) = F_{ST}$ (fixation index) of colony and F_{ST}

$$= F_t$$

since $1 - F_t = \left(\frac{1}{1 - 2N}\right)^t (1 - F_0)$

$$F_t = 1 - \left(\frac{1}{1 - 2N}\right)^t \text{ when } F_0 = 0.0$$

Thus, $1 - F_{30} = 1 - \left(\frac{1}{2N}\right)^{30}(1 - F_0)$

$$= \left(1 - \frac{1}{40}\right)^{30} \text{ since } F_0 = 0 \text{ because foundation population}$$

was large

$$= 0.468$$

So, Ft = 0.532

Thus, there had been substantial inbreeding even though the mating was random and the genotypic frequencies within the colony follow HW law. The inbreeding did not result from actual non random (assortative) mating but from the fact that the population was small in size.

9.6. Assume that the mouse population in four barns, each has about the same sample size. The estimated values of F_{ST} for genes were 0.10, 0.16 and 0.11 with an average of 0.12. Estimate how long it will take from random genetic drift to result a value of $F_{ST} = 0.12$ in the ideal situation (assuming no migration) taking N = 20 and N = 100

Hint: $\qquad 1 - F_t = \left(1 - \dfrac{1}{40}\right)^t \qquad\qquad$ with $F_t = 0.12$ and $N = 20$

$$= \frac{\ln(0.88)}{\ln(0.975)} = 5 \text{ generations}$$

Similarly, $t = 26$ generations for $N = 100$

Chapter 10
Change of Genetic Structure Non Random Mating – I: Inbreeding

This chapter covers the effect of inbreeding on change of population structure. This will cover the genotypic distribution in an inbred population, properties of equilibrium population and recurrent relations of F under regular systems of inbreeding.

10.1 Inbreeding Increases Homozygosity

The primary effect of inbreeding is that it increases the homozygosity. The frequency of homozygous genotypes is increased at the expense of the frequency of heterozygous genotypes. The inbreeding converts a proportion of heterozygote into identical homozygote.

Therefore, the heterozygosity in an inbred population $(\mathbf{H_I})$ is expected to be less than in random mating population (Ho = 2pq). The magnitude of $\mathbf{H_I}$ depends on the rate of inbreeding. The degree of inbreeding is measured in terms of the proportionate reduction in heterozygosity in the inbred population (Ho – H_I) relative to that in a random mating population (base population, Ho = 2pq). This degree of inbreeding is denoted by F and estimated as:

$$F = \frac{(H_O - H_I)}{H_O}$$

.... Eq. 10.1

Where,   Ho is the heterozygosity in base population $=2pq$

H_I is the heterozygosity in inbred population

The quantity $\left[\dfrac{(H_O - H_I)}{H_O} \right]$ defines the effect of inbreeding and called as the inbreeding coefficient, denoted by **F.**

The actual frequency of heterozygous genotype in inbred population (H_I) in terms of F from above relation (10.1) can be written as-

$$Ho - H_I = Ho\,F$$
$$H_I = Ho - Ho\,F$$
$$= Ho\,(1 - F)$$
$$= 2p_0 q_0\,(1 - F) \qquad \text{................. Eq. 10.2}$$

where,   F = Probability of identical homozygote,

$1 - F = H_I / H_0$ = Heterozygosity

H_I = heterozygosity in inbred population.

Fraction of original heterozygote (Ho) that have not become identical as yet.

The above relation indicates that the frequency of heterozygotes in an inbred population is decreased in proportion to $1 - F$ of the heterozygosity in base population. Therefore, the proportion of heterozygote in any generation (t) that remains present under inbreeding $[H_{I(t)}]$ can be expressed in terms of the fraction of heterozygote in base population (Ho) as:

$$H_{I\,(t)} = Ho\,(1 - F_t) \qquad \text{................. Eq. 10.2 (a)}$$
$$= 2p_0 q_0\,(1 - F_t).$$

$$1 - F_t = \dfrac{H_t}{H_O} \qquad \text{................. Eq. 10.2 (b)}$$

$= $ *Panmictic index* (P_t) called by Wright (1951).

10.2 Consequences of Homozygosity

The increase in homozygosity due to inbreeding has the following consequences:

(i) Genetic Structure

The inbreeding changes the *genetic structure* of the inbred population by changing the genotypic frequencies. With complete inbreeding (F = 0), the heterozygotes are completely eliminated from the population and the whole inbred population contains only the homozygotes. The frequencies of homozygotes for two alleles (dominant and recessive) become equal to the allelic frequencies of base population.

The above relation, Eq. 10.2 (a), $H_I = 2p_0 q_0 (1 - F)$, indicates that the frequency of heterozygote in an inbred population is equal to $2p_0 q_0 (1 - F)$. Thus, the change in the frequency of heterozygote due to inbreeding is $-2\,p_0 q_0\,F$. This is the loss of heterozygote with inbreeding. The heterozygote lost due to inbreeding $(2\,p_0 q_0 F)$ is converted into identical homozygote for both the alleles. Thus, the rate of increase in homozygosity is $2pqF$ in each generation. The conversion of heterozygote into homozygote is equal to $p_0 q_0 F$ for each of the two alleles (A and a). Therefore, the increase in AA homozygote per generation is equal to pqF and the increase in aa homozygote is also equal to pqF.

Estimation of Frequency of each Homozygote under Inbreeding

The increase in identical homozygote for the two alleles (AA and aa) in an inbred population can be estimated, separately.

The frequency of allele A is represented by p and frequency of AA genotype is represented by D. The $p = D + \frac{1}{2} H$ and $H_1 = 2pq\,(1 - F)$.

The *frequency of AA genotype in an inbred population* will be:

$$p_0 \quad\quad = D_0 + \tfrac{1}{2}\,H_0$$

$$D_0 \quad\quad = p_0 - \tfrac{1}{2}\,H_0$$

$$D_{(AA)\,I} = p_0 - \tfrac{1}{2}\,[2p_0 q_0\,(1 - F)] \quad\quad\quad \text{Under inbreeding}$$

$$= p_0 - p_0 q_0\,(1 - F) = p_0 - p_0 q_0 + p_0 q_0 F$$

$$= p_0\,(1 - q_0) + p_0 q_0 F$$

$$= p_0^2 + p_0 q_0 F \quad\quad\quad\quad\quad\quad\quad\quad\quad\quad \text{Eq 10.3 (a)}$$

or$\quad\quad$ $p_0 - p_0 q_0\,(1 - F) = p_0 - p_0(1 - p_0)\,(1 - F)$

$$= p_0 - p_0 + p_0^2 + p_0 F - p_0^2 F$$

$$= p_0^2\,(1 - F) + p_0 F \quad\quad\quad\quad\quad\quad\quad\quad \text{Eq 10.3 (b)}$$

The equation 10.3 (a) has indicated that the genotype AA after inbreeding has two component parts *viz.* $p_0^2 + p_0 q_0 F$. The first component part (p_0^2) of inbred genotype $[D_{(AA)I}]$ is the original part of homozygous genotype whereas the second component part $(p_0 q_0 F)$ is due inbreeding.

The equation 10.3 (b) above has also partitioned the inbred genotype $[D_{(AA)I}]$ in two component parts *viz.* $p_0^2\,(1 - F)$ and $p_0 F$. However, both component parts $[p_0^2\,(1 - F) + p_0 F]$ of inbred genotype $[D_{(AA)I}]$ are homozygote but with a difference that first part is the independent or random component of allozygous alleles (*i.e.* alleles identical by state) and the second part $(p_0 q_0 F)$ corresponds to increased homozygosity due to inbreeding (alleles identical by descent).

The *frequency of aa homozygote in an inbred population* will be obtained similarly as –

$$R_{(aa)\,I} = q - \tfrac{1}{2}\,H$$

$$= q_0 - \tfrac{1}{2}\,[2p_0 q_0\,(1 - F)]$$

On solving/simplification, this becomes as –

$$R_{(aa)\,I} = q_0^2 + p_0 q_0 F \quad\quad\quad\quad\quad \text{.................. Eq. 10.4 (a)}$$

$$= q_0^2\,(1 - F) + q_0 F \quad\quad\quad\quad \text{.................. Eq. 10.4 (b)}$$

Therefore, the frequencies of 3 genotypes present under random mating $(p_0^2, 2p_0q_0, q_0^2)$ are changed after inbreeding as under:

Table 10.1: Genotype Frequencies for a Locus with Two Alleles under Inbreeding

Geno-types	Random Mating (F = 0)	With inbreeding coefficient F			Complete Inbreeding (F = 1)
		Original +	Change Due to Inbreeding	Allozygous + Autozygous (Identical)	
AA	p_0^2	$= p_0^2 +$	p_0q_0F	$= p_0^2(1-F) \quad + p_0F$	p_0
Aa	$2p_0q_0$	$= 2p_0q_0 -$	$2p_0q_0F$	$= 2p_0q_0(1-F)$	
aa	q_0^2	$= q_0^2 +$	p_0q_0F	$= q_0^2(1-F) \quad + q_0F$	q_0

The fraction of identical homozygote equals to F and hence, F is the probability of identical homozygote.

Component Parts of Identical Homozygote

It is an important point to consider that the inbreeding coefficient of subsequent generations is made up of two parts *viz.* an increment in F due to inbreeding (ΔF) and the reminder part attributable to the previous inbreeding (F_{t-1}) having the inbreeding coefficient of the previous generation. Thus, the cumulative F has two parts which are new F (ΔF) and F from previous generation (F_{t-1}). The new inbreeding (ΔF) brings together the genes that were replicated in the grand parent generation. These two parts are the components of identical homozygote which are called as new inbreeding (increment in inbreeding, ΔF) and the old inbreeding (F_{t-1}). Therefore, the value of F is cumulative and every generation identical homozygote arises by new replication of genes and by previous replication of genes. This characteristic of F is helpful in comparing the inbreeding effects of different breeding systems.

The consequence of inbreeding is to produce an excess of homozygote and deficiency of heterozygote. However, the reasons of the differences may be others like subdivision of population into sub groups known as stratification principle or Wahlund effect, selection favouring homozygote, assortative mating for homozygote, and presence of silent recessive alleles. Therefore, the breeding structure of the population (migration, selective value of genotypes) should be exactly known to conclude the cause of the discrepancy and to interpret the deviations from the square law. This is because many evolutionary forces may conspire to reduce F to zero which leads the genotypes into confirmation of HWE, *viz.* selection in favour of heterozygote will counteract the effect of inbreeding (and the reduction of heterozygote by inbreeding will not be appeared).

Homozygosity Under different Systems of Inbreeding

The rate of decrease in heterozygosity depends upon the intensity of inbreeding. The rate of decrease in heterozygosity and consequent increase in homozygosity (F) per generation with full sib mating and also with parent-offspring mating is ¼ which means that ¼ of the total non-identical genotypes are made identical homozygous and hence F = 0.25 among the progeny produced by full sib mating and parent-offspring mating. Under half- sib mating, $\frac{1}{8}$ of the non- identical genotypes are made identical and hence F = 0.125 among the progeny of half sibs.

The net amount of increase in homozygosity is more in first generation and in early generations than in subsequent generations under any system of inbreeding. However, the rate of increase is same in all generations.

(ii) Frequency of Recessive Traits

The most important feature of inbreeding is that it increases the frequency of recessive traits that are rarely present in a random mating population. This is because the frequency of recessive homozygous genotype is increased due to inbreeding. Many recessive genes, being paired with dominant genes remain hidden in out-bred population, are brought in homozygous condition by inbreeding. The inbreeding thus brings the recessive genes, present in rare frequency in a random mating population, to light by increasing the frequency of homozygous recessive individuals in the population. The recessive genes have unfavourable effect and hence the homozygous recessive individuals are undesirable.

This is well known for inherited diseases controlled by recessive genes in homozygous condition. This can be seen by comparing the recessive genotype (R) under inbreeding [$R_1 = q^2 (1-F) + qF$] with that in random mating population [$R_0 = q2$]. This ratio of $R_1 : R_0$ is increased with the decrease in the frequency of recessive allele and with the increase in the degree of inbreeding (F). Therefore, the incidence of the disease/defect is increased among the progeny produced by mating of more closely relatives. The risk of an affected progeny under inbreeding relative to that from a mating of non-relatives (random mating) will be $\dfrac{\left[q^2(1-F)+qF\right]}{q^2} = (1-F)+\left(\dfrac{F}{q}\right)$.

The risk will be increased with the increase in the degree of inbreeding and with the decrease in the frequency of recessive allele. The inbreeding has thus greater effect when the frequency of deleterious recessive allele is rare in the base population. Therefore, more intense selection by culling less desirable individuals from the herd is required and hence a large population is needed to develop a superior line.

The probability of the genotype *aa* is q^2 (1-F) + qF in an inbred population. If *a* denotes the rare deleterious recessive allele, then among the progeny of first cousin mating (inbreeding) the frequency of *aa* genotype is

$$q^2(1-F)+qF = q^2\left(1-\frac{1}{16}\right)+q\left(\frac{1}{16}\right) \text{ because } F = \frac{1}{16} \text{ for these progenies where as the}$$

frequency of recessive homozygote with random mating is q^2. Therefore, the risk of an affected offspring from a first cousins mating relative to random mating will be:

$$\frac{q^2(1-F)+qF}{q^2} \qquad = (1-F)+\left(\frac{F}{q}\right) = 0.9375+\left(\frac{0.0625}{q}\right)$$

$$= 1.56 \qquad\qquad \text{for } q = 0.1$$

$$= 2.18 \qquad \text{for } q = 0.05$$
$$= 7.18 \qquad \text{for } q = 0.01$$

Therefore, the inbreeding has greater effect when the frequency of the deleterious recessive allele is rare.

(iii) The inbreeding leads to *gene fixation*, increases *prepotency* and also increases the *phenotypic similarity* among relatives. The homozygosity is equally increased for dominant genes, thereby increasing the frequency of homozygous dominant animals which are more desirable than homozygous recessive animals. These inbred parents homozygous for dominant genes are more potent to transmit their characteristics to their progeny than non-inbred parents. This results the progeny to resemble their parents.

(iv) The inbreeding leads to *genetic differentiation between lines and genetic similarity within line*. The inbreeding has an effect on heritability to reduce it within lines because of decrease in additive genetic variance within line on inbreeding

Inbreeding and Gene Frequencies

The inbreeding does not change the gene frequencies, inspite of changing the genotype frequencies in favour of the homozygote. This has been shown above. Therefore, the F is independent of gene frequencies.

10.3 Properties of Inbreeding Equilibrium Population (Effects of Inbreeding on Population Structure)

(1) Wright's Equilibrium – Zygotic Proportions Under Inbreeding

The genotypic frequencies for a single locus with two alleles under inbreeding has been given in table 10.1

These genotypic frequencies remain constant with constant value of F from generation to generation. This is called as Wright's Equilibrium Law. The gene frequencies are not changed along the change in F but the genotypic frequencies are changed with a change in F. Thus F is independent of gene frequencies and gives an indication of the association of genes into pairs (genotypes).

Change in genotypic proportions with different values of F with p = q = 0.5.

		Genotype Frequencies		
F	p	D $(p^2 + pqF)$	H $2pq\,(1 - F)$	R $(q^2 + pqF)$
0	0.5	0.25	0.50	0.25
0.25	0.5	0.3125	0.375	0.3125
0.50	0.5	0.375	0.25	0.375
0.75	0.5	0.4375	0.125	0.4375
1.0	0.5	0.50	0.0 0.50	

The above genotypic frequencies with some degree of inbreeding are intermediate between the zygotic frequencies in a random mating population (p^2, $2pq$, q^2) and those occurred in a completely inbred population (p, o, q) for any value of gene frequency. Thus the Wright's proportions of genotypes can be expressed as deviation from random mating proportions (p^2, $2pq$, q^2) and as deviation from the case of complete inbreeding (Table 10.1). There is also another way to represent the genotypic proportions under inbreeding. This is as given in Table 10.1

Random (panmictic) component: $(1-F)$ $(p^2, 2pq, q^2)$ = Allozgous

plus identical component: $F(p, 0, q)$ = Autozygous

Thus, the total genotypic proportions including random and identical components are: $(1-F)$ $(p^2 + 2pq + q^2) + F(p + 0 + q)$. The random component consists of $(1-F)$ of the whole population and represents allozygous while the identical or completely inbred or fixed component consists of F of the whole population and represents the autozygous.

(2) Relation between Heterozygote and Homozygote

The property an equilibrium population states that the proportion of heterozygote is twice the square root of the product of the two types of homozygote.

$H = 2\sqrt{DR}$ and hence, $H^2 = 4DR$

This property is used as a test of equilibrium, is independent of gene frequencies, and relates the values of D, H. R under random mating. In a random mating population,

$4DR - H^2 = 0$ and

$$\frac{D}{\left(D+\frac{1}{2}H\right)} + \frac{R}{\left(R+\frac{1}{2}H\right)} = \frac{D}{p} + \frac{R}{q} = 1.0$$

In an inbred population, the frequencies of both the homozygote are increased at the expense of the frequency of heterozygote. Therefore, in an inbred population, $4DR - H^2 > 0$ and similarly $D/p + R/q > 1.0$. The excess amount represents the inbreeding coefficient. Therefore, in an inbred population,

$$\frac{D}{\left(D+\frac{1}{2}H\right)} + \frac{R}{\left(R+\frac{1}{2}H\right)} = \frac{D}{p} + \frac{R}{q} = 1.0 - F$$

Under random mating, $H = 2pq$ and hence $H^2 = 4p^2q^2 = 4DR$. Therefore, $4DR - H^2 = 0$. However, this expression ($4DR - H^2$) will be greater than zero under inbreeding. This can be verified by substituting the genotypic frequencies under inbreeding into this expression as:

$4DR - H^2$ $= 4 (p^2 + pqF) (q^2 + pqF) - [2pq (1-F)]^2$.

$= 4 p^2q F + 4 p q^2 F + 8 p^2 q^2 F$

$= 4 pqF$

(3) Equilateral Triangle Property

Any population (D, H, R) under random mating may be represented by a point (P) in an equilateral triangle. The points representing different populations in equilibrium condition lie on the parabola and thus any equilibrium population corresponds to a point on the parabola. A perpendicular from the point P to the base divides the base in two segments which are proportional to gene frequencies. This property holds true for any equilibrium population with different gene frequencies.

In an inbred population under continuous inbreeding the F is increased and hence the genotypic frequencies are changed but without changing the gene frequencies. The genotypic frequencies of an inbred population can also be represented by a point P inside the equilateral triangle either with fixed value of F for various gene frequencies in different populations or with changing F in an inbred population. As the gene frequencies do not change along change in F, so the point P representing the genotypic frequencies in inbred population for different values of F, should be located anywhere on the perpendicular (projection) drawn from P to the base of triangle instead of changing the location of P on the parabola. Therefore, the inbreeding moves the point P, representing inbred populations with same gene frequencies with changing F. along the perpendicular drawn to the base of the triangle. The frequency of heterozygote is represented by perpendicular distance from the point P to the base and in inbred population the frequency of heterozygote is less than under random mating. Therefore, the inbreeding press the parabola down towards the base of the triangle and with complete inbreeding (F = 1) the parabola coincides with the base. Thus inbreeding moves the point P towards the base in a vertical direction along a projection to the base because there is no change in gene frequencies under inbreeding while the point P moves along the parabola with change in gene frequencies due to any force like selection. The change in position of P in a vertical direction on the perpendicular represents the equation of the parabola is: $4DR - H^2 = 4 F pq$.

(4) Frequencies of Mating

The heterozygous mating (Aa x Aa) are twice as frequent as those between the two different homozygote (AA x aa and aa x AA) in an equilibrium population. This relation is entirely independent of the gene frequencies in the population. This relationship holds true for any random mating population or with any degree of inbreeding in the population and for any kind of equilibrium population. Therefore, f (Aa x Aa) = 2f (AAx Aa) = 2 f (AA x aa + aa x AA). Fisher (1918) noted this property of equilibrium population while working on the corelations between relatives on the supposition of Mendelian inheritance. The reason has already been explained in Chapter 3 under point 3 of section 3.2.3.

The frequencies of parental mating are used to estimate the genotypic frequencies of offspring generation. The mating of 3 genotypes in all combinations produces the progeny in the proportion as outlined under section 3.2.3.

(5) Change in Population Mean on Inbreeding

It is well known that inbreeding has harmful effects on reproduction and vigour and hence it is avoided as far as possible, except for some specific purposes *viz.*

development of inbred lines (genetically uniform) for using them in bioassay and research work as well as for crossing the lines to take the advantage of hybrid vigour.

The inbreeding changes the genetic structure of population (genotype frequencies). It is now important to see the effect of these changes in genotypic frequencies on the quantitative traits. The population mean of productive traits is reduced due to inbreeding and this reduction is known as *inbreeding depression.* The population mean of a random mating population for single locus two alleles is: $M_o =$ a (p-q) + 2pqd.

The M_0 has two components attributed to the homozygotes [a (p-q)] and to the heterozygotes (2pqd). The proportion of two types of homozygotes in an inbred population is increased equally and hence do not contribute to the population mean whereas the proportion of heterozygotes is reduced to 2pq (1-F) in an inbred population from 2pq of the random bred population. The population mean under inbreeding will be:

$$M_I = a (p-q) + 2pqd (1-F)$$
$$= a (p-q) + 2pqd - 2pqdF$$
$$= M_0 - 2pqdF$$

This can be verified from weighted average of genotypic values, *i.e.* weighting the genotypic values with their frequencies as:

Genotypes	Freq. in Inbred Population	Genotypic Values	Freq. x Value
A_1A_1	$p^2 + pqF$	a	$a (p^2 + pqF)$
A_1A_2	$2pq (1-F)$	d	$d[2pq (1-F)]$
A_2A_2	$q^2 + pqF$	$- a$	$- a (q^2 + pqF)$

$$\text{Total} = M_I = a (p^2 + pqF) - a (q^2 + pqF) + d[2pq (1-F)]$$
$$= ap^2 + apqF - aq^2 - apqF + 2pqd - 2pqdF$$
$$= a (p^2 - q^2) + 2pqd - 2pqdF$$
$$= a (p-q) + 2pqd - 2pqdF$$
$$= M_0 - 2pqdF$$

(6) Change of Variance on Inbreeding

The inbreeding besides reducing the mean value also changes the variance. The inbreeding influences both genetic as well as environmental variance.

(i) Genetic Variance

The inbreeding differentiates the base population into distinct lines with extreme values of gene frequencies as 0 or 1.0, as a result of gene fixation. The different alleles become homozygous in different lines arising from base population. This results a decrease in the genetic variance within lines or families on inbreeding and the genetic differences between lines become more and the total additive variance (between and within, lines) increases. This means that the inbreeding leads to genetic differences between lines and genetic similarity within lines. The genetic variance within lines decreases because the gene frequencies at extreme values reduce the genetic component of variance. Redistribution of genetic variance is therefore one of the consequence of inbreeding leading to the increase of genetic component between the means of lines and a decrease of component within the lines.

(a) No Dominance

When there is no dominance (d=0), the variance is due to additive genes and the complete genetic variance is explained by the additive variance.

In a random mating population, the total genetic variance is:

$V_{G.T(0)} = \sigma^2_{A0} = 2p_0q_0a^2$ which is equal to a^2 times the frequencies of heterozygotes.

In an inbred population, the *total genetic variance* is: $V_{G.T(I)} = 2pq(1 + F)$. This is the variance of whole population. Thus, F is also a measure of the percentage increase of genetic variance due to inbreeding. The total genetic variance in the whole population with complete inbreeding (F = 1.0) will be doubled to that of the genetic variance in the base population (random mating). Thus, $V_{G.T(I)} = 2\,V_{G0}\,F$.

This total genetic variance represents the *between line variance,* because the within line variance ($V_{G.W}$) with complete inbreeding becomes zero ($V_{G.W} = 0$) as the inbred lines become completely homozygous. Thus, the total genetic variance in the whole population under inbreeding is the between line genetic variance which is as:

$V_{G.T(I)} = 2\,V_{G0}\,F = V_{G.B}$

The *within line genetic variance* ($V_{G.W}$) on inbreeding can be obtained from $V_{G0} = V_A = 2p_0q_0a^2$. The frequency of heterozygotes in an inbred population is equal to $2pq$ (1-F) and hence it is reduced by an amount equal to $2pqF$. This also reduces the genetic differences within line and hence the genetic variance within line can be obtained as:

$$V_{G.W} = 2p_0q_0a^2(1\text{-}F)$$
$$= V_{G0}(1\text{-}F).$$

Thus, the genetic variance within line ($V_{G.W}$) under inbreeding is reduced equal to $V_{G0}F$. This genetic variance within line is reduces to zero with complete inbreeding. Thus, there is no genetic variance in a complete inbred line.

The break up of the total genetic variance is into between line genetic variance (2 V_{G0} F) and within line genetic variance [$V_{G0}(1\text{-}F)$]. This is as under-

$$V_{G.T} = V_{G.B} + V_{G.W}$$
$$V_{G0}(1\text{+}F) = 2\,V_{G0}\,F + V_{G0}(1\text{-}F).$$

(b) Dominance

The change of genetic variance on inbreeding depends on initial gene frequencies with any degree of dominance unlike the change of genetic variance due to additive genes. It is thus difficult to generalize the situation. The effect of inbreeding on variation is due to recessive genes. The within line variance increases in first few generations of inbred up to F = 0.5, remains more or less constant till F approaches 1.0 and the increase is associated with the relation of gene frequency and the variance due to dominant gene. The between line variance and total genetic variance increase with the increase in rate of inbreeding.

(ii) Environmental Variance

The genetic variance in inbred lines as well as in their hybrids (F_1) is negligible and hence the difference in phenotypic variance between them represents the environmental part of variance. The environmental variance differs between inbred and hybrids. The inbred are more susceptible to environmental factors than hybrids and hence the inbred individuals show more environmental variance than non-inbred. The environmental variation may be induced or variation may be in adaptability of individuals to different environments. There are some characters like body temperature which are not influenced by environmental variations. This restriction of variation is known as homeostasis. There are some other characters like amount of sweat which vary with variation in ambient temperature. The relation of these two types of characters with fitness is different. The individuals for homeostatic characters are fittest by regulating their physiological functions in different environments while the individuals for second category of characters are fittest by varying according to environmental conditions. The homeostasis, which may be under the control of certain genes, may be reduced by inbreeding and hence it may leads to an increase in environmental variance of inbred. Secondly, the heterozygotes produce two enzymes which provide a biochemical diversity making the heterozygotes to be well buffered to different environments while the homozygotes produce only one enzyme.

10.4 Genetic Causes of Inbreeding Depression

The amount of change in population mean on inbreeding (– 2pqdF), called the inbreeding depression, indicates the followings:

☆ There is reduction in mean of an inbred population compared to the mean of a random mating population and it equals to the amount of 2pqdF.

☆ The reduction in population mean is a function of gene frequencies, the degree of inbreeding and dominance among alleles.

(i) The change in mean due to inbreeding is greatest at intermediate gene frequencies (p = q = ½). This is because the inbreeding depression depends on the frequencies of heterozygotes which are maximum when p = q = ½. Therefore, if inbreeding is started in a completely heterozygous population (crossbreds produced by crossing two breeds or pure line), inbreeding depression will be maximum compared to that started in a population with high or low gene frequencies.

(ii) The inbreeding depression is linear to the degree of inbreeding, provided there is dominance. This is because inbreeding depression equals – 2pqdF.

(iii) The change in population mean under inbreeding depends on the type of gene action *viz.* additive or non-additive gene action (dominance, over-dominance and epistasis).

(a) In case of **additive effect,** there will be no change of mean on inbreeding. Therefore, no change in mean due to inbreeding is thus an indication of the additive gene action. *It is thus said that inbreeding is not always harmful.* The inbreeding is not harmful or detrimental for traits affected by additive gene action. Additive genes are made homozugous without regard to their effect. The additive genes are thus least affected by increase in homozygosity. Thus, homozygosity has no meaning for genes that act additively. The merit of the population is increased till the genetic variation is fully exhausted, provided there is selection in favour of superior individuals. The selection plays an important role. The selection increases the mean value whereas no selection results no decline in mean value under inbreeding, in case of additive gene action. The proportion of the total variation in a trait controlled by additive gene action is measured by heritability. The traits controlled mostly by additive gene action have high heritability estimates. Therefore, the amount of inbreeding depression in a trait is inversely related to the size of heritability.

(b) In absence of dominance among alleles ($d = 0$), there will be no change in mean on inbreeding. This is because the inbreeding depression equals -$2pqdF$. Further, in case of polygenic traits, the dominance is not sufficient cause of inbreeding depression but it is the directional dominance. The inbreeding depression will occur only if the dominance effect of all or most of the loci are in the same direction (**directional dominance**). The dominance in both the directions in equal amount will not change the mean on inbreeding. The inbreeding will reduce the mean if favourable genes are dominant over their alleles which are not favourable. The reduction in mean of an inbred population is further due to the expression of recessive alleles, coming into homozygous condition, which remain hidden by dominant alleles in a non- inbred population. This results the average value of the population to reduce towards the value of recessive genotype. The selection against recessive genotype can counteract the effect of inbreeding on population mean. Ina case of complete homozygosity for dominant alleles that increase the value of the trait there will not be any decrease in the mean value of the character.

(c) The reduction in mean value is more in case of **overdominance** when heterozygotes exceed to that of the better homozygote. Since inbreeding increases the homozygosity at the expense of heterozygosity, a reduction in mean value of a trait affected by over-dominance of alleles is likely to occur if there has been no selection for more desirable individuals. The selection for desirable individuals means the selection in favour of heterozygotes and hence the increase in homozygosity will be at a lower rate in the inbred population. The inbreeding leads to a decline when dominance is positive (alleles with positive effects are dominant). This makes the heterozygotes to be superior compared to either homozygotes. Therefore, as long as **d** is positive, the inbreeding will produce a decline in mean value of the inbred population. Thus, the positive dominance (favourable alleles to be dominant, directional dominance) and over-dominance are the two possible causes of reduction in mean value on inbreeding.

(d) For polygenic traits, the **epistasis** without dominance does not produce a decrease in the mean. However, the dominance and overdominance with no epistasis decrease the mean on inbreeding proportional to F. The inbreeding effect may be quadratic in F if there is both dominance and epistasis. There is no inbreeding effect without dominance whether or not there is epistasis.

10.5 Physiological Bases of Inbreeding Effect

The inbred are more susceptible to change in environment than outbreds. There is in general reduction in growth rate and fertility but an increase in death rates and susceptibility to diseases among inbred. These effects seem to be the consequence of the combined effect of many pairs of recessive genes rather than at particular locus. The inbreeding changes the genotypic frequencies in favour of homozygotes and it leads to an increase in more pairs of recessive genes among inbred individuals, though the frequency of recessive gene does not change but they appear more often as homozygotes. The reason of detrimental effect of homozygous recessive genotypes may be the deficiency of essential enzymes that could have been produced by their dominant alleles or due to the production of abnormal proteins by recessive homozygotes. Not only this, but there could be some imbalance of some hormones among inbred.

10.6 Regular Systems of Inbreeding

The mating of relatives of the same degree of relationship in each succeeding generation is called the regular systems of inbreeding. As the same mating system is practiced in all generations under regular system of inbreeding, all the individuals in the same generation have the same inbreeding coefficient. Under these systems, the F increases in a regular and predictable fashion. Such systems include selfing, sib mating (full sibs, half sibs), parent-offspring mating, mating of cousins of various degree of relationship, repeated back cross with parent (line breeding) which may be highly inbred or random bred.

The *purpose of regular systems of inbreeding* is to produce rapid inbreeding for which the mating of close relatives is made. It is often useful to know how rapidly the inbreeding coefficient increases under regular system of mating. The method of computing inbreeding coefficient from pedigrees can be used to derive recurrent relations for inbreeding coefficient in successive generations under regular systems of inbreeding. The recurrent equation relates the inbreeding coefficient in any generation (t) to its previous generations (t-1, t-2) under any regular system of inbreeding. The generation of interest for practical purposes is indicated by t, the previous one generation by t-1 and likewise t-2, t-3 going far back.

The F in successive generations can be calculated from co-ancestries before actual mating is done. Thus, it is important to understand about the co-ancestry, its method of computation and the basic co-ancestries of different mating systems.

10.7 Co-Ancestry

The co-ancestry is the degree of relationship by descent between the two individuals and it is identical with the inbreeding coefficient of their progeny if they are mated. Therefore, the co-ancestry of two individuals is the probability that two gametes taken at random, one from each, carry alleles identical by descent.

The inbreeding coefficient of an individual depends on the amount of co-ancestry of its two parents. The inbreeding coefficients in successive generations can be estimated from the co-ancestries of the pedigrees of real population, known as *pedigreed population*. The computation of inbreeding coefficient from co-ancestry is more convenient and used in solving many problems. The calculation inbreeding coefficient from co-ancestry is mainly used in planning of the mating to avoid inbreeding. The method of co-ancestry for calculating the inbreeding coefficient is not different from path coefficient method used in pedigreed population. However, it differ in the sense that this method works based on forward calculation to know the inbreeding coefficient of the progeny that will be produced from a particular mating whereas the path coefficient method work by tracing from the present back to the common ancestors. This is because the inbreeding coefficient of the progeny depends on the amount of common ancestry of the mated pair.

10.7.1 Computation of Co-ancestry

The co-ancestry or the coefficient of co-ancestry of two individuals is computed in two ways, depending on the generation to which they belong *i.e.* whether they belong to the same generation or to different generations.

(i) Co-ancestry of Two Individuals of same Generation

It is taken as the average relationship of the parents of one individual with the parents of the other individual. Consider the following pedigree of Z individual with its parents X and Y which are not related and hence have their 4 parents (A and B are the parents of X while C and D are the parents of Y).

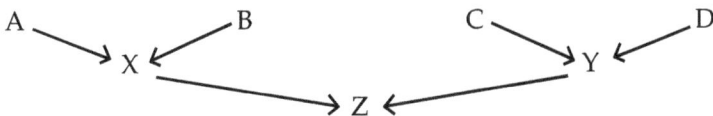

Figure 10.1

The co-ancestry of X and Y (f_{XY}) in the above pedigree is taken as the average of the 4 co-ancestries of their parents taking:

X = ½ A + ½ B and Y = ½ C + ½ D

Therefore, f_{XY} $= f\left(\dfrac{1}{2}A + \dfrac{1}{2}B\right)\left(\dfrac{1}{2}C + \dfrac{1}{2}D\right)$

$$= \frac{1}{4}\left(f_{AC} + f_{AD} + f_{BC} + f_{BD}\right)$$

$$= F_Z$$

And hence, the coefficient of co-ancestry between two individuals equals the average of the coefficient of co-ancestry between their respective parents.

(ii) Co-ancestry of Two Individuals of different Generations

It is taken as the average of the co-ancestry of any one individual with parents of the other individual as:

(a) *Co-ancestry of X with parents of Y:*

$$Y = \frac{1}{2}C + \frac{1}{2}D \qquad \text{Thus,}$$

$$f_{XY} = f_{X\left(\frac{1}{2}C + \frac{1}{2}D\right)} = \frac{1}{2}f_{XC} + \frac{1}{2}f_{XD}$$

$$= \frac{1}{2}f_{XC} + \frac{1}{2}f_{XD}$$

$$= F_Z$$

(b) *Co-ancestry of Y with parents of X:*

$$X = \frac{1}{2}A + \frac{1}{2}B \qquad \text{Thus,}$$

$$f_{XY} = f_{Y\left(\frac{1}{2}A + \frac{1}{2}B\right)} = \frac{1}{2}f_{YA} + \frac{1}{2}f_{YB}$$

$$= \frac{1}{2}f_{YA} + \frac{1}{2}f_{YB}$$

$$= F_Z$$

According to this procedure of co-ancestry of two individuals of different generations, the co-ancestry of X with parents (C and D) of other individual (Y) belonging to different generations can be computed as:

$$f_{XC} = f_{C\left(\frac{1}{2}A + \frac{1}{2}B\right)} = \frac{1}{2}f_{AC} + \frac{1}{2}f_{BC} = \frac{1}{2}\left(f_{AC} + f_{BC}\right)$$

$$f_{XD} = f_{D\left(\frac{1}{2}A + \frac{1}{2}B\right)} = \frac{1}{2}f_{AD} + \frac{1}{2}f_{BD} = \frac{1}{2}\left(f_{AD} + f_{BD}\right)$$

$$f_{AY} = f_{A\left(\frac{1}{2}C + \frac{1}{2}D\right)} = \frac{1}{2}f_{AC} + \frac{1}{2}f_{AD} = \frac{1}{2}\left(f_{AC} + f_{AD}\right)$$

$$f_{BY} = f_{B\left(\frac{1}{2}C+\frac{1}{2}D\right)} = \frac{1}{2}f_{BC} + \frac{1}{2}f_{BD} = \frac{1}{2}\left(f_{BC} + f_{BD}\right)$$

Now, the f_{XY} can be computed either as the average of the f_{XC} and f_{XD} or as the average of the f_{YA} and f_{YB}:

$$f_{XY} = \frac{1}{2}\left(f_{XC} + f_{XD}\right)$$

$$= \frac{1}{2}\left(\frac{1}{2}f_{AC} + \frac{1}{2}f_{BC} + \frac{1}{2}f_{AD} + \frac{1}{2}f_{BD}\right)$$

$$= \frac{1}{4}\left(f_{AC} + f_{BC} + f_{AD} + f_{BD}\right) = Fz$$

or $$f_{XY} = \frac{1}{2}\left(f_{YA} + f_{YB}\right)$$

$$= \frac{1}{2}\left(\frac{1}{2}f_{AC} + \frac{1}{2}f_{AD} + \frac{1}{2}f_{BC} + \frac{1}{2}f_{BD}\right)$$

$$= \frac{1}{4}\left(f_{AC} + f_{AD} + f_{BC} + f_{BD}\right) = Fz$$

10.7.2 Basic Co-ancestries

The most important co-ancestries are the co-ancestry of an individual with itself and with its parents, and of sibs (FS and HS).

(i) Co-ancestry of Individual with Itself (Selfing, f_{XX})

Consider an individual which carries two alleles (A_1 and A_2) at a locus. The probability that the two gametes produced by this individual, taken at random, are both A_1 or both A_2 is ½ and the probability that one is A_1 and the other is A_2 is also ½ but then the probability that A_1 and A_2 are identical by descent is the F of the progeny. Therefore, the total probability that the two gametes (A_1 and A_2) taken at random carry identical alleles is ½ + ½ F_X and so:

$$f_{XX} = \frac{1}{2} + \frac{1}{2}F_X = \frac{1}{2}\left(1 + F_X\right) \qquad \text{................ Eq. 10.5}$$

$$= \frac{1}{2} \qquad \text{when } F_X = 0$$

This is the coefficient of co-ancestry of an individual with itself (f_{XX}) which implies that the individual carries alleles identical by descent. This is the inbreeding coefficient of an offspring by selfing. Thus, F of an individual becomes as:

$$f_{XX} = \frac{1}{2}(1+F_X) \text{ and hence}$$

$$2f_{XX} = 1 + F_X$$

$$\text{Thus, } F_X = 2f_{XX} - 1$$

(ii) Co-ancestry of Parent-Offspring (f_{PO})

The co-ancestry of an individual X with its parent A (f_{XA}) is computed considering that A and B are two parents of X which are uncorrelated:

Parent offspring: When, Z = A + X and X = A + B

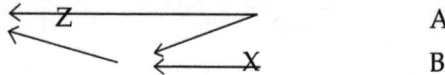

$$f_{AX.} = \text{Average co-ancestry of A with both parents of X which are A and B}$$

$$= f_{A\left(\frac{1}{2}A+\frac{1}{2}B\right)}$$

$$= \frac{1}{2}f_{AA} + \frac{1}{2}f_{AB}$$

$$= \frac{1}{2}\left[\left(\frac{1}{2}\right)+f_{AB}\right] \qquad \text{since, } f_{AA} = \frac{1}{2}(1+F_A) = \frac{1}{2}(1+0) = \frac{1}{2}$$

$$\text{and } f_{AB} = 0 \text{, since A \& B are uncorrelated}$$

$$= \frac{1}{4} = F_Z \qquad\qquad\qquad \text{..............} \text{Eq. 10.6}$$

Thus, co-ancestry of PO is ¼ which is F of their progeny (Fz).

(iii) Co-ancestry of sibs

The sibs belong to the same generation.

(a)   *Full sibs:* When, $Z = \frac{1}{2}X + \frac{1}{2}Y$; and $X = Y = \frac{1}{2}A + \frac{1}{2}B$

$$Fz = f_{XY}$$

$$= f_{\left(\frac{1}{2}A+\frac{1}{2}B\right)\left(\frac{1}{2}A+\frac{1}{2}B\right)}$$

$$= \frac{1}{4}f_{AA} + \frac{1}{4}f_{AB} + \frac{1}{4}f_{AB} + \frac{1}{4}f_{BB}$$

$$= \frac{1}{4}f_{AA} + \frac{1}{2}f_{AB} + \frac{1}{4}f_{BB}$$

$$= \frac{1}{4}\left(\frac{1}{2} + 0 + \frac{1}{2}\right) \qquad \text{when A and B are not correlated}$$

$$= \frac{1}{4} \qquad\qquad\qquad \text{................. Eq. 10.7}$$

or $\qquad$ = Average co-ancestry of X with parents of Y

$$= f_{X\left(\frac{1}{2}A + \frac{1}{2}B\right)} = \frac{1}{2}_{XA} + \frac{1}{2}_{XB}$$

$$= \frac{1}{2}(f_{XA} + f_{XB}) = \frac{1}{2}\left(\frac{1}{4} + \frac{1}{4}\right) \qquad \text{Since X and A are PO}$$

$$= \frac{1}{4}$$

Thus, co-ancestry of FS is $\dfrac{1}{4}$ which is the F of their progeny (Fz).

(b) Half sibs: When, Z = X + Y; X = A + B and Y = A + C

Fz $\qquad = F_{XY}$

$\qquad$ = Average co-ancestry of 4 parents of X and Y

$$= f_{\left(\frac{1}{2}A + \frac{1}{2}B\right)\left(\frac{1}{2}A + \frac{1}{2}C\right)}$$

$$= \frac{1}{4}f_{AA} + \frac{1}{4}f_{AC} + \frac{1}{4}f_{AB} + \frac{1}{4}f_{BC}$$

$$= \frac{1}{4}(f_{AA} + f_{AC} + f_{AB} + f_{BC})$$

$$= \frac{1}{4}\left(\frac{1}{2} + 0 + 0 + 0\right)$$

$$= \frac{1}{8} \qquad\qquad \text{................. Eq 10.8 with no previous inbreeding}$$

or $\qquad$ = Average co-ancestry of X with parents of Y

$$= f_{X\left(\frac{1}{2}A + \frac{1}{2}C\right)} = \frac{1}{2}(f_{XA} + f_{XC})$$

$$= \frac{1}{2}\left(\frac{1}{4} + 0\right)$$

$$= \frac{1}{8}$$

Thus, the co-ancestry of half sibs is $\frac{1}{8}$ which is the F of their progeny (Fz).

10.8 Recurrence Relations of F and H Under Various Systems of Inbreeding

The close inbreeding breaks the population into groups or isolates of size N depending upon the mating system of close inbreeding. The isolate sizes are N=1 under complete selfing, N = 2 under full sib mating, N = 4 under double first cousin mating, N = 8 under quadruple second cousin mating etc. The isolate size N = 2^K for more distant cousins.

Recurrence Equations of F and H

The recurrence equations to relate the F in one generation to the previous generations under different inbreeding systems (close inbreeding and cousin mating) can be formulated from the pedigree of the individual produced by a particular system of inbreeding.

10.8.1 Close Inbreeding (Selfing, Parent-offspring and Sib mating)

(i) Selfing

The selfing gives the most rapid inbreeding maximum possible, approaching the F as 0.999 after 10 generations. The recurrence relation under selfing can be computed, considering t – 2, t – 1 and t generations with respect to individuals of these generations (X, Y and Z0 as under –

Generations	Individuals
t–2	X
t –1	Y
t	Z

Figure 10.2: Selfing: The individuals are shown by letters and gametes by dotes.

The inbreeding coefficients of individuals of different generation can be calculated as:

$$F_{X(t-2)} \quad = 0 \text{ Since parents are non-inbred}$$

$$F_{Y(t-1)} \quad = f_{XX}$$

$$= \frac{1}{2}(1+F_X) = \frac{1}{2}(1+F_{Xt-2}) = \frac{1}{2}$$

$$F_{Z(t)} \quad = f_{YY}$$

$$= \frac{1}{2}(1+F_{t-2})$$

$$= \frac{1}{2}(1+F_{t-1}) \qquad \text{since Y belong to } t-1 \text{ generation}$$

$$= \frac{1}{2}\left(1+\frac{1}{2}\right) = \frac{3}{4}$$

Thus, in t generation, the recurrence equation of F under selfing becomes as:

$$F_t = \frac{1}{2}(1+F_{t-1})$$

The above equation of F_t indicates that homozygosity is increased each generation of selfing. The rate of increase in inbreeding (F) equals ½ and remains constant, going to 0.999 in 10th generation.

The consequent heterozygosity in t generation (Ht) can be estimated from equation 10.2 (a) of $H_t = H_o(1 - F_t)$ by putting the value of Ft = ½ (1 + F_{t-1}) as:

$$H_t \qquad = H_o(1-F_{t-1})$$

$$= \frac{1}{2}H_{t-1}$$

$$= \left(\frac{1}{2}\right)^2 H_{t-2}$$

$$= \left(\frac{1}{2}\right)^t H_0$$

and $H_{t-1} = \frac{1}{2}H_{t-2}$

Thus, the heterozygosity is decreased in each generation by half of that present in previous generation.

(ii) Full Sib Mating

Consider the pedigree of an individual X produced from mating of full sibs (P and Q) whose parents were A and B. The grand parents of individual X possess four alleles (A_1, A_2, A_3, A_4). Any of these 4 alleles may become identical homozygote in the individual X.

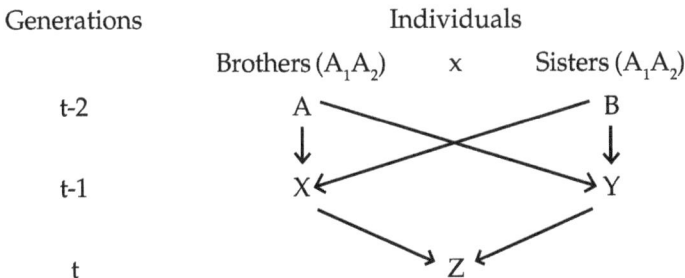

Generations   Individuals

Brothers (A_1A_2)   x   Sisters (A_1A_2)

t-2   A   B

t-1   X   Y

t   Z

The F_t can be obtained as:

$$F_Z = F_t = F_{XY} = \frac{1}{4}\left(f_{AA} + f_{BB} + 2f_{AB}\right)$$

Since, $f_{AA} = F_{BB} = \frac{1}{2}(1+F_A)$ and $f_{AB} = F_X = F_{t-1}$

Therefore, $F_t \qquad = \frac{1}{4}\left[\frac{1}{2}(1+F_{t-2})+\frac{1}{2}(1+F_{t-1})+ 2F_{t-1}\right]$

$$= \frac{1}{4}+\frac{1}{2}F_{t-1} +\frac{1}{4}F_{t-2}$$

This is the recurrence relation (equation) of F under full sib mating.

The recurrence relationship of heterozygosity can be obtained from F_t by converting F recurrence statement into H series as:

$$H_t \quad = H_0(1 - F_t)$$

$$= H_0\left(1-\frac{1}{4}-\frac{1}{2}F_{t-1}-\frac{1}{4}F_{t-2}\right) \quad \text{since} \quad F_t =\frac{1}{4}+\frac{1}{2}F_{t-1}+\frac{1}{4}F_{t-2}$$

$$= \frac{1}{2}H_{t-1} +\frac{1}{4}H_{t-2}$$

(iii) Other Systems of Close Inbreeding

Similarly, the recurrence equations of F and H for other systems of close mating (Parent-offspring mating, half sib mating) can be obtained from the co-ancestry of parent-offspring and of half sibs, respectively. (see Table 10.3)

The recurrence relations can be used to compute the F under different regular systems of inbreeding for subsequent generations. These have been given as under:

Table 10.2: Inbreeding coefficient under different systems of inbreeding

Inbreeding Generation	Selfing	Full Sib Mating	Parent-offspring Mating		Half sib Mating
			Younger Parent	Repeated to Same Parent	
0	0	0	0	•0	0
1	0.5	0.25	Same	0.25	0.125
2	0.75	0.375	as	0.375	0.219
3	0.875	0.50	for	0.438	0.305
4	0.938	0.594	full	0.469	0.381
5	0.969	0.672	Sibs	0.484	0.449

Inbreeding Generation	Selfing	Full Sib Mating	Parent-offspring Mating		Half sib Mating
			Younger Parent	Repeated to Same Parent	
6	0.984	0.734		0.492	0.509
7	0.992	0.785		0.496	0.563
8	0.996	0.826		0.498	0.611
9	0.998	0.859		0.499	0.654
10	0.999	0.886			0.691
15		0.961			0.827
20		0.986			0.903
Infinite	1	1		0.50	1

The relative increase of homozygosity or decrease of heterozygosity can be used to compare the different regular systems of inbreeding. The number of generations required for a comparative loss of heterozygosity can be estimated as

$$\text{Loss}_S = \text{Loss}^t_{FS} = \text{Loss}^{t'}_{HS}$$

Where,   S, FS, and HS indicate selfing, full sibs mating and half sib mating,

t, t' are the number of generations.

The loss of heterozygosity by one generation of selfing is ½ and equivalent to 3.27 generations of full sib mating or 5.95 generations of half sib mating. Thus, 1.82 generations of half sib mating are equivalent to one generation of full sib mating.

Gene Fixation

It may be of interest to know the probability of gene fixation due to inbreeding instead of inbreeding coefficient. It may be of interest to know that after how much time, all the individuals of a line are expected to become homozygous for the same allele at a particular locus. The number of alleles and their arrangement in the initial mating of the line determines the probability of gene fixation. The probability of fixation is more when the numbers of alleles are less. In a sib mated line there are maximum of four alleles and the probability of fixation at any one locus is 0, 0.063, 0.172, 0.293, 0.409, 0.5 12, 0.601, 0.675, 0.736, and 0.785 in generations first through ten under full sib mating. The probability of fixation becomes only a little less than the F after the first few generations *e.g.* the probability of fixation is 0.925 and the F is 0.961 in fifteenth generation while these are 0.975 and 0.986 in twentieth generation of full sib mating.

With continuous close inbreeding in a line, it is expected that the line becomes highly inbred and may be called as pure line which implies for the degree of purity of a line. The pure line concept is based on the probability of fixation at all loci or the proportion of the complete genome expected to be fixed. This is also known as the probability of total fixation which depends upon the total map length. The probability of total fixation can not be obtained. The complete purity of any line is virtually not attained. The probability of fixation of the locus depends, however, on the fixation of a locus linked to it. If one locus is fixed the other linked locus also become fixed. It takes long time for the total fixation than required for fixation of one locus. No individual is virtually expected to become completely homozygous for all loci and also no line totally gets fixed even after 20 generations of full sibs mating. It requires about 50 generations of sib mating to result in 95 per cent individuals to become completely homozygous and about 5 per cent of the genome is still expected to be heterozygous after 50 generations and the probability of total fixation is nearly the same after this period.

10.8.2. Cousin Mating

The offspring of sibs are termed as cousins. These offspring may be from full sibs or half sibs. Thus, the cousins are those individuals whose parents are sibs. In case of cousins from full sibs, parents of cousins may belong to a single family (called as ordinary or single first cousins) or to two separate families (called as double first cousins) or to four families of sib-ship (called as quardruple second cousins) or to eight families of sib-ships (called as octuple third cousins).

(i) Cousins from Two or more Sib-ships

    (a) *Double-first cousin mating*: The individuals whose parents belong to two sib-ships (full sibs of two families) are known as double first cousins. The individuals P and Q are double first cousins. Fathers of the cousins are full sibs as well as the mothers. Two full brothers are married with full sisters of another family. When only the double first cousins are mated in every generation, a number of separate lines of descents, called as isolates, are formed and each isolate has four individuals of two sib-ships whereas in case of sib mating each line of descent consist only two individuals of one sib-ship. Thus each breeding unit under the system of double first cousin mating consists of N = 4 individuals of two sib-ships. The mating within a group of four individuals in each generation is not random and hence the possible mating between full sibs and the selfing among the four individuals is excluded. Thus, the most distant relationship among these four individuals is that of double first cousins. It requires 3 generations before progeny of cousin mating could be produced. The rate of decrease in H is 8 per cent per generation.

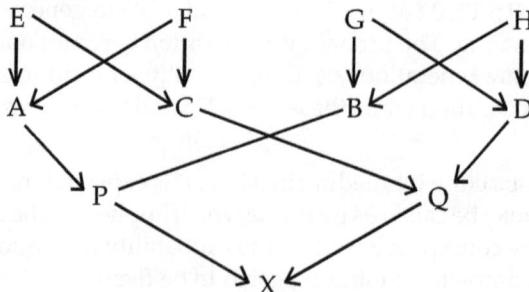

(b) *Quadruple-second-cousin mating*: This mating system breaks up the population into isolates of size N = 8 wherein the grand parents belong to four sib-ships. Among these 8 individuals the mating other than this system is excluded. The rate of decrease in H is 3.5 per cent per generation.

(c) *Octuple third cousin mating*: The continued exclusive octuple third cousin mating will give rise to isolate of size N = 16 wherein the grandparents belong to eight sib-ships. The eventual rate of decrease in H is 1.7 per cent per generation.

(ii) Cousins from One Sib Ship

Progeny from one full sib-ship: The progeny of full sibs of single family are called as single first cousins or first cousins or full cousins or simply cousins. The progeny of these single first cousins is known as single second cousin. In case of continued single first (or second) cousin mating, the limiting value of H is not necessarily zero if the mates are too distantly related.

(a) *Ordinary or single first cousin mating*: The inbreeding coefficient of the progeny produced by single first cousin mating can be obtained from the co-ancestry of the parents (single first cousins). P and Q are single first cousins. The grand-parents of single first cousins are considered as unrelated and hence $F_{t-3} = 0$. Therefore, the inbreeding coefficient of the children of single first cousins is $1/16 = 0.625$.

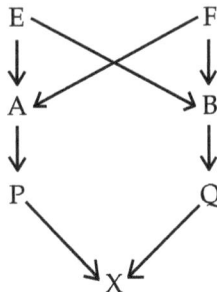

(b) *Single second cousin mating*: The progeny of single first cousins are termed as second cousins. These are thus the individuals whose only two out of eight grand-parents are full sibs. The value of F remains constant from generation to generation as long as the second cousin mating is continued. Thus, the limiting value of F is not unity. Therefore, even when all mating in a population are between relatives for an indefinite period it does not lead to complete homozygosis but to equilibrium condition with a constant F. The equilibrium value is nearly equal to that in a random mating population.

(c) *Half first cousins – Progeny from half sib-ship*: The half first cousins are the progeny of half sibs. The half first cousins are the mates in the next generation under the system of continued half-first cousin mating. The continued mating of this system leads to an equilibrium condition other than complete homozygosis. Therefore, the situation for continued mating between half first cousins is very similar to the continued mating between single second cousins.

In summary, the continued mating between relatives more remote than first cousins (single) cause only an insignificant decrease in heterozygosis of the population. Therefore, from population composition point of view such mating system can be hardly considered as inbreeding.

The *homozygosity and heterozygosity recurrence equations* for other close relative mating systems can be obtained in the similar way. These equations for different systems of inbreeding have been given here:

Table 10.3: Homozygosity and heterozygosity recurrence equations for different systems of inbreeding.

Sl.No.	Mating	Systems F_t Recurrence	H_t Recurrence
1.	Selfing	$\dfrac{1}{2}\left(1+F_{t-1}\right)$	$\dfrac{1}{2}H_{t-1}$
2.	Full sibs	$\dfrac{1}{4}+\dfrac{1}{2}F_{t-1}+\dfrac{1}{4}F_{t-2}$	$\dfrac{1}{2}H_{t-1}+\dfrac{1}{4}H_{t-2}$
3.	Parent-offspring:		
	(i) With younger parent	Same as for full sib	Same as for full sibs
	(ii) Repeatedly to one parent		
	(a) Parent inbred	Same as for selfing	Same as for selfing
	(b) Parent not inbred	$\dfrac{1}{4}+\dfrac{1}{2}F_{t-1}$	$\dfrac{1}{4}H_0+\dfrac{1}{2}H_{t-1}$
4.	Half sibs		
	(i) Sire x half sisters	$\dfrac{1}{8}+\dfrac{3}{4}F_{t-1}+\dfrac{1}{8}F_{t-2}$	$\dfrac{3}{4}H_{t-1}+\dfrac{1}{8}H_{t-2}$
	(ii) Sire x two half	$\dfrac{3}{16}+\dfrac{1}{2}F_{t-1}+\dfrac{1}{4}F_{t-2}$	$\dfrac{1}{2}H_{t-1}+\dfrac{1}{4}H_{t-1}$
	sisters which are full sibs	$+\dfrac{1}{4}F_{t-3}$	$+\dfrac{1}{16}H_{t-1}$
5.	Double first cousins	$\dfrac{1}{8}+\dfrac{1}{2}F_{t-1}+\dfrac{1}{4}F_{t-2}$	$\dfrac{1}{2}H_{t-1}+\dfrac{1}{4}H_{t-2}+\dfrac{1}{8}H_{t-3}$
		$+\dfrac{1}{8}F_{t-3}$	

Contd...

Table 10.3–Contd...

Sl.No.	Mating	Systems F_t Recurrence	H_t Recurrence
6.	Quadruple second cousins	–	$\frac{1}{2}H_{t-1} + \frac{1}{4}H_{t-2} + \frac{1}{8}H_{t-3}$ $+ \frac{1}{16}H_{t-4}$
7.	Octuple third cousins:	–	$\frac{1}{2}H_{t-1} + \frac{1}{4}H_{t-2} + \frac{1}{8}H_{t-3}$ $+ \frac{1}{16}H_{t-4} + \frac{1}{32}H_{t-5}$
8.	Single first cousins	$\frac{1}{16} + \frac{1}{16}F_{t-3}$	
9.	Single second cousins	$\frac{1}{64}\left(1 + \frac{1}{8}F_{t-2}\right.$ $\left. + \frac{1}{32}F_{t-3} + \frac{1}{64}F_{t-4}\right)$	$\frac{13}{32} + \frac{1}{8}H_{t-1} + \frac{1}{32}H_{t-2}$ $+ \frac{1}{64}H_{t-3}$
10.	Half first cousins	$\frac{1}{32} + \frac{1}{8}F_{t-2} + \frac{1}{32}F_{t-3}$	$\frac{13}{32} + \frac{1}{8}H_{t-2} + \frac{1}{32}H_{t-3}$

10.9 Increment in F and Decrease in H

The recurrence statements were expressed in terms of additive fractions of previous generation homozygosity or heterozygosity. It is needed to express the recurrence equations in terms of an increase in F (ΔF) and decrease in heterozygosity (ΔH) so as to correlate the loss of heterozygosity with the isolate size (N) in small populations. This is done by expressing the H recurrence in another form as a difference which is obtained by substracting successive terms.

Increment in F (ΔF)

The rate of increase in F is obtained by substracting the earlier generation F (F_{t-1}) from the later generation F (F_t). The increment in F (Δ F) with regular full sib mating will be as:

$$F_t = \frac{1}{4} + \frac{1}{2}F_{t-1} + \frac{1}{4}F_{t-2}$$

$$F_{t-1} = \frac{1}{4} + \frac{1}{2}F_{t-2} + \frac{1}{4}F_{t-3}$$

Now substracting the F_{t-1} from F_t will give the (Δ F) as:

$$(\Delta F) = F_t - F_{t-1} = \frac{1}{2}F_{t-1} - \frac{1}{4}F_{t-2} - \frac{1}{4}F_{t-3}$$

Likewise, the increment in F (Δ F) for any regular system of close inbreeding can be obtained.

Decrease of Heterozygosity (ΔH)

The change in heterozygosity (ΔH) is also expressed as a difference of H recurrence of two successive generations. This is done by tracing H recurrence one generation back and dividing it by 2 before substracting it (H_{t-1}) from H_t.

The recurrence relation of H for any regular system of mating can be obtained in alternate form and these have been given below:

Regular mating system	*H in t generation*
Selfing	$H_{t-1} - \left(\dfrac{1}{2}\right)^2 H_{t-2}$
Full sibs	$H_{t-1} - \left(\dfrac{1}{2}\right)^3 H_{t-3}$
Double first cousins	$H_{t-1} - \left(\dfrac{1}{2}\right)^4 H_{t-4}$
Quadruple second cousins	$H_{t-1} - \left(\dfrac{1}{2}\right)^5 H_{t-5}$
Octuple third cousins	$H_{t-1} - \left(\dfrac{1}{2}\right)^6 H_{t-6}$
More distant cousins	$H_{t-1} - \left(\dfrac{1}{2}\right)^{2+K} H_{t-(2+K)}$

Chapter 11
Change of Genetic Structure Non Random Mating – II: Out Breeding

The mating of unrelated individuals is called a out breeding and it is opposite or complementary to the inbreeding. The out breeding is of many types. The details of the different forms of out breeding have been discussed in later chapter. In this chapter have been discussed mainly the genetic and phenotypic consequences of out breeding on population structure.

11.1 Genetic Effect of Outbreeding

The out breeding is opposite to inbreeding and hence its effects on the genetic structure of population as well as on population performance are also opposite to inbreeding.

The out breeding tends to increase heterozygosity because the mated pairs are genetically unrelated having different alleles or the same alleles with their different frequencies. The important and peculiar characteristic of out breeding is that the maximum heterozygosity is attainted in first generation outcrosses and goes on decreasing in subsequent generations produced by random mating of out bred. The decrease in heterozygosity in subsequent generation is due to the segregation of genes which consequently increases the homozygosity. The two parents are homozygous (AA and aa) and their F_1 progenies are all heterozygous (Aa) while the F_2 progenies are produced in a ratio of AA : 2 Aa : aa. Further the crossbreds of F_1

generation are likely to be uniform in traits related to physical fitness particularly when the parents are homozygous for different alleles of a particular pair. However, the out bred can not breed true because of heterozygosity and hence the selection is less effective among out bred.

11.2 Change of Mean on Crossing – Heterosis

The progeny produced by crossing inbred lines or purebred populations, is called the out bred or crossbred. The out bred progeny show an increase in the value of characters which are affected by inbreeding, showing inbreeding depression. Thus, the fitness reduced in terms of reproduction and vigour due to inbreeding is restored on crossing the inbred or purebred populations. This increase in value of characters of crossbreds produced by crossing inbred lines is called as hybrid vigour or *heterosis* which is opposite or complementary to the phenomenon of inbreeding depression. Thus, the phenomenon of heterosis is reverse to the phenomenon of inbreeding depression. The amount of heterosis is the difference between the mean performance of the crossbreds and inbred.

The out bred are heterozygotes in which the effects of undesirable recessive genes are hidden by the effect of favourable genes (dominant). There-fore, the out bred are superior to the average of their parents. This superiority of out bred/crossbreds over the average of their parents is called the heterosis or hybrid vigour. The hybrid vigour is the opposite to the phenomenon of inbreeding depression.

The heterosis is the measure of the effect of outbreeding. This is the phenomenon by which crossbred progenies are better than the average value of the two purebreds used to produce crossbred progeny. The heterosis is caused by heterozygosity created due to crossing two purebred populations with different gene frequencies. The cause of heterosis, like inbreeding depression is the non-additive gene action (dominance, overdominance and epistasis) to be discussed in subsequent section.

The **heterosis** is defined as the amount by which the mean of F_1 generation, produced by crossing two breeds, exceeds to its better parent. Thus, the heterosis (H) is indicated as: $H = F_1 > P_1 > P_2$.

11.3 Estimation of Heterosis

Mainly there are two approaches to estimate the heterosis *viz.* quantitative approach for estimation of heterosis shown by quantitative characters and second is the theoretical approach based on gene frequency.

1. Quantitative Estimation

The amount of heterosis is quantitatively estimated by comparing the mean value of purebred and crossbred animals as:

Heterosis = mean of F_1 progeny – mean of parental breeds

This can also be expressed in terms of percentage as:

$$\text{Per cent heterosis} = \frac{\text{Mean of } F_1 \text{ progeny} - \text{Mean of parent breeds}}{\text{Mean of parent breed}} \times 100\%$$

2. Theoretical Estimation: Gene frequency and gene effect method:

Theoretical basis of heterosis can be better taken in terms of gene frequencies in the two lines or breeds. The lines differ in gene frequencies because the inbreeding causes the dispersion of gene frequencies. The two lines are crossed to produce hybrids (F_1) and then F_2 are produced by inter-se mating of F_1. The heterosis observed in F_1 and F_2 is measured as the deviation of F_1 performance from the mind parent value which is the difference of F_1 and F_2 from the mean of the two parental lines crossed to produce F_1. The heterosis can only be shown by hybrids if their parental populations differ in gene frequencies. Therefore, to explain the heterosis in terms of difference of gene frequencies between the two parental populations, let the gene frequencies, for a locus with two alleles, be p and q in one population, and p′ and q′ in second population.

The difference in gene frequencies is represented by y so that $y = p - p' = q'-q$, then the gene frequencies p′ and q′ in the second generation will be as p′ = (p − y) and q′ = (q + y). The population mean in first (M_1) and second (M_2) population will be:

$$M_1 = a (p - q) + 2 d pq$$
$$M_2 = a [(p - y) - (q + y)] + 2 d (p - y) (q + y)$$
$$= a (p - y - q - y) + 2 d [pq + y (p - q) - y^2]$$
$$= a (p - q - 2 y) + 2 d [pq + y (p - q) - y^2]$$

The average value of two populations (M_p) will be:

$$M_p = \tfrac{1}{2} (M_1 + M_2)$$
$$= a (p - q - y) + d [2 pq + y (p - q) - y^2] \quad \text{................. Eq. 11.1}$$

The random mating of animals of the two populations will produce 3 genotypes (A_1A_1, A_1A_2 and A_2A_2) in F_1 generation with their frequencies as:

Table 11.1: Genotype Frequencies

		Gametes from I Population	
		$A_1(p)$	$A_2(q)$
Gametes from	A_1 (p − y)	A_1A_1 [p (p − y)]	A_1A_2 [q (p − y)]
II population	A_2 (q + y)	A_1A_2 [p (q + y)]	A_2A_2 [q (q + y)]

Total Genotypes (F_1) =	A_1A_1	$[A_1A_2 + A_1A_2]$	A_2A_2
Genotype frequency (F_1) =	p (p − y):	[q (p − y) + p (q + y)]:	q (q + y)
	= p (p − y):	[2 pq + y (p − q)]:	q (q + y)
Genotypic values =	a	d	−a

Mean genotypic value (F_1) = a p (p − y) − a q (q + y) + d [2 pq + y (p − q)]

(freq. x value)
$$= a(p^2 - py - q^2 - qy) + d [2pq + y (p - q)]$$
$$= a (p - q - y) + d [2pq + y (p - q)]$$
$$\text{................. Eq.11.2}$$

Now, the amount of heterosis (H_{F1}) will be obtained as the difference between the mean of F_1 and mid-parent value (M_P). This will be obtained by substracting equation 11.1 from equation 11.2 as:

$$H_{F1} = M_{F1} - M_P = (Eq. 11.2) - (Eq. 11.1)$$
$$= dy^2$$

The combined effect of all loci will not change this equation of heterosis. The contribution of separate loci combines additively and thus the heterosis in F_1 is (H_{F1}):

$$H_{F1} = \Sigma dy^2 \qquad\qquad .... Eq. 11.3$$

11.4 Genetic Basis of Heterosis

The hybrid vigour is the opposite to the phenomenon of inbreeding depression. Thus, the heterosis is caused by heterozygosity created due to crossing of two purebred populations with different gene frequencies. The *magnitude of heterosis depends on two factors viz.* the genetic diversity of the mated pairs and the type of gene action.

1. The *genetic diversity* among mates decides the rate of heterosis. The more distantly unrelated mates have fewer genes in common and hence the out bred progeny is more heterozygous. The line bred progeny produced by two lines of the same breed is expected to be slightly more heterozygous (genetically divergent) than that of the average heterozygosity of the breed in general. The genetic diversity is more in F_1 progeny produced by mating of animals of two breeds. Further, the genetic diversity between a Zebu and European breed is more than the genetic diversity among different Zebu breeds of cattle or among different breeds of European cattle. Therefore, the crossbreds produced from European and Zebu breeds will be more heterozygous than the crossbred produced from mating between any two Zebu breeds or between any two European breeds. The magnitude of heterosis will be according to the genetic distance between mates. The equation of heterosis $H_{F1} = \Sigma dy^2$ indicates that the amount of heterosis depends on the difference of gene frequency (y^2) between the two populations to be crossed. Therefore, the amount of heterosis increases with the degree of genetic differences between the two mated populations but is limited by the barrier of inter-specific sterility.

Regarding the effect of difference of gene frequency between two lines, it is evident that the amount of heterosis to be observed will entirely be specific to the particular cross depending upon the genes by which the two lines differ and hence the heterosis will be different in different crosses. This is because the different pairs of lines will have different values of Σdy^2.

The effect of the difference of gene frequencies of two lines on the amount of heterosis is not universal, particularly for the populations which have adapted to local conditions. Such populations which differ in gene frequencies through adaptation to local conditions may fail to show heterosis and the F_2 generation may have low fitness. The epistatic interaction may be the reason for this. The fitness or adaptation is a complex trait which involves many characters and hence depends on the interrelation of many functions of the organism. Therefore, the adaptation is the result of genes at many loci that are selected under local conditions. Thus, the adaptation is more a function of the epistatic interactions at many loci. In view of this, the crossbreds (hybrids) produced, from two such populations which are adapted to different local conditions, may not adapt to either of the local conditions. Moreover, the favourable combinations of genes are broken due to segregation in production of F_2 generation.

2. The *non-additive gene action* (dominance, over dominance and epistasis) causes the heterosis, like inbreeding depression. No heterosis is observed for traits governed by additive gene action. The traits showing heterosis are called often as **heterotic traits**.

When additive gene action affects the character, the mean of F_1 progeny is exactly the same as the mean of the parents if environmental variations are not taken into account. Thus, this type of gene action is not responsible for heterosis. The mean of F_1 progeny differ from the mean of the parents, if non-additive gene action is important. In this case the mean of the F_1 may even be higher than the better parent or lower than the inferior parent. When F_1 exceed the better parent it is called useful heterosis.

(i) Dominance Hypothesis

The degree of heterosis depends upon the type of trait and type of mating. The early expressed traits, like survival and growth rate to weaning are more influenced. The traits which are more adversely affected by inbreeding also show greatest degree of heterosis. The mating of unrelated individuals (mating of inbred, two purebreds) shows heterosis in their offspring. There are two reasons for this.

The mated unrelated individuals are homozygous for different alleles. The animals of one purebred will be homozygous for some loci and the animals of other group (lines, purebred) will be homozygous for other loci. The crossing of lines or breeds (homozygous for different gene) produces the heterozygous offspring. The favourable dominant genes in the offspring will mask the unfavourable recessive. Thus the performance of the hybrid offspring will exceed to that of the average of the parents and sometimes exceed even to that of better parent. This is because each purebred will be homozygous for some loci (for favourable genes at some and for unfavourable genes at other). In case if one line or breed complements the other, the hybrid progeny will have more favourable genes than either parent. The effects of favourable genes are generally dominant to those of unfavourable genes. Thus, the performance of the hybrid progeny is superior to that of parental line. For example, for polygenic traits, one line or breed may be homozygous dominant for some pairs and homozygous recessive for another like AA, bb, CC and DD whereas the other breed may be respectively homozygous recessive and dominant at other loci aa, BB, cc, dd. On crossing them the resulting progeny (F1) will carry dominant alleles at all loci and would be superior to both parents for that trait.

Secondly, the crosses between two lines or breeds having different gene frequencies (p and q) produce a lower frequency of recessive than the average of the two parents. This is because the frequency of the recessive in the cross will be qq instead of ½ ($q^2 + q'^2$). For example if q = 0.2 and q' = 0.6, then qq' = 0.12 and ½ ($q^2 + q'^2$) = ½ (0.04 + 0.36) = 0.20. This is always true except for equal gene frequencies and so the performance of the hybrid is superior to the average of the parents.

The heterosis depends on the dominance. Thus, loci with no dominance (d=0), which means additive gene action, will not cause heterosis. Further, the dominance must be directional otherwise the effect of equal dominance (some loci are dominant in one direction to increase the value of traits and others are dominant in other direction to decrease the value of the trait) will be cancelled out. Thus, the heterosis is like that of inbreeding depression which also depends on directional dominance. From this it can be inferred that absence of heterosis does not mean that the individual loci do not show dominance, because heterosis will occur only when the dominance is directional.

(ii) Over Dominance Theory

The over dominance is the interaction between genes that are alleles and it results in the heterozygous individual being superior to the best homozygous parent. The crossbreeding result in superior animals if over dominance is important for the reason that the animal produced by crossbreeding has a maximum number of heterozygous loci. For example, for a gene locus, there will be three different genotypes such as A_1A_1, A_1A_2, and A_2A_2. If over dominance is present, the alleles A_1 and A_2 coming together (A_1A_2) produce a reaction which is not produced by them separately. The over dominance may be an important factor in heterosis for some character and in some species. Crow (1952) suggested that the dominance hypothesis can account for only 5 per cent of the increase in performance in crosses of lines of corn. Thus, the dominance theory appears to be insufficient to explain heterosis in corn. However, heterosis observed in corn can be only due to over dominance at least at few loci affecting corn yield.

(iii) Epistatic Effects

The epistasis is a phenomenon of interacting of genes which are not alleles. The epistasis is the effect of genes resulting from the new combination of genes from different loci. The different genes coming together in the hybrid interact with each other and produce greater effect than when they are alone in different parents. For example in plant, one dominant gene governs the length of internodes (long) and the other dominant gene governs the number of internodes. When these two dominant gene pairs are present in a single hybrid, they show their multiplication effect and result in offspring taller than expected from the average height of parental types having few but long internodes and having many but short internodes.

11.5 Physiological Basis of Heterosis

It has been concluded on the basis of some studies that crossbreds have a more efficient metabolic system. This may be due the reaction produced by the presence of genes in different combinations.

The heterotic effect seems to be the consequence of the combined effect of many pairs of genes rather than at particular locus. The out breeding changes the genotypic frequencies in favour of heterozygotes and it leads to an increase in more pairs of heterozygous genes among out bred individuals and decrease in recessive homozygotes. The reason of beneficial effect of heterozygous genotypes may be through the production of essential enzymes or normal proteins that could have been produced by the dominant alleles.

11.6 Heterosis versus Inbreeding Depression

(i) These are two genetic phenomena which are reverse to each other. The inbreeding depression is a consequence of inbreeding whereas the heterosis or hybrid vigour results from crossing of inbred lines or different races, breeds or varieties differing in gene frequencies.

(ii) The inbreeding tends to reduce the mean phenotypic value of characters closely connected to fitness in animals and lead to loss of general vigor and fertility. This loss or reduction in mean performance is known as inbreeding depression. The outbreeding (crossing the inbred lines) restores the reduced fertility and vigour. The progeny produced on crossing inbred or purebred lines (known as F_1) show an increase in performance of those traits that suffered a reduction from inbreeding.   (iii) The inbreeding depression is caused due to the increased homozygosity while the heterosis is the effect of increased heterozygosity.

(iii) *The heterosis equals inbreeding depression in amount but with opposite sign.* The inbreeding depression equals $-2pqdF$ and the amount of heterosis is dy^2 where *d* is the non-additive gene effect and y is the genetic diversity of mated parents ($y = p_1 - p_2 = q_2 - q_1 =$ difference in gene frequency). The y^2 should be equal to $2pqF$ to prove the heterosis equal to inbreeding depression. This can be proved from variance of gene frequency ($\sigma^2 q$) among lines as:

$$\sigma^2 q = \frac{pq}{(2N)} = pq\,F \qquad \text{since,} \quad \frac{1}{(2N)} = F$$

Taking a population subdivided into many lines and that the pairs of lines are crossed at random, the mean squared difference of gene frequency between pairs of lines (y^2) will be equal to twice the variance of gene frequencies among the lines. Thus, $y^2 = 2\sigma^2 q = 2pqF$. Therefore, the amount of heterosis (dy^2) equals to the inbreeding depression ($-2pqdF$) with opposite sign. The observed inbreeding depression is linear to F. When lines are crossed at random, the average coefficient of inbreeding (F) in the crossbred progeny reverts to that of the base population. Thus, the mean value of any trait in the crossbred progeny is expected to be the same as the mean of base population.

In view of the fact that heterosis is reverse to inbreeding depression, it can be said that inbreeding followed by crossing of inbred lines in a large population can not make a permanent change in the population mean, in the absence of selection. The mean gene frequencies in an inbred population do not change without selection. The average inbreeding coefficient in crossbred population reverts back to that of the base population and the genotype frequencies are same to that of the base population. Therefore, the mean value of a character in crossbred progeny that showed inbreeding depression on inbreeding, is expected to be the same what it was in the base population. Further, if the random mating is followed in crossbred population continuously in subsequent generations, the population mean will remain equal to the mean of base population.

Robert (1960) conducted an experiment on mice to test this theoretical expectation of the equivalence of the effects of two phenomena (inbreeding depression on inbreeding and heterosis on crossing), in the absence of selection, for the litter size as a character. He recorded the mean value of litter size in base (random mating) population, in inbred lines produced by inbreeding, in crossbred population produced by crossing inbred lines and again in a population produced by random mating of crossbred population. He observed that inbreeding depression and heterosis were nearly equal within the limits of experimental error.

(iv) The effect of inbreeding depends on dominance effect, gene frequencies and the degree of inbreeding (- 2pqdF). If additive gene effects only influence a trait (d = 0), no heterosis or inbreeding depression occurs. Thus, the loci without dominance and the traits which are highly heritable show no heterosis or inbreeding depression. Further a change in the direction of more recessive alleles and the genes with intermediate gene frequencies (p = q = 0.5) have the greatest effect on the change of mean. However, it is not only the dominance effect but it is the directional dominance which influence heterosis. The absence of heterosis does not indicate the absence of dominance because the amount of heterosis depends on directional dominance. If some loci show dominance in one direction and others in other direction, their effects are cancelled out and as a result no heterosis is observed. The same is true for inbreeding depression. No heterosis is observed if the mated lines do not differ in their gene frequencies. Maximum heterosis is exhibited if one allele is fixed in one line and the other in other line which make the difference maximum in gene frequencies.

(v) The amount of heterosis increases with the degree of genetic differences between the two mated population and is limited by the barrier of inter-specific sterility. The amount of inbreeding depression, on the other hand, increases with the degree of genetic similarity between two populations mated.

11.7 Genetic Variance of Crossing

The knowledge of the variance between crosses is important in order to predict the magnitude of improvement expected from crossing inbred lines. This is important to relate the inbreeding coefficient with the between cross variance because it provides the amount of gain by increasing the intensity of inbreeding. The idea of genetic variance between crosses can be better conceived under the assumptions that

☆ A large number of inbred lines are produced from the base population without selection and these lines have the same inbreeding coefficient.

☆ These inbred lines are crossed at random, each cross being made from many individuals of the parent lines and the parents within their lines are not related to each other.

The inbreeding does not change the gene frequencies and hence the gametes produced by inbred lines will be the same as those produced by base population. Therefore, all the genotypes will be formed among the crosses and any crossbred progeny will have any genotype of the base population. This will result the genetic variance after crossing equal to that of the base population. This is because on crossing the fully inbred lines [$P_{1(AA)}$ x $P_{2(aa)}$], there is no genetic variance within the cross [due to having similar genotypes by all the crossbred progeny as: $F_{1(Aa)}$] and thus the between cross variance will be equal to the genetic variance of the base population. When the lines crossed are partially inbred, some genetic variance will appear within the cross and the between cross variance will be less than it was between crosses produced from fully inbred lines.

The crossbred individuals of a cross (F_1) can be considered as a family with same degree of relationship between them depending upon the F of the parental inbred lines. The components of variance between crosses are the covariance of the related individuals. The composition of the covariance of relatives of any type is given in terms of the genetic components (additive and dominance) and the coefficients of relationship (r and u) a given below. The coefficients of relationship (r and u) can be estimated from coancestries of following individuals of two lines, where two individuals (A and C) belong to one parental line and other two individuals (B and D) belong to other parental line, producing two F_1 individuals (X and Y):

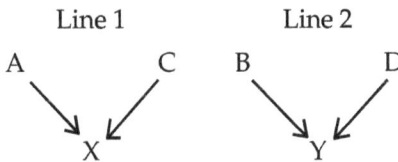

$$r = 2\,f_{XY} \text{ and } u = f_{AC}\,f_{BD} + f_{AD}\,f_{BC}$$

The procedure to compute co-ancestry has been given in detail in last chapter under regular systems of inbreeding (section 6.3).

$$\text{Cov} = r\,V_A + u\,V_D \qquad \text{For single locus}$$

$$= r\,V_A + u\,V_D + r^2\,V_{AA} + ru\,V_{AD} + u^2\,V_{DD}$$

$$+ r^3\,V_{AAA} + r^2u\,V_{AAD} + r\,u^2\,V_{ADD} + u^3\,V_{DDD} \qquad \text{For more loci}$$

The fraction coefficient 'r' concerns the additive variance and is the coefficient of relationship (genetic correlation) between relatives and it is twice the inbreeding coefficient of their progeny ($r = 2F$). The u is the fraction or coefficient of dominance variance and represents the probability that relatives have the same genotype through identity by descent. This is the probability that both alleles at a locus in an individual are identical to those in another relative. Thus u is zero unless the relatives have paths of co-ancestry through both of their parents like FS and double first cousins.

The two coefficients of relationship (r and u) can be estimated from the co-ancestries and these two coefficients can be expressed in terms of F (inbreeding coefficient) as:

$$r = 2fxy = F \text{ and }$$

$$u = F^2.$$

The components of genetic variance between crosses (σ^2_X) can be expressed as:

$$\sigma^2_X = F V_A + F^2 V_D + F^2 V_{AA} + F^3 V_{AD} + F^4 V_{DD}$$

This expression of between cross genetic variance has two terms which are the inbreeding coefficient (F) of the individual of the next generation of the lines and the variance in the base population due to additive and dominance variance. It is assumed that all lines have same F (equally inbred) and there is no relationship between the lines. The genetic variance within the lines $[(1 - F) V_A + (1 - F^2) V_D]$ is fully responded within crosses. It can be seen that the contribution of additive variance increases linearly with F while the dominance and interaction component increase in proportion to the square or higher power of F. Therefore, the crosses are more different genetically with an increase of the level of inbreeding. The cross is genetically equivalent to a full sib family in the base population when F = 0.5 but whole of the genetic variance appears between crosses when F = 1.0.

11.8 Combining Ability: GCA and SCA

Observational Components of Genetic Variance between Crosses

The total genetic variance between crosses (σ^2_X) was obtained considering that each line was used in one cross only. Further, this genetic variance contained the additive and interaction components of variance with their coefficients in terms of F. These two variance components (additive and interaction) can be estimated in terms of observational components of variance to be expressed as combining ability which is of two types (general and specific) corresponding to the two causal components (additive and interaction). The concept of GCA and SCA was introduced by Sprague and Tatum (1942).

The estimation of the observational components of variance in term of G.C.A. and S.C.A., requires the crossing of a number of inbred lines in all possible combinations which is called a *"diallel cross"*. Thus in diallel cross, each line is crossed with every other line. This is the commonly used experimental design for crossing inbred lines. The analysis of a diallel cross provides the information on the nature and amount of genetic parameters as well as on the GCA of parents (lines) and the SCA of the crosses.

The crossing of a line with several lines will give an estimate of the mean performance of the line based on all crosses made by crossing this line with all other lines in all possible combinations. The mean performance of this line expressed as a deviation from mean of all crosses (μ), is called as the *general combining ability (G.C.A.)* of the line. Thus, each line will have its G.C.A. Therefore, the GCA of a line is the average value of the F_1's produced by crossing a line with several other liens and expressing it as a deviation from the over all mean of all the possible crosses (μ).

Now, any particular cross of two lines should have its expected mean value equal to the sum of the G.C.A. of two lines. However, it may not be true but this cross may have its expected mean value different from the sum of the G.C.A. of two lines. This deviation of the mean value of a particular cross from the sum of G.C.A. of two lines is called the *specific combining ability* of the cross (S.C.A.). Thus, each cross will have its S.C.A. The SCA is thus the mean performance of a particular cross of two lines expressed as deviation of this cross from the GCA of the two lines.

The GCA's are the main effects due to genic values which cause differences in GCA. The SCA is due to the interaction effect (dominance, over dominance and epistasis) which causes differences in SCA. This is the genetic basis of SCA.

The deviation of true mean of a cross (X_{ij}) between any two lines (i^{th} and j^{th}) contain the sum of their GCA's and SCA. Thus,

$$X_{ij} - \mu = \text{Genotypic value of a cross } (X_{ij})$$

$$= GCA_i + GCA_j + SCA_{ij}$$

where, μ = Overall mean of all possible crosses

(Involving all lines in all possible combinations)

= General mean of all crosses in a diallele cross

$$GCA_i = X_i - \mu$$

$$GCA_j = X_j - \mu$$

$$SCA_{ij} = X_{ij} - (\mu + GCA_i + GCA_j)$$

The between cross genetic variance (total) will thus be as:

$$\sigma^2_X = \sigma^2_{GCAi} + \sigma^2_{GCAj} + \sigma^2_{SCAij}$$

$$= 2\sigma^2_{GCA} + \sigma^2_{SCA}$$

The GCA's and SCA are uncorrelated.

The variance of GCA is the additive genetic variance $(V_A + V_{AA})$ in the base population which is due to differences in additive gene effects whereas the variance of SCA $((V_D + V_{AD} + V_{DD})$ is due to the non-additive gene effects

Further the variance of GCA increases linearly with F while the variance of SCA is expected to increase with higher powers of F and so the variance of SCA is more important as a cause of variation among crosses at higher degree of inbreeding (F). Therefore, it is advisable to use highly inbred lines for selection among crosses to be most effective. This means that when non-additive gene action has more influence on a trait, the most effective procedure of improvement is to produce highly inbred lines and then crossing them to find that which lines combine best.

The analogy between the causal components and observational components of the genetic variance making up the between cross variance is given here as:

Causal Components of Variance	*Observational Components of Variance*
Additive genetic variance	
$= F V_A + F^2 V_{AA} + \dots$	$GCA = \sigma^2_{GCA}$
Non-additive genetic variance	
$= F^2 V_D + F^3 V^{AD} + F^4 V_{DD} + \dots$	$SCA = \sigma^2_{SCA}$

The variance of GCA and the variance of SCA are the two components of the total genetic variance between crosses. These two components can be estimated directly from observations on phenotypic values and hence these are the observational components.

The measurement of GCA is important because the utilization of variance of GCA is applied as a method of improvement by crossing. By comparing the GCA of different lines, the best lines are selected which are most likely yield the best cross among all the crosses of the available lines. The correlation between performance of parental inbred lines and the crossbred progeny is generally high for traits with high GCA and large additive gene effects. Thus prediction of cross performance with reasonable accuracy for such traits can be made from performance of the parental lines.

11.9 Estimation of GCA and SCA

1. Progeny Performance

The GCA of the two lines do not provide a reliable guide to the performance of their cross if much of the variation between crosses is due to SCA. The SCA is measured by making specific crosses between the lines. The method of *diallel cross* is used in poultry breeding by crossing a number of inbred lines in all possible combinations.

Besides this, the *polycross method* in plants and *top crossing* in animals is used. In top crossing the individuals from the line under test are crossed with the individuals from the base population. The mean value of their progeny measures the GCA of the line. This is because the gametes of individuals from the base population are genetically equivalent to the gametes of a random set of inbred lines derived without selection from the base population.

Without making and testing a particular cross, the SCA of that cross can not be measured. This requires a large number of crosses to be made and tested to achieve a reasonably high intensity of selection for SCA. The superior combining ability can also be built into the lines by selection. The selection creates the differences in gene frequencies in two lines at all loci that affect the character and show dominance. The directed process of selection for producing differences of gene frequency is more effective and economical than by the random process of inbreeding. The recurrent selection and reciprocal recurrent selection have been devised based on this idea.

2. Covariance Method

The GCA and SCA variance components can be taken in terms of covariances of full sibs and half sibs. The variance due to differences between maternal or paternal parents is the covariance of half sib families and represents the GCA. The SCA variance is the interaction between maternal and paternal parents which can be taken as the difference between the total variation among progeny family means and the sum of the variances due to differences among maternal and among paternal parents or by substracting twice the covariance of half sibs from covariance of full sibs. Thus, assuming that reciprocal crosses are equal, $SCA = Cov_{FS} - 2\,Cov_{HS}$.

The four **basic mating systems** used to estimate GCA and SCA are the single pair mating, nested design, factorial design, and diallel cross.

(i) **Single pair mating**: This design is used between two breeding lines (P_1 and P_2) for multiparous animals such as pigs, poultry, and mice. The sires and dams are selected from the reference population (non inbred random mating population) and mated in pairs to produce progeny families each of n size tested in r replicates of randomized block experiment,

(ii) **Nested or hierarchical design**: Each sire (S) is mated to several different dams (d) and each mating produces several full sibs progeny tested in replicates of a randomized block experiment. This is most suited to large animals.

(iii) **Factorial experiment**: Each sire is mated to every dam. Thus S sires and D dams are crossed in all possible combinations and each mating produces several full sib progeny which are evaluated in r replicates of a randomized block experiment. This is difficult with animals as the females can not be mated to several males simultaneously. The nested and the factorial designs were used by Comestock and Robinson (1952) and known as North Carolina design 1 and 2, respectively.

(iv) **Diallel design**: This involves the crossing of number of lines among themselves in all possible combinations. Such a cross is known as diallel cross. The analysis of diallel crosses (known as diallel analysis) is useful to estimate the nature and amount of genetic parameters and to estimate the GCA of parents and the SCA of their crosses. The diallel theory (based on the concept of D, H components of variation used by Mather) was developed in 1960's by Junks and Hayman (1953), Jinks (1954, 1956), and Hayman (1954, 1957, 1958). A worked example of the technique was given by Aksel and Johnson (1963). Later on, Mather and Jinks (1971) described the recent developments about the technique of diallel analysis.

The experimental designs are primarily classed as the single mating and multiple mating programmes. The multiple mating programmes include the diallele analysis (full and partial) proposed by Hayman (1954) and Griffing (1956), triallel or three way cross and quadriallel (double cross or four breed crosses) analysis given by Rawlings and Cockerham (1962), and line x tester analysis after Kempthorne (1957). The other types of designs are the North Carolina Design 1, 2 and 3 after Comstock and Robinson (1948, 1952) which are also used to estimate the additive and dominance variance after producing FS and HS progenies from biparental mating in F_2 generation of a cross between two pure lines.

The multiple mating designs are not used in large livestock breeding but mostly used in poultry and plant breeding. The interested readers may consult the book of Biometrical Methods in Quantitative Genetcs by Singh, R.K. and Chaudhary, B.D. (1985).

Chapter 12

Change of Genetic Structure: Phenotypic Assortative Mating

The classification of mating systems based on phenotypes of the mated pairs is done on the basis of direction and magnitude of correlation between the phenotypes of the mates (r_m) which depends on the similarity or dissimilarity in phenotypes of mated pairs. This is then called as the phenotypic assortative or phenotypic disassortative mating.

12.1 Classification of Mating System Based on Phenotypes

Similarity in phenotypes of mates causes the positive correlation and the mating system is called *positive phenotypic assortative mating*. The positive correlation may be perfect $(r_m = 1.0)$ or incomplete < 1.0. Depending upon the magnitude of correlation between phenotypes of mates the positive phenotypic assortative mating is of two types *viz.* complete positive pheno-typic assortative mating when $r_m = 1.0$ and the incomplete or partial positive phenotypic assortative mating when $r_m < 1.0$. This is a mixture of random mating and the positive phenotypic assortative mating. Thus r_m may take any positive value.

The dissimilarity in phenotypes of mates causes negative correlation and the mating system is called *negative phenotypic assortative mating*. This is also called *phenotypic disassortative mating*. The negative correlation may be perfect $(r_m = -1.0)$ when the phenotypes are dissimilar for all the mates and called as the complete phenotypic disassortative mating. The negative correlation may also be less than 1

$(r_m = -1.0)$ and the mating system is called incomplete phenotypic disassotiative mating. This system is a mixture of random mating and disassortative mating. Thus r_m may take any negative value.

Table 12.1: Classification of Mating Systems Based on Phenotypes

Types of Mating Based on Phenotype	Phenotypes of Mates	Correlation (r) among phenotypes of mates
1. Positive assortative:	Similar	Positive
(i) Complete	Completely Similar	1.0
(ii) Incomplete	Mixed	< 1.0
(mixture of assortative and random mating)		
2. Negative assortative		
or disassortative:	Different	Negative
(i) Complete	Completely different	− 1.0
(ii) Incomplete	Mixed	< − 1.0
(mixture of disassortative and random mating)		

12.2 Positive Phenotypic Assortative Mating

The mated pairs are made according to the external resemblance of individu-als and the mating is of "like with like". Thus mating occurs between individuals of similar phenotypes.

The flowering time in plants is a trait with positive assortative mating. The plants flowering early in the season are pollinated by other early flowering plants and likewise late flowering with late flowering. The positive assortative mating also occurs for some traits to some extent in human beings like height, body colour, intelligence, etc. The examples in cattle are the mating of polled with polled, homed with horned; red with red, roan with roan, white with white.

The consequences of positive assortative mating are complex and depend on a number of factors *viz.* correlation between mates (m) which decides the type of assortative mating (complete, incomplete), the proportion of population mating assortatively, gene action (dominance and no dominance), and number of gene loci affecting a trait. The dominance, decrease in m and an increase in number of gene loci decrease the rate of decline in heterozygosity per generation.

This type of mating, also simply called as assortative mating, is of two types *viz.* complete and incomplete. The consequence for the genotypes in both types of mating is the reduction in heterozygosity with a consequent increase in homozygosity without affecting the gene frequencies.

The rate of decrease in heterozygosity is one half each generation under complete phenotypic positive assortative mating and at equilibrium there is complete elimination of heterozygotes. In case when the phenotypic positive assortative mating is incomplete, the rate of decrease in heterozygosity is less than complete assortative mating depending upon the magnitude of r_m and at equilibrium the heterozygotes have non-zero value because of the occurrence of random mating to some extent. The effects of two types of positive phenotypic assortative mating have been shown here:

12.2.1 Complete Positive Phenotypic Assortative Mating

All the mating occur between individuals of the similar phenotypes having r_m = 1.0. The individuals with dominant phenotype mate with individuals of dominant phenotype and recessives with recessives only. There is no mating between dominants and the recessives.

Under complete phenotypic assortative mating, the frequencies of heterozygotes are reduced and consequently the frequencies of homozygotes are increased. The population ultimately has only two extreme phenotypes (AA and aa for two allelic system; and AABB and aabb under two loci case). This effect of fixing only two phenotypes even for two loci case is in contrast to the effect of inbreeding which leads to fixation of all the 4 homozygous phenotype. At equilibrium, the frequencies of homozygotes are equal to the initial frequency of the allele contained in the homozygote. At equilibrium the heterozygotes do not exist in population. However, the gene frequencies remain unchanged.

Further, the dominance of alleles, low allelic frequencies and more number of loci affecting a trait reduce the rate of decrease in the frequency of heterozygote.

When there is no dominance, the mating is like to like and identical to selfing and close inbreeding. But when there is dominance, the effect is little different than in case of codominance.

(i) Codominance

For single locus two alleles (A and a), there will be three genotypes (AA, Aa and an) with their frequencies as p^2, $2pq$ and q^2 in an equilibrium population. The mating under complete assortative mating system will occur between AA x AA, Aa x Aa and aa x aa.

The frequency of heterozygotes are reduced to half whereas the frequencies of both the homozygotes are increased equally on the expense of the' heterozygotes, very identical to the consequences of the inbreeding. The frequency of heterozygotes is reduced to half because of the limited scope of uniting two alleles together to produce heterozygote. The frequency of any of the two alleles did not change.

At equilibrium the heterozygotes do not exist in population. However, the gene frequencies remain unchanged.

(ii) Dominance

When there is dominance, the results are little different. Consider two alleles at a locus (A and a) where the allele A is dominant over allele a. This will produce only two phenotypes *viz*. dominant and recessive phenotypes because the heterozygous individuals will express the dominant phenotype. Now, the mating will be between the individuals with similar phenotype *viz*. dominant x dominant and recessive x recessive. There will be no mating of AA x aa and Aa x aa. However, at genotypic level there will be three kinds of mating between dominant x dominant individuals which are AA x AA, AA xAa and Aa x Aa.

Now consider the initial population with random mating genotype frequencies as D for AA, H for Aa and R for aa genotype. The total frequency of Dom. x Dom. type mating will be $(D + H)^2$ or $1 - R$ while of rec. x rec. mating will be R among all mating.

In this case, the mating of AA x Aa is positive assortative at phenotypic level but it is actually the diassortative mating at genotypic level. This will produce the progeny which will all have dominant phenotype but genotypically they will.be homozygous dominants and the heterozygous in equal proportions. Due to this type (AA x Aa) of extra mating under this condition of dominance, some more heterozygous individuals over the condition of no dominance will be produced, although the overall proportion of heterozy-gotes will be lesser than under random mating. Thus, *the rate of decrease in heterozygosity is much less* in this type of mating with dominance than in close inbreeding or complete phenotypic asortative mating. However, there is no change in gene frequency under complete positive phenotypic assortative mating with dominance too.

The rate of change (decrease) in heterozygosity depends upon the allelic frequency. The change (decrease) is more rapid when the allelic frequency (q) is large than when the frequency is small.

The heterozygosity is reduced to zero at equilibrium under complete positive assortative mating. However, the equilibrium is delayed for some more generations under the condition of dominance. The frequency of homozygote (AA) at equilibrium is equal to the initial frequency of A allele.

12.2.2 Incomplete Positive Phenotypic Assortative Mating

This is the mating system with some amount of heterogamy when mating also occur between the individuals of different phenotypes but in very lower proportion than the mating between individuals of the similar phenotypes. Thus, random mating also occurs to some extent in addition to positive assortative mating. This makes the correlation between phenotypes of mates though positive but less than one and hence $r_m = \; < 1.0$.

This type of mating occurs when heterozygotes can not be distinguished from phenotypes for qualitative trait (in case of dominance) as discussed above, and in case of additive gene action for quantitative traits. The complete positive phenotypic assortative mating is not possible because in such cases some of the mating also occur between heterozygote and recessives and hence the mating occur in all possible combinations of the phenotypes for the traits affected by polygenes. Thus, random mating also occurs to some extent. Therefore, these cases are covered under incompletely positive phenotypic assortative mating. This type of mating is a mixture of random and the assortalive mating, depending upon the correlation of the phenotypes between mates. The assortative and random mating may be in any proportion but definitely the frequency of assortative mating is more than random mating. Thus, the correlation between the phenotype of mates is positive but less than 1.0 (r = < 1.0).

The equilibrium for heterozygosity in the population will be non-zero value which means that some heterozygosity will persist in the population after infinite number of continuous generation of incomplete positive assortative mating. The heterozygosity will be less at equilibrium when the correlation between mates is higher.

The heterozygosity remained present in the population at equilibrium is higher with dominance than with no dominance under incomplete positive assortative mating. The heterozygotes are thus not completely eliminated from the population but remain present at equilibrium. The frequency of heterozygotes is decreased with the increase in the proportion of the population that mates assortatively (m). For example, if the frequency of A allele is $p = \frac{1}{2}$ the value of heterozygosity at equilibrium (H) for different values of m will be as under:

m	0	0.25	0.50	0.75	0.90	1
H	0.5	0.45	0.39	0.30	0.05	0

When the frequency of heterozygotes in the initial population is low than the frequency of heterozygotes at equilibrium, the incomplete assortative mating increases the heterozygosity.

Dangers of the Assortative Mating

The assortative mating has its dangerous effect. With assortative mating, the individuals with the same phenotype mate together and have no effect on the change of gene frequency but tend to increase the frequency of homozygotes with a consequent decrease in the frequency of heterozygotes. Therefore, the incidence of the disease is increased in the population caused by homozygous condition of alleles. This can be illustrated for a disease caused due to a recessive gene with its frequency as $q = 0.2$. The equilibrium frequencies of heterozygotes (H) and of recessive homozygotes (R, causing the disease) will be as:

m	0	0.10	0.25	0.50	0.75	0.9	1.0
H	0.32	0.314	0.302	0.278	0.232	0.163	0
R	0.04	0.043	0.049	0.061	0.084	0.119	0.200

Therefore, under random mating (m = 0) the incidence of the disease is low (4.0 per cent) whereas the incidence of the disease is increased with the increase in proportion of assortative mating (m) in the population.

Two or More Loci Case of Assortative Mating

The genotypic changes become complicate, for traits affected by two or more gene loci, if all genotypes are not distinguishable, in which case the assortment is equivalent to selfing. For a trait controlled by two gene loci with two alleles and each locus having duplicate additive action without dominance (A = B. and Aa BB. = AABB.) there will be five phenotypes from nine genotypes. The nine genotypes will be grouped into the phenotypic classes as AABB; AaBB = AABb; AaBb = aa BB = AAbb; aaBb = Aabb; and aabb. The choice of mates will depend upon the phenotypes. *The reduction in heterozygosity is less compared to single locus case.* Each phenotypic set is changed into extremes only and ultimately *the population will have only two extreme phenotypes (AABB and aabb)* under complete assortative mating for a trait instead of

Therefore, this mating system maintains both the alleles in the population and hence it is capable to oppose the effect of selection or random drift which leads to make population homozygous.

(ii) Codominance

When there is no dominance between the two alleles at a locus all the three genotypes will be distinguished from phenotypes and with complete disassortative mating system, the mating will occur as D x H, D x R, H x R. Among these three kinds of crosses the two crosses *viz.* D x H (AA x Aa) and H x R (Aa x an) will not change the distribution of genotypes in the progeny as they will produce the parental type genotypes in equal proportions. However, the D x R mating (AA x aa) will produce only the heterozygotes and hence it will increase the amount of heterozygosity in progeny generation. In this system other 3 types of mating (D x D, H x R, R x R) do not occur and hence the relative frequencies of the rest 3 types of mating which occur under this system must be normalized by dividing their frequencies with total (T = 1 $- D^2 - H^2 - R^2$)

The proportion of both the homozygotes is reduced and the heterozygosity is increased in successive generation. At equilibrium all the three genotypes exist. In successive generations, the homozygotes become proportional to the ratio of H/T. The ratio of D/R does not change in any generation as well as at equilibrium (Dt/Rt $= D_{t-1}/R_{t-1}$). This system maintains all the three genotype at equilibrium without fixation.

The three genotypes approach to equilibrium with higher heterozygosity than present in initial population (random mating). This means that heterozygotes have higher frequency and hence stores higher genetic variability. Thus, this system is used as a source of germ plasm conservation.

12.3.2 Incomplete Negative Phenotypic Assortative Mating

This is the mating system when in addition to negative assortative mating some fraction of population mate at random. Therefore, the effect of this mating system on the genetic composition of progeny generation can be estimated in terms of the proportion of population having negative assortative mating (m) and rest of the proportion of the population as random mating (1- m).

Now consider that among the dominants there are homozygous dominants (D) and heterozygous dominants (H). The mating within the dominant group are at random. The genotypic frequencies and gene frequencies change from generation to generation. Diasassortative mating, complete or incomplete, leads to a change in gene frequency.

It can also be noted that when the dominants are half (D + H = ½), $p_1 = p$ irrespective of the value of m and hence there is no change in gene frequency. When dominants are > ½, p decreases but when dominants are < ½, p increases, Thus, there is an equilibrium when D + H (dominants) = ½ which means that R = ½ and p = ½. This is a stable equilibrium.

Now taking dominants (D + H) = R = ½, the final gene frequency (equilibrium gene frequency, p) depends on *m*, though the change in *p* is very less with the changing value of *m*. However, the changes in genotypic frequencies are more with changing **m**. With an increase in **m** the frequency of AA genotype is reduced and approach to zero when **m** = 1.0. The frequency of *aa* genotype remains constant whereas the frequency of heterozygous genotype increases and become equal to the frequency of recessive when m = 1.0.

The important point to consider is that the dominants and recessives remain equal in proportion, whatever the value of m is (even when the negative assortative mating is incomplete). The phenotypic mating frequencies at equilibrium are:

Dom. x Dom.   = ¼ (1 – m)

Dom. x Rec. = ½ (1+ m)

Rec. x   Rec.   = ¼ (1 – m)

Thus, the two types of mating between individuals of the similar phenotypes (AA x AA, aa x aa) are equal in frequency whatever the value of m is. The *m* measures the degree of negative assortativeness (r_m).

Chapter 13
Genetic Load

Mutant genes are part of the genetic variation. The maintenance of genetic variability is, of course, advantageous but many of the mutant genes are deleterious to their carriers. Each population contains mutant genes most of which harm their homozygous carriers. The individuals carrying deleterious genes have low fitness values. Therefore, individuals with different genotypes have their different fitness values. The variation in fitness of genotypes in a population gives rise to the concept of genetic load.

13.1 Definition of Genetic Load

The terms genetic load and "load of mutations" were first used by Muller (1950) to describe the effect of mutant genes on human population to alert the people to the dangers of hereditary diseases and to the threat of high energy radiations which induce gene mutations. He concluded that 10 per cent or more of all germ cells carry a newly arisen mutation and that 20 per cent of all human deaths have an ultimate genetic cause.

Muller (1950) called the genetic load as the change in an average fitness associated with maintaining variability in the population and the load was taken as a burden measured in terms of reduced fitness but felt in terms of death, sterility, illness, pain and frustration. The fitness of some individuals carrying deleterious mutants is reduced to various degree and this results in reduction of the average fitness of the population (W) than the fitness of the most fit genotype in the population (W_{max}, taken as unity). This *reduction in average fitness of the population is known as 'genetic load" of the population*. The individuals with low fitness are present in all populations to varying degree. A population having some individuals with low fitness is called genetically imperfect. Thus, no population is having a perfect genetic constitution but genetically imperfect. The individuals carrying unfavourable genes are eliminated through natural or artificial selection and hence they leave the population without making their genetic contribution to future generation. This is known as *'genetic death"*. A population is genetically perfect if there is no genetic death in the population. *The proportion of genetic imperfection (genetic death) of a population is called the genetic load.* Thus, the genetic load of a population is accompanied by a loss of a portion of its individuals through their genetic death in terms of sterility, inability to mate and to become parents.

The *"genetic load"* has been defined by Crow (1958) as the proportional amount by which the average fitness (or any other measurable trait) of a population (**W**) is reduced relatives to that of the optimal genotype of the population. The optimal genotype is that which has maximum fitness value. Thus a population with genetic variation in fitness (or other character) should have a genetic load. Alternatively, the genetic load is defined as the proportional amount by which the average fitness of a population is reduced by genetic process relative to the fitness of the population in which the process is absent. For example, in estimating the mutation load (genetic variability arises due to mutation) the reference population (optimal genotype) is the one which has no mutation. Likewise, when the segregation load is taken, the reference population (optimal genotype) is a non-segregating population at equilibrium. Therefore, the genetic load is taken as:

Genetic load, $L = (W_{max} - W)/W_{max}$

where, W_{max} is the fitness of reference population (fittest genotype) usually taken as 1.0;

W is the average fitness of the whole population.

Assigning the value of W max = 1.0, the genetic load becomes as under:

$L = 1 - W$

Thus, the genetic load is a quantity computed by prescribed mathematical rules rather than a collection of deleterious mutant genes or lethal genes etc.

13.2 Mathematical Illustration of Genetic Load

As a result of genetic imperfection (low fitness of individual carrying deleterious alleles) the individuals with low fitness are culled. This results a loss in the frequency of such individuals having low fitness. This loss of individuals is the incurred genetic load. This can be better understood by the following example. Suppose the gene *a* is completely recessive and deleterious in homozygous condition and some of the individuals which are homozygous for this gene (aa) are culled, the coefficient of selection (loss of fitness) being equal to S. Therefore, the fitness of homozygotes (aa) is $W = 1 - S$. Now the frequency of recessive homozygotes after selection will be:

Genotypes	AA	Aa	aa
Frequency	p^2	$2pq$	q^2
Fitness	1	1	$1 - S$
Frequency after selection:	p^2	$2pq$	$q^2(1-S)$

Average fitness: $W = p^2 + 2pq + q^2 - sq^2$

$$= 1 - sq^2$$

The fitness of the reference population (Wm) is one. Therefore, the genetic load will be:

$$L = \frac{(W_{max} - W)}{W_{max}}$$

$$= \frac{[1 - (1 - sq^2)]}{1}$$

$$= -sq^2$$

The loss in fitness of individuals is equal to Sq^2 which is the genetic load in a random mating population. This is the mutational genetic load because the allele *a* was produced by mutation. If the population is having N individuals before selection, the total number of individuals which will be eliminated from the population due to genetic imperfection is equal to Sq^2N. This is equal to genetic death because these individuals equal to Sq^2N could not become the parent and hence could not make any genetic contribution towards the gene pool of the next generation.

13.3 Types of Genetic Load

The total load may be classified as the expressed load and the hidden load. The load which is expressed under random mating system is called the expressed load whereas the hidden load is concealed by heterozygosis and brought to expression by inbreeding.

The average fitness of a population (**W**) is decreased due to the presence of unfavourable genes or gene combinations. The unfavourable genes arise due to mutation and come to their phenotypic expression as a result of segregation, recombination, inbreeding, migration, incompatibility of mother and foetus etc. Therefore, the genetic load may arise by any of these factors. The different types of genetic loads are thus named after the factor which leads to a change (reduction) in the average fitness of the population. The most important are the mutation load and the segregation load. However, every source of genetic variation can be cited as the basis for its own genetic load.

1. Mutation Load

The mutation is an essential part of evolution and constitutes a part of genetic load of a species. Both types of mutations (deleterious mutation producing deleterious genes and the beneficial mutation producing beneficial genes) produce genetic load. No doubt that the deleterious genes produced by mutation will be eliminated because of their low fitness. It is interesting that beneficial genes produced by mutation also produce the genetic load because they replace the older genes which now have become "transitional and deleterious" compared to the newly produced beneficial genes. The genetic load due to mutation is $Sq^2 = u$ and the number of genetic deaths will be equal to Sq^2N. Most of the mutants are deleterious and therefore, an increase in mutation rate (u) will increase genetic load as well as an increase in genetic death whereas low rate of mutation will decrease the genetic load as well as a decrease in genetic death.

The expressed genetic mutation load in a population with random mating or inbreeding can be obtained. Taking the population with inbreeding coefficient, F the zygotic frequencies and their fitness will be

Genotypes	AA	Aa	aa
Frequency	$p^2(1-F) + pF$	$2pq(1-F)$	$q^2(1-F) + qF$
Relative Fitness	$w_{11} = W_{max}$	$w_{12} = W_{max}(1-hs)$	$w_{22} = W_{max}(1-S)$

Where,   S = Homozygote selective disadvantage or selection coefficient

hs = Heterozygotes selective disadvantage

The genetic load L $= 1 - \mathbf{W}$

$$= hs\,[2pq\,(1-F)] + S\,[q^2\,(1-F) + qF]$$

In random mating population, the $F = 0$ and hence the mutation load will be:

$L = 2pqhs + sq^2$

(i) For Complete Recessive Allele (h = 0)

The mutation load will be $L = Sq^2$.

This is equal to the reduction in fitness as a result of mutation. In case of complete recessive the total proportion of the population remained after selection (average fitness) is:

$\mathbf{W} = 1 - Sq^2$ taking the fitness of AA and Aa as 1.0.

Thus the genetic load in this case is Sq^2.

Since $q^2 = \dfrac{u}{S}$, the incidence of affected individuals in a population under

selection and mutation equilibrium for recessive, because if an allele is completely

recessive its equilibrium frequency (q) is $\sqrt{\dfrac{u}{S}}$ and hence the mean fitness of the

equilibrium population is: $W = 1 - S\left(\dfrac{u}{S}\right) = 1 - u$

Therefore, the genetic load of equilibrium population is:

$L = 1 - \mathbf{W}$

$= 1 - (1 - u) = u$

This is the genetic load that has its existence to recurrent mutation. Therefore, the mutation load in case of a recessive allele equals the rate at which the allele arise by mutation (u) and is independent of the effect of the allele in fitness. This was pointed out by Haldane (1937). Thus, the frequency of genetic death (Sq^2) at equilibrium depends on the mutation rate (u) alone since $L = Sq^2 = u$ and not affected by the degree of harmfulness (fitness) of the allele (S). This is because more harmful genes come to equilibrium at low frequencies.

(ii) For Incompletely Recessive Allele (h = 0.5, no dominance)

The mutation load will be:

$$L = 2pq\,hS + Sq^2$$
$$= pqS + Sq^2 \qquad \text{(since, h = ½)}$$
$$= Sq$$

When the allele is dominant to an appreciable degree (incomplete recessive) its equilibrium frequency by recurrent mutation equals $\dfrac{u}{hs}$ and hence taking h = 0.5,

$$q = \frac{u}{hs}$$

$$= \frac{2u}{S} \qquad \text{(taking h=0,5)}$$

Thus, the mutation load for incomplete recessive allele is

$$L = Sq$$

$$= S\left(\frac{u}{hs}\right)$$

$$= 2\,u \qquad\qquad \text{(taking h = 0.5)}$$

This is the effect of mutation (incomplete recessive) on the average fitness of the population. In this case also the mutation load is independent of the effect of the mutant allele upon its carriers but it is equal to the twice of the mutation rate.

The mutant alleles are either completely recessive or incompletely, so the mutation load lie between u and 2u. The mutations are seldom completely recessive and hence the mutation load is nearly equal to 2u (twice the mutation rate).

In an inbred population (F = 1), the mutation load will be:

$$L_1 = hS[2pq(1-F)] + S\,[q^2(1-F) + qF]$$
$$= Sq \text{ (taking F = l)}$$

The inbred population (F = 1) will become homozygous for AA or aa without affecting gene frequencies. Thus there will be u/hs homozygous aa individuals and each affected individual represents a loss of fitness equal to S. The average fitness of the population will be lowered as:

$$Sq = S\left(\frac{u}{hS}\right)$$

$$= \frac{u}{h}$$

Thus, inbred load (genetic load of homozygous population) is

$$L = Sq = \frac{u}{h}$$

Therefore, the load is equal to the mutation rate, in general, if the mutant is completely recessive or if there is enough inbreeding to eliminate the mutant genes as homozygotes. But the load is twice the mutation rate when h is appreciable (incomplete recessive mutant). Thus, partially dominant mutants produce about twice the load compared to recessive. This can be explained based on genetic extinction or genetic death (Muller, 1950) which is pre-adult death or failure to reproduce. When the mutant allele is recessive, the genetic death eliminates two genes per extinction among 2N genes in a diploid population of N size but if the mutant is dominant, then the genetic death eliminate only one mutant. This will held true only in case of rare dominant mutants because when their frequency will be higher it will be eliminated as homozygote resulting two eliminations.

The mutation load is 1.5 u for sex linked recessive with equal mutation rates in the two sexes. But when the mutation rate differs in the two sexes, the mutation load is:

$$L = \frac{(u_m \pm 2u_f)}{2}$$

Secondly, all the eliminations are through genetic death of males for sex linked recessive mutant.

It is thus evident that the genetic load (number of genetic extinctions per gene eliminated) for dominant, recessive and sex linked recessives is in the ratio of 2:1:1.5. In an inbred population with high F, the eliminations are through homozygotes and so it is like recessive mutant.

Load Ratio

Now, the ratio of inbred load (L_I, when F = I) to the random mating load (L_R, when F = 0) can be obtained taking h = 0 (complete recessive):

$$\frac{L_I}{L_R} = \frac{Sq}{Sq^2} = \frac{1}{q}$$

$$= \frac{\left(\dfrac{u}{h}\right)}{u} = \frac{1}{h}$$

and taking h as the dominant term

$$\frac{L_I}{L_R} = \frac{\left(\dfrac{u}{h}\right)}{2u}$$

$$= \frac{\left(\dfrac{u}{h}\right)}{\left(\dfrac{1}{2u}\right)}$$

$$= \frac{1}{2h}$$

Therefore, with increase in *h*, the ratio is reduced and if *h* is small, the mutation load is increased by inbreeding.

2. Segregation Load: Balanced Polymorphism

This is also known as balanced load. This occurs when the fittest genotype is heterozygous (when the heterozygotes are superior to both the homozygotes). Thus, the fitness of heterozygote is taken as unity while that of dominant homozygote as 1- S_1 and of recessive homozygote as $1 - S_2$. The Mendelian segregation produce homozygotes which are inferior in fitness compared to heterozygotes. This load is known as segregation load (Crow 1958) or **balanced load** (Dobzhansky *et al*, 1960).

The segregation load is the decrease in fitness compared to the fittest heterozygote which produce homozygous progeny (with low fitness) by Mende-lian segregation. When the heterozygotes are superior than both the homozygotes, the relative fitness of the three genotypes are 1- S_1(AA), 1.0 (Aa), and $(1 - S_2)$ (aa). Therefore, the average fitness of the population will-be:

$$W = p^2(1 - S_1) + 2pq + q^2(1 - S_2)$$
$$= 1 - S_1 p^2 - S_2 q^2$$
$$= 1 - (S_1 p^2 + S_2 q^2)$$

Thus, the population would suffer a loss in fitness by $S_1 p^2 + S_2 q^2$. This loss in fitness of the population is the segregation load. Therefore, the segregation load is:

$$L = 1 - W$$
$$= S_1 p^2 + S_2 q^2$$

The reduction in fitness (load) equals $S_1 p^2$ for AA genotype and $S_2 q^2$ for the aa genotype.

In equilibrium population the segregation load can be obtained by taking the frequencies of alleles A and a at equilibrium as:

$$P_{(A)} = \frac{S_2}{(S_1 + S_2)} \text{ and}$$

$$q_{(a)} = \frac{S_1}{(S_1 + S_2)}$$

Now substituting the equilibrium gene frequencies of both the alleles in the segregation load equation will result in the segregation load of an equilibrium population as:

$$L = S_1 p^2 + S_2 q^2$$

$$= \frac{S_1 S_2}{(S_1 + S_2)}$$

This is the loss in average fitness of the population at equilibrium and is due to segregation of genes, called as the segregation load. Thus, at equilibrium in a polymorphic population (balanced polymorphism or heterozygous superiority) the genetic load (due to segregation) is $S_1 S_2 / (S_1 + S_2)$ which equals the disadvantage of a given homozygote (S_1) multiplied by the frequency of that particular alleles (p_i). Therefore,

$$\frac{S_1 S_2}{(S_1 + S_2)} = S_1\, p \qquad \text{Since} \quad p = \frac{S_2}{(S_1 + S_2)}$$

$$\text{or} \quad \frac{S_1 S_2}{(S_1 + S_2)} = S_2\, q \qquad \text{Since} \quad q = \frac{S_1}{(S_1 + S_2)}$$

Therefore, the segregation load $\left[\dfrac{S_1 S_2}{(S_1 + s_2)}\right] = S_i p_i$

Where, S_i is the selective disadvantage of ith homozygote,

                p_i is the frequency of that i^{th} allele forming the ith homozygote.

The gene frequencies do not change at equilibrium and therefore the average disadvantage suffered by each allele at a given locus regardless of the total number of alleles must equal that suffered by all others and these must equal the segregation load of the population.

The average fitness of a polymorphic population is maximum when the responsible genes are at their equilibrium frequencies. Thus for individu-als of the genotypes AA, Aa and aa whose relative fitness are 1- S_1, 1, and 1- S_2, the average fitness can be written as

$$1 - S_1\left[\frac{S_2}{(S_1 + S_2)}\right]$$

Thus, the average fitness is greater than $1 - S_1$ or $1 - S_2$. Therefore, the average fitness of the equilibrium population is higher than of the population homozygous for either of the two alleles.

The relative fitness of 3 genotypes can be interpreted as:

For every daughter left by a heterozygous female (Aa), the AA female leaves only $1 - S_1$ daughter and the aa female leaves only $1 - S_2$. The average female in the population, consequently, leaves only $1 - \left[\dfrac{S_1 S_2}{(S_1 + S_2)} \right]$ daughter for each daughter left by a heterozygous female.

It is thus evident that segregation load can be computed from information on only one allele and its homozygous effect on fitness. This is also true for multiple alleles. Secondly, the allele with the least selective disadvantage produce large segregation load.

However, the segregation load will be less if the number of multiple alleles are more. The segregation load is inversely proportional to the number of alleles in the population: $L = S/n$

Where,   S is the harmonic mean of the homozygous disadvantages,

n is the number of alleles.

The minimum estimate of the segregation load for multiple alleles is the product of the frequency of that allele and its homozygous selective disadvantage relative to the best genotype.

The multiple loci, which are independent in inheritance and in their effect on fitness, will have their collective segregation load roughly equal to the sum of individual load. And the linkage between loci reduces the segregation load.

The Segregation Load is Greater than Mutation Load

When the abnormal gene is maintained by heterozygote advantage, the genetic load is larger than when the abnormal gene is determined by recurrent mutation. The mutation load is equal to the rate of mutation (u) which is definitely less than the segregation load.

Effect of Inbreeding on Mutational and Segregation Load

The effects of the mutation load and of segregation load is reversed by inbreeding. Consequently the mutational load causes greater depression of fitness than the segregation load. This is because the inbreeding reduces the proportion of heterozygotes and complete in-breeding eliminates them completely leaving only the homozygotes in the population in the proportions p AA: q aa. A deleterious recessive mutation in a completely inbred population will cause a load equal to Sq, the selection coefficient for aa genotype being S. Therefore, a ratio between mutational load in an inbred and in a random mating population will be:

$$\frac{L_{I(M)}}{L_{R(M)}} = \frac{Sq}{Sq^2} = \frac{1}{q}$$

Thus, when q is low the load upon inbreeding will be increased.

In case of segregation load upon inbreeding taking exclusively the segregation load, the increase in load will depend upon the selective values of the two types of homozygotes (S_1 and S_2). Thus, on inbreeding the segregation load will be $S_1p + S_2q$ which becomes as segregation inbred load or segregation load in an inbreed population after substituting the equilibrium values of p and q as:

$$S_1 p + S_2 q = \left[\frac{S_1 S_2}{(S_1 + S_2)} + \frac{S_1 S_2}{(S_1 + S_2)} \right]$$

$$= \frac{2 S_1 S_2}{(S_1 + S_2)}$$

Now the ratio of segregation load in an inbred and in a random mating population can be taken as:

$$\frac{L_{I(M)}}{L_{R(M)}} = \frac{\left[\dfrac{2 S_1 S_2}{(S_1 + S_2)} \right]}{\left[\dfrac{S_1 S_2}{(S_1 + S_2)} \right]}$$

$$= \left[\frac{2 S_1 S_2}{(S_1 + S_2)} \right] \left[\frac{(S_1 + S_2)}{S_1 S_2} \right]$$

$$= 2$$

This ratio of segregation load is quite small than the ratio of 1/q produced by the mutation load with inbreeding. Therefore, mutation load causes greater depression of fitness than segregation load in an inbred population. Thus inbreeding cause a reversal of the effects of the two types of load.

In most natural populations, both types of load (mutational and segregation) occur but it is difficult to distinguish and determine their relative importance. This is because of the heterozygous expression of the mutational load and multiple allelic systems in segregation load. The effect of mutational load on inbreeding may cause a change less than 1/q when some heterozygous expression of genes will appear under random mating because all genes are not fully recessive. Secondly, there will be an increase in segregation load in multiple allelic systems because the frequency of deleterious homozygotes will be increased upon inbreeding than random mating.

3. Recombination Load

The recombination produces a decrease in fitness by increasing the inferior types. For example, if two chromosomes (AB and Ab) are favoured on the average by natural selection in various zygotic combination into which they enter, but the other two types aB and ab are disfavoured. As a result of recombination the inferior types will be increased leading to a decrease in fitness and hence a genetic load.

4. Migration Load

Every individual perform better in its original habitat and if migrated to another place its fitness is reduced in the new environmental conditions. This is because an individual carries genes, which are selected in its original habitat, may not be equally favourable in the new area. The migration, to a new area may therefore, reduce the average fitness of the population. This reduction in average fitness of the population due to introduction of less favourable immigrant genes is called as the migration load. Thus, migration load is caused by migrants entering a new environment.

5. Population Size and Genetic Load

The consequence of small population is to drift away the gene frequencies from equilibrium. The population fitness is highest at equilibrium proportions. Thus, the genetic drift away from equilibrium frequencies will reduce the fitness leading to a genetic load. This is called as finite population load or drift load.

6. Incompatibility Load

Sometimes, there is incompatibility of alleles contributed by male parent with the genotypes of the mother. The individual (usually the mother and the unborn child, foetus) of different genotypes interact unfavourably. As a result there is probability of death of the embryo neonatally. This is known as incompatibility of mother and foetus. The best known example is Rh + child from Rh – mother. The heterozygous baby (Rh rh) from Rh negative women (rh rh) suffered from hemolytic disease which may cause death of the child rather than the baby is born to heterozygous or Rh positive mother. Therefore, the heterozygous children born to recessive mothers than born to heterozygous or Rh + mothers have low fitness and thereby causing a genetic load. Further, the genetic load is influenced by the inbreeding of the mother or child. The incompatibility load is increased in proportion to the F of the mother but decreased in proportion to the F of the child.

7. Meiotic Drive Load or Gametic Selection Load

This is caused by preferential segregation of deleterious alleles. Non-Mendelian segregation, meiotic drive or segregation distortion is a term used to explain the exception to Mendal's law of segregation. This is an example of gametic selection which occurs when part of the gametes are inviable or ineffective in fertilization. This occurs when one of the gametes produced by heterozygous genotype is either lethal or unable to follow the usual meiotic segregation pattern and this phenomenon is termed as meiotic drive. Therefore, meiotic drive is a mechanism (generally associated with various kinds of chromosomal structural changes in heterozygous form) which may affect the genetic composition of a population via inequalities in chromosomal transmission during meiosis. Regardless of their individual selective advantage or disadvantage the genes in a chromosome favoured by preferential segregation make a disproportionate contribution to the gene pool of the next generation. The meiotic drive is an exception to the rule of 1:1 recovery of segregating allele in heterozygous organism. This is the result of the unequal frequencies of recovery of the two kinds of gametes produced by heterozygotes and probably no specific genetic factors are involved in the non random assortment of chromosomes. The heterozygotes produce gametes in a ratio deviating from the expected ratio of 1:1 (Mendelian ratio) because the gametes having one of the two alleles is either not formed or fail to function properly. Thus, this deviation in gametic ratio is the property of heterozygous genotype and not of the gametic pool of the population for which it differs from gametic selection. Therefore, meiotic drive is a force capable of changing gene frequencies in population depending upon the nature of meiotic division producing two kinds to gametes from a heterozygote in a ratio different from 1:1.

Meiotic drive can result in increased frequency of alleles despite their selective advantage or in decreased frequencies of alleles that would otherwise be selectively favoured. Thus the mechanisms leading to meiotic drive are themselves subject to selection to reduce the fitness and hence genetic load.

The typical examples of meiotic drive are the t alleles (tailless allele) in male mice, and that involving a dominant segregation distorter (SD) gene in Drosophila. The segregation distortion occurs in male mice at t locus bearing t- alleles (the t alleles are recessive lethal) and causes the heterozy-gous male to transmit tailless t alleles in frequencies as high as 99 per cent compared to the normal allele. This occurs due to the difference in the fertilizing capacity of two types of sperms produced by heterozygotes which may be due to the specific antigens produced by t alleles on the surface of the sperm. The sperms carrying t allele get advantage.

The SD gene (segregation distortion locus) in Drosophila is the best known example of meiotic drive. This locus causes the malfunction of sperm carrying the SD$^+$ chromosomes in male (SD/SD$^+$) heterozygotes. When SD chromosome is present in male, it instructs its homologue (SD$^+$) to self destruct so that the only SD carrying sperms function. Consequently, the SD chromosome tends to increase in the population. Thus SD chromosome produces functional sperm while its SD$^+$ homologue is mostly lost in dysfunctional sperm. The males heterozygous for SD gene may transmit the SD carrying chromosome to more than 95 per cent of offspring while SD is without any effect in the females. The SD locus causes break on the homologous chromosome at correspond-ing point during synapsis. This results in sister strand fusion and the formation of chromatid bridge, producing nonfunctional gametes carrying SD$^+$ chromosome while SD carrying chromosome produce normal gametes.

Another system in Drosophila involving segregation distortion is called recovery distorter (RD). The RD distorts the sex ratio in favour of females. Males from RD lines may produce offspring up to 65 per cent females due to a reduction in recovery of Y chromosome. The RD is without effect in the female. This is also called as sex ratio factor (SR gene) present on X chromosome which causes complete degeneration of the Y chromosomes.

The PK locus (pollen killer gene) in wheat and tobacco causes the death of gametes carrying normal alleles producing a ratio different from 1:1.

Meiotic drive is typically found in male sex only as explained above. Its effect is like gametic selection.

8. Heterogenous Environment or Dysentric Load

The different genotypes respond differently in different environments leading one allele to be favoured in one environment while another allele in other environment and thus the selection coefficient is influenced causing the reduction in average fitness and hence genetic load. The individuals of a population are well adapted, though not perfectly, to their way of life under certain environment. Thus, the genes are selected according to the environment and such genes are better adapted ones. The environment is changing one. As a consequence of the change in environment the selected better adapted genes in earlier environment become ill adapted in the changed environment and replaced by the alleles more fitted to the new environment. This replacement leads to genetic load known as substitution load. This load occurs with the change of environment.

9. Hybrid Load

This is caused by hybridization of separate populations.

13.4 Significance of Genetic Load

Environmental conditions are changed with time and accordingly the advantages of different genotypes are changed. As a result of rapid change in environment the population with genetic perfection (little or no genetic death) becomes genetically imperfect in new environment. On the contrary, in a new environment the genetically imperfect population (with genetic death or genetic load) having deleterious genes improves its average fitness because the formerly deleterious genes may have better fitness in new environment. The presence of genetic load in terms of genetic variability may thus be of greater significance in new environment than the absence of genetic load. The optimum genotype with maximum fitness ($W_{max} = 1$) may change with time, place, and for different reason at the same place (*e.g.* division of labour into males and females). In the presence of genetic load, measured in terms of departure from the optimum genotype with maximum fitness, the advantage of genetic variability can be taken in the newly developed environment. Therefore, in terms of evolution the optimum genotype has its little or limited evolutionary value.

In the long run, the presence of a variety of mutant alleles in a population increases its ability to respond adaptively to an ever changing environment. The ability to evolve requires a genetic load.

Part II
Quantitative Genetics

Chapter 14
Quantitative Inheritance

In population genetics the characters are classified on the basis of their mode of inheritance, (number gene loci controlling the character), type and causes of variation among individuals of a population. Accordingly, the characters are grouped as qualitative and quantitative characters.

14.1 Qualitative and Quantitative Characters

Some characters are controlled by one or few pairs of genes with their major effects which are not affected by environment, in general, making possible to classify the genotypes accurately based on phenotypes and hence show discontinuous variation expressed in Mendelian ratios. The phenotypes of such aharacters are easily distinguished one from another. Such characters are called as **qualitative characters.** There is another category of characters controlled by many gene pairs (poly genes) with their minor effects which are modified by the environment and show continuous variation. The phenotypes of such characters have so small differences that simple observation can not make distinction between different phenotypes. Such characters are called as **quantitative characters** or **metric traits.**

These two types of characters (qualitative and quantitative) differ from each other with respect to the way the characters are measured, number of gene loci affecting the character and the extent of the effect of gene on the character, modification of gene's effect by the environment, type of variation shown by the character, description of a population for the character, inheritance pattern and the method of study used for the character.

1. Qualitative Characters

These characters are also called as *attributes*. They have the following characteristics-

☆ The characters are simply *measured/recorded with naked eyes or by chemical test* or other test. There is no quantitative measurement for these characters. Such characters are called as qualitative traits or attributes. The observation on an individual is called the phenotype. The phenotype is assigned a rank or value to each individual according to the phenotype of the individual.

☆ These characters are *controlled by one or few pairs of genes* with major effect of each gene and hence these genes are called as major genes. Each pair of gene has an effect large enough to cause discontinuity even in the presence of segregation of genes at other loci. Such genes have their effect involving varying degree of *dominance and epistasis*. It is easy to estimate the effect of evolutionary forces, mating system and population size on changing the genetic structure of population for traits governed by such genes.

☆ These characters are *usually not affected by environment*, but only in very few cases. The classical examples of environmental modification are the flower colour of Chinese Primrose, colour pattern in rabbit, sex limited and sex influenced characters, occurrence of diabetes, etc.

☆ These characters show *discontinuous variation*. The major effect of gene and no effect of environment to modify the genotypic value of the character cause discontinuity in phenotypic values. The data collected on these characters is binomially distributed as the individuals of a population belong to different distinct classes. This is because the individuals are recognized as belonging to one or the other group without use of special measuring tools *viz.* black or red or white coat colour animals; spotted cows or not; horned or polled cows; droopy or erect ears in pigs; tall and dwarf plants etc. This makes it possible to classify the phenotypes accurately and all the individuals of a population are grouped into discrete classes.

☆ A population is described for a qualitative character by estimating the percentage or proportion (ratios or frequencies) of individuals of each genotypic/phenotypic class. This is done by summarizing the raw data collected on different individuals (black and white coat colour of sheep) after counting the numbers of animals according to the phenotypic class *viz.* black or white colour.

☆ *Mendelian analysis* is applied to study the inheritance pattern of these characters. This is because the Mendelian ratios are expressed by these characters. The study of inheritance pattern of these characters is called as Mendelian genetics. The chi-square test of association is applied between the observed and expected ratios based on Mendelian inheritance to test the significance of departure in observed and expected ratios.

2. Quantitative Characters

These characters are also called as *metric traits*. They have the following characteristics:

✰ The characters are *measured in metric units* like gm., kg, cm, days. These are the quantitative measurements to measure the character in a quantitative way assigning a numerical value to the phenotype of the character. Thus, the observation recorded on an individual in metric unit is called as phenotypic value and the character is called as quantitative or metric trait.

✰ These characters are controlled by *many gene pairs* (*i.e.* genes present at many loci). They are also called as polygenes because the genes are many in numbers to influence a character. The characters controlled by polygenes are also called as polygenic characters. Each gene has small effect and such genes are called as minor genes for their minor effect. Some genes add to or make positive contributions to the character, others do not. The value of the character is increased by the genes that make positive contribution and hence such genes are called *additive genes* and this kind of gene action is called *additive gene action* which is in contrast to dominance and epistasis (called as *nonadditive gene action*),

✰ All these characters are affected by *environmental factors* which cause modification in genotypic value assigned by the genes to the character. For example, milk production is affected by the diet given to a cow.

✰ The characters show *continuation variation* in phenotypic values of different individuals. The continuation variation is caused by the segregation of genes at many loci affecting the character and environmental modification of genotypic value of the character, for example, milk production, lactation length, body weight, wool production etc. The distribution of individuals follows the normal distribution.

✰ A population is described for a quantitative character by estimating the population parameters *viz.* the mean, variance and covariance.

✰ The *statistical methods* are applied to study the inheritance pattern of these characters due to the continuous variation. Mostly, the analysis of variance is conducted to test the significance of differences attributed to different genetic and environmental factors. As a result a new branch of genetics has been developed to study the inheritance pattern and it is called as quantitative genetics or biometrical genetics.

The genetics of quantitative characters in a population is called as **Quantitative Genetics.** This deals with the study of the inheritance of quantitative characters by applying the statistical methods to estimate the genetic parameters *viz.* mean, variance and covariance. These parameters characterize the genetic variation in any quantitative character in a population and the changes that take place from time to time.

14.2 Quantitative Inheritance

Mendelian's laws of inheritance were founded on the basis of clear cut differences in phenotypic values of individuals belonging to different genotypic classes. These differences were qualitative (tall and short plants, round and wrinkled seeds, green and yellow pods, etc) and accounted for by distinct genes. On the other hand, the quantitative differences follow a normal distribution from low to high values with continuity in values of different individuals without sharp distinction and hence called continuous variation. At that time it was difficult to analyse genetically the continuous variation that could be accounted for by distinct genes. It was therefore considered that environmental differences between genetically identical individuals may cause the continuous variation in phenotypic values. Thus, the early geneticists (Bateson and De Vries) proposed that continuous variation is not produced by genes but by the environment and hence not inherited.

14.2.1 Development of Multiple Factor Hypotheses

Galton (1889), a cousin of Charles Darwin, tried to explain the origin of observable differences between humans for physical and mental characteristics. He observed that these differences were small and appeared to be inherited. The correlation and regression techniques were invented to measure the degree to which such characters are inherited. The biometricians tried to demonstrate statistically that there was likeness between relatives for continuously distributed quantitative characters and *blending inheritance theory* was proposed indicating that individuals seem to be a mixture of parental characteristics which were in turn the mixture of their grand parents, etc.

Yule (1906) proposed that continuous variation may be the result of small effect of a multitude of individual genes on the character.

Johannsen (1909) formulated his *pure line theory* based on the breeding experiment for *seed weight of beans* ranging from 15 to 90 centigrams and demonstrated that many genetic differences really existed for seed weight. The bean is highly self-pollinated plant and hence he established 19 pure lines from 19 seeds of different weight. It was concluded that a population of individuals showing continuous variation consist of a number of genetically different groups and each group has a range of values due to environmental differences between individuals. Thus, this experiment was found useful to explain that the continuous variation results from both genetic and environmental factors.

Nilsson-Ehle (1909), Scandavian geneticist, supported the hypoth-esis of Yule and Johannsen by experimental evidence on *seed colour in wheat*. He reported three gene pairs (Aa Bb Cc) responsible for grain colour in wheat showing dominance-recessive relationship and segregat-ing in Mendelian fashion. Any of the three gene pairs when segregating alone produced F_2 progeny in a ratio of 3 red: 1 white, two gene pairs segregating at the same time produced F_2 ratio of 15 red: 1 white and likewise a cross between heterozygotes for all the 3 gene pairs produced F_2 ratio of 63 red: 1 white. All the three gene pairs appeared to act similarly and hence it made little difference that which of the red gene (A, B or C) was segregating. It was obvious that red grained plants of F_2 population were of various genotypes which were shown in F_3 families. Some of them produced all red, some in ratio of 3 red: 1 white, others 15 red: 1 white and still others produced 63: 1 ratio. Thus a variety of red genotypes occur having different number of red genes and the intensity of red colour depends on the number of dominant alleles present. The plants having either less or more number of red genes will have extreme phenotypes for red colour with low frequency whereas those plants having intermediate number of red genes will have intermediate phenotype with high frequency. Such a phenotypic distribution from segregation of three independent genes each with definite effect looks like normal distribution which is a characteristic of a quantitative trait.

Further breeding experiment in support of quantitative inheritance was reported by East (1916) for *flower length of tobacco plant*. He made a cross of two self-pollinating varieties which had been long inbred and hence homozygous having the flower length of 40.5 mm and 93.3 mm. But there was variation within each variety which indicated environmental variation. The F_1 flowers were intermediate in size (63 mm) to both the parents as expected for the genes having quantitative additive effects. Further the variability in F_1 was similar to each parent which indicated that the F_1 genotypes were probably genetically uniform, *i.e.* uniformly heterozygous for the same genes. Therefore, the variability in F_1 was assigned to environmental effects as in the parental lines. When F_1's were crossed, the F_2 generation showed wider continuous distribution than F_1 and parental varieties. This indicated that the differences in F_2 were not only environmental but also genetic resulted from segregation and recombination of genes. Further evidence of genetic difference was observed in F_3 generation produced from different F_2 individuals. The mean value of each F_3 group depended upon the F_2 individuals crossed. This indicated that F_2 generation was a mixture of many genotypes. Thus, East presented the conclusive evidence that quantitative characters are governed by many gene pairs with small additive effects.

14.2.2 Gene Numbers and Phenotypic Classes with their Ratios

The different kinds of gametes produced by heterozygous individual for **n** genes are 2^n that are distributed according to the coefficients of the binomial expanded to the nth power $(\frac{1}{2} + \frac{1}{2})^n$. For three independent segregating genes, the expansion of the binomial $(\frac{1}{2}$ red $+ \frac{1}{2}$ white$)^3$ will produce 8 types of gametes from one individual in the ratio of $1/8$ (3 red genes): $3/8$ (2 red genes): $3/8$ (1 red genes): $1/8$ (no red genes). For the mating of two such heterozygotes the distribution of colour differences among the zygotes will be:

$(\frac{1}{2}$ red $+ \frac{1}{2}$ white$)^3$ x $(\frac{1}{2}$ red $+ \frac{1}{2}$ white$)^3$ = $(\frac{1}{2}$ red $+ \frac{1}{2}$ white$)^6$.

This will produce the ratio of zygotes as:

No of individuals   1 : 6 : 15 : 20 : 15 : 6 : 1 = 64

No. of red genes   6   5   4   3   2   1   0

The *number of phenotypic classes* of the quantitative traits increases in arithmetic way with an increase in the number of gene pairs (n) on the assumption that the genes are segregating independently (no linkage) with additive and cumulative effects, have equal gene frequency and not affected by environment. However, a number of different genotypes can produce the same or similar phenotype due to additive relation among genes and absence of dominance between alleles. The information given in Table 14.1 below is useful.

Table 14.1: Numbers of Phenotypic Classes in F_2 Generation in Relation to Numbers of Gene Pairs

No. of Gene Pairs (n)	No. Gametes Produced by F_1	No. of Genotypes in F_2	F_2 Size $(F_1 \times F_1)$ for All Combinations	Phenotypic Classes (Numbers)	Ratio of Phenotypic Classes in F_2 Generation
n	2^n	3^n	4^n	$2n + 1$	$\left[\dfrac{2n!}{k!}(2n-k)!\right]\left(\dfrac{1}{2}\right)^{2n}$
1	2	3	4	3	1:2:1
2	4	9	16	5	1:4:6:4:1
3	8	27	64	7	1:6:15:20:15:6:1
4	16	81	256	9	1:8:28:56:70:56:28:8:1
5	32	243	1024	11	1:10:45:120:210:252:210:120:45:10:1
6	64	729	4096	13	1:12:66:220:495:792:924:792:495:220:66:12:1

Where,   k = number of contributing genes in the genotype

      3^n = no. of homozygotes + no. of heterozygotes

      = $2^n + (3^n - 2^n)$

The quantitative traits are controlled by many gene pairs (factors) called as multiple factors and the inheritance of these factors is called as multiple *factor inheritance*. Mather has proposed the term polygenes for these multiple factors. The increase in number of polygenes affecting a trait produces the continuity of measurements (phenotypic values).

From the information given in Table 14.1 above, the number of genes involved can be estimated if the ratio and number of phenotypes is known.

14.2.3 Illustration of Polygenic Inheritance

The polygenic inheritance involves many gene pairs and the environment also modifies the genotypic values and hence the phenotypic values making the distribution of phenotypic values in to normal distribution. To illustrate the polygenic inheritance, some assumptions have to be made like additive effect of genes ignoring the gene interaction effect, no linkage, no environment effect, equal gene frequncies and that each gene is a contributing gene adding its effect to the phenotypic value.

The coat colour in HF cattle is controlled by many gene pairs producing the variation in spotting of coat from little white (almost black) to almost white. To simplify the illustration, let only two pairs of genes are involved. These gene pairs are A and a at A locus and E and e at E locus. Consider the genes A and E are the contributing genes that add to the amount of spotting (White colour) each equal to 20 percent white surface of the animal body while their alleles *a* and *e* are the neutral genes that do not affect spotting of animal surface. Let the assumptions mentioned above (no dominance between alleles, no epistasis among genes, no linkge, no environment effect and equal gene frequencies) hold true to understand easier the concept. Thus the genotype *aaee* is the neutral genotype producing minimum amount of white and called as the *basic genotype* while the genotype AAEE will produce the maximum amount of white spotting. Let further the basic genotype *aaee* to produce only 10 percent white spotting on body surface.

There will be produced 9 genotypes for two gene pairs among F_2 population produced by crossing F_1 dihybrid (*AaEe*) which were in turn produced by crossing animals of genotype *aaee* (animals with minimum amount of white) with animals of genotype *AAEE* (animals with almost white surface of body). According to the number of contributing genes, the 9 genotypes can be grouped into 5 types of genotypes *viz.* aaee; Aaee and aaEe; AAee, aaEE and AaEe; AAEe and AaEE; and AAEE. Under the assumption of equal gene frequencies, the maximum frequency of animals will be of those having 50 percent white and 50 percent black surface of the body compared to other combinations of spotting. This will be partly because there will be more numbers of genotypes out of total 16 genotypes (6/16) for the phenotype having 50 percent white and 50 percent black animals.

The total results of dihybrid cross according to the numbers of contributing genes in different 5 categories of genotypes in F_2 population with respect to degree of spotting can be illusted better in a tabular form as under:

No. of Contributing Genes	No. of Possible Genotypes as per Contributing Genes	Phenotypic Ratio	Degree of White Spotting (per cent)
0	aaee	1	10 (almost black)
1	Aaee, aaEe	4	30
2	AAee, aaEE, AaEe	6	50
3	AAEe, AaEE	4	70
4	AAEE	1	90 (almost white)

It is important point here to consider that if the assumptions made to understand the principle may not hold true, it may then leads to certain implications. The important is that any two phenotypes of the character will not be distinguished clearly.

14.2.4 Phenotypic Effect of Increase in Numbers of Polygenes

The genotypes are not important but phenotypes become much more important with increase in numbers of polygenes. This is because a number of different genotypes produce the same or similar genotype. For example, in case of a character for spotting of HF cows controlled by 2 gene pairs, the cows having 50 percent white body colour may have any of the 3 genotypes (AAee, aaEE and AaEe). The numbers of genotypes with the same or similar phenotypic effect are increased with the increase in number of gene pairs affecting a polygenic trait.

Secondly, plotting the coefficients of the expanded binomial on graph paper and connecting the points by a smooth line results a curve in conforming the shape of the curve of normal distribution which is known as bell shape population curve. Further, the increase in the number of polygenes affecting a trait increases the number of phenotypes, results into small increments between phenotypes, increase in the number of bars on histogram representing a separate phenotype point on the curve, and sometimes the difference between two phenotypes become indistinguishable when the number of phenotypes increase and the increments between them is decreased.

Thirdly, the increase in number of polygenes results to a phenomenon called as *transgressive variation* wherein some of the exceptional individuals are observed among the F_2 generation which exceed in their performance beyond the range of variation of both the parents.

14.3 Possible Estimate of Number of Gene Pairs

The following methods can be used to estimate the approximate number of *polygenes* involved in controlling a quantitative character.

1. Phenotypic Variability and Number of Loci

The phenotypic variability exists even in a group of individuals having identical genotype and all of this is environmental in origin. The phenotypic variability is all environmental in genetically uniform hybrid produced by crossing two pure lines. But among the F_2 individuals, produced by mating F_1 individuals, new gene combinations will be formed. As a result F_2 generation is expected to have much more variability than the F_1 and the F_2 generation will be between the means of the two parental lines. Assuming the environment as constant from generations to generation, the variation in F_1 and F_2 due to environment will be approximately the same. And so the increased phenotypic variability in F_2 over the F_1 population will be the genetic variability. Therefore, the difference between the phenotypic variability of F_2 and F_1 will represent the genetic variability of the F_2 population.

2. F_2 Ratio Method of Estimating the Number of Genes

The F_2 generation is more variable because of gene segregation. Some of the F_2 individuals are alike in phenotype as that of one of the pure parental individuals/ strains. The proportion of such F_2 individuals with extreme phenotype depends upon the number of gene pairs affecting the trait. The relation between the number of gene pairs and the fraction of extreme F_2 individuals gives a rough estimate of the number of gene loci controlling the trait. The estimate is rough because the multifactor traits are also affected by the environmental factors.

The genes segregate and recombine. As a result with the increase in number of segregating gene pairs, the relative proportion of F_2 individuals, exactly like their parents, decreases. This has been shown in Table 14.1. For example, for one, two, three, four, five gene pair differences in a trait, the ratio of F_2 progeny having a particular parental genotype falls to ¼, 1/16, 1/64, 1/256 and 1/2024, respectively. East (1916) raised 444 F_1 plants of tobacco to study the Corolla (flower) length and he could not find any plant of the parental genotype, indicating that more than four gene pairs are involved in controlling this trait.

3. Total Response and Number of Loci

The total response achieved through selection depends on the genetic variation of the base population. To establish the relation between total response (R_T) and additive genetic variance (σ^2_A) requires some assumptions *viz.* all loci controlling a trait have equal effect on the character, have equal frequencies (0.5) and the alleles with opposite effects (favourable and unfavourable) are fixed in two inbred lines (associated genes). The equal effect of all genes on the trait make $R = \Sigma 2a = 2na$ with **n** as the number of gene loci each having a homozygote difference of 2a. The σ^2_A with the assumption of equal frequencies and equal (additive) effect of genes will become as:

$$\sigma^2_A = 2pq[a + d(q-p)]^2$$
$$= \tfrac{1}{2}\,na^2 \text{ No dominance: } p = q = 0.5$$

Now expressing the range in terms of additive genetic standard deviation $\left(\dfrac{R}{\sigma_A}\right)$ and squaring leads to:

$$\frac{R^2}{\sigma_A{}^2} = \frac{(2na)^2}{\tfrac{1}{2}na^2} = \frac{4n^2a^2}{\tfrac{1}{2}na^2} = 8n$$

Therefore, $8n = \dfrac{R^2}{\sigma_A{}^2}$;

$$n = \frac{R^2}{8\sigma^2_A}$$

Thus, the total response relative to the initial genetic variance $\left(\dfrac{R}{\sigma^2_A}\right)$ depends primarily on the number of loci contributing to the variation. When the number of loci will be more the response will be more in relation to the original variance. However, the violation of the assumption in obtaining the number of gene loci from total response and the genetic variance either underestimate or overestimate the number of gene loci. The failure of equal effect and equal gene frequencies underestimate while the violation of third assumption (associated genes) overestimate the number due to the reason that will be less in this case. The third condition can be met by estimating the σ^2_A from F_2 and subsequent generations.

4. Marker Chromosome

A technique using marker chromosomes in Drosophila to identify some genes having fairly large effect on bristle number has been developed. However, it is still quite difficult to identify *polygenes* with small effect.

14.4 Mode of Inheritance of Quantitative Traits

The quantitative characters show the following mode of inheritance, In other words, the essential features of the multiple factor hypothesis or quantitative inheritance or the polygenic inheritance are as under:

1. The quantitative characters are inherited. This means that they are controlled by genes.
2. The inheritance pattern of these characters is of Mendelian type. This means that the genes controlling these characters are nuclear born.
3. These characters are controlled by many gene pairs called as *polygenes* or minor genes.
4. Such characters are affected by environmental factors.
5. These characters show continuous variation,

The effect of *polygenes* and the environmental factors cause continuously graded series of phenotypic values from one extreme to the other within the range. This is called as continuous variation. However, very few individuals are found to have the extreme phenotypic values and progressively more individuals have their phenotypic value nearer to the average value of the population. This type of symmetrical distribution of phenotypic values is bell shaped and called *normal distribution*.

The evidences in support of the above characteristic features of quantitative inheritance are well documented and discussed below.

1. The Phenotypic Value for a Quantitative Trait is Inherited

The quantitative characters are controlled by genes and hence the continuous variation is inherited. This is well evidenced from the following facts:

(i) Different breeds, lines and strains within a species show different mean performance for quantitative characters even if they are raised together and given the same environment.

(ii) The relatives show resemblance or similarities to each other compared to unrelated individual for the quantitative characters.

(iii) These characters respond to selection and show inbreeding depression.

(iv) The other evidences relating the gene and quantitative characters have been discussed under section 14.5.

2. The Poly Genes are Nuclear Born

The genes controlling the quantitative characters are inherited in Mendelian fashion. Such genes are many in number which means that many gene pairs called as *polygenes* affect a single quantitative character. These genes have their effect similar to each other, supplementing each other and sufficiently small compared to total variation or to the non-heritable variation.

Secondly, the effect of *polygenes* is easily modified by the variation in environment. As such the Mendelian ratios are not exhibited by the quantitative characters. Thus such *polygenes* can not easily be identified individually. As a result the inheritance of individual gene of a polygenic system cannot be followed by Mandelian method.

Inspite of the above essential features of the multiple factor hypotheses, it is true based on the following evidences that *polygenes* are borne on the chromosomes and follow the Mendelian inheritance.

(1) Reciprocal Crosses

Based on nuclear heredity (discontinuously variable character or qualitative characters) the two parents contribute equally to the genotype of the offspring due to the halving nature of inheritance. In other words, equal inheritance from the two parents is expected under Mendelian inheritance but unequal contribution of two parents if the inheritance is of other type. The quantitative characters behave like qualitative characters with respect to reciprocal crosses.

(2) Properties of Nuclear Borne Genes

The segregation and linkage of genes are the two properties characteristic to the nuclear borne genes. The usual methods are not enough to observe the segregation and linkage of polygenes. The evidences to observe segregation and linkage of polygenes are as under:

(i) Segregation of Polygenes

The necessary test of segregation is the relative variation of the different generations following crossing. The two true breeding lines or strains and their F_1 generation show only the environmental variation due to the reason that all the individuals within each population (two true breeding lines, and F_1 population) are genetically uniform. When F_2 generation is produced from inter-se-mating of F_1 individuals, the nuclear genes which are different in the parents (two true breeding lines) will segregate in F_2 generation and the genetic segregation leads to the genetic variation. Thus the variability in F_2 generation is more than the parental generation and F_1. Thus the frequency distribution is broader and flatter. The F_2 generation is expected to be equally affected by the environment as the F_1 and parental generations. The excess part of variability in F_2 generation compared to F_1 and parental generation can be explained due to segregation and recombination of genes resulting in genetic variability. According to the Mendelian inheritance, half of the F_2 individuals are homozygous for the genes at each locus *viz.* $\frac{1}{4}$AA, $\frac{1}{4}$aa, $\frac{1}{2}$Aa. Thus the segregation occurs in F_3 families, though only for half the gene pairs on average. Therefore, the average variation of F_3 families is between F_2, and parents and F_1, with the differences in F_3 families among themselves to the extent that some families will have extreme variances while others and mostly of them will have intermediate. The mean phenotypes of the F_3 families will differ due to the homozygous genes for which the F_2 individuals differ and these mean phenotypes are correlated with the phenotypes of the F_2 parents. Greater variation in F_2 generation is observed than either F_1 or the parental generation even when the parental lines are not nearly true breeding. The magnitude of differences among F_3 families depends upon the number of genes segregating and controlling the character. The extreme variation in F_3 families is produced by homozygous individuals. The homozygosity is increased with continued selfing in successive generations. This leads to reduced genetic variability within the family but greater variability between families. This gives rise to differences between the means of the F_3 families which are correlated with the mean of the F_2 parents. The results of relative variation in different generations following crossing with respect to qualitative characters have accorded with the expectation of nuclear borne genes. Thus the polygenes show segregation and hence they are nuclear borne.

(ii) Linkage Shown by Polygenes

The linkage of nuclear genes is their second property. The test of linkage is difficult for the reason that polygenes have small and supplementary effect and further their effect is modified by the environment. There are evidences which have proved that polygenes show linkage with major genes as well as among themselves.

Linkage Relationship between Major Genes and Polygenes

This can be tested in two ways. The first way is to test the significance of differences among the mean phenotypic values of quantitative traits corresponding to the phenotypic classes of qualitative traits. The linkage between major genes and *polygenes* has been reported in many cases. Two early examples can be cited to support the linkage relationship between *major genes* and *polygenes*.

(a) The evidence of linkage between *major gene* and *polygenes* was first given by Sax (1923). The colour of seed in bean (phaseolus vulgaris) is controlled by a single gene pair whereas the seed size showed continuous variation. He crossed a strain having coloured large sized seeds with another strain with white small seeds. The F_2 generation gave a ratio of 3 coloured: 1 white seeded plant. He found that the average weight of seeds was proportional to the number of dominant genes affecting the seed colour. The average seed weight was 30.7 for the plants with PP genotypes, 28.3 for Pp genotypes and 26.4 for pp genotype. The differences in seed weight of three genotypes were found to be significant. This experiment was in the direction to show linkage between major gene affecting pigmentation (seed colour) and polygenes affecting seed size, but this did not rule out the possibility of pleiotropic effect of *major gene*.

(b) Another experiment was conducted by Rasmusson (1935) on garden pea considering flower colour controlled by *major genes* and flowering time controlled by *polygenes*. The flower colour and flowering time in 4 varieties of garden pea are as under:

Sl.No.	Varieties (parents)	Flower Colour (Major gene)	Flowering Time in Days (Deviation from av. flowering time of standard varieties)
1.	Gj	Coloured	8.5 days (late)
2.	Bism	White	–9.3 days (Early)
3.	HRT – II	Coloured	–6.1 days (Early)
4.	St	White	Late

The mean flowering time of F_2 plants with coloured and white flowers recorded is given as under:

Cross	Mean Flowering Time		Dfference	Linkage Relationhip
	Coloured Flowers	White Flowes		
G$_j$ x Bism	5.37	2.11	2.36*	Present
HRT x Bism	– 7.97	– 8.30	0.33	Incomplete
HRT x St.	– 1.24	1.83	– 2.87	Reverse

* significant difference

The cross between coloured – late and white-early flowering varieties (Gi and Bism, respectively) showed that F_2 plants with coloured flowers had significantly late flowering than white flower plants. This showed an association between pigmentation gene (*major gene*) and the *polygenes* responsible for the flowering time. But this association may be due to pleiotropic action. The pleiotropic gene action produces linkage always. Therefore, if the two characters (flower colour and flowering time) are produced due to pleiotropic gene effect, there would have been association in all the other crosses *viz.* HRT x Bism and HRT x St crosses.

The flowering time difference associated with flower colour was not observed in the cross of HRT x Bism which were both early flowering varieties but with coloured and white flowers. Had the two characters been produced due to pleiotropic gene action there could have been difference in flowering time of plants with coloured and white glowers because the genes responsible for pigmentation should have also been responsible for late flowering in case of pleiotropism. But in this cross both coloured and white flowered plants have nearly equal mean flowering time. This ruled out the possibility of pleiotropic gene action of coloured gene and gave the evidence of linkage between coloured gene and polygenes (affecting flowering time) in Gj x Bism cross. There was no association between two types of genes in second cross of HRT x Bism because linkage was broken down.

The relation between two characters in a third cross of HRT x St (coloured early flowering and white late flowering varieties) was reversed which is expected from the linkage.

Evidence of Linkage among the Polygenes

The following evidences are available —

(a) Mather and Harrison (1949) used the chromosome assay technique for the distribution of genes affecting the number of abdominal chaetae on the chromosomes of Drosophila.

The linkage among *polygenes* is evident from the different trends of genetic correlation and correlated response in the trait (s) not under selection as a result of selection for a trait genetically correlated with other trait (s). Mather and Harrison (1949) practiced selection for increase in number of abdominal chaetae on Drosophila from a cross between the Oregon and Samarkand stocks. The parental stocks had 36 and 32 number of chaetae. The F_1 and F_2 had 36 numbers. The average number of chaetae increased till 20 generations but the fertility decreased. When selection was reversed the chaetae number decreased and the fertility improved. In the second phase of selection, there was no correlated response in fertility and the relaxed selection did not decrease chaetae number. The results are summarized below:

	Selection Ccheme	*Chaetae Number*	*Fertility*	*Result*
I.	Selection	Increased	Decreased	Correlation
	Relaxation	Decreased	Increased	Correlation (Re-association)
II.	Selection	Increased	No response	No correlation
	Relaxation	No decrease	—	—

Such an association, re-association and no association must follow due to recombination on the assumption of linkage. In second selection for high chaetae number the association of high chaetae number with low fertility was broken and therefore no correlated response in fertility was observed. The correlated response in other trait (s) due to selection in one trait gives an indication of the linkage relations between different polygenic systems when the correlated response is not always observed. On the other hand, if the correlated response is always observed it is an indication of the pleiotropic gene action.

(b) It has been observed that the economic characters showing continuous variation in farm animals show different trends of genetic correlation among the traits and the correlated response in different herds and even in the same herd in different generations. Such a different trend ruled out the possibility of pleiotropic gene action and indicates the linkage of polygenes, affecting different traits, which is breakable in successive generations.

3. Quantitative Characters are Controlled by Polygenes

The chromosome assays in Drosophila (the use of major genes for markers) has shown that the genes for continuous variation are nuclear born and that all the three major chromosomes carry polygenes affecting the abdominal chaetae number. Mather and Harrision (1949) interpreted their results of chromosomal assays on abdominal chaetae number that at least eight genes on all the three chromosomes; (two polygenes in chromosome II, at least three in chromosome – Ill and probably three in the X chromosome), are responsible for the abdominal chaetae number. Breese and Mather (1957, 1960) have shown that at least six genes present on Chromosome – III are responsible for this character of abdominal chaetae number. Thus there are eleven as the minimum number of genes in this system affecting the number of abdominal chaetae. They have observed that the polygenes affecting chaetae number and viability are distributed along the length of chromosome – III.

Wigan (1949) had shown that the genes determining the number of sterno-pleural number are widely distributed along the X chromosome.

At least twenty polygenes have been estimated by Student (1934) to be responsible for the control of oil content in maize and hypothesized that the number of polygenes should be about two hundred. The litter size in mice was found to be controlled by about eighty genes. The different members of the polygenic system affecting abdominal chaetae number were distinguished only by their linkage relation.

4. The Quantitative Characters are Influenced by Environment

The effects of polygenes affecting the quantitative characters are highly susceptible and prone to environmental changes. The genotypic values determined by the effect of genes are modified by the variation in environment. The evidence of the environmental effect on the phenotypic expression of the genotype come from the fact of the differences in the phenotypic values for a metric trait of the same individual at different ages or under different environmental conditions (*viz.* feeding regime etc.). The genotype is fixed at zygotic stage but an individual after its birth receives different environments at its different ages. It is daily observation that body weight changes from time to time depending upon the diet; a dairy cow produces different amount of milk on different days in the same lactation; the growth and yield of plants depends upon the fertility level of soil, temperature and other climatic factors and on the cultural practices etc. With a fixed or constant genotype of the individual throughout the life and different measurements of the same character at different times under different environmental circumstances determine the extent to which the inherited tendency of quantitative traits is expressed in terms of the phenotypic value. Therefore, the environmental conditions control the expression of polygenes.

5. The Quantitative Characters show Continuous Variation

There is a continuously graded series of phenotypic values, of the quantitative traits, from one extreme to the other within the range. This continuous variation in phenotypic values of different individuals for a quantitative trait is caused by the effect of polygenes and by the effect of non-genetic causes (environmental factors). The simultaneous segregation of many genes affecting a quantitative trait creates many genotypes and hence many expressions (phenotypes) of the character. The environmental factors further modify the expression of polygenes (genotypes) and produce many phenotypes of the character.

The number of phenotypic classes (the phenotypic values) depends upon the number of genes affecting a character, number of alleles at a locus, and the interaction between genes present at the same or different loci.

14.5 Relation between Gene and Character (Genetic Basis of Characters)

The existence of genes to play their role in controlling the development and expression of character is inferred from the effects of genes to cause differences in the expression of the character by changing the phenotype or phenotypic value. However, the genes do not produce the character directly but via some specific biochemical reactions. The primary function of a gene is to produce a specific protein which often acts as an enzyme or more precisely a polypeptide. The enzyme has an effect to catalyze a specific biochemical reaction that leads to the development and expression of the character. Thus, enzyme production is the primary function of a gene while the development and expression of a character is the ultimate function of a gene through intermediary biochemical reactions. However, such relation between these functions of a gene is known only for a very few characters.

The following principles have emerged to establish the relation between gene and character.

1. Like Begets like and Dissimilarities

This means that every newly formed or developed living individual has the characteristics similar and common to its species, breed, race or line. Thus, in plant kingdom, the plants of a species give rise to the plants of its own species *viz.* a mango give rise to mango tree, wheat to wheat plant and so on whereas the different animal species produce the animals having the similar and common characteristics of their own species, such that the cats beget cat, dogs produce dogs, human to human.

There exist *genetic differences* between different breeds, strains/race/lines. The different breeds of a species show genetic differences *viz.* the animals of two breeds have distinctive genetic differences in color, appearance and other physical characteristics like horn pattern, body size and body weight. Likewise, the mean performance for a quantitative trait (body weight, milk yield) is different for different breeds, lines and strains within a species. These are the indications of the genetic differences among breeds, strains and lines.

There also exist *genetic variations* between the animals of a breed/strains/lines as well as between any two closely related individuals belonging to the same sire – dam families, even if they are raised together under the same environment, especially for quantitative traits.

There is some *resemblance* (*similarity*) between genetically related individuals compared to unrelated individuals within a breed/race. Not only this, but the progeny resemble to their parents, though the resemblance among relatives in not exact. This indicates that genetically related individuals within a breed/strain/line share common genes responsible for producing the similarities among relatives.

The quantitative characters show *response to selection* which indicates the genetic differences among different individuals (selected and culled).

The quantitative characters also show *inbreeding depression* on crossing the closely related individuals and its converse *hybrid vigour* on crossing the individuals with different genetic background.

2. Joint Effect of Genotype and Environment to Produce Phenotype

The principle that the phenotype is the joint product of genotype and environment was first given by Johannsen. The variation among individuals within a breed as well as between any two closely related individuals even of the same sire-dam family (full sibs) and the within individual variation for a character measured at different times on the same individual can be viewed in support of this principle.

(i) Individual Variation

The different individuals of a population even the related individuals belonging to the same sire-dam family (full sibs) have different phenotypic values for a quantitative trait, *e.g.* the amount of milk produced is different by different cows of the same breed, of the same family (full sisters) and of the same age residing in the same herd kept under the similar feeding, management and other environmental conditions. Likewise, the body weight and size of cows, the age at maturity/first calving, the duration (days) for how long the cows remain in milk in a lactation (called as the lactation length), the duration (days) for how long the milk production is interrupted between two calving (called as dry period), the duration in days from calving to exhibition of first heat (post-partum breeding interval) or to conception (service period) are different in different cows of the same sire-dam family kept under similar conditions. There exist in all the characters such individual variations within a population even of relatives kept under similar environment.

The individuals of a population in the same environment differ from each other in their phenotypic values of a character under reference. These differences are called individual variations. There are two reasons of individual variation *viz.* genetic and environmental. The first is that the individual variation can be ascribed due to differences in the genetic make up of different individuals. It is well known that the genes carried by a cow (individual) are different from those carried by another cow of the same breed, herd and family because they are the progeny of different ancestry (great grand parents, grand parents, and parents). Thus, a cow may be high or low producer because of its ancestry having high or low producing genes.

Secondly, the individual variations also exist due to the reason that all the individuals of a population do not receive the same amount and quality of feed and fodders, the same management and the same other environmental conditions. The environment received by different cows is different *e.g.* they may calve at different times (months, seasons) of the year when the fodder availability and the climatic conditions are different or their age and body condition at the time of calving may be different or they may receive different management practices etc. The environment influences the gene's expression to develop the character. The environment includes climatic factors, geographical locations, quantity and quality of food, age and size or body condition of the animal, disease incidence, management practices and any kind of stress etc.

Therefore, any variation in either genotype (ancestry) or environment causes the variation in the development and expression of the character. The genotype determines the genotypic values for a character and the environment modifies the genotypic value before the final expression of the character as phenotypic value.

(ii) Within Individual Variation

There are some characters which are repeatable at different times in the life of an animal *e.g.* milk production, lactation length, dry period, wool production, egg production etc. The phenotypic values of a character recorded on the same individual at different times (age) are different, *e.g.* a dairy cow produces different amount of milk on different days of a lactation and in different lactations. Likewise, the body weight differs at different time (age) depending upon the nutrition level, health, age, stress condition and other environmental factors which have a changing nature at different times. An individual is subjected to a varied environment factors day to day. This explains the differences in a day to day milk production of a cow in the same lactation and indifferent lactations. This type of variation between different records of the same individual on the same character recorded at different times (age of the animal) is known as within individual or intra-individual variation and these are due to change in the environmental conditions from time to time otherwise the genotype of an individual is determined and fixed at zygotic stage before its birth and does not change throughout the life. Therefore, the genotype cannot cause variation in repeated measurements of a character whereas the environmental factors have a changing nature from time to time.

The environment is different for different individuals and at different times for the same individual. The environment changes the expression of genes. For example, as long as a cow receives balanced ration, its milk production will be high and as soon as the feeding of balanced ration is stopped to the cow, its milk production goes down. A man losses in its body weight when goes on hunger strike or during illness or living in. any stress condition. Thus, the change in environment results in a change in the phenotypic value of the character recorded on the same individual at different times and hence the expression of a character is changed due to change in environment. Therefore, the environment received by an individual during the course of development and expression of the character play a very important role to modify the phenotypic value of metric traits.

The phenotypic variation in a character can not be observed simply by observation of the phenotypic values and it is not possible to assign the nature and amount of differences in any character, like milk production simply by recording the milk yield. The breeding test and statistical analysis of the data can partition the components of variation.

3. Genetic Systems Affecting the Characters

The genes as the hereditary material is evidenced from their effects to cause differences *in* the expression of the phenotype of a character of an organism, Depending upon the nature, relation and the magnitude of the effect of genes to produce heritable variation in a character, the genes are categorized as major genes and minor genes.

(i) Major Gene System

There are some genes whose effects are large enough to cause discontinuous variation (to produce different phenotypes of a character) even in the presence of segregation of genes at other loci and under different environmental factors. The characters controlled by these genes are little affected by other genes (basic genotype or genetic background) or by the environment. These genes are known as *oligo-genes.* The characters controlled by the *oligo-genes* are called qualitative characters. Such genes are also called *major genes* for the reason of their major effect and hence to cause major differences among individuals of a population. The change produced in the phenotype of a character by such major genes can be distinguished by making simple observations. Mostly, one or two pairs of such genes are responsible for the expression of the character *e.g.* Mendelian characters and qualitative characters like flower colour in plants, eye colour in Drosophila, coat colour in Short horn breed of cattle etc. Likewise, the difference between sickle cell haemoglobiri and normal haemoglobin (Hb) is due to a change in single gene in which the glutamic acid of normal Hb is replaced by valine at a specific place in the globin part of the molecule and produces the sickle cell hemoglobin.

(ii) Polygenic System

The second category of genes controlling a character are the members of a polygenic system. The effect of such genes is small or minor and hence called as *minor genes*. Such genes affecting a character are many in number and hence called as *polygenes*. These *polygenes* have their small, similar and supplementary effects. They can neither be recognized nor can be counted as individual genes but as a polygenic system and hence they all may be the members of the polygenic system. The characters produced by *polygenes* are called as quantitative characters. The development of these characters is very much affected by the genetic background and by the environment. The examples are the genes affecting the abdominal chaetae and minute bristles in Drosophila, and all the quantitative characters showing continuous variation. It has been well established that the polygenes causing continuous variation are inherited and they are nuclear born transmitted in a Mendelian fashion.

(iii) Combined Effect of Major and Minor Genes

The differences in a character may be partly due to major gene differences and partly to a polygenic system. Thus the major genes and polygenes may cause the differences partly in the same character, for example, dwarf and normal stature in man. The dwarfs have clear distinctions from the normal and are due to specific major gene differences. Among normal the variation in their height is continuous and assumes the polygenic variation. The abdominal chaetae number in Drosphila show continuous (polygenic) variation among wild type individuals but the number is drastically changed by major genes.

(iv) Similar Phenotypes by Different Genes

Further evidence of the relation between genes and characters comes from the fact that similar phenotypes is caused by different genes in same case. The breeding tests have shown that the large coloured spots observed to be alike on the petals of two species of cotton (Gossypium hirsutum and G. barbadense) are similar but the genes affecting them are different. A single gene is responsible for short tail on the hind wings of the butter fly in some races whereas in other types the character is due to polygenes. The sex determination in different species of plants and animals is governed by different sets of genes.

4. Pleiotropic Gene Action

The effect of a gene is not restricted to only one character but a gene may control more than one character. This manifold effect of a gene to control two or more characters is called the pleiotropic gene action and the phenomenon is called as the pleiotropism. Cocks (1954) had reported pleiotropic effect of a gene H in Drosophila which removes some of the major bristles of the head and thorax, also reduces the number of abdominal chaetae and the sterno-pleural chaetae. He has also observed that another gene Sc remove major bristles from scutellum and reduces the abdominal chaetae to more extent than gene H but Sc gene has little effect on the number of sternopleural chaetae and the effect of another gene *Sp* is to nearly double the number of sternopleurals but hardly affects the number of abdominal chaete.

The pleiotropic effect of a gene are very complex and may be due to a single initial action which changes the general course of development and may leads to a number of abnormalities. Gruneberg (1963) published the inherited skeletal disorders in rats and mice. He stated that varied patterns of effects in rats and mice are the consequence of single gene changes. A recessive gene is known in rat which kills the rats soon after birth and these rats show a wide range of peculiarities especially in the circulatory and respiratory systems and also appear in the form of snout, the occlusion of incisor teeth, and the inability to suckle and all these effects are arisen from an initial breakdown of cartilage. However, the complexity of effects, which arise from a simple change, depends on the chain of events (multiplicity of stages) between the action of the gene and its final expression in the phenotype. The longer is the chain the greater is the complexity of effects.

14.6 *Polygenes* and *Major Genes*

(i) The polygenes can not be recognized or counted as individuals. They are recognized as groups associated in a segment of chromosome instead of individuals. The *major genes* (oligogenes) can be recognized individually.

(ii) The polygenes have effects on the character similar to each other, supplementing each other and sufficiently small compared to the total or non-heritable variation. As a result smooth continuous variation of the phenotypes appeared.

Simultaneous segregation of *polygenes* produces many genotypes and many expressions of the character (phenotypes or phenotypic values). Taking equal effect of *polygenes* of the $system_1$ on the character, each will have a small effect (small amount of variation will be contributed by each) and can not produce discontinuity in the phenotypic distribution. The fact that each of the polygene contributes a small portion of the variation can be well evidenced by estimating the average effect of each gene substitution. This can be estimated by dividing the difference in phenotypic values of the two extreme phenotypes with the estimated number of *polygenes* involved in the system. For example, in the experiment of Mather and Hanson (1949) the two extreme lines differed by 34.2 abdominal chaetae. Now taking a minimum of eleven gene pairs involved in controlling the variation in the character, the average effect of each gene substitution is around three chaetae. This average effect of each polygene is nearly equal to the non-heritable standard deviation of about 2.8 in this character. This average effect will be smaller than non-heritable component of variation if eleven is a low estimate of the number of polygenes affecting the chaetae number.

The different *polygenes* must have similar and supplementary effect because neither a single chromosome nor a single gene could produce the differences in chaetae number observed by Mather and Harrison's lines, but all the chromosomes and all the genes had their more or less equal effects in producing differences. Supplementary effect between genes acting in the same direction implies a balancing effect between genes acting in opposite direction. Due to this balancing effect the polygenic systems have a great capacity to hide or store variability even with phenotypic similarity (uniformity) and this capacity is increased as (n-1)/n with the increase in number of genes (n) in the system affecting a trait.

A major gene has large and specific effect because the role played by the *major gene* cannot be duplicated by other genes. This means that the deficiency of a *major gene* cannot be gained by other genes of the nucleus. The *polygenes* cannot match with *major genes* regarding the specifications of their action.

(iii) The *polygene* is one member of a system whose parts are interchangeable in development. The individual effects of *polygenes* are small but all the members of the polygenic system may act together to produce big differences *viz.* the phenotypes of the extreme genotypes. The *polygenes* may act against each other to produce similar phenotypes from different genotypes. They have their conditional advantage in selection over the other. This means that the advantage or disadvantage depends on the alleles present at other loci of the system.

(iv) *Polygenes* produce continuous variation whereas the major genes produce discontinuous. Different methods are used to establish them. Ratio method is used for discontinuous variation (major genes) whereas the variance and correlation computed from continuous distribution of phenotypic values are used for *polygenes*. These familiar techniques are used to distinguish the two types of inheritance. Sometimes a confusion is raised in their distinction with the difference in statistical methods. The variances and correlations produced by the single gene difference (major gene) can be considered to handle the major genes which produce discontinuous variation. Likewise the polygenes with relatively small and non-specific effect can be handled by the methods used in Mendelian genetics provided the hidden effect of segregation of other genes is erased by suitable breeding method, the environmental variance is reduced to the maximum possibility by rigorous control of environment and recourse had to extensive progeny testing.

All the characters of a living being except the antigenic characters are subject to both continuous and discontinuous variation and hence both polygenic and major gene difference are inferred from them. For example, the major gene differences distinct the dwarf men from the normal but the variation in stature among normal men shows continuous variation. Likewise, the abdominal chaetae number in Drosophila is a polygenic trait among wild type individuals and among scute individuals but the major gene **Sc** can drastically change the abdominal chaetae number (Clocks, 1954).

Besides the major genes and polygenic system there is some evidence to show that gene changes of intermediate effect between major and polygenic system occur through intermediate, among induced mutations affecting viability in Drosophila, are less common than either those of the small effect or those that produce complete lethality.

The relatively small and interchangeable effects of the polygenes give rise to the special properties of the polygenic variation in selection explained here.

(v) A polygene, which acts as a major gene to affect another character, can not have the properties of a polygenic system for its total action because it can not be replaced. Therefore, such a polygene will act as a major gene in selection which means that it will respond to selection as a major gene effect.

(vi) Polygenes are of more concern to the animal and plant breeder for genetic improvement. The polygenes are also the system of smooth adaptive change and of speciation. They provide the most necessary genetic skeleton, the variation of fine adjustment and encasing the whole into fine shape for natural selection.

14.7 Measures of Gene Action

Based on the properties of a population for metric trait (Mean, variance and covariance) the gene action can be identified by two genetic phenomenon displayed by metric characters *viz.* the inbreeding depression with its opposite hybrid vigour or heterosis, and the resemblance between relatives in terms of heritability.

1. Additive vs Non-Additive Gene Action

(i) Inbreeding Depression or Heterosis

The inbreeding depression and heterosis can be measured by comparing means, *e.g.* means of generations, parents with their crosses, and so on. The inbreeding tends to reduce the mean level of all characters closely related to fitness and in consequence lead to loss of general vigour and fertility which are restored on crossing different lines. The magnitude of inbreeding depression and heterosis indicate the degree of the effect of non-additive gene action (NAGA) on the character.

Heterosis is absent when traits are influenced only by additive gene action. In other words, if AGA only influences a trait (no dominance, d = 0) no Inbreeding depression or heterosis occurs. Thus heterosis and inbreeding depression depends on the occurrence of dominance. Traits with inbreeding depression and showing dominance in crosses are called the heterotic traits. The loci with additive gene action (AGA), *i.e.* without dominance (d = 0) cause neither inbreeding depression nor heterosis.

The inbreeding depression and heterosis depends on directional dominance and thus absence of heterosis or inbreeding depression is not a proof to conclude that individual loci show no dominance or epistasis. This is because some loci may have dominance and epistacy in one direction and some in other so as their effects are cancelled out, resulting no heterosis in spite of the dominance and epistasis being shown by individual loci.

(ii) Magnitude of Heritability

The second genetic phenomenon is the resemblance between relatives. It is well known that relatives tend to resemble each other and the extent of relationship determines the extent of resemblance: closer the relationship the closer is the resemblance. The genes and the environmental circumstances commonly shared by the relatives cause the resemblance between them. The degree of resemblance provides the means of estimating the amount of additive genetic variance which is expressed in terms of heritability. The magnitude of heritability indicates the type of gene action. If the h^2 of a character is high the additive gene action is indicated but if it is low the non- additive gene action is important while the intermediate value of h^2 indicates both types of gene action. The h^2 is the most reliable measure of gene action as it is based on functions of squares of gene effects, though its estimation requires enough number of relatives.

2. Additive and Multiplicative Gene Action

The two types of gene action are differentiated from the shape of distribution (normal vs skewed), mean values of F_1 and parents, and from the variance of the population.

(i) Test of Distribution

The characters governed by additive gene action show normal distribution of phenotypic values. On the contrary, the traits governed by multiplicative gene action tend to be skewed into an asymmetrical curve in F_2 segregating population. This skewed distribution if caused by multiplicative gene action can be converted into a normal distribution by simply transforming the data on log scale. This gives the evidence of multiplicative gene action.

The effect of multiplicative genes increases in a multiplicative increment and form a geometric series such as 2, 4, 8, 16 representing the contribution of 1, 2, 3, 4 active alleles, respectively rather than in arithmetic or additive increment (which is in case of additive gene action). For example, the geometric mean of 1.4 and 3.6 is $\sqrt{1.4}$ x 3.6 = 2.24 forming the geometric series 1.4, 2.2, 3.6, 5.7 which is increasing by a multiple increment of 0.6. The arithmetic mean of 1.4 and 3.6 is $(1.4 + 3.6)/2 = 2.5$ forming arithmetic series 1.4, 2.5, 3.6, 4.7 which is increasing by an additive increment of 1.1. Some examples of multiplicative gene action are known in some crosses of tomato for mean fruit weight (Power, 1950).

(ii) Test of Mean Performance

Two strains/lines/varieties/breeds differing in their mean performance are crossed to produce the F_1 progeny. The expected arithmetic and geometric mean of the two strains/lines/breeds and F_1 are calculated and compared with the observed mean of the F_1 progeny. A close agreement between the F_1 observed mean and the expected arithmetic mean (based on two parental means) indicates the additive gene action. But if the observed F_1 mean is close to the expected geometric mean of the two parents, it then indicates the multiplicative gene action.

(iii) Variance Test

In case of additive gene action, the variance is independent of mean. Different strains/lines/varieties differing in their mean values for a trait may have same or different coefficient of variation. With the increase in mean value, the variance may be increased proportionately or in different extent which results the C.V. constant or different in two cases. When the C.V. is different in the two populations it indicates the additive gene action. This is because variance is independent of mean for normal distribution caused by additive gene action. When the C.V. is constant or same it indicates the multiplicative gene action. This is because the variance is dependent of mean in this case.

14.8 Sources of Variation

The phenotypic expression of a metric character is under the control of genotype of the individual, the environmental circumstances experienced by the individual, and the scale of measurement used to measure the character.

14.8.1 Genetic Variations

The different sources of genetic variation can be grouped as:

(1) Primary Level and Ultimate Sources at Individual Level

There are some genetic factors which shape and change the genetic structure of the individual. These include the chromosomal variation and extra chromosomal variation.

(a) The *chromosomal variation* includes the existing genetic variation, variation arising from segregation and recombination of genes during meiosis, variation within individual arising from gene action and the future variation caused due to change in genetic materials. The genetic variation thus exists and occurs due to the following causes:

☆ Existence of genes in pairs at all loci in every diploid individual,

☆ Existence of multiple alleles at a locus,

☆ Number of gene loci (polygenes) affecting a character,

☆ Gene action or expression *viz.* additive and non additive gene action,

☆ Genetic recombination (crossing over, segregation and recombination),

☆ Change in genetic material (Gene mutation and chromosomal aberrations).

☆ Sex linked gene.

The genetic variation due to gene action constitutes most of the part of genetic variation for quantitative characters. The existing genetic variation and that arising from gene recombination are considered basic causes of genetic variation although all types of genetic variations are basic.

Maintenance of genetic variability: The Mendelian populations have plasticity in terms of the store of great amount of genetic variability. There are a number of factors with great importance in conserving the genetic variation. The existence of genetic variability is very well evident from response to selection, inbreeding depression or appearance of recessive traits on inbreeding, balanced polymorphism due to superiority in fitness of interme-diate phenotype, greater variability of F_2 population and production of three genotypes from heterozygous mating for one gene pair, etc. There are a number of mechanisms which preserve the genetic variability and these are listed as:

1. Mutation
2. Genetic recombination
3. Inversion and reciprocal translocation heterozygosity
4. Meiotic drive
5. Superiority of heterozygotes
6. Genetic and phenotypic disassortative mating
7. Complex interaction of opposing forces like mutation-selection balance, and artificial selection opposed by natural selection.
8. Differential environmental preference of different genotypes and adaptation to local environment.
9. Population size – random genetic drift.

(b) The *extra chromosomal variation* involves the plasmatic factors called as plasma genes or cytogenes or plasmids. The inheritance due to cytoplasmic factors is called as *cytoplasmic inheritance.* The cytoplasmic factors do not contribute to genetic variation in metric traits. Therefore, the variation in metric traits due to cytoplasm is not important.

(2) Secondary Level of Processes

Creating genetic variation at *population level*: These processes change the genetic structure of population rather than of the individual. These are population size, mating systems, selection, migration, mutation and geographical isolation. These processes are capable of molding the genetic make up of a population into new species in conformity with the environment and ecology of species.

The genetic variations produced by either level of process are ultimately fixed. The isolating mechanism either geographical or reproductive helps in the fixation of genes.

14.8.2 Environmental Variations

Some environmental factors cause variations in gene expression. The term environment includes all the non-genetic factors other than genes effect that influence the phenotypic value of the character. The gene expression is environment specific. The environmental factors play an important role in the expression of genotype in the form of a character (phenotypic value) and cause variation in gene expression among individuals. The differences caused by environmental factors are known as environmental variations which are not heritable but limited up to the individual.

Evidences

The evidences of the effects of environmental factors to influence the performance (phenotypic value) of individuals are observed daily in our life *viz.* variation in body weight, milk production, work capacity, etc. The environmental conditions are not similar but changing every time in the life of an individual and between different individuals. The environmental conditions are thus different for different individuals of a population, even in the same herd, in spite of the best effort of the owner. This may be due to the differences in age, climatic (cold and heat stress, humidity, etc) and nutritional factors, physical condition, thermo-regulatory mechanism and genotypes, etc. Temperature affects the morphological and physiological expression of animals and plants. The climatic and nutritional factors are different to the animals born in different years and seasons.

The environment modifies the genotypic value of a character during the course of its development but before it is expressed and measured in the form of phenotypic value on an individual. For example, the genotype of the cow is fixed and hence the genotypic value for milk yield is also fixed but the amount of milk produced by a cow on different days is different. The milk yield produced by a cow is increased or decreased depending on the amount and quality of ration fed to the cow. Thus, the environment (amount and quality of ration) changes the milk yield of the cow by modifying the genotypic value of cow for milk yield.

Classification of Environmental Factors

The environmental factors have been classified on different basis *viz.* known or unknown causes, duration of their effect, and internal or external to the individual.

(i) Known (Tangible) and Unknown (Intangible) Causes

The known causes of environmental factors are the feeding levels, age, climatic factors, farm effect, management factors *viz.* open versus close housing, weaning practice, frequency of milking, floor versus battery system. These environmental factors causes major effect and their effects can be partly reduced by designing proper experiment. The effect of some environmental factors are beyond control, like maternal effect arises in mammals due to sharing common environment by relatives during prenatal and postnatal period, mainly due to nutrition of the mother. The common intra-uterine environment of litter mates, milk yield and mothering ability of sows also provide a common environment to the piglets. Moreover, some variation is caused due to error in recording the observations either due to carelessness involved in recording as human error or machine error (balance for recording body weight and milk yield) or due to error in recording the score characters (judging of animals, carcass quality characters, organolaptic quality, etc). The environment variance caused by tangible factors can be eliminated statistically by adjusting the data.

Unknown factors (intangible causes) also cause variation in phenotypic values of quantitative traits, though the variation due to them is small (micro-environmental effects), *viz.* variation between monozygotic twins.

(ii) Permanent versus Temporary Environmental Factors

The examples of these environmental factors have been given in the chapter of repeatability. The effect of these two types of factors can be separated off by partitioning the total phenotypic variance into variance within individual and between individuals by analysis of variance

(iii) Random and Fix Environmental Factors

The environmental effects which are *internal to the individual* and vary between individuals of a population influencing the individual records of animals (for which called as *variable effects*) are categorized as *random effects*. These factors affect the individual alone and not the whole population. The examples of random or internal environmental factors are hormone level, sex hormone, diet of the animal, sex, lameness and minor infection, chance accident, social dominance, age, reproductive status (pregnancy or lactation effect), maternal effect (age and weight of dam, type of birth), sire of animal, inbreeding level of individual. The random environmental factors cause a large share of the total variation.

The other category of environmental factors is the *fix effects* which includes those factors which *affect the whole population*, and are constant for a group of animals. These factors include climatic factors (temperature, humidity, season, sun light), years, regions, feeding level, husbandry practices and other factors which affect all the animals.

The occurrence of disease affects both individual as well as population as a whole and hence taken accordingly.

14.8.3 G–E Interaction

The genes also interact with the environment besides being interacting among them-selves. Please see chapter 17 of this book.

14.8.4 Scale Effect

The biological processes are responsible for the expression of characters in living organisms. The characters are measured in some units of measurements. The units are quantitative *viz.* gm, cm, days, numbers etc.

The scale of measurement is not important for qualitative characters because the population is grouped into various classes depending upon the expression of the character and the grouping has genetical base (foundation). The character is completetly described by the frequencies of different classes and the analysis needs no assumption about the material relations of the classes. The grouping of the individuals of a population requires a genetical significance if imposed naturally *viz.* number of positive alleles and the gene action.

On the contrary, the grouping of individuals of a population for characters showing continuous variation if made would be artificial with no genetical foundation. This is because the continuous variation is the result of the action of polygenes and the environment factors. Therefore, there is no genetic significance to describe and analyze the continuous variation in terms of frequencies of different classes but the continuous variation is described and analysed in terms of some biometrical quantities *viz.* mean and variance. The normal distribution is assumed to analyse the continuous variation and the variance as independent of mean. This means that the variance should not be changed with change of mean.

1. Proper Scale to Measure a Polygenic Character

The change of scale may change the values of biometrical quantities (mean and variance) and that the change is unequal for measurements of different magnitudes. Thus, the validity of the description and analysis of continuous variation depend on the scale of measurement of the trait. The scale of measurement of a trait should not be a cause of the change of variance following change of population mean. However, if the scale of measurement of a trait becomes the cause of change of variance following the change of population mean, it is called the *scale effect*. Therefore, the choice of an appropriate scale is the first step in the analysis of polygenic variation.

The transformation of scale is a statistical tool used to simplify the analysis of data and to draw valid conclusions and interpretation of results. However, if the transformation is not done but required, it then gives rise to the phenomenon or an effect called the *scale effect*. The scale effect disappears when the original data is transformed into an appropriate scale. Thus the purpose of scale transformatiom is to remove the scale effect.

It is charming to suppose that every character has its natural scale of measurement but it is misleading. The example to be cited in this context may be the growth which is a geometrical rather than an arithmetic process and thus a geometric scale to measure the growth is the most natural. Therefore, the growth measured originally in arithmetic scale needs to be transformed into logarithms which is most appropriate.

Regarding growth as a trait, the biological significance is not the same for an equal amount of increase in body weight of two individuals which differ significantly in body weight *e.g.* 1 kg increase in body weght of an individual weighing 20 kg and a similar amount of increase (1 kg) in body weight of another individual weighing 200 kg. However, the biological significance is same if the increase in body weight of two individuals is same in percentage.

The scale of measurement is used which is convenient to measure the trait based on experience. Thus, the data are recorded in the most convenient scale to measure the trait *e.g.* the phenotypic values are recorded in gm, cm, inches, numbers, days or any unit which is most convenient. Such a scale which is most convenient to measure the trait may not be especially appropriate to represent the character for the purpose of genetic analysis. The scale used to measure the character should not be supposed appropriate for the purpose of genetic analysis due to the followings

(a) A single scale can not reflect equally the peculiarity of nature of all the genes affecting a trait. Some genes have additive as well as the non-additive nature to influence a trait while others may have their multiplicative effect by increasing the value of a trait in multiplicative increment forming a geometric series rather than in arithmetic or additive increment as in case of additive effect of gene.

(b) There are some factors which control the discontinuities in a meristic trait and those factors may not have any scale relation to the action of genes mediating the underlying continuous distribution of potential manifestation of the trait.

(c) The scale appropriate to represent the variation in a trait for one set of individuals under one set of conditions may not be equally appropriate to represent the same character in different set of individuals or under different conditions.

One scale may not be appropriate for all the populations and for all the components (genetic and environmental) of the variation. Power (1950) analyzed the character 'weight per locule' in tomato for a number of crosses and found that in some crosses the arithmetic scale was appropriate while in others the geometric scale was appropriate as well as the genetic and environmental variation required separate scales in some crosses of F_2 generation.

Therefore, it is not possible to choose a priori scale to measure variation in a trait. The scale to measure a trait should be such which facilitates both analysis and interpretation of data and the use of resulting statistics.

2. Reasons of Scale Transformation

The scale transformation is done to remove scale effect for the following three main reasons:

1. To make the distribution normal
2. To make the variance independent of mean
3. To remove or minimize the non-additive interactions.

Normal distribution is taken as the main criterion to analyse the continuous variation. The necessity to transform the data is indicated when the distribution of phenotypic values are not distributed normally but are markedly asymmetrical or skewed. Sometimes the transformation is also required when the data are distributed normally but considering the main criteria that the variance should be independent of mean. These scale effects of non-normality of data and dependence of variance on mean disappears by appropriate transformation.

(i) Normal Distribution

The amount of variation in relation to mean (C.V.) affects the normal distribution. The degree of asymmetry depends on the coefficient of variation. The higher is the coefficient of variation more will be the degree of skewness. The transformation of scale leads to a difference in the shape of the distribution curve if the coefficient of variation is fairly high, say 20 percent or more. Therefore the transformation is not required when the coefficient of variation is low compared to that when it is high. This criterion is applicable to all kinds of transformation.

(ii) Independence of Variance on Mean

The second point to consider regarding the transformation of scale is the independence of variance on mean. The change of variance following a change of the population mean (dependence of variance on mean) is another important and commonest scale effect. There are some characters like body height which need scale transformation to make the variance independent of mean, though the distribution may be normal for different populations separately. The example of two way selection experiment on body weight may be cited here. Mac Arther (1949) conducted a two way selection experiment for 60 days body weight in mice. He observed that the standard deviation of small strain was less than the base population and standard deviation of large strain was more than the base population. The three population *viz*. small, base and large strain had 1.71, 2.56 and 5.10 standard deviation with their mean as 11.97, 23.16 and 39.85. Thus there was an increase in variance with an increase in mean and vice versa. However, the coefficient of variation of three strains was nearly equal (14.3, 11.1 and 12.8 per cent) and remains constant or unchanged. Moreover, all these three strains (populations) did not seem to be sufficiently asymmetrical (non-normal) and hence there was no need for scale transformation but the transformation is still needed to make the variance independent of mean.

The coefficient of variation provides the criteria to the appropriateness of a log transformation in a way that if two populations have the same variance on a log scale, then the coefficient of variation will be the same on arithmetic scale. Thus if the coefficient of variation is constant then the variance will be constant on log scale. Therefore, in order to compare the variances it is better to simply compare the coefficient of variation rather than taking the variance on log scale. In this example, the change of variance due to selection can thus be attributed largely to the scale of measurement because on log scale the variance did not change.

In two way selection experiment, the selection differential and response to selection will also be changed if the variance changes with the change of mean. The response will be asymmetrical. The probable reason of asymmetry in response could be assigned to scale effect if the response is symmetrical on transforming the data to log scale. The scale effect can be eliminated by taking the response to selection as a ratio of the selection differential (realized heritability which is very little affected by scale effect, Falconer, 1954).

The effect of scale in relation to variance and mean complicates the comparison of the variances of two populations whose means also differ like the comparison of variances of inbred and hybrids. The genetic variances of inbred as well as of F_1 hybrids are almost negligible. The inbred are more susceptible to environment than hybrids and thus the inbred have reduced homeostatic power (power to remain stable) making them more variable. Thus the difference between the variances of the inbred and their F_1's (hybrids) is due to environment component. If for example, the homeostatic power is responsible to a difference of variance, then the scale effect, in relation to the difference of mean, is not expected for a similar difference.

(iii) Nature of Genetic Variance

The scale effects have their influence on the occurrence, direction and degree of interaction effect of genes

(a) Change of Occurrence, Direction and Degree of Dominance and Epistasis

Mather and Jinks (1982) have illustrated this phenomena by taking the expression of the character associated with three genotypes aa, Aa and AA as 1, 4 and 9 recorded on some scale (say direct scale) and then transforming these values on log as well as on square root scale as:

Table 14.1: Hypothetical Example

Genotypes		aa	Aa	AA	mean
	DS	1	4	9	5
Bb	LS	0	0.602	0.954	0.478
	SS	1	2	3	2
	DS	4	9	16	10
Bb	LS	0.602	0.954	1.204	0.903
	SS	2	3	4	3
	DS	9	16	25	17
BB	LS	0.954	1.204	1.398	1.176
	SS	3	4	5	4
	DS	5	10	17	11
m	LS	0.478	0.903	1.176	0.827
	SS	2	3	4	3

DS = Direct scale, LS = log scale, SS = Square root scale

The *dominance is indicated* when heterozyzote (Aa) is not exactly intermediate (mid point) between two homozygotes.

The *interaction effect (epistasis) is indicated* when the effect of substituting an allele for one gene pair is different in the presence of different genotypes of other gene pair, *e.g.* the effect of substituting A allele for allele *a* on direct scale in Table 11.1 above is:

3 units in the presence of bb or 5 units,

5 units in the presence of Bb or 7 units, and

7 units in the presence of BB or 9 units.

Direct Scale

(1) *There is dominance*: The allele *a* is dominant over A and *b* over B

(2) *There is Interaction effect*: The effect of substituting A for *a* is less in the presence of bb than of Bb and greatest of all in the presence of BB. The relations of A-a and B-b are reciprocal.

Log Scale

(1) *Dominance has reversed*: The A allele has become dominant over *a* and likewise B allele has become dominant over *b* allele.

(2) *Interaction effect has also been reversed*. The effect of substituting A allele for *a* allele is greater with bb genotype (0.602), intermediate with Bb genotype (0.352) and least with BB genotype (0.254).

Square Root Scale

(1) *Absence of dominance effect*. Heterozygote did not deviate from mid point for either gene.

(2) *Absence of interaction*: The effect of substitution of A for *a* allele is equal in the presence of all the 3 genotypes at other locus *viz*. bb, Bb and BB.

The above example has illustrated that the occurrence, direction and magnitude of dominance effect as well as interaction effect depend on the scale used to measure the character.

King (1955) studied the effect of *pygmy gene* (*major gene* affecting body size) in small and large strain mice. The homozygote carrying *pygmy gene* was much reduced in size. The pygmies of small strain were about 7 gm smaller than normal whereas of the larger strain the pygmies were about 14 gm smaller than normal. This indicated the epistatic interaction of *pygmy gene* with genes at other loci influencing body size. However, expressing the effect of pygmy gene in proportion, it was found constant and independent of the other genes present for body size (small and large body size strain). The pygmies were about half the weight of their normal litter mates in both the strains. Thus comparison on log scale, there was no interaction effect.

(b) Interchange of Gene Effect by Change in Scale

The change of scale may lead to a change of the non-allelic interaction to allelic interaction. This can be illustrated by an example cited by Mather and Jinks (1982) as under:

Table 14.2

Genotypes		aa	Aa	AA	mean
bb	Direct Scale (DS)	1	2	3	2
	Log Scale (LS)	0.0	0.30 1	0.477	0.218
Bb	DS	2	4	6	4
	LS	0.301	0.602	0.778	0.519

Genotypes		aa	Aa	AA	mean
BB	DS	3	6	9	6
	LS	0.477	0.778	0.954	0.715
Mean	DS	2	4	6	4
	LS	0.218	0.519	0.715	0.466

Direct Scale

(1) Dominance is absent: Neither of the allele of either locus is dominant.

(2) Non allelic interaction is present: The effect of substituting A for a is least with bb (one unit), intermediate with Bb (2 units) and greatest with BB (3 units)

Log Scale

(1) Dominance appeared: The A becomes dominant over *a* and B over *b*.

(2) Non allelic interaction has vanished: The effect of substituting A for *a* is equal for all the genotypes at B locus (0.301 and 0.176).

It is thus very much obvious that the degree of dominance is influenced by the scale of measurement and hence the amount of dominance variance is affected proportionately. Secondly, the scale of measurement also influences the amount of interaction variance. In general, a scale transformation may remove or minimize the interaction variance which may be taken as a scale effect. The scale transformation which removes or minimizes the interaction effect is useful in drawing the conclusion from an analysis conducted and the assumption of the absence of interaction effect.

The scale effect may also give rise to G – E interaction which may be removed or reduced by scale transformation. However, the effects due to gene interaction and G – E interaction can not be removed or reduced always by scale transformation particularly when there is change in rank order of genotypes in different environments.

3. Transformation of Scale

The raw data recorded on a scale which is most convenient to measure the trait based on experience is the direct scale. The point to consider is whether the original units of measurement require their transformation into another scale before analysis *e.g.* logarithms, reciprocals or square root, depending on the aim of using the data. This is called the *"scale-transformation"*. The choice of scale and its transformation is mostly subjective. However, it requires some objective criteria. The most common and useful transformation is the logarithmic transformation. This converts the arithmetic scale into a geometric scale. The log transformation is done when the upper end of the scale requires foreshortening. The growth is a geometric phenomenon and hence the log transformation is appropriate.

The scale transformation is done to each record. However, it is not necessary always in case of log transformation. Wright (1968) had suggested the following formulae to convert the mean and variance:

Log x = log x – ½ log (1 +C²)

Var. log x = 0.4343 log (1 + C²)

where,   C = Coefficient of variation computed from arithmetic values

             Logs = To the base 10.

4. Tests of Suitable Scale

The followings are two tests to judge a suitable scale to reverse the interaction effects:

(i) Comparison of the Effects of a Specific Factor

The specific factor may be genetic or environmental. The example of the effect of *pygmy gene* in mice on body weight in different genetic background (small and large size strain for body weight) may be cited here. By comparing the effect of a single gene (pygmy) in small and large strain for body size, it was observed that the gene had additive effect in both the strains on a log scale but the gene indicated the epistatic interaction with other genes affecting body size on direct scale. Thus the scale transformation to log scale removed the interaction effect and hence the log transformation is a suitable scale.

(ii) Comparison of Observed and Expected Means of different Generations

Two populations with different means are crossed to produce F_1, F_2, B_1, B_2 generations. In the absence of epistatic interactions the means of the F_2 and back crosses are expected as under:

$F_2 = $ ½ $(F_1 + P)$

$B_1 = $ ½ $(F_1 + P_1)$

$B_2 = $ ½ $(F_1 + P_2)$

This has been shown in chapter 12 under section 12.6.2. The scale on which the observed means are closest to their expectation is taken as the best scale.

5. Problems in Choice of a Scale

To give description of the genetic properties of the population is the first aim of an experiment in quantitative genetics. A scale transformation creates doubts instead of enlightening the description. Therefore, scale transformation should not be done without good reason. It was mentioned that scale transformation is essentially a statistical tool applied to simplify the analysis of the data to draw valid conclusions from the analysis and sometimes to interpret the results.

The scale transformation is done to remove or reduce the epistatic interaction effects which are the essential part of the description of the population. It is better to conclude that a character is influenced by epistasis, if it is found, rather than considering as a scale effect. When the epistasis disappears on scale transformation it could be concluded that the loci combined their effect by multiplication rather than by addition. Likewise, if a difference of variance can be attributed to a scale effect based on valid reasons it then does not require more complicated genetic explanation. Regarding the interpretation of result, the choice of scale is problematic and the scale transformation should be based on some criteria other than the property (like epistasis) about which the conclusion is to be drawn. If there is no independent criterion for scale transformation, then there is no meaning to distinguish between a scale effect and other interpretation.

Solved Examples

Example 14.1

The mean level of two varieties was observed to be 20 and 170 units respectively and of their F_1 progeny as 56 units. Which type of gene action can be suggested?

Solution:

Arithmetic mean = $(20 + 170)/2 = 95$ units

Geometric mean = $\sqrt{20 \times 170} = 58.3$ units

The F_1 mean is close to the geometric mean of parents. Therefore, multiplicative gene action is indicated.

Example 14.2

A strain has a mean value of 45 units and σ^2 28 units^2, another strain as 15 units with σ^2 3.2 units^2. Interpret the results in terms of gene action and find out the expected mean of their F_1 progeny based on the finding of the result.

Solution

$$C.V._{(1)} \quad = (\sigma_p/\mu) \times 100$$
$$= (\sqrt{28})/45 \times 100 = 11.76 \text{ per cent}$$
$$C.V._{(2)} \quad = (\sigma_p/\mu) \times 100$$
$$= (\sqrt{3.2})/15 \times 100 = 11.93 \text{ per cent}$$

The C.V. for the two populations are almost similar and therefore multiplicative gene action is indicated. The expected mean of their F_1 progeny will be close to their geometric mean = $\sqrt{45 \times 15} = 25.98$ units and not equal to their arithmetic mean = $(45 + 15)/2 = 30$ units.

Example 14.3

Assuming the multiplicative gene action, predict the mean and variance of back cross progeny produced by crossing F_1 whose mean value is 60 units with 200 units^2 variance with the parental strain having a mean of 160 units.

Solution

Based on multiplicative gene action, the expected mean of back cross progeny will be equal to the geometric mean of the two parents with the same CV as that of F_1 progeny.

Expected mean (backcross) = $\sqrt{60 \times 160} = 97.98$ units

CV (F_1) = $\sqrt{(200)}/60 = 0.24$

$\sigma_{P(B)}$ = CV $\times \mu = 0.24 \times 97.98 = 23.09$

Therefore, $\sigma^2_{P(B)} = (23.09)^2 = 533.3$ units^2.

Chapter 15
Determinants of Phenotypic Value

The phenotypic expression (phenotype) of a metric trait is called as the phenotypic value and it is developed by the joint action of the genotype of the individual and the environmental circumstances under which the individual lived during the course of development and expression of the trait. The principle that the phenotypic value of a quantitative character is a joint product of genotype (gene effects) and environment was first given by Johannsen.

The expression of a genotype is called the phenotype. The genotype determines the genotypic value of an individual for the trait and the environment modifies this genotypes value causing a deviation in the genotypic value in either direction depending upon the type of environment (favourable or unfavourable). This deviation results continuous variation in metric traits caused partly by heritable and partly by non-heritable (environmental) factors. The heredity and environment are therefore considered two main factors and the only determinants of the phenotypic value for metric traits. Therefore, any change either in genotype or in environment would result a change in the phenotypic value of individual for the quantitative trait.

The observable or measurable differences among individuals of a population for a particular character (phenotypic values) are called as *phenotypic variation*. The variation in genotype and environment gives rise to the variation in phenotypic values.

15.1 Components of Phenotypic Value (P)

The variability in phenotypic values due to gene's effects and environmental effects can not be separated by simple observations but it requires the statistical analysis of data. The division of phenotypic value into its component parts attributable to different factors (genotype and environment) is essentially required to know how the population parameters are influenced by the properties of genes for metric trait and how these parameters can be utilized for genetic improvement of livestock.

1. Genotypic Value (G)

The genes controlling a character have their effect on the development of the character of an individual and confer a certain value to the character. This value of the character conferred by the genotype attributed to the effect of genes is called as the genotypic value, denoted by the letter G. The effect of genotype is studied in terms of the genetic differences between different genetic groups of individuals. These genetic groups may be different breeds of a species (breed differences), different herd of a breed (herd differences or strain or line differences) and sire differences based on different families (half-sib families) of a sire or likewise dam families in a herd.

2. Environmental Deviation (E)

The evidences that environmental factors modify the genotypic value and the classification of various environmental factors have been given in last chapter. There are two determinants (components) of the phenotypic value (P) corresponding to the value assigned by the genotype called as genotypic value (G) and the deviation caused in genotypic value by the environment called as environmental deviation (E). The phenotypic value has thus its component parts as-

$$P = G + E$$

where,

P = Phenotypic value

G = Genotypic value (a part of P due to the gene's effect).

E = Environmental deviation in genotypic value.

Mean environmental deviation is zero: The individuals of a population are exposed to different environmental conditions normal for a population, like different feeding regimes, different seasons of the year, etc. These different environments have their different effect on gene expression. The better environment favours the full expression of the genotype while the poor environment does not. As a result, the phenotypic value is expected to be higher under favourable environment (say, balanced diet) but to be lower under poor environment (say, deficient diet). Therefore, the environmental effects are cancelled in taking the average of the phenotypic values of all the individuals exposed to different environmental effects, and thus the mean environmental deviation in the population as a whole is zero (Σ E = 0). This is because the environmental effects are measured as deviation and the sum of mean deviation is always zero in a normal population. *Therefore, the environmental deviations (effects) do not contribute to the population mean.* This results the mean phenotypic value (P) equal to the mean genotypic value (G) and represents the population mean (M). In other words, the population mean refers equally to the mean phenotypic value as well as to the mean genotypic value.

3. Genotype – Environment Interaction (I_{GE})

The partitioning of phenotypic value into genotypic value and environmental deviation assumes that these two effects are additive and independent in their effect to produce the phenotypic value. The additive effect means that the environmental effect is associated irrespective of the genotype on which it acts while the independent effect means that there is no correlation between these two effects of genotype and environment. Under the assumptions of additive and independency of genetic and environmental effects in their action, the relative performances of two genotypes should remain the same in a changed environment. However, different genotypes (breeds) may perform differently in different environments. This means that a specific difference in environment produces different effects on different genotypes. Thus, the genotype and environment are not independent to develop a phenotype (phenotypic value) and hence the effects of two factors are not additive in producing the phenotypic value. Therefore, these two assumptions do not hold true in practical situation.

The G-E interaction is based on the logic that different sets of genes express under different environments and this is also the basis of adaptability of different breeds (genotypes) of a species under different environments. In population genetics, the G-E interaction is taken in terms of the performance of two genotypes under two environments. All the genotypes are affected by change in environment but to a different degree. A specific difference of environment (say, change in any environmental effect like temperature) has its different effect on different genotypes (native and exotic breeds reared under native environment) for the reason that *different genes (genotypes) express themselves differently in different environments*. The genes interact among themselves and also interact with the environment both internal and external to the individual to produce their effects on phenotypic value. Thus, a genotype fails to give the same response in different environments. *The differential response of different genotypes under different environments is called the G-E interaction by a **biologist**.*

A naturalist considers the response in terms of adaptability. Thus, the *differential adaptability of different genotypes (breeds) in different environmental conditions* is called as the *G-E interaction* by a **naturalist**.

As a result of genotype – environment interaction the *genetic and environmental factors do not combine their effects linearly (additively)* to produce the phenotypic value. This means that the phenotypic value is not simply the sum of the effects of genotype and environment but an additional component is associated to phenotypic value. This is the meaning of G – E interaction to a **statistician and animal geneticist** (Breeder). The additional part of phenotypic value is represented as I_{GE}. This makes the mathematical model of phenotypic value as: $P = G + E + I_{GE}$

15.2 Estimation of Components of Phenotypic Value

The different components of the phenotypic value are estimated based on a number of genotypes, say *n* genotypes (n = 1, 2, ...i....,n) measured in a number of environments, say *m* environments (m = 1, 2, ...j,....m).

Table 15.1: Phenotypic Values (p_{ij}) of n Genotypes Measured under m Environments

Genotypes	Environments					Mean Genotypic Value $\left(\overline{G}_i = \overline{P}_i\right)$
	1	2	3	j	m	
1	P_{11}	P_{12}	P_{13}	P_{1j}	P_{1m}	$\overline{P}_{1.}$
2	P_{21}	P_{22}	P_{23}	P_{2j}	P_{2m}	$\overline{P}_{2.}$
3	P_{31}	P_{32}	P_{33}	P_{3j}	P_{3m}	$\overline{P}_{3.}$
.						
.						
i	P_{i1}	P_{i2}	P_{i3}	P_{ij}	P_{im}	$\overline{P}_{i.}$
.						
.						
n	P_{n1}	P_{n2}	P_{n3}	P_{nj}	P_{nm}	$\overline{P}_{n.}$
Envron. Deviation $ej = \overline{P}_j - \overline{P}_{..}$	$\overline{P}_{.1}$	$\overline{P}_{.2}$	$\overline{P}_{.3}$	$\overline{P}_{.j}$	$\overline{P}_{.m}$	$\overline{P}_{..} = u$

P_{ij}	=	$G_i + E_j + I_{Gi\,Ej}$. It is the phenotypic value of ith genotype under jth environment,
G_i	=	Genotypic value of ith genotype
$\overline{P}_{i.}$	=	It is the average of phenotypic values of ith genotype over all environments,
E_j	=	Environmental deviation for jth environment
$\overline{P}_{.j} - \overline{P}_{..}$	=	It is the environmental deviation, due to j$_{th}$ environment for all the genotypes, taken as deviation of the mean of all genotypes in jth environment ($P_{.j}$) from population mean $\left(\overline{P}_{..}\right)$
$I_{Gi\,Ej}$	=	$P_{ij} - (G_i + E_j)$
$P_{ij} - (P_{i.} + P_{.j})$	=	It is the interaction component between ith genotype with jth environment. This is estimated as the difference of the phenotypic value of ith genotype measured under jth environment (P_{ij}) from sum of the genotypic value of ith genotype and jth environmental deviation.

When a particular genotype is measured under different normal environmental conditions, the mean over all environments is the mean genotypic value of that genotype and the deviation of mean phenotypic value under one environment from the mean genotypic value is the environmental deviation (e). The mean of all environmental deviations would be zero. ($\Sigma\ e_j = 0$). This has been made clear in solved example 15.1

15.3 Genotypic Value (G) and its Components

The genes constituting the genotype of a character may have their independent and individual effect (additive gene effect) and also they may produce their effects by interacting with each other (interaction effect). The interaction effect may be allelic (dominant effect) or it may be non-allelic (epitatic or more commonly called as interaction effect).

Models of genotypic value: The genotypic value is accordingly partitioned to the corresponding additive effect and non additive effects of genes (interaction effect). The absence of interaction effect of genes means that the genes concern act additively within locus or between loci. The additive gene action with reference to genes at one locus means the absence of dominance whereas with reference to genes at different loci means the absence of epistasis. However, the genes have their both types of effects on the character.

(1) Additive-Dominance Model of Genotypic Value

When there is independent effect of two or more loci, which means no epistasis, there are only two kinds of gene effects *viz.* additive and dominance. Thus, the genotypic value is described by the additive (A) and dominance effect (D) of genes as:

$$G = A + D$$

This is the additive-dominance model of genotypic value and has the following characteristics:

(i) This model represents either the single locus effect or taking all loci together affecting a trait as the sum of the values for additive and dominance effect of genes for individual loci,

(ii) The additive genetic value has two parts corresponding to the additive effect of two different alleles at a locus with no relation between them because average value of any one part is zero and their covariance is also zero,

(iii) The mean dominance deviation is zero,

(iv) The A and D parts of genotypic value are not correlated, and

(v) The genotypic value equals additive genetic value in the absence of dominance effect of genes at a locus as: $G = A + 0$

This model of genotypic value with additive dominance components can be illustrated taking a trait governed by single locus with two allele *viz.* A_1 and A_2 The population will have three genotypes (A_1A_1, A_1A_2, A_2A_2). It is assumed that the A_1 allele is favourable allele (having positive effect on the character) whereas A_2 allele is undesirable (with negative effect on the phenotypic value). The effect of gene difference on the phenotype is specified by two parameters (**a** and **d**) which describe the additive and dominance effects. The genotypic value of a genotype, carrying i^{th} and j^{th} allele and denoted by (G_{ij}), is measured in units of the character as the deviation of the phenotypic value of G_{ij} genotype from the mid point of the phenotypic values of two homozygotes. The average of the two homozygotes is called as the *mid point (m)* or as the point of origin (o).

The following *assumptions* are taken to estimate the genotypic value and its components as well as the population mean:

☆ The population is in H.W. equilibrium,

☆ There is no effect of environment,

☆ There is no measurement error and

☆ The character is affected by single locus with two alleles (A_1 and A_2).

☆ The A_1 allele increases the value while A_2 allele decreases the value of the character.

With the above specified conditions, the genotypes, their frequencies and values, and their phenotypic values can be represented as:

Genotypes	Frequency	Phenotypic Value (P_{ij})	Genotypic Value $(G_{ij} = P_{ij} - m)$
A_1A_1	p^2	$P_{11} = m + a$	$G_{11} = P_{11} - m = a$
A_1A_2	$2pq$	$P_{12} = m + d$	$G_{12} = P_{12} - m = d$
A_2A_2	q^2	$P_{22} = m - a$	$G_{22} = P_{22} - m = -a$

m = *Mid Parent Value* = ½ $(P_{11} + P_{22})$ = ½ $(P_{A1A1} + P_{A2A2})$

= Average of phenotypic values of two homozygotes

a = *Additive gene effect* = ½ $(P_{11} - P_{22})$ = ½ $(P_{A1A1} - P_{A2A2})$

= Average of the difference in phenotypic values of two homozygotes

d = *Dominance effect* = $P_{12} - m$

= Deviation of heterozygote phenotypic value (P_{ij}) from the mid parent value **(m)**.

The *m* is independent on the distribution of genes between the genotypes and thus **m** is the natural zero point from which measurements can be expressed as deviations. The value of **m** is constant depending on the action of genes not under consideration and taken as the basis of measurement of two parameters (**a** and **d**). However, both *a* and *d* are independent of **m**.

The **a** indicates the gene's contribution to the additive genetic effect among the individuals of a population whereas **d** indicates the dominance effect of the gene. Therefore, the value of **d** depends upon the degree of dominance between two alleles. The degree of dominance is taken as **d/a**. The relationship of **d** to a *i.e.* degree of dominance (**d/a**) defines the kind of dominance *viz.* complete dominance of A_1 or complete dominance of A_2, no dominance or codominance between two alleles, overdominance of A_1 or overdominance of A_2, incomplete dominance of A_1 or incomplete dominance of A_2.

The parameters **a**, **d** and **–a** are also taken as the arbitrarily assigned values of genotypes, used to describe the effect of gene difference on the phenotype. The arbitrary assigned genotypic values (**a**, **d** and **-a**) are helpful to obtain general formulae of values, mean, and variance of a population for a trait. The **a** represents an increment in a constant direction whereas **d** represents a change in either direction depending upon the dominance of either increasing or decreasing allele. The genotypic values a and d are estimated as deviation of phenotypic value of a particular genotype from mid point between to homozygotes.

(2) Interaction Model of Genotypic Value

When the different loci interact together to produce the genotypic value of a quantitative character, it means the effects of genes at different loci are dependent on each other and this is called as epistasis. In such a case, an additional component, known as interaction effect between loci, also influence the genotypic value. This represents the epistatic effect or epistatic deviation or the interaction effect of genes between loci, denoted by I. Thus, the genotypic value of all loci becomes as:

$$G = A + D + I$$

15.4 Population Mean

The population mean (M) for a quantitative trait is the mean of phenotypic values of all the individuals of different genotypes in a population. However, the population mean in quantitative genetics is expressed as a deviation from mid parent value or mid point (m) as $M = P - m$.

1. Single Locus

Now considering a trait being controlled by a single locus with two alleles, there will be three genotypes in the population assuming their frequencies in H.W. proportions.

The *population mean (M) in absolute term* will be:

$$M = P^2 P_{11} + 2pq\, P_{12} + q^2\, P_{22}$$
$$= p^2\,(m + a) + 2pq\,(m + d) + q^2\,(m - a) \text{ taking } P_{ij} = m + g_{ij}$$
$$= p^2 m + p^2 a + 2pq\, m + 2pq\, d + q^2 m - q^2 a$$
$$= m\,(p^2 + 2pq + q^2) + a\,(p^2 - q^2) + 2pq\, d$$
$$= m + a\,(p - q) + 2pq\, d$$

The *population mean (M)* as a *deviation from mid point (m)* will thus be:

$$M = \overline{P} - m = a\,(p - q) + 2pq\, d$$

The *m* is the mid point between two homozygotes and it is a fixed part of the population mean. The rest quantity *[a (p – q) + 2pq d]* is the population mean (M) taken as a deviation from the mid value of two homozygote (*m*). The *population mean (M) as a deviation* from mid point is the weighted average of the genotypic values and obtained as the sum of product of the assigned value of each genotype with its frequency as shown in Table 15.2.

The population mean (M) is the mean genotypic value $\left(\overline{G}\right)$ and the mean phenotypic value of the population $\left(\overline{P}\right)$ for the character concerned. Thus, the population mean $(M) = \overline{P} = \overline{G}$. The genotypic values **a** and **d** are deviations in phenotypic values from the mean *value of two* homozygotes (m). However, the population mean is expressed as a deviation from mid point of two homozygotes (m) and it is the weighted average of genotypic values as: **[a (p – q) + 2 pq d].**

Table 15.2: Population Mean

Genotypes	Frequency	Value	Freq. x Value
A_1A_1	p^2	a	p^2 a
A_1A_2	2pq	d	2pq d
A_2A_2	q^2	–a	$-q^2$a
		Sum = Mean =	a (p – q) + 2 pq d = M

The population mean has two parts *viz.*

a (p – q) attributable to homozygotes and

2pqd attributable to heterozygote.

Therefore, the gene effect (a and d) and the gene frequency (p and q) are the two factors affecting the population mean.

The gene effects influence the population mean in a way that:

M = a (p – q) + 2pq d $\qquad$ when there is incomplete dominance,

M = a (p – q) = a (1 – 2q) $\qquad$ when there is no dominance (d=0) and

M = a (1 – 2q²) $\qquad$ when there is complete dominance (d= a).

The *effect of gene frequency* on the population mean can be understood taking one of the two alleles as fixed in the population (*i.e.* either p = 1.0 or q = 1.0). The population mean will then be as under-

M = a when the allele A_1 is fixed (p= 1) and

M = -a when the allele A_2 is fixed (q= 1).

Therefore, the total range of values attributable to the locus is **2a** in the absence of overdominance but the mean will be found beyond this range in case of overdominance in an unfixed population (no allele is fixed in the population).

2. Two or more Loci

Several loci affect the quantitative trait. Thus, the population mean is the sum of the effects of separate loci as:

M = Σ a (p – q) + 2 Σ pqd

In this case the point of origin from which the mean value is measured is the mid point of the total range which is equal to the average mid homozygote point of all loci separately. The total range in the absence of overdominance is 2 Σ a. In a line fixed for

A allele, the mean will be $+ \Sigma$ a whereas for a line in which is fixed for *a* allele the mean will be $- \Sigma$ a.

The population mean with one locus (A) is represented as M_A and for another locus (B) as M_B. The mean considering both loci together will be $M_A + M_B$. The mid point between two double homozygotes (O) will be the point of origin from which the mean is measured. Thus, the population mean $= O + M_A + M_A$. The M_A and M_B are calculated separately for two loci as a $(1 - 2q)$ when there is no dominance. The a_A and a_A are taken as the mean between the two homozygotes for the respective loci.

15.5 Estimation of Genotypic Value

The genotypic values of three genotypes are measured as a deviation of the assigned genotypic values (a, d, – a) from population mean. The arbitrarily assigned genotypic values of three genotypes are **a, d** and **–a**, whereas the population mean (M) is $[a (p - q) + 2pq \, d]$. The genotypic values of three genotypes as a deviation from population mean will be as under:

Table 15.3: Genotypic Values of 3 Genotypes

Genotypes	Assigned Value	Genotypic Values*
A_1A_1	a	a – M = a- [a (p – q) + 2pqd] = 2q (a – pd)
A_1A_2	d	d – M = d- [a(p – q) + 2pqd] = a (q – p) + d (1 – 2pq)
A_2A_2	– a	– a – M = -a- [a (p – q) + 2pq d] = -2p (a + q d)

*Taken as deviation from population mean, M = a (p – q) + 2 pq d

Mean Genotypic Value is Zero

Since the genotypic values are taken as deviations from population mean, the mean genotypic value of the population would be zero. This can be verified by multiplying the genotypic value of each genotype with its frequency and summing the cross product for 3 genotypes. This is because the sum of the cross products of the value with its frequency is the mean. This sum which is the mean is zero.

15.6 Estimation of the Components of Genotypic Value

There are two models to describe the genotypic value. These are additive-dominance model used for singe locus two alleles system and interaction model used for two or more loci. The components of genotypic value are estimated by two methods:

(i) Theoretical estimation from gene effect and gene frequency and

(ii) Quantitative estimation from generation means.

15.6.1 Theoretical Estimation: Gene Effect and Frequency

This consider single locus with two alleles (A and a) to estimate additive and dominance components as given here below:

I. Additive Component of Genotypic Value (Breeding Value)

This is the first and most important part of genotypic value and it depends on the *average effect of genes*. The sum of the average effect of the genes affecting a character and carried by an individual is called by various names *viz. additive genetic value* or *additive genetic merit* or *breeding value (B.V.) of genotype (individual)*. This is because the B.V. is caused by additive gene effect (average effect of genes) irrespective of the presence or absence of another gene at one locus or many loci. The average effect of gene is a fixed part of genotypic value, represented by "A" and it is transmitted to the progeny as such.

The breeding value is taken in two ways *viz.* in terms of the average effect of genes carried by the individual and second in terms of measured value of the progeny of the individual. However, both these ways are related to each other because the mean value of the progeny of the individual depends on the sum of the average effect of genes carried by the parent.

(i) Breeding Value Estimated from Progeny Performance

The most accurate and practical method of estimating the B.V. of an individual is the mean performance of its large number of progeny. The mean value (performance) of the progeny is due to the average effect of genes carried by the parent. The progeny performance of any parent deviates from the population mean and this deviation is called as the **transmitting ability** of the parent. *Twice the transmitting ability is the B.V.* for the reason that the progeny contains only a sample half of the genes of the parent, due to the halving nature of inheritance.

The B.V. of different individuals though may be taken as absolute value but is generally taken as the deviation from population mean in order to know the relative superiority of different individuals under testing. The B.V. is the property of the individual and the population to which the individual belongs.

(ii) Breeding Value Estimated from Average Effect of Gene

The B.V. represents the *sum of the average effect of genes of all loci affecting a character.* The magnitude of the average effect of gene has two characteristic features. The first is that it depends on the gene frequency. The second is that it is related to the genotypic value, **a** and **d**, used to express the population mean. Thus, it is the property of genes and the population.

The average effect of genes, the transmitting ability and the breeding value (B.V.) of the genotypes (individuals) can be estimated by taking a male parent either with genotype A_1A_1 or A_2A_2 at a locus mated to the females of all the 3 genotypes. The mean value of progeny of the male parent of genotype A_1A_1 taken as deviation from population mean is the average effect of the gene A_1. This is because it will introduce the A_1 gene and will replace the A_2 gene.

(a) Average Effect of A_1 Gene

This can be estimated by mating A_1A_1 individuals with females of 3 genotypes as shown below:

	Genotypes of		Genotype Frequency among progeny	Genotypic Value
Male Parent	Female Parent	Progeny		
A_1A_1	A_1A_1	A_1A_1	p	a
A_1A_1	A_1A_2	A_1A_2	q	d
A_1A_1	A_2A_2	—	0	0

This mating has introduced the A_1 allele in place of A_2 allele. The expected mean of the progeny produced from A_1A_1 male (P_{11}) is the sum of cross product of genotypic value with its frequency as:

$$P_{11} = p\,a + q\,d$$

The deviation of progeny mean (P_{11}) from population mean (M) is the *transmitting ability of a male parent*. Thus, A_1A_1 *male* will have its transmitting ability ((T_{11})) as:

$$
\begin{aligned}
T_{11} &= P_{11} - M \\
&= p\,a + q\,d - [a\,(p-q) + 2pq\,d] \\
&= q\,a + q\,d - 2pq\,d \\
&= q\,a + q\,d\,(1-2p) \\
&= q\,[a + d\,(q-p)] \\
&= q\,\alpha = \alpha_1
\end{aligned}
$$

The quantity $q\,[a + d\,(q-p)]$ which is the transmitting ability of A_1A_1 genotype, is also called the *average effect of A_1 gene denoted by α_1*. The B.V. of A_1A_1 male is twice of its transmitting ability as-

$$
\begin{aligned}
B.V._{11} &= 2\,T_{11} \\
&= 2q\,\alpha = 2q\,\{a + q\,(q-p)\} = 2\,\alpha_1.
\end{aligned}
$$

(b) Average Effect of A_2 Gene

This can also be estimated by the similar method used to estimate the average effect of A_1 gene. The A_2A_2 male is mated to the females of 3 genotypes of the population:

	Genotypes of		Genotype Frequency among progeny	Genotypic Value
Male Parent	Female Parent	Progeny		
A_2A_2	A_1A_1	—	0	0
A_2A_2	A_1A_2	A_1A_2	p	d
A_2A_2	A_2A_2	A_2A_2	q	−a

This mating has introduced the A_2 gene in place of A_1 gene. The expected mean of progeny (P_{22}) produced from A_2A_2 male is the sum of cross product of genotypic value with its frequency as: $P_{22} = p\,d - q\,a$

The *transmitting ability of A_2A_2 male (genotype)* denoted as T_{22} taken as deviation from population mean will be-

$$T_{22} = P_{22} - M = pd - qa - [a(p-q) + 2pqd]$$
$$= -ap + pd - 2pqd$$
$$= -p[a + d(-1 + 2q)]$$
$$= -p[a + d(q-p)]$$
$$= -p\alpha$$
$$= \alpha_2$$

The quantity $-p[a + d(q-p)]$ is the transmitting ability of A_2A_2 genotype and also the *average effect of A_2 gene* denoted by α_2. The breeding value of A_2A_2 genotype is equal to twice of the transmitting ability as:

$$\text{B.V.}_{22} = 2T_{22}$$
$$= -2p\alpha = -2p[a + d(q-p)]$$
$$= 2\alpha_2$$

(c) B.V. of A_1A_2 Genotype

The B.V. of heterozygous genotype is estimated by adding the average effect of both the gene as:

$$\text{B.V.}_{12} = \alpha_1 + \alpha_2 = q\alpha + (-p\alpha)$$
$$= (q-p)\alpha = (q-p)[a + d(q-p)]$$

It is obvious from the above that the B.V. of an individual is the sum of the average effect of genes carried by the individual. The B.V. is the function of gene frequencies and genotypic values, and hence population specific.

Summary

The different values *viz.* average effect of two genes, transmitting ability and breeding values of 3 genotypes can be summarized as:

Average effect of A_1 gene = Transmitting ability of A_1A_1 genotype = $\alpha_1 = q\alpha$

Average effect of A_2 gene = Transmitting ability of A_2A_2 genotype = $\alpha_2 = -p\alpha$

Transmitting ability of A_1A_2 genotype = $\frac{1}{2}[\alpha_1 + \alpha_2] = \frac{1}{2}(q-p)\alpha$

B.V. of A_1A_1 genotype = $2\alpha_1 = 2q\alpha$

B.V. of A_1A_2 genotype = $\alpha_1 + \alpha_2 = (q-p)\alpha$

B.V. of A_2A_2 genotype = $2\alpha_2 = -2p\alpha$

Average Effect of Gene Substitution

The change in population mean is described by the average effects of two genes at a locus when one allele (A_1) replaces the other allele (A_2). This change in population mean is indicated by the difference in the average effect of two alleles at a locus (A_1 and A_2) *viz.* $\alpha_1 - \alpha_2$. Therefore, the *difference in the average effect of two alleles is called as the average effect of gene substitution*, denoted by the letter α. The average effect of gene substitution (α) can be estimated in either of the following ways:

(i) The average effect of gene substitution (α) is equal to the difference in the average effect of two alleles.

$= \alpha_1 - \alpha_2 = \alpha =$ Average effect of gene substitution

(ii) The average effect of gene substitution (α) is equal to the difference in B.V. of heterozygote from the B.V. of either homozygote:

$= \text{B.V.}_{\cdot 11} - \text{B.V.}_{\cdot 12} \text{ or } BV_{12} - BV_{22}$

$= 2q\,\alpha - (q-p)\,\alpha = 2q\,\alpha - q\,\alpha + p\,\alpha$

$= \alpha\,(q+p) = \alpha$

$=$ Average effect of gene substitution

Mean B.V. Equals Zero

The mean breeding value can be obtained by multiplying the BV with the frequency of each genotype and summing them all. This will equal zero.

II. Non Additive Component of Genotypic Value (Gene Combination Value)

The non additive gene effect is due to the effect of genes when combined to form the genotype and show interaction. Thus, let it be denoted as the *gene combination value* (G. C. V.) which is a value produced by gene combination.

(i) Dominance Deviation (D)

This is within locus interaction and called as *allelic interaction* or *intra allelic interaction*. The dominance effect arises when the phenotypic value of heterozygote deviates from the average phenotypic value of two homozygotes. The dominance effect arises because the effect of gene substitution is not additive for all genotypes in the population.

This can be understood in another way, that when two alleles unite to form the genotype, they interact with each other and produce an additional effect which is not accounted for by the effect of two alleles taken singly. The genotypic value deviates from the sum of the average effect of genes. This deviated value is called the interaction effect. This is the value of gene combination in the genotype produced due to gene interaction. Thus, the dominance deviation can be defined as the gene combination value of the genotype at a locus.

This dominance deviation is added to the BV of genotype to obtain the genotypic value. Thus, $G = A + D$. Therefore, in the absence of dominance, the BV and genotypic value are equal and hence the difference in BV and genotypic value of a particular genotype indicates the dominance deviation (D). In other words, *the deviation of genotypic value from BV for a locus is called dominance deviation*. This is the meaning of dominance deviation or dominance effect. According to additive-dominance model of genotypic value, the genotypic value (G) is taken as:

$G = A + D$ and so, $D = G - A$.

Thus, dominance deviation can be estimated by difference as:

$[D_{ij} = G_{ij} - (\alpha_i + \alpha_j)]$ as given under:

Table 15.4: Dominance Deviations of Three Genotypes

Genotypes	Genotypic Values (G_{ij})	Breeding Values (A_{ij})	Dominance Deviations (D_{ij})
A_1A_1	$2q\ (a - pd)$	$2q\ \alpha$	$-2q^2d$
A_1A_2	$a\ (q - p) + d\ (1 - 2pq)$	$(q - p)\ \alpha$	$2\ pqd$
A_2A_2	$-2\ p\ (a + qd)$	$-2\ p\ \alpha$	$-2p^2d$

Where, $\alpha = a + d\ (q - p)$

It is clear that all the dominance deviations are functions of gene frequency and *d*. This is because the average effect of genes, BV and genotypic values depends on the gene frequency. The dominance deviations are zero when the alleles do not show dominance (d = 0) and in this case the genotypic values and BV will be equal as:

$G = A + D$

$= A + 0 = A$

Mean Dominance Deviation is zero

This is based on the fact that mean BV and mean G.V. are equal to zero. It can also be proved by multiplying the dominance deviation by the frequency of each genotype and summing the cross products.

BV and Dominance Deviation are not Correlated

This can be verified by multiplying the two values (**A** and **D**) with frequency of each genotype and summing the cross products over all the 3 genotypes.

(ii) Interaction Deviation (I): Two Loci Case

This is between loci interaction. In addition to the additive (A) and dominance (D) effects of genes present on same locus, the genes present on different loci also interact. It is generally referred as the interaction deviation denoted by I. The interaction effects are caused by interaction between genes present on two or more loci and known as *non-allelic* or *inter allelic interactions* which are generally called as *epistasis*. This is indicated when the sum of the gene's effect of all loci deviate from the phenotypic or genotypic values. The aggregate genotypic value for two loci taken together (G_{AB}) can be defined as:

$G_{AB} = G_A + G_B + I_{AB}$

where, $\mathbf{G_A}$ and $\mathbf{G_B}$ are genotypic values of two loci (A and B) combining the A and D effects together in G_A and G_B.

$\mathbf{I_{AB}}$ is the interaction effect of two loci indicating the deviation from additive combination of genes.

The interaction effect (I) are indicated when the additive-dominance effects are not sufficient to account completely the genotypic value. The genotype can be defined as:

$G = M + A + D + I$

The interaction component (I_{AB}) can be obtained as a difference:

$I \quad = G - A - D$

$= G - (A + D)$

The kind of interaction depends on the mode of gene action of loci which mean whether the interaction is involved between additive or dominance deviation. This can be seen in two loci (A and B) case as:

$I_{AB} = I_{AA} + I_{AD} + I_{DD}$

where, I_{AB} is the interaction effect of genes between two loci (A and B),

I_{AA} is the interaction between additive values of two loci,

I_{AD} is the interaction between additive value of one locus and dominance deviation of other locus or vice versa,

I_{DD} is the interaction between dominance deviations of two loci.

Indication of Interaction Effect of Two Loci (I_{AB})

The magnitude of epistasis is indicated by the difference between two homozygotes for one locus with respect to genotype for the other locus. When these differences (between two homozygotes) at one locus are independent of the genotype of the other locus, it then indicates that the two loci act additively (independently) and they do not interact. In this case, the difference between two homozygotes for one locus will be equal for each genotype of other locus. For example, the difference in phenotypic value between two homozygotes (A_1A_1 and A_2A_2) or between heterozygote and one homozygote (A_1A_2 and A_2A_2 or A_1A_2 and A_1A_1) will be of equal size for B_1B_1, B_1B_2, and B_2B_2 genotypes. Similarly, the difference between any two genotypes for B locus will be similar for any genotype at A locus (A_1A_1, A_1A_2 and A_2A_2). On the contrary, if the differences are not equal but vary for different genotypes of other locus, it then indicates that the effects of the two loci are dependent on each other and hence shows that they do not act additively but interact with each other showing epistasis. Therefore, *the epistasis is indicated when the phenotypic expression of any genotype at one locus is dependent upon the genotype of the other locus.*

15.6.2 Quantitative Estimation: Estimation of Components of Genotypic Value from Generation Means

The components of genotypic values are estimated quantitatively from the means of different generations produced by crossing two purebred lines/strains. The genetic components are estimated separately for the characters controlled by single locus or by more loci. This requires the knowledge of the expected generation means in term of the genetic components and the relationship among means of different generations, considering single locus and two loci case differently.

I. Single Locus Case

When a character is controlled by single locus, there are only two genetic parameters *viz.* additive and dominance. The composition of means of different generations in terms of these two genetic components has been given here:

(1) Expected Generation Means: Additive and Dominance Components

A true breeding line is homozygous for all the loci affecting a trait. However, some of the loci may have favourable (positive) effect to increase the value of the trait while, others may decrease the value of the trait. The genes having positive and negative effect influence the average measurement of the trait (m, the mid point or zero point) and hence the genes effect is measured as deviation from mid point (m) which is constant depending on the action of gene not under consideration (basis genotype or genetic background) and of the environmental effects.

1. True Breeding Strain

The phenotypic value of a true breeding strain will be as

$m + \Sigma a^+ - \Sigma a^-$

where, Σa^+ indicates the sum of effects of favourable genes,

Σa^- indicates the sum of effects of unfavourable genes,

m is the mean of two straits which is the natural zero point used to express the measurements as deviation from it. The *m* is independent of the pattern of the distribution of positive and negative alleles in two straits.

Suppose one strain designated as P_1 has all the favourable (positive) alleles with genotype as AA while the other strains (P_2) has all the negative (unfavourable) alleles with its genotype as aa. The phenotypic mean of these two strains will be as:

$\overline{P}_{1(AA)} = m + a$

$\overline{P}_{2(aa)} = m - a$

The *a* represents the additive effect of gene and can be estimated by comparing' the two strains for their mean phenotypic value by substracting the mean of the smaller strain (S_2 or P_2) from the mean of longer strain (S_2 or P_1) and taking into account the genes for which the two strains differ. The mean phenotypic value of two strains will differ as:

$S_1 - S_2 = \overline{P}_1 - \overline{P}_2$ $= (m + \Sigma a^+ - \Sigma a^-) - (m + \Sigma a^+ - \Sigma a^-)$

$= 2(\Sigma a^+ - \Sigma a^-)$

However, the distribution of genes between the two strains influences the difference between their mean phenotypic values. In case of iso-directional distribution of genes (all positive alleles are present in one strain and all negative in the other strain), the difference in mean phenotypic values of two strains will be:

$\overline{P}_1 - \overline{P}_2 = 2 \Sigma a^+ = 2 Ka$

When $a_A = a_B = a_C = ... = a_K$

where, K represents the number of loci.

Generally, the genes with positive and negative effects are dispersed in the two strains. Thus, the difference between strain means can be represented by the measure of the gene distribution between strains denoted by r which indicates the degree of association of genes of similar effect. Now taking K as the number of gene loci affecting a trait for which the two strains differ, K' as the number of genes with positive effects present in one strain with $k - k'$ as the number of genes with negative effects and vice versa for the other strain. When $a_A = a_B = a_C = ... = a_K = a$, the difference between the mean phenotypic value will be:

$$\overline{P}_1 - \overline{P}_2 = 2(K—2K')a$$

$$= 2\,r\,Ka$$

where, $r = (K - 2K')/K$

               $r = 1$ when all the positive genes are present in one strain with equal distribution in two strains.

Taking the effect of each A gene as a + instead of 1 for all K genes, the difference can be represented as:

$$\overline{P}_1 - \overline{P}_2 = 2\,r\,\Sigma\,a = 2\,\Sigma a^+$$

2. F₁ Generation

The F_1 is produced from two strains and is heterozygous for all the K genes whether the genes are associated or distributed. The F_1 mean deviates from m by

$= \Sigma\ d$ when $d_A = d_B = ... = d$ K taking sign into account. When there is no dominance or the d increments are balanced by the dominance of positive and negative genes, then $\Sigma d = 0$ and the F_1 mean is equal to m. Therefore,

$\overline{F}_1 = m + \Sigma d$ When there is dominance

     $= m$ When there is no dominance

The average dominance of genes is measured by a ratio of the amount by which the F_1 deviates from m ($d = F_1 - m$) to half of the difference among parents (a). Thus, this measure is

$$\frac{d}{a} = \frac{\Sigma d}{r\Sigma a}$$

This ratio with equal effects of the genes is Ka/rkd. The use of this ratio (average dominance of genes) assumes that the genes of similar effect are associated in one parent ($r = 1$) and that the dominance is unidirec-tional for all loci (all d increments have same sign).

3. Subsequent Generations

The expected mean of any genera-tion in terms of the genetic parameters a and d as a deviation from m can be written if the relative frequencies of three genotypes for each gene pair are known for that population. The expected means of the generations derived by selfing, sib mating and back crossing can be obtained as under.

(i) F_2 Generation

The F_2 generation is produced by inter-se- mating of F_1 individuals and the expected ratio of three genetic classes of F_2 individuals is ¼ AA: ½ Aa: ¼aa for one gene pair. Thus half the F_2 generation individuals are heterozygotes and another half are homozygotes of two types in equal ratio having positive and negative alleles. The contribution of two types of homozygotes in F_2 mean will be cancelled out by their positive and negative effects of equal size. The heterozygotes which constitute 50 per cent of F_2 population will only contribute to F2 mean and hence the F_2 mean will be:

$$\overline{F_2} = m + \tfrac{1}{2} \Sigma\, d$$

(ii) F_3 and Subsequent Generation Produced by Selfing (Fn)

The proportion of heterozygotes is reduced to half in each successive generation produced by selfing. Therefore, any generation (Fn) produced from F_1 will have a proportion of $(\tfrac{1}{2})^{n-1}$ heterozygotes and a proportion of $\tfrac{1}{2}[1 - (\tfrac{1}{2})^{n-1}]$ homozygotes of each type. Thus Fn mean will be:

$$\overline{Fn} = m + (\tfrac{1}{2})^{n-1} \Sigma\, d$$

$$\overline{F_3} = m + (\tfrac{1}{2})^{3-1} \Sigma\, d$$

$$= m + \tfrac{1}{4} \Sigma\, d$$

(iii) Sib Mating Generations (Sn)

The first generation produced by sib mating of F_1 will have its mean (S_2) equal to the mean of F_2 generation $\left(\overline{F_2}\right)$ and hence $\overline{S_2} = \overline{F_2} = m + \tfrac{1}{2}\Sigma d$. But the expected generation mean of the subsequent generations produced by sib mating are different to those produced by selfing. This is because the frequencies of heterozygote in sib mating generations are different from selfing series. The frequency of heterozygotes in n^{th} generation of sib mating can be obtained from Fibonacci series starting from fn = 2 (the $F_2 = S_2$) as ½, 2/4, 3/8, 5/16, 8/32, 13/64, etc. instead of $(1/2)^{n-1}$ of the selfing series. The frequency of homozygotes of each type will be cancelled out. Thus, the heterozygotes will contribute to generation mean and hence the expected mean of nth generation of sib mating will be:

$$\overline{S_n} = m + fn\, \Sigma d$$

(iv) Back Cross Generations

The crossing of F_1 with either of the parent (P_1 or P_2) is called backcross. Thus, there are two backcrosses of first generation *viz.* backcross to superior parent (B_1) and backcross with inferior parent (B_2). For a single locus with two alleles only two genotypes *viz.* heterozygote and one of the two homozygotes are produced. The frequency of heterozygotes in n^{th} generation of repeated back cross with one of the either parent (say, B_n) is $(\tfrac{1}{2})^n$ where as the frequency of the homozygote is $1 - (\tfrac{1}{2})^n$. Therefore, the expected generation means will be:

$$\bar{B}_1 = m + (\tfrac{1}{2})^n + \tfrac{1}{2}\,\Sigma d$$

$$\bar{B}_{1n} = m + [1 - (\tfrac{1}{2})^n]\,\Sigma a + (\tfrac{1}{2})^n\,\Sigma d$$

$$\bar{B}_2 = m - \tfrac{1}{2}\,\Sigma a + \tfrac{1}{2}\,\Sigma d$$

$$\bar{B}_{2n} = m - [1 - (\tfrac{1}{2})^n]\,\Sigma a + (\tfrac{1}{2})^n\,\Sigma d$$

(2) Relationship among Expected Means of Generations

The relationships and level of inheritance among means of different generations can be obtained on the basis of assuming the additive dominance model and absence of differential viability and fertility as given below in table.

Table 15.5: Relationship among Generation Means

Generations	Cross made to Produce Generations	Relation among Generations	Level of Inheritance of P_1 Parent
F_1	$P_1 \times P_2$	$\tfrac{1}{2}\,\bar{P}_1 + \tfrac{1}{2}\,\bar{P}_2 = m$ (no dominance) $= m + \Sigma d$ (dominance)	$\tfrac{1}{2}$
F_2	$F_1 + F_1$	$\bar{F}_2 - m = \tfrac{1}{2}(\bar{F}_1 - m)$ $= \bar{F}_2 - \tfrac{1}{2}(\bar{P}_1 + \bar{P}_2) = \tfrac{1}{2}[\bar{F}_1 - \tfrac{1}{2}(\bar{P}_1 + \bar{P}_2)]$ $\bar{F}_2 = \tfrac{1}{2}\,\bar{F}_1 + \tfrac{1}{4}(\bar{P}_1 + \bar{P}_2)$	$\tfrac{1}{2}$
F_3	$F_2 + F_2$	$\tfrac{1}{2}\,\bar{F}_2 + \tfrac{1}{4}(\bar{P}_1 + \bar{P}_2)$	
F_n	$F_{n-1} \times F_{n-1}$	$\tfrac{1}{2}\,\bar{F}_{n-1} + \tfrac{1}{4}(\bar{P}_1 + \bar{P}_2)$	$\tfrac{1}{2}$
B_1	$F_1 \times P_1$	$\tfrac{1}{2}\,\bar{F}_1 + \tfrac{1}{2}\,\bar{P}_1 = \tfrac{1}{2}[\tfrac{1}{2}\,\bar{P}_1 + \bar{P}_2) + \tfrac{1}{2}\,\bar{P}_1$ $= \tfrac{3}{4}\,\bar{P}_1 + \tfrac{1}{4}\,\bar{P}_2$	$\tfrac{3}{4}$
B_2	$F_1 \times P_2$	$\tfrac{1}{2}\,\bar{F}_1 + \tfrac{1}{2}\,\bar{P}_2 = \tfrac{1}{2}[\tfrac{1}{2}\,\bar{P}_1 + \bar{P}_2) + \tfrac{1}{2}\,\bar{P}_2$ $= \tfrac{3}{4}\,\bar{P}_2 + \tfrac{1}{4}\,\bar{P}_1$	$\tfrac{1}{4}$
B_{11}	$B_1 \times P_1$	$\tfrac{1}{2}[\tfrac{1}{2}\,\bar{F}_1 + \tfrac{1}{2}\,\bar{P}_1) + \bar{P}_1] = \tfrac{1}{4}\,\bar{F}_1 + \tfrac{3}{4}\,\bar{P}_1$	$\tfrac{7}{8}$
B_{12}	$B_1 \times P_2$	$\tfrac{1}{2}[\tfrac{1}{2}\,\bar{F}_1 + \tfrac{1}{2}\,\bar{P}_1) + \bar{P}_2] = \tfrac{3}{4}\,\bar{F}_1 + \tfrac{1}{4}\,P_2$	$\tfrac{3}{8}$
B_{21}	$B_2 \times P_1$	$\tfrac{1}{2}[\tfrac{1}{2}\,\bar{F}_1 + \tfrac{1}{2}\,\bar{P}_2) + \bar{P}_1] = \tfrac{1}{4}\,\bar{F}_1 + \tfrac{1}{4}\,\bar{P}_2 + \tfrac{1}{2}\,\bar{P}_1$ $= \tfrac{3}{4}\,\bar{F}_1 + \tfrac{1}{4}\,\bar{P}_1$	$\tfrac{5}{8}$
B_{22}	$B_2 \times P_2$	$\tfrac{1}{2}[\tfrac{1}{2}\,\bar{F}_1 + \tfrac{1}{2}\,\bar{P}_2) + \bar{P}_1] = \tfrac{1}{4}\,\bar{F}_1 + \tfrac{1}{4}\,\bar{P}_2 + \tfrac{1}{2}\,\bar{P}_2$ $= \tfrac{1}{4}\,\bar{F}_1 + \tfrac{3}{4}\,\bar{P}_2$	$\tfrac{1}{8}$

The expectation of F_2 mean can also be taken in terms of the mean of backcrosses as:

$$\overline{F_2} = \tfrac{1}{2}(\overline{B_1} + \overline{B_2}) = \tfrac{1}{2}[\tfrac{1}{2}\overline{F_1} + \tfrac{1}{2}\overline{P_1} + \tfrac{1}{2}\overline{F_1} + \tfrac{1}{2}\overline{P_2}]$$

$$= \tfrac{1}{2}(\overline{F_1} + \tfrac{1}{2}\overline{P_1} + \tfrac{1}{2}\overline{P_2})$$

$$= \tfrac{1}{2}\overline{F_1} + \tfrac{1}{4}(\overline{P_1} + \overline{P_2})$$

$$\overline{F_2} = \tfrac{1}{4}(\overline{B_{11}} + \overline{B_{12}} + \overline{B_{21}} + \overline{B_{22}})$$

$$\overline{F_3} = \tfrac{1}{2}(\overline{B_{11}} + \overline{B_{22}})$$

(3) Estimation of Additive and Dominance Components

The mean parental value or the mid point (m), additive effect (a) and dominance (d) components in the absence of non-allelic interaction can be estimated as:

$$M = \tfrac{1}{2}(\overline{P_1} + \overline{P_2}) = \text{Mid- parent value}$$

$$a = \tfrac{1}{2}(\overline{P_1} - \overline{P_2}) = \text{Average gene effect}$$

$$\mathbf{d} = \tfrac{1}{2}(\overline{F_1} - m) = \text{Dominance effect of gene}$$

However, these parameters have been estimated by Jinks and Jones (1958) using the following formulae:

$$m = \tfrac{1}{2}\overline{P_1} + \tfrac{1}{2}\overline{P_2} + 4\overline{F_2} - 2\overline{B_1} - 2\overline{B_2}$$

$$= \tfrac{1}{2}(\overline{P_1} + \overline{P_2}) + 2(\overline{F_2} - \overline{B_1} - \overline{B_2})$$

$$a = \tfrac{1}{2}(\overline{P_1} - \overline{P_2})$$

$$d = 6(\overline{B_1} + \overline{B_2}) - 8\overline{F_2} - \overline{F_1} - 3/2(\overline{P_1} + \overline{P_2})$$

With their variance as:

$$Vm = \tfrac{1}{4}(V_{\overline{p}1} + V_{\overline{p}2}) + 4(V_{\overline{F}2} + V_{\overline{B}1} + V_{\overline{B}2})$$

$$Va = \tfrac{1}{4}(V_{\overline{p}1} + V_{\overline{p}2})$$

$$Vd = 36(V_{\overline{B}1} + V_{\overline{B}2}) + 64\,V_{\overline{F}2} + V_{\overline{F}1} + 9/4(V_{\overline{p}1} + V_{\overline{p}2})$$

and the standard errors as:

S.E.(m) = $\sqrt{Vm}$

S.E.(a) = $\sqrt{Va}$

S.E.(d) = $\sqrt{Vd}$

The t test of significance is applied as:

$$t = \frac{\text{Value of the parameter}}{\text{S.E. of the parameter}}$$

e.g. $t(m) = m/\text{S.E.}(m)$

The variance of mean like V_{P1} etc. and the S.E. are estimated as:

Variance of sample mean = Variance/n

$$\text{S.E.} = \sqrt{\frac{\text{Variance}}{n}}$$

where, n is the number of observations.

(4) Testing of Additive Dominance Model: Scaling Tests

Two tests are available to test the expected relationship between generation means depending on the additive and dominance effect in absence of linkage and non-allelic interaction effects of the genes. These are the scaling tests given by Mather (1949) and the joint scaling test devised by Cavalli (1952).

(i) Scaling Tests

Mather (1949) proposed the scaling tests to calculate some relationship among generation means such as, A $2B_{1-} P_1 - = 0$ assuming the additive dominance model. These tests use only a few combinations of families. It is necessary to test the absence of non allelic interaction. He proposed the following four quantities/tests:

$$A = 2\overline{B}_1 - \overline{P}_1 - \overline{F}_1$$

$$B = 2\overline{B}_2 - \overline{P}_2 - \overline{F}_1$$

$$C = 4\overline{F}_2 - 2\overline{F}_1 - \overline{P}_1 - \overline{P}_2$$

$$D = 4\overline{F}_3 - 2\overline{F}_2 - \overline{P}_1 - \overline{P}_2$$

$$= 2\overline{F}_2 - \overline{B}_1 - \overline{B}_2$$

The values of the quantities A, B, C and D should be equal to zero within the limits of their standard error. If any of the scale (A, B, C and D) is significantly different from zero, it then indicates the presence of non-allelic interaction as

A and B scales give evidence on i, j and I type of gene interactions

C indicates '1' type of gene interaction.

D is an indication of 'i' type of gene interaction.

These scaling tests require the data on 6 families which are the two true breeding strains (P_1 and P_2), their first two crossbred generations (F_1 and F_2), and backcross generations (B_1, and B_2). The values of these scales are tested for their significant departure from zero by estimating their variances as:

$$V_A = 4 V_{\bar{B}1} + V_{\bar{P}1} + V_{\bar{F}1}$$

$$V_B = 4 V_{\bar{B}2} + V_{\bar{P}2} + V_{\bar{F}1}$$

$$V_C = 16 V_{\bar{F}2} + 4 V_{\bar{P}1} + V_{\bar{P}1} + V_{\bar{P}2}$$

$$V_D = 4 V_{\bar{F}2} + V_{\bar{B}1} + V_{\bar{B}2}$$

The standard errors of the above tests are estimated by taking the square root of the respective variances of the scales, *e.g.*

Standard error of $A = \sqrt{V_A}$

The variance of mean of any generation $V_{\bar{P}1}$ is estimated as:

Variance of P_1 mean ($V_{\bar{P}1}$) = Variance/n

where, n is the number of observations.

Now, the t values are estimated for each scaling test as:

$t_{(A)} = $ Value of $A/S.E._{(A),}$ and so on.

The calculated values of t are compared with the tabulated t values at 5 per cent level of significance for the degree of freedom equal to the sum of the degree of freedom of different generations used to apply the test. For example, the degree of freedom for scaling test A will be equal to:

D.F. for $A = $ d.f. of $V_{\bar{B}1}$ + d.f. for $V_{\bar{P}1}$ + d.f. for $V_{\bar{P}2}$

The degree of freedom for any generation is equal to the number of observations minus one.

(ii) Joint Scaling Test

Cavalli (1952) devised the "joint scaling test". This test can combine any combination of generations at the same time. The test also estimates the genetic parameters (m, a, and d) of the model and makes the comparison of observed generation means with that expected on the basis of these parameters (m, a, and d). To estimate three parameters, a minimum of three types of generations are required. However, there should be a perfect agreement between the observed and expected generation means and this provides no test of the goodness of fit. But four or more numbers of generations are required to provide the test of goodness of fit. Thus the joint scaling test can test the goodness of fit when the data on more than three generations (families) are available.

II. Two Gene Pairs

With two pairs of genes, each with two alleles (A – a and B – b) in a diploid population, the expectation of means of different generation can be obtained based on the different phenotypes in term of the genetic parameters *viz.*

(i) Mid point (m)

(ii) Additive effect of both loci (a_A and a_B),

(iii) Dominance effect of two loci (d_A and d_B), and

(iv) Interaction effect of non-allelic gene (i, j and l)

There are two kind of crosses for two gene pairs depending on the association of increasing alleles in one parent (coupling phase) or their distribution in two parents (repulsion phase). The association and dispersion of genes affect the sign of the effect of the genetic component (except m) of both the parent and both of the backcrosses whereas the signs of the coefficients of genetic parameters of other crosses are independent of genes distribution in the absence of linkage.

(1) Expected Generation Means (Two loci)

The expected generation means for two loci case in terms of genetic components for different generations based on their genotypes have been given in table 15.7.

F_2 Generation

The details of the procedure to get the expected genetic components based on different genotypes of F_2 generation have been given here. There will be nine genotypes of F_2 generation and the complete description of the differences among genotypes can be given by eight genetic parameters which are as:

2 additive effects of genes for two loci designated as a_A and a_B,

2 dominance effects of genes for two loci designated as d_A and d_B

4 non-allelic interaction effects of genes designated as

$i\,(a_A\,a_B),\ j\,(a_A\,d_B)$ or $\ j\,(d_A\,a_B),\ l\,(d_A\,d_B)$

The different genetic components of nine genotypes of F_2 generation can be represented as given in Table 15.6 below:

Table 15.6: Different Genotypes and the Genetic Components of
F_2 Generation for Two Gene Pairs

Genotypes	1 BB	2 Bb	1 bb	F_2 Mean
1 AA	$a_A + a_B + i$	$a_A + d_B + j$	$a_A - a_B - i$	$a_A + \frac{1}{2} d_B + \frac{1}{2} j$
2 Aa	$d_A + a_B + j$	$d_A + d_B + l$	$d_A - a_B - j$	$d_A + \frac{1}{2} d_B + \frac{1}{2} l$
1 aa	$-a_A + a_B - i$	$-a_A + d_B - j$	$-a_A - a_B + i$	$-a_A + \frac{1}{2} d_B - \frac{1}{2} j$
F_2 Mean	$\frac{1}{2} d_A + a_B + \frac{1}{2} j$	$\frac{1}{2} d_A + d_B + \frac{1}{2} l$	$\frac{1}{2} d_A - a_B - \frac{1}{2} j$	$\frac{1}{2} d_A + \frac{1}{2} d_B + \frac{1}{4} l$

Thus, the F_2 mean is composed of $\frac{1}{2} d_A + \frac{1}{2} d_B + \frac{1}{4} I$. The coefficients of dominant effects of both genes are $\frac{1}{2}$ and of interaction component is $\frac{1}{4}$ l. Looking at F_2 column of table 15.6, the a_A and $- a_A$ are cancelled with each other and the mean is $\frac{1}{2} d_A$ because the heterozygotes among F_2 generation constitute half of the population. The coefficient of interaction parameters are obtained in all cases as the products of the coefficients of the corresponding a and d components taking sign into account directly.

The three components of non-allelic interaction are denoted as:

$$I = I_{AA} + I_{AA} + I_{AA}.$$

$$\text{or} = i(a_A a_B) + j(a_A d_B) + l(d_A d_B)$$

Table 15.7: Coefficients of Genetic Components for Digenic Crosses

Generations	m	a_A	a_B	d_A	d_B	i_{AA}	j_{AD}	j_{DA}	l_{DD}
(i) Gene association: AABB x aabb									
P_1	1	1	1	–	–	1	–	–	–
P_2	1	– 1	– 1	–	–	1	–	–	–
F_1	1	–	–	1	1	–	–	–	1
$F_2 = S_2$	1	–	–	½	½	–	–	–	¼
F_3	1	–	–	¼	¼	–	–	–	$^1/_{16}$
F_{n+1}	1	–	–	$(½)^n$	$(½)^n$	–	–	–	$(½)^{2n}$
S_3	1	–	–	½	½	–	–	–	¼
B_1	1	½	½	½	½	¼	¼	¼	¼
B_2	1	– ½	– ½	½	½	¼	– ¼	– ¼	¼
(ii) Gene dispersion: AAbb x aaBB									
P_1	1	1	–1	–	–	–1	–	–	–
P_2	1	–1	1	–	–	–1	–	–	–
(The coefficients are same for F_1, F_2, F_3, F_{n+1} and S_3 generations)									
B_1	1	½	– ½	½	½	– ¼	¼	– ¼	¼
B_2	1	– ½	½	½	½	– ¼	– ¼	¼	¼

Second Backcross Generations

The expected means of second backcross generations according to their genotypes in the presence of digenic interactions will be as under:

$$B_{11} = m + ¾\,a + ¼\,d + {}_{9/16}\,i + {}_{3/16}\,j + {}_{1/16}\,l$$

$$B_{12} = m - ¼\,a + ¾\,d + {}_{1/16}\,i - {}_{3/16}\,j + {}_{9/16}\,l$$

$$B_{21} = m + ¼\,a + ¾\,d + {}_{1/16}\,i + {}_{3/16}\,j + {}_{9/16}\,l$$

$$B_{22} = m - ¾\,a + ¼\,d + {}_{9/16}\,i - {}_{3/16}\,j + {}_{1/16}\,l$$

The magnitude and sign of coefficients of interaction components depends on the magnitude and sign of the non-interacting genetic components and obtained as the products of the corresponding a and d parameters.

(2) Estimation of Genetic Components for Digenic Crosses

The effect of non-allelic interactions on the generation means along with the estimates of their magnitude can be estimated provided the means of six generations are available.

(i) Six Parameter Model

Jinks and Jones (1958) proposed the following 6 parameter model:

m = Similar as given earlier for single locus

a = Similar as given earlier for single locus

d = Similar as given earlier for single locus

$$i = 2\overline{B}_1 + 2\overline{B}_2 - 4\overline{F}_2$$

$$j = 2\overline{B}_1 - \overline{P}_1 - 2\overline{B}_2 + \overline{P}_2$$

$$l = \overline{P}_1 + \overline{P}_2 + 2\overline{F}_1 + 4(\overline{F}_2 - \overline{B}_1 - \overline{B}_2)$$

The variances and standard errors of these estimates can be calculated as outlined under section 15.6.2(3) for single looks and the significance is also tested by 't' test.

Hayman (1958) proposed the following six parameter model

$$m = mean = \overline{F}_2$$

$$a = \overline{B}_1 - \overline{B}_2$$

$$d = \overline{F}_1 - 4\overline{F}_2 - \tfrac{1}{2}(\overline{P}_1 + \overline{P}_2) + 2(\overline{B}_1 + \overline{B}_2)$$

i = Similar as proposed by Jinks and Jones (1958),

j = Similar as proposed by Jinks and Jones (1958),

l = Similar as proposed by Jinks and Jones (1958).

The calculations of variances and standard errors, and the t test are obtained as given above.

(ii) Five Parameter Model

A five parameter model was given when B_1 and B_2 generations are not available but F_3 generation is available. The model is given by Hayman (1958) as under -

$$m = \overline{F}_2$$

$$a = \tfrac{1}{2}(\overline{P}_1 - \overline{P}_2)$$

$$d = \tfrac{1}{4}\overline{F}_1 + \tfrac{3}{4}\overline{F}_2 - \overline{F}_3$$

$$j = \overline{P}_1 - \overline{F}_2 + \tfrac{1}{2}\overline{P}_1 - \tfrac{1}{2}\overline{P}_2 + \tfrac{1}{2}d - \tfrac{1}{4}l$$

$$l = 1/3(16\overline{F}_3 - 24\overline{F}_2 + 8\overline{F}_1)$$

The calculations for variances, standard errors of the estimates and t test are obtained as given above.

The evidence of the presence of non-allelic interactions is indicated when there is a failure of the relationship (goodness of fit) between observed and expected generation mean on additive – dominance model. This can be tested either by using the test of goodness of fit (χ^2 test) or by the individual scaling tests or joint scaling test.

Numerical Solved Examples

Example 15.1

Birth weights are given below for 4 genetic groups of calves born during 4 seasons. Find out the major components of phenotypic value and test their values for the second group calves born in first season.

Genetic/Seasons Groups	S_1	S_2	S_3	S_4	Total	$G_{i.}$ = Mean
G_1	18	20	20	22	80	20.00
G_2	17	19	18	20	74	18.50
G_3	19	18	19	19	75	18.75
G_4	17	19	20	19	75	18.75
Total	71	76	77	80	304	
Mean ($E._j$)	17.75	19.0	19.25	20.0		19.0
= e_j	−1.25	0.0	0.25	1.0		

Solution

Population Mean = 19.0

(i) **Genotypic values-** These are the mean birth weight of the corresponding genetic group over all the environments ($G_{i.}$): G_1= 20.0; G_2= 18.5; G_3= 18.75 and G_4= 18.75 Kg.

(ii) **Environmental Deviations-** These are the deviations of the mean of all genotypes under one environment from the population mean viz. e_j = M − $E._{j,}$
E_1 = 17.75 – 19.0 = -1.25; E_2 = 19.0 – 19.0 = 0.0;
E_3 = 19.25 – 19.00.25 and E_4= 20.0 – 19.0 = 1.0 Kg. (Note that $\Sigma e_j = 0$)

(iii) **G-E interaction –** These will be 4 x 4= 16 in numbers corresponding to the P_{ij}.
$I_{G2\ EI}$ = $P_{21} - (G_{i.} + E_j)$
$I_{G2\ EI}$ = 17 – (18.5 – 1.25) = 17 – 18.5 + 1.25
= 18.25 – 18.5
= – 0.25 Kg.

(iv) **Expected Phenotypic value (P_{21})** = G_2. + $E._1$ + I_{G2EI}
= 18.5 – 1.25 – 0.25
= 18.5 – 1.5 = 17.0

The genotypic values for the different genotypes can also be expressed as deviation from the population mean (19.0 Kg in this example).

The genotypic worth of the second genetic group was to produce the calves weighing 18.5 Kg (G_2=18.5 Kg) but when this genotype (G_2) was measured in different environments the birth weight of valves born in different seasons varied from 17 to 20 kg. The environment in different seasons experienced by the animals of this genotype modified the genotypic value in both the sides of the genotypic value of 18.5 kg.

In this example, it can be observed that mean environmental deviation equal to zero.

$$E_j = -1.25 + 0 + 0.25 + 1.00$$

The same is true for the environmental deviations for each genotype. For example, the mean phenotypic value for the second genetic group (G_2) is 18.5 which is the population mean or the mean genotypic value for this genotype (G_2). The environmental deviations for the first through fourth environments (seasons) are -1.5, 0.5, -0.5 and 1.5, respectively whose sum is zero. Therefore, the environment has no contribution to the population mean.

Now considering a breed as a single genotype, for example take 2nd breed as a single cow which produced calves sired by same bull in different lactations (example 10.1) with birth weight of 4 calves as 17, 19, 18 and 20 kg, respectively during different lactations. The average birth weight of 4 calves produced by this cow is 18.5 kg which is the population mean or mean phenotypic value or the mean genotypic value of this cow which was modified by the effect of lactation number (environment). Thus 18.5 kg birth weight was the genotype value for birth weight of 2nd cow in this example.

Example 15.2

The following is a random mating population with phenotypic values of 3 genotypes and the numbers of individuals of each genotype.

Genotypes	No. of Observations	Phenotypic Values (P_{ij})
A_1A_1	27	50
A_1A_2	36	36
A_2A_2	12	18

From the information about the above population estimate the following population parameters: Gene frequencies of two allele, population mean, average effect of gene substitution, average effect of two alleles, genotypic values, breeding values and dominance deviation of 3 genotypes.

Solution

(i) Gene frequencies: $p = (27 \times 2 + 36)/75$ (2)

                                                $= 90/150$

                                                $= 0.60$ and

          $q = 1 - 0.6 = 0.4$

(ii) Mid point (m = o) = Mean of two homozygote

= ½ (50 + 18)

= 34 = Effect of basic genotype

(iii) Dominance effect (d) = heterozygote – mid point

= 36 – 34 = 2

(iv) Gene effects and Genotypic values of 3 genotypes (**a, d** and **–a**):

Genotypic value of G_{11} = Av. effect of dom. allele (**a**)

= Av. of the diff of 2 homozygote

= ½ (50 – 18) = 16

Genotypic value of G_{12} = dominance effect(d)

= Heterozygote – mid point

= P_{12} – m

= 36 – 34

= 2

Genotypic value of G_{22} = Av. effect of recessive allele (**- a**)

= Equal to **a** but with –ive sign

= – 16

These genotypic values indicate the additive effect of **A** and **a** allele, and the dominance effect (**d**).

or, Genotypic values of 3 genotypes (**a, d** and **–a**) estimated as a deviation of the respective phenotypic value (p_{ij}) from mid point (**m**) value as:

G_{ij} = P_{ij} – **m**

a = 50 – 34

= 16;

d = 36 – 34

= 2

(v) Population mean (Absolute mean) = Arithmetic average

= [Sum of cross product of phenotypic values and numbers of individuals]/ total number of individuals

= [(27 x 50) + (36 x 36) + (12 x 18)]/75

= 38.16

Population mean (M) = Arithmetic mean as deviation from mid point (**m**)

= Arithmetic Av. – mid point

= 38.16 – 34.0

= 4.16

Population mean (M) = Weighted average of all genotypic values

$$= \text{Sum of product of genotypic freq. x}$$
$$\text{assigned genotypic values } \textbf{(fv)}$$
$$= (0.36 \times 16) + (0.48 \times 2) + (0.16 \times -16)$$
$$= 5.76 + 0.96 - 2.56$$
$$= 4.16$$

Population mean in absolute terms

$$= m + \Sigma fv$$
$$= 34.0 + 4.16$$
$$= 38.16$$

Average effect of gene substitution (α)

$$= a + d(q - p)$$
$$= 16 + 2(0.4 - 0.6)$$
$$= 15.6$$

Average effect of A_1 allele (α_1)

$$= q[a + d(-p)]$$
$$= q\alpha$$
$$= 0.4 \times 15.6$$
$$= 6.2$$

Average effect of A_2 allele (α_2)

$$= -p[a + d(q - p)]$$
$$= -p\alpha$$
$$= -0.6 \times 15.6$$
$$= -9.36$$

Genotypic value of A_1A_1 genotype

$$= 2q(a - pd)$$
$$= 2 \times 0.4(16 - 0.6 \times 2)$$
$$= 11.84$$

Genotypic value of A_1A_2 genotype

$$= a(q - p) + d(1 - 2pq)$$
$$= 16(0.4 - 0.6) + 2(1 - 0.48)$$
$$= -2.16$$

Genotypic value of A_2A_2 genotype

$$= -2p(a + qd)$$
$$= -2 \times 0.6(16 + 0.4 \times 2)$$
$$= -1.2 \times 16.8$$
$$= -20.16.$$

The genotypic values can also be obtained as deviation of assigned genotypic values from mean (4.16) *viz.*

$g_{11} = a - m$; $g_{12} = d - m$; and $g_{22} = -a - m$.

Similarly, the breeding values and dominance deviation of 3 genotypes can also be estimated by putting the numerical values in their respective formulae.

Example 15.3: Two Loci Case

Find out the population mean from the given means of four genotypes for a character controlled by two loci having complete dominance for $M = a(1 - 2q^2)$, with frequency of genotype *aa* as $(q^2_A) = 0.2$ and frequency of genotype *bb* as $(q^2_B) = 0.4$. The genotypic frequencies are given in parenthesis below.

	B – (0.6)	bb (0.4)	Difference of Homozygotes $(2a_B)$
A – (0.8)	75	70	5
aa (0.2)	28	24	4
Difference $(2a_A)$	47	46	

Solution

The population mean can be estimated in two ways:

(i) *From gene effect and gene frequencies:*

Mid point (m) $= \frac{1}{2}[(A - B-) + (aa\ bb)]$

      $= \frac{1}{2}(75 + 24)$

      $= 99/2 = 49.5$

Effect of A allele (a_A) $= 70 - 24 = 46/2 = 23$

      or $= 75 - 28 = 47/2 = 22.5$.

Effect of B allele (a_B) $= (28 - 24)/2 = 2$

      or $= (75 - 70)/2 = 2.5$

The difference between B – and bb for A – genotype is same as it is for aa genotype (about 4) and similarly the difference between A – and aa genotype for B – genotype is same as for bb genotype (about 46). This indicates that both loci act additively and do not show interaction.

Moreover, the difference between composite genotype having dominant allele (A – B -) and having no dominant allele (aa bb) is $75 - 24 = 51$ which is equal to $2a_A + 2a_B = 46.5 + 4.5 = 51$.

The joint effect of two loci on population mean can be worked out from separate effect of two loci as:

M_A $= a(1 - 2q^2_A)$ in case of complete dominance when $d = a$

   $= 23(1 - 2 \times 0.2) = 23 \times 0.6 = 13.8$

M_B $= a(1 - 2q^2_B)$

   $= 2(1 - 2 \times 0.4) = 2 \times 0.2 = 0.4$

Mean $= M_A + M_B = 13.8 + 0.4 = 14.2$

Absolute mean $= m + M_{(A + B)} = 49.5 + 14.2 = 63.7$

(ii) *From frequencies and values of genotypes* as:

Genotypes	Frequencies	Values	Cross Product
A – B –	0.48 (= 0.8 x 0.6)	75	36.00
aa B –	0.12 (= 0.2 x 0.6)	28	3.35
A – bb	0.32 (= 0.8 x 0.4)	70	22.40
aa bb	0.08 (= 0.2 x 0.4)	24	1.92

$$\Sigma = 63.68 = \text{Mean}$$

Example 15.4: Two Loci Case with Interaction Effect of Loci

Find out the population mean, additive effects and interact effect of two loci from the following information:

(i) Complete dominance for both loci

(ii) $q^2_A = 0.4$ and $q^2_B = 0.2$

(iii) Phenotypic values for different genotypes as under:

	A –	aa	Difference	Freq.
B –	15	8	7	0.8
bb	10	8	2	0.2
Difference	5	0		
Freq.	0.6	0.4		

Solution

The phenotypic values of 4 phenotypes showed dependence because the values of B – and bb genotypes in combination with aa genotype is same (8 and 8) but differ in combination with A – genotype (15 and 10) and the values of A – and aa genotypes are different in combination with either B – genotype (15 and 8) or with bb genotype (10 and 8). Therefore, the difference in phenotypic values between A – and aa genotypes for B – genotype at B locus is different (7) than the difference for bb genotype (2) and similarly the difference in phenotypic values between B – and bb genotype for A – genotype at A locus is different (5) than the difference for aa genotype (0). Thus, the two loci have interacted to produce the phenotypic values.

Mid point (m) = ½ (15 + 8) = 11.5

Population mean = Sum of cross product of frequency x values

$$= (0.48 \times 15) + (0.12 \times 10) + (0.32 \times 8) + (0.08 \times 7)$$

$$= 7.20 + 1.20 + 2.56 + 0.56$$

$$= 11.52$$

Genotypic values (G_A and G_B): Genotypic values for a single locus is expressed as deviation from population mean with complete dominance as -

$$= 2a_A \, q_A^2 \text{ and } 2a_B \, q_B^2 \text{ for two dominant genotypes combined and}$$

$$- 2a \, (1 - q_A^2) \text{ and } - 2a \, (1 - q_B^2) \text{ for recessive genotypes.}$$

For dominants:

Mean genotypic difference of A locus = $2 \, a_A = 7 \times 0.8 + 2 \times 0.2 = 6.0$

Average genotypic value of A – genotype irrespective of the other locus

$$= G_A \text{ for A – B – as well as for A – bb genotype}$$

$$= 2a_A q_A^2 = 6 \times 0.4 = 2.4$$

Mean genotypic difference for B locus = $2a_B = 5 \times 0.6 + 0 \times 0.4 = 3.0$

Average genotypic value of B – genotype irrespective of the other locus

$$= G_B \text{ for A – B – as well as for aa B- genotype}$$

$$= 2a_B q_B^2 = 3 \times 0.2 = 0.6$$

For recessive homozygotes:

Mean genotypic difference of A locus = $2 \, a_A = 7 \times 0.8 + 2 \times 0.2 = 6.0$

Average value of aa genotype irrespective of the other locus

$$= G_A \text{ for aa B – as well as for aa bb genotype}$$

$$- 2a_A(1 - q_A^2) = - 6.0 \times 0.6 = - 3.6$$

Mean genotypic difference for B locus = $2a_B = 5 \times 0.6 + 0 \times 0.4 = 3.0$

Average value of bb genotype irrespective of the other locus

$$= G_B \text{ for A – bb as well as for aa bb genotype}$$

$$- 2a_B(1 - q_B^2) = - 3 \times 0.8 = - 2.4$$

Genotypes	Mean Genotypic Difference $= 2a_A \text{ or } 2a_B$	Frequency $q^2 \text{ or } (1 - q^2)$	G.V. $= 2a \, q^2 \text{ or}$ $- 2a \, (1 - q^2)$
A –	6.0	0.4	$6 \times 0.4 = 2.4$
aa	6.0	0.6	$- 6 \times 0.6 = - 3.6$
B –	3.0	0.2	$3 \times 0.2 = 0.6$
bb	3.0	0.8	$- 3 \times 0.8 = - 2.4$

where,

q^2 is the frequency of dominants and

$1 - q^2$ is the frequency of recessive homozygote,

$2aq^2$ is the genotypic value for dominants and

-2a $(1 - q^2)$ is the genotypic value for recessive homozygotes.

Interaction component (I_{AB}): It is taken by difference as –

$I_{AB} = G - (G_A + G_B)$ Where, $G = M + G_A + G_B + I_{AB}$

Genotypes	Frequency	Observed value (P)	P – M = G	G_A	G_B	$G_A + G_B$	I_{AB}
A – B –	0.6 x 0.8 = 0.48	15	3.48	2.4	0.6	3.0	0.48
A – bb	0.6 x 0.2 = 0.12	10	– 1.52	2.4	– 2.4	0.0	– 1.52
aa B –	0.4 x 0.8 = 0.32	8	– 3.52	– 3.6	0.6	– 3.0	– 0.52
aa bb	0.4 x 0.2 = 0.08	8	– 3.82	– 3.6	– 2.4	– 6.0	2.48

Verification of the results: Verify the genotypic values by the following equation-

$G = M + G_A + G_B + I_{AB}$

Chapter 16
Heterosis

The allelic (dominance) and non-allelic interaction effects are measured by a combined estimate, when the animals of different genetic backgrounds (lines, strain, breeds) are mated. This type of mating is called the line crossing or crossbreeding. The crossbred progeny so produced from mating of animals of different genetic background show increased vigour relative to their purebred parents.

16.1 Definition of Heterosis

The term *heterosis* was coined by Shull (1914) to describe the increased vigour of crossbreds over its parents. The heterosis (H) in terms of increased vigour is defined as the amount by which the mean of F_1 generation exceeds to its better parent.

$$H = \overline{F}_1 > \overline{P}_1 > \overline{P}_2$$

Positive and Negative Heterosis

The better parent is taken as the one having greater mean. In earlier section, the P_1 was been taken as a better parent, having positive alleles. However, it is not the magnitude of the mean that decides the better parent but the decision rests on the character concerned. There are some characters for which the better parent has low mean, like age at first calving (AFC), service period, etc. The cow with low AFC or short service period is a better cow. The F_1 should have greater yield than its P_1 parent $\left(\overline{F}_1 > \overline{P}_1\right)$ when P_1 is a better parent (milk yield) whereas when the P_2 is the better parent (AFC), the F_1 should have lower mean than its P_2 parent. Therefore, F_1 should have lower mean than P_2 for heterosis to occur. The heterosis is positive in the first case $\left(\overline{F}_1 > \overline{P}_1\right)$ whereas the heterosis is negative in the second case $\left(\overline{F}_1 < \overline{P}_2\right)$.

In animal breeding, the heterosis is defined as the amount by which the F_1 population mean exceeds the mid-parent value.

$$H = \overline{F}_1 > \frac{\left(\overline{P}_1 + \overline{P}_2\right)}{2} = \overline{F}_1 - P$$

16.2 Hybrid Vigour Lost on Inbreeding is Restored on Crossing

This can be invariably said that the hybrid vigour is the undoing of the accumulated inbreeding depression. This can be verified from the changes occurred in mean breeding values, gene combination values and genotypic values when a base population is changed into inbred lines which are then line crossed.

The base population may be taken as a wild species of domestic breeds before domestication which is random bred and hence had the hybrid vigour. During-the passage of time the base population got divided into a number of subpopulations of small size (breeds/lines) under natu-ral conditions or deliberately. These sub populations underwent inbreeding and hence differentiated in gene and genotype frequencies and also in their average breeding values, gene combination values and overall genotypic values. However, when these sub populations (breeds, lines, inbred lines) are crossed together they have the hybrid combinations (heterozygosity) at all or most of the loci and hence show the hybrid vigour. This can be illustrated by the hypothetical numerical example cited below: -

Consider a base population which is in HWE for one locus having two alleles (A and a) with equal frequencies and independent effect on the character, the A allele contributes 4 units while a allele contributes -2 units. In estimating the G, the complete dominance is taken and it causes the heterozygotes to have 8 units.

Genotypes	Freq.	G	B.V.	G.C.V. = G − BV
I. Base Population				
AA	0.25	8	8	0
Aa	0.50	8	2	6
aa	0.25	4	4	0
Mean of Base		5	2	3
Population (= Freq. x Value)				
II. Mean of two homozygotyes				
(inbred lines)	–	2	2	0
III. Line Crosses				
AA x AA = AA	–	8	8	0
aa x aa = aa	–	4	4	0
AAx aa = Aa	–	8	2	6
aa x AA = Aa	–	8	2	6
Mean	–	5	2	3

The base population has the mean G.V. of 5 units, out of which the mean BV was 2 units and the mean gene combination value of 3 units. When this base population is divided into inbred lines, the respective mean values for two inbred lines (AA and aa) were 2, 2 and 0, indicating the inbreeding depression for genotypic values which was due to nil contribution of gene combination value (a cause of inbreeding depression). However, when two inbred lines were crossed among themselves in all the four ways, the mean B.V., mean G V and mean gene combination value equal to that of the base population which was entirely due to the contribution of gene combination value – a cause of heterosis. It is important to note here that three out of the four line crosses performed better than the average animal of the base population and two of these three (Two heterozygous types of line crosses) have better gene combination value (more hybrid vigour). This suggested that better performance and more hybrid vigour can be achieved by breeding and using just the superior line crosses than that of the original base population. This is the principle of exploiting the gene combination value (non additive genetic variance).

16.3 Specification and Estimation of Heterosis

The parental generation means and F_1 mean are specified and estimated in terms of genetic parameters (components) and similarly the expected magnitude of heterosis can be specified. The model of Mather and Jinks (1971) can be used to describe the purebred and crossbred populations, to define the genetic components of heterosis and their derivation. The model include the additive effects of genes (a), the dominance effects (d), and non-allelic interaction effects of genes (i, j and *l*), defined earlier. The two components *viz.* a and i are fixed while others are not fixed but contribute to the heterosis.

The definition and specification of the components of heterosis requires some *assumptions viz.* two gene pairs each with two alleles (A-a, B-b), additive gene effects, gene interaction (allelic and non allelic), free recombination, absence of sex linkage, maternal and paternal effects and G-E interaction, and the parental populations with associated alleles of both pairs (AABB x aabb) and with dispersed alleles of both pairs (AAbb x aaBB).

1. Heterosis as a Deviation from Superior Parent

The heterosis can be specified by two models *viz.* additive-dominance model when epistasis is absent and the interaction model in the presence of epistatic effects of genes.

(i) Additive-Dominance Model

The expected magnitude of heterosis can be specified as under:

$$\text{Heterosis} = \overline{F_1} - \overline{P_1} = (m + d) - (m + a) \qquad \text{for positive heterosis}$$

$$= d - a$$

$$\text{or} \quad = \overline{F_1} - \overline{P_2} = (m + d) - (m - a) \qquad \text{for negative heterosis}$$

Therefore, the **d** must be positive and greater than **a** for heterosis to occur in case of positive heterosis. On the other hand, for negative heterosis, the heterosis will occur only when **d** is negative and greater than **a**. Thus for both the positive and negative heterosis to occur, the **d** must be greater than **a**. The **d** will be greater than **a** under either of the two or both of the following conditions -

(a) Degree of dominance (d/a): There should be over-dominance (d/a> 1) for all or some loci.

(b) Degree of association of genes: There should be dispersion of completely or incompletely dominant genes.

Moreover, the heterosis is more likely to occur when the dominance is unidirectional so that the **d** is not subjected to internal cancellation. However, the two causes of heterosis can not be distinguished from analysis of generation mean and this requires the analysis of variance. This model has some advantage. It requires only 3 families (P_1, P_2 and F_1) to estimate three parameters. Secondly, it gives a perfect estimate of heterosis, if the means of more generations are available.

(ii) Heterosis with Interaction Model

The specification of heterosis is more complex when additive dominance model is inadequate. When there is significant contribution of non-allelic interactions, the magnitude of heterosis is specified as

Heterosis = $\overline{F}_1 - \overline{P}_1$ = d + l - a + i for positive heterosis

$$= \overline{F}_1 - \overline{P}_2 = d + l - (-a + i) \text{ for negative heterosis}$$

The (d + l) must be positive and greater than (a + i) for the occurrence of positive heterosis. However, either one of the two interaction components of F_1 (d or l) and not both may be negative but their balance effect must be positive and greater than (a + i). Further, the value of **a** will be positive whereas **i** may be positive or negative within the same restrictions. For negative heterosis, the balance effect of (d + l) must be negative and greater than (- a + l).

The heterosis is more likely to occur when the gene interaction is predominantly of complementary type which makes the d and l of the same sign and/or the interacting gene pairs are dispersed.

2. Heterosis Measured as Deviation from Mid Parent Value

The heterosis as deviation from mid parent value can be estimated in the following three ways:

(i) When Parental Information is Known

The complete description (specification) of the genetic model of different generations in terms of genetic components and their coefficients *viz.* contribution of additive gene effects and the components of heterosis (dominance and epistatic effects) have been given by Jinks and Jones (1958) and presented in Table 15.7. The heterosis in terms of dominance and epistatic components for different crossbred generations

$(F_1, F_2, B_1, B_2, B_{11}, B_{22}, B_{12}, B_{21})$ can be estimated as the difference between the mean of a particular crossbred generation and the parental mean generation ($\overline{P}_1$ and $\overline{P}_2$). The heterosis so estimated contains its various components of different size as shown under:

$$H_{F1} = \overline{F}_1 - \tfrac{1}{2}(\overline{P}_1 + \overline{P}_2) \qquad\qquad = d - i + l$$

$$H_{F2} = \overline{F}_2 - \tfrac{1}{2}(\overline{P}_1 + \overline{P}_2) \qquad\qquad = \tfrac{1}{2}d - i + \tfrac{1}{4}l$$

$$H_{B1} = \overline{B}_1 - (\tfrac{3}{4}\overline{P}_1 + \tfrac{1}{4}\overline{P}_2) \qquad\quad = \tfrac{1}{2}d - \tfrac{3}{4}i + \tfrac{1}{4}j + \tfrac{1}{4}l$$

$$H_{B2} = \overline{B}_2 - (\tfrac{1}{4}\overline{P}_1 + \tfrac{3}{4}\overline{P}_2) \qquad\quad = \tfrac{1}{2}d - \tfrac{3}{4}I - \tfrac{1}{4}j + \tfrac{1}{4}l$$

$$H_{B11} = \overline{B}_{11} - (7/8\,\overline{P}_1 + 1/8\,\overline{P}_2) \qquad = \tfrac{1}{4}d - {}_{7/16}i + {}_{3/16}j + {}_{1/16}l$$

$$H_{B22} = \overline{B}_{22} - (1/8\,\overline{P}_1 + 7/8\,\overline{P}_2) \qquad = \tfrac{1}{4}d - {}_{7/16}i - {}_{3/16}j + {}_{1/16}l$$

$$H_{B12} = \overline{B}_{12} - (3/8\,\overline{P}_1 + 5/8\,\overline{P}_2) \qquad = \tfrac{3}{4}d - {}_{15/16}i - {}_{3/16}j + {}_{9/10}l$$

$$H_{B21} = \overline{B}_{21} - (5/8\,\overline{P}_1 + 3/8\,\overline{P}_2) \qquad = {}_{3/4}d - {}_{15/16}i + {}_{3/16}j + {}_{9/16}l$$

(ii) When Performance of Purebred Parents is not Known

The biometrical approach given above to estimate the heterosis requires the mean performance of both the purebred parents. But in large livestock crossbreeding programme, the performance level of exotic breed is not available. Therefore, it is not possible to estimate heterosis in crossbreed-ing programme of dairy cattle from the above equations. In such situation, two procedures are used to estimate heterosis, namely statistical method and biometrical method.

In *statistical approach,* the means of different grades of crossbred population are taken as dependent variable while the mean of sires bred, dam's bred and level of heterozygosity are taken as independent variables (Parekh, 1973 and Parmar and Dev, 1978). However, this approach assumes the single locus with two alleles to obtain the value of heterozy-gosity which is not valid for polygenic traits and the dependent variables have no relationship with the parameters of the biometrical genetic model.

The *biometrical approach* to estimate heterosis is based on fitting of genetic model in terms of gene effects (additive, dominance and epistatic) to the means of crossbred generations. Nitter (1978) estimated the heterosis as twice the difference F_1 and F_2. Thus

$$H_{F1} = 2(\overline{F}_1 - \overline{F}_2) = d + {}_{3/2}l$$

However, the H_{F1} can also be estimated as:

$$H_{F1} = 2\overline{F}_1 - (\overline{B}_1 + \overline{B}_2) \qquad \text{since } \overline{F}_2 = \tfrac{1}{2}(\overline{B}_1 + \overline{B}_2)$$

$$= d - \tfrac{1}{2}i + {}_{3/2}l$$

(iii) Gene Frequency Method

When the two parent breeds differ in their gene frequency the procedure to estimate the heterosis has been given in Chapter 11.

16.4 Loss of Hybrid Vigous in Subsequent Generations

In animal breeding the hybrid vigour is measured as the difference between the average performance of crossbred (F_1) and the average performance of their purebred parent lines/breeds as:

$$H.V. = \overline{F}_1 - (\overline{P}_1 + \overline{P}_2)/2$$

$$= \overline{F}_1 - \overline{P}$$

and expressed as the percentage of the average perfor-mance of the parental breeds -

$$\text{per cent H.V.} = \frac{\left(\overline{F}_1 - \overline{P}\right)}{P} \times 100$$

(i) F_1 Hybrid

The hybrid vigour is maximum in the first cross (F_1) and attributed to the gene combination value by increasing heterozygosity. This is called as F_1 hybrid vigour. This F_1 hybrid vigour is reduced in F_2 generation to the extent of 50 per cent. The hybrid vigour shown in later generations is called the retained hybrid vigour which is commonly expressed as a proportion of F_1 hybrid vigour. The loss in hybrid vigour can be estimated under certain assumptions *viz.* dominance model for hybrid vigour taking only marginal rate of epistasis and secondly that the hybrid vigour is linearly related to heterozygosity. This can be illustrated in a better way considering one locus case, though the metric traits are polygenic, and by crossing two lines A and B with different gene frequencies as:

Breed A: $p_T = 0.3$ and $q_t = 0.7$

Breed B: $p_T = 0.7$ and $q_t = 0.3$

and further assuming that both breeds are in H.W.E. Therefore, the heterozygosity (H) in both breeds is equal as:

$$H_A = 2pq = 2\,(0.3)\,(0.7) = 0.42$$

$$H_B = 2pq = 2\,(0.7)\,(0.3) = 0.42$$

$$H = \frac{\left(H_A + H_B\right)}{2} = 0.42$$

The F_1 population will have more heterozygosity (0.58). This can be verified from the random union of gamete frequencies of two breeds *viz.* $(0.3 + 0.7)\,(0.7 + 0.3) = 0.21 + 0.09 + 0.49 + 0.21$ in which two middle terms are the frequencies of heterozygous genotype in the F_1 progeny making the total of 0.58. Thus, there was an increase in heterozygosity by $(0.58 - 0.16) = 0.16$ in F_1 generation compared to average heterozygosity of the two breeds. Therefore, assuming dominance, the increased heterozygosity will lead to the hybrid vigour.

(ii) F_2 Generation

The F_1 hybrid vigour (H_{F1}) is reduced to half in F_2 generation.

$$H_{F2} = M_{F2} - M_P$$
$$= \frac{1}{2} dy^2 = \frac{1}{2} H_{F1}$$

The gene frequencies after random mating of two breeds to produce F_1 generation becomes equal ($p = q = 0.5$) in the F_1 (see that $p = P + \frac{1}{2}H$ and $q = R + \frac{1}{2}H$). The *inter-se mating* of F_1s reduces the heterozygosity among F_2's to 0.50, indicating a decrease in the level of heterozygosity of F_1s. The heterozygosity in F_2 generation is the average heterozygosity of the two pure breeds and of F_1s. Therefore, the hybrid vigour in F_2 generation (H_{F2}) is halved to that exhibited by F_1 population. This shows that the F_2 will regress and expected to be half way from F_1 mean in the direction of mid-parent value. The regression of F_2 value is due to the homozygosity at some loci produced by *inter se mating of F_1's*. The animals of F_2 and F_3 population produced by *inter-se* mating are expected to be homozygous for alleles of inferior parent (*e.g.* Zebu alleles for milk production) at some loci.

Considering the joint effect of all loci affecting a character, the H_{F2} will be half to that of H_{F1} provided the epistatic interaction is absent. This is because the genotypes at more loci will not attain HWE value in the F_2 but will attain it in subsequent generation.

(iii) F_3 and Subsequent Generation

There is a constant level of retained hybrid vigour in F_3 and subsequent generations provided there is no inbreeding and as well as the G.C.V. is retained. This is because the heterozygosity does not change from the level of heterozygosity of F_2 generation.

The F_2s are actually in HWE and so will be the subsequent generations (F_3, F_4, F_5 and so on). Therefore, the offspring of F_2 and further generations should show half of F_1 hybrid vigour. Thus, there is a constant level of retained hybrid vigour in subsequent generations provided there is no inbreeding and the dominance model of heterosis is adequate. However, the dominance model may not work always. The crossing of two pure breeds break up the favourable epistatic combinations that are fixed due to long term selection in purebred population provided the favourable epistatic genes are located either on different chromosomes or on the same chromosome located distantly. Thus, the entire loss of gene combination value is reflected in the level of F_1 hybrid vigour.

However, the situation is different when the loci with epistatic effects are linked. The favourable epistatic combinations are broken up gradually by crossing over phenomena over a number of generations. This causes a further loss of retained hybrid vigour in F_3 and subsequent generations till the population attain HWE. This loss in retained hybrid vigour is called as the *recombination loss* which is caused by recombination of linked loci and reflected through the loss in gene combination value. Therefore, the recombination loss is a loss in gene combination value caused by the gradual breaking up of favourable epistatic combination of linked loci in subsequent generations of hybrids.

Recombination Effect

It is known that $H_{F2} = \frac{1}{2} H_{F1}$. However, the relationship between the estimated heterosis F_1 and F_2 generations in terms of its components as shown under point 2 of section 16.3 based on $H_{F2} = \frac{1}{2} H_{F1}$ is as under:

$$H_{F2} = \frac{1}{2} H_{F1}$$
$$\frac{1}{2}d - i + \frac{1}{4}l = \frac{1}{2}d - \frac{1}{2}i + \frac{1}{2}l$$

The F_2's are actually in HWE proportions and remains so in subsequent generations. Therefore, the F_2 and further generations should show half of F_1 hybrid vigour. However, the favourable epistatic combinations are broken up gradually by crossing over phenomenon over a number of generations. This causes a further loss of hybrid vigour in subsequent generations till the population attains HWE proportions. This loss in retained hybrid vigour is called as the *recombination loss* caused by recombination of linked loci and reflected through the loss in G.C.V. Thus, the recombination loss is a loss in G.C.V. caused by the gradual breaking up of favourable epistatic combination of linked loci in subsequent generations. This recombination loss is seen to be a combination of the effects of interaction between pairs of genes both at the same locus (dominance) and at different loci (epistasis). The situation is different in backcross generations which are like that of graded progenies in which the homozygosity is continuously increased due to increase in the level of inheritance of either of the two parental breeds. This results in the retained hybrid vigour to disappear gradually with continuous back crossing.

It is obvious that dominance components of the two sides of equation are equal. Whereas i component is twice and l the component is half in H_{F2} than in $\frac{1}{2} H_{F1}$ (assumed heterosis in F_2). This difference between actual and assumed H_{F2} is what is called the recombination effect or epistatic loss. This is the loss in epistatic superiority of pure breeds due to recombination in gametes produced by crossbred parents and denoted by r (Dickerson, 1972). This intends to measure deviation from linear association of heterosis with the degree of heterozygosity and describes the average fraction of independently segregating pairs of loci in gametes from both parents which are expected to be non-parental combinations. The recombination effect is the change in epistatic effects in F_2 individuals, relative to those of the F_1, from gamete recombination between chromosomes of the parental population (P_1 and P_2)) described by Dickerson (1969) and represent an epistatic loss in H_{F2} compared to H_{F1}. Following Dickerson (1969) it has become common to use the term recombination loss to describe interaction effects among loci. The r = 0 in purebreds and in F_1 because the gametes derive from parental combinations but r = $\frac{1}{2}$ in F_2 and r = $\frac{1}{4}$ in backcrosses. The recombination loss is seen to be a combina-tion of the effects of interaction between pairs of genes both at the same locus (dominance) and at different loci (epistasis). The term recombination loss implies that coupling and repulsion heterozygotes are different. For example, when the genes are associated (AABB, aabb) in purebreds, an F_2 individual receiving the coupling phase gametes (AB, ab – produced from inter se mating of F_1 in which both parents produce AB, Ab, aB and ab gametes in equal frequency) suffered no recombination loss in contrast to one that inherits the repulsion gametes (Ab and aB).

(iv) Backcross Generations

The continuing back crossing of cross breds with either of the parental pure breed is like that of grading up and hence the backcross progenies after some generations become homozygous for the genes present in parental breed with a consequent decrease in heterozygosity continuously in each generation. This results in the retained hybrid vigour to disappear gradually with continuous back crossing.

16.5 Types of Hybrid Vigour

Dickersion (19.73) had described the various types of heterosis as individual, maternal and paternal heterosis on the basis that some of the traits have three genetic components viz, direct (individual), maternal and paternal.

The direct component of a trait is due to the effect of an individual's gene on its performance. *Individual heterosis* is the improvement in performance of an individual animal, relative to the mean of its parents, which is not attribut-able to maternal, paternal or sex linkage effects. It is caused by individual genotype (heterozygosity) and is the *heterosis in progeny*. The survival rates of heterozygous embryos and fetuses in pigs are increased in all species resulting in more number of live births and it is due to heterosis. An increase in birth rates in sheep and cattle (in terms of number of calves and lambs per 100 females bred) has also been observed when crossbreds are produced from purebreds. Moreover, the birth weights, survival rates in ealy life, growth rates and efficiency of gains of crossbred progeny than purebreds are also increased. Thus, there is heterosis in progeny (crossbreds).

The *maternal component* is due to the effect of genes in the dam (of the individual) which influence the individual's performance via the environment provided by the dam. Maternal heterosis (heterosis in dam) is the heterosis in a population due to the use of crossbred dams instead of purebred *e.g.* milk production, improved prenatal environment, larger litter size, etc. The heterosis in dam increases the number of progeny per dam by increasing the ovulation rate, providing better uterine environment and the inherent ability of the embryos and fetuses to survive. The intra-uterine environment of crossbred dams helps to produce more progeny at birth, particularly in litter bearing animals. The crossbred dams also produce more milk which affects the weaning weights in pigs, sheep and cattle. Thus, crossbreeding is advantageous in pork, mutton and beef production.

The *paternal component* is like that of maternal component but due to the effects of genes of the sire (of the individual) that influence the individual's performance via the environment provided by the sire. Paternal heterosis (heterosis in sires) is the advantage of using the crossbred versus purebred sires on the performance of the progeny. The male transmits to its no more than half of its genes in the progeny. The crossbred males are not able to transmit hybrid vigour and they are not as prepotent as inbred sires. Therefore, the crossbred sires look better but can not breed better. On the contrary, the superiority of inbred sires is fixed in the homozygous state and is not due to heterozygosity. Therefore, the inbred sires can breed better than they look.

All the traits have direct component while the maternal and paternal components are trait specific. However, each component has the potential for hybrid vigour for which the hybrid vigour is termed as individual, maternal and paternal hybrid vigour corresponding to three components.

The maternal and paternal effects arise where the mother or fa-ther makes a contribution to the phenotype of their progeny above that one which results from the genes they contribute to the zygote. Therefore, the maternal and paternal heterosis is observed in such traits which are conditioned by the maternal and paternal effects like the traits con-nected with reproduction, pre and postnatal growth.

The heterosis in F_1 is attributable to the individual effects and the maternal effect is zero whereas in F_2 the individual effect is lost about half the heterosis in F_1 but the maternal component show the full heterosis.

The three types of hybrid vigour have the following characteristics and can be better explained by citing the example of fertility (conception rate).

Sl.No.	Characteristics	Individual Hybrid Vigour	Maternal H.V.	Paternal H.V.
1.	**Cause**: Effects of genes or gene contributions of the:	Embryo: that affects its survival	Dam: ability to conceive	Sire: ability to make pregnant to the female
2.	**Generation**:	Current generation (embryo)	Previous (dam)	Previous (sire)
3.	**Indication:** (Indicated by better performance of) –	Crossed progeny over its parents	Crossbred dams (as mothers)	Crossbred sires
4.	**Examples:**			
	Dairy Cattle	All traits	Fat per cent	Conception rate
	Beef Cattle	All traits	Birt wt. Weaning wt. Yearling wt	Conception rate No.weaned/ 100 cows, WeaningWt/cow
	Sheep	All traits	No. born Weaning wt. Lambs weaned /ewe	Conception rate Lambing rate, Lambs weaned /ewe
	Poultry	All traits	Hatchability	—
	Pig	All traits	No. born, No. weaned, Litter wt., Back fat thickness	Conception rate
		Hybrid pigs survive better and grow faster	Hybrid sows produce larger and heavier litters	Hybrid boars increase the conception rate

16.6 Estimation of the Cause of Heterosis

This requires two steps *viz.* to determine the model of heterosis and estimation of the components of the model. The scaling tests are applied to determine the model so that the proper specification of heterosis can be given. With the scaling tests the adequacy of the interaction model including digenic or higher order interactions or linkage of interacting genes or the additive-dominance model is determined. After the model is determined, the second step is to estimate the component parameters of the model from the means of different generations by the procedure expalined in Chapter 15.

16.7 Effect of Linkage on Heterosis

The spepcification of heterosis is not affected by linkage because the linkage, even of interacting pairs of genes, does not affect the specifications of parental and F_1 means. However, the linkage biases the estimate of the heterosis components and affects the interpretation of the cause of heterosis by distorting the relative magnitudes of the components of heterosis.

The d, i and *l* components of heterosis are biased with linkage of genes while the component *a* remains unbiased. Assuming the dispersed genes linked in repulsion phase, the magnitude of heterosis will remain constant but the estimates of the different components of heterosis will change with a change in the recombination percentage (r). The true values of the three components (d, i and l) will not change but the apparent value of d will rise while those of i and *l* will fall with fall in recombination percentage. With complete linkage (no recombi-nation) the **d** becomes the sole component of heterosis. This is as per expectation that the two gene pairs are indistinguishable from a single gene with the summed effects of the individual genes when there is complete linkage. Thus the non-allelic interactions become domi-nance effect. The same is true for linkage of genes in coupling phase as well as for more pairs of linked genes. Therefore, linkage always leads to an overestimate of the contribution of the non-allelic interac-tion components to the magnitude of heterosis.

16.8 Norm of Reaction of Genotype under Varying Environment

There is norm of reaction of genotypes which creates the relationships between phenotype and environment. The norm of reaction of any genotype is the distribution of phenotypes that result when the genotype undergoes growth and development in a range of environments. If the behaviour of different genotypes of a particular locus (AA, AA', A'A') are observed in a range of environments it would be found that the allele A may show favourable effect and may also be dominant over its allele A' in one environment but under the changed environment the allele A' may be favourable and the dominance relation between the alleles may be lost. Thus the values of a and d are changed, when the population is shifted from one environment to another.

The importance of norm of reaction lies in the fact that it decides the genetic architecture of traits in terms of estimates of the genetic parameters *viz.* a and *d* used to describe a trait. Consequently the response to selection which depends upon the heritability is also affected by the norm of reaction. Not only this but this norm of reaction also affects the performance of the improved (selected) population under changed environmental conditions.

The norms of reaction of viability of various genotypes were studied by Dobzhansky and Spassky (1944) under two temperatures. The various genotypes contained chromosomes taken from natural population of Drosophila psudoobscura. The relative viabilities for two chromosomes designated as A and B were obtained as under:

Genotypes	Temperature (°C)	
	16.5	25.5
AA	0.92	0.32
AB	1.0	1.00
BB	0.71	0.75

At low temperature, the estimates are

m = ½(0.92 + 0.71) = 0.815,

a   = ½(0.92 – 0.71) = 0.105,

d   = 1.00 – 0.815 = 0.185

At high temperature, the estimates are:

m = ½ (0.32 + 0.75) = 0.535,

a = ½ (0.32 – 0.75) = – 0.215,

d = 1.00 -. 0.535 = 0.465

In this example, the chromosome **A** had greater viability at low temperature than that of B chromosome and hence A was favourable but with a change in environment (high temperature) the viability was reversed because the B chromosome had greater viability than A. Thus, at high temperature B was found to have favourable effect on the viability.

16.9 Effect of Environment on Heterosis

The heterosis is a function of the environment which implies that the magnitude of heterosis depends upon the environment.

The homozygotes show a greater interaction with the environment than do the heterozygotes. This is an evidence of the **G-E** interaction which comes from the fact that the estimates of **d** differ significantly in two environments. The G-E interaction model should be fitted if it is observed that the model assuming no G-E interaction is inadequate. The necessity of inclusion of interaction parameter comes from the fact when the estimate I_{ae} is significant and that the estimate of I_{de} is small and not significant although **d** is as great or greater than *a* in magnitude. All these show that homozygotes are more prone (sensitive) to the environment than do the heterozygotes.

When the parents and their F_1's are measured in a number of environments, the expectations of the magnitude of heterosis (j^{th} environment), with additive – dominance model, can be written as:

Heterosis $= \overline{F}_{1j} - \overline{P}_{1j}$

$$= d - a - I_{ae} + I_{de} \qquad \text{positive heterois}$$

or $= \overline{F}_{1j} - \overline{P}_{2j}$

$$= d - (-a) + I_{ae} + I_{de} \qquad \text{negative heterosis}$$

The change in the magnitude of heterosis in different environments can be predicted from the relative magnitudes of **d** and **a** as well as from the relative magnitude of $I_{ae} + I_{de}$. When a = d or $I_{ae} = I_{de}$ in **all** environments, the heterosis remains constants in all environments. When **a** is greater than **d,** the heterosis is decreased with an improvement in environment.

Therefore, the heterosis is more in poor environment when a > d but the heterosis is more in better environment when a < d.

The amount of heterosis shown in the cross decides the method of cross breeding to maintain a crossbred population *viz.* terminal crossing and rotational crossing. In terminal crossing the crossbred progeny are not used for further breeding and hence not used for dairy animals but it is important for meat animals. The terminal crossing is of two type *viz.* commercial crossing and three way crossing. In commercial crossing the F_1 animals are produced in each generation and slaughtered. In three ways crossing wherein the crossbred dams are used for breeding to exploit their maternal ability. The crossbred dams may be either backcrossed to the sire's breed or to a third breed. The rotational crossing also called as the reciprocal back crossing or criss crossing involves the use of sires of two or more breeds in alternate generations. The criss crossing with two breeds exploits 67 per cent heterosis whereas with three breeds (rotational crossing) exploits 87 per cent and the commercial crossing exploit 100 per cent heterosis. However, when complementarity is important than heterosis the *interse* mating is used which utilizes only half the heterosis of the first cross.

The amount of heterosis is more for the followings:

(i) For the characters related to "fitness" which have been under the influence of natural selection for a long time and therefore have low heritability.

(ii) In a poor environment than in good environment.

In a poor environment the improved exotic breed cannot exploit its genetic potential fully and hence differ in production performance to a lesser extent from the local adapted breed. Therefore, on crossing, the F_1 show high performance indicating the heterosis to a greater extent.

Whereas in a better environment the situation is different in the sense that the exotic breed exploits its genetic potential fully and differ significantly in production from the local breed. The F_1 produced in better environment thus shows improved performance by an intermediate amount slightly above the mid-parent value and hence the heterosis is less.

Such a model for different amount of heterosis and additive effects of two breeds in poor and good environment was given by Cunningham (1981). He explained that the difference between the F_1 and the local breed is largely due to heterosis in poor environment but due to additive genetic effects (differences) between two breeds in good environment. The model can be illustrated digrammatically as under —

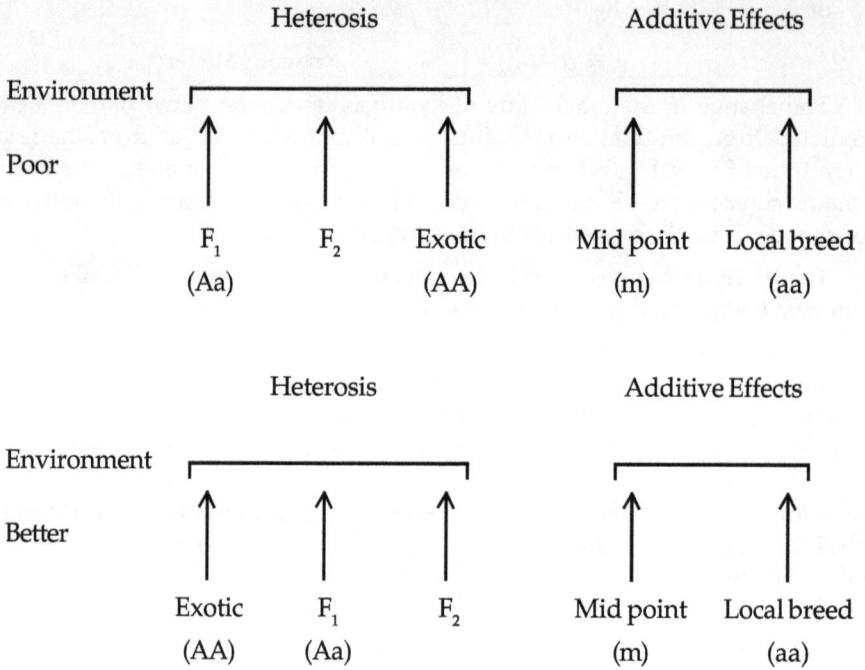

	Heterosis			Additive Effects	
Environment					
Poor					
F_1	F_2	Exotic		Mid point	Local breed
(Aa)		(AA)		(m)	(aa)

	Heterosis			Additive Effects	
Environment					
Better					
Exotic	F_1	F_2		Mid point	Local breed
(AA)	(Aa)			(m)	(aa)

Chapter 17
Genotype-Environment Interaction

In a very simple language, the interaction of genes with external environment *viz*. climatic, nutritional, management factors etc. is called the genotype-environment interaction. The genes and environment may interact in a number of different ways:

(i) The environment may affect the genetic composition of a population by pressure of selection and this leads to evolutionary changes.

(ii) The environment may distort the segregation and recombination expected on genetic theory.

(iii) It may change the genetic material as mutagenic effects of radiation and various chemical substances, and also as conditioning effect and para-mutation. Thus, the first effect of environment in changing the genetic material is through artificially induced mutation. The second is **a** different kind of effect of the environment on the genetic material discovered by Durrant (1958) by observing that certain varieties of flax plants not only show the effects of certain treatments combinations of fertilizer (nitrogenous, phosphate and potash) on their growth but the effect is transmitted to their progenies of next and later generations through pollen and egg. Such an effect was called *conditioning effect* by him which resemble to para-mutation in maize (Brink, 1960). Such conditioning effects have also been observed by Highkin (1958) in peas and by Hill (1967) in Nicotiana rustica.

(iv) The environment may interact with genotypes to produce differences in phenotypic values of the individuals of a population. This is the most important and of immediate concern arising from interplay of genetic and environmental effects.

The best possible genotype will not exhibit to its full potentiality unless it gets proper environment. Likewise, the best possible environment is also not sufficient enough to develop a superior individual unless the proper genotype is present in the individual. Thus, the proper genotype and proper environment are not independent to develop a phenotype (phenotypic value). The animals of a certain genotype (breed) may perform better in one environment than in other. One environment may permit the expression of a genotype into phenotype or phenotypic value while another does not. For example, various herds or breeds show different performance in different environments. Thus differential phenotypic responses/expressions are observed for different genotypes with changed environment. Therefore, each genotype has its specific adaptability for which the genotype-environment interaction is responsible and it cannot be explained by the additive model. Under the two assumptions of additivity and independency of genetic and environment effects in their action, the relative performance of two genotypes should remain the same in a changed environments. However, a genotype performs differently in different environments. This implies that a specific difference in environment produces different effects on different genotypes.

The concept and definition of G – E interaction has already been given under point 3 of section 15.1.

17.1 Types of G-E Interaction

To be more illustrative about the G – E interaction, it is better to understand the types of G – E relationship with a simple case of 2 genotypes (G_1 and G_2) reared in two environments (E_1 and E_2). Haldane (1946) had given six different relationships between the four phenotypes produced. These relationships are basically linear and non-linear. Mather and Jones (1958) have given the description of G – E interaction in continuous variation. The types of G – E interaction based on the relative magnitude of differences between genotypes and between environments have also been given by Mc.Bridge (1958), and Dunlop (1962).

Two 2 genotypes under 2 environments produce 4 different phenotypes which show 4 types of interactions on the basis of the distinction made between two types of environmental differences (micro and macro environment) and also between intra and inter population genotypic differences as shown here.

	Micro Environment *(Small Difference)*	*Macro Environment* *(Large Difference)*
Intra Population genotypes (Small differences) *e.g.* within herd, flocks	Type A	Type B
Inter Population geno-types (Large differences) *e.g.* between strains, breeds.	Type C	Type D

The intra-population genotypes includes small differences in genotypes forming a continum for genetic merit within a population like single herd of dairy cattle or flock of sheep, poultry etc.

The inter-population includes large genetic differences like several lines, strains, breeds or crosses.

The micro environment includes small differences in the envi-ronment like antibiotic feeding, behaviour pattern, individual vs group housing, birds housed on floor vs. cages. These are the differences within herd.

The macro environment includes large differences in environ-ment like two planes of nutrition, temperate vs tropical climate, different climatic conditions created under controlled conditions, different cultural practices, different dates of hatching, battery vs floor rearing, sire-herd etc.

1. Linear or Additive Relationship

This is grouped as *type A interaction*. When there is no change in the phenotypic values between 2 genotypes in either environment and it indicates the linear relation between genotype and environment. The phenotypic values of 2 genotypes may be either increased or decreased equally, with similar change, in the same direction under changed environment (E_2). Thus, there was *no change in the rank* order of two genotypes under changed environment. This occurs when the animals of a single herd/flock with small genetic differences (being intra population genotypes, of the same herd or flock) are kept and tested in two environments with small differences (micro-environment), like antibiotic feeding, individual versus group housing, birds housed on floor versus cages. This type of relation indicates that some genes (genotypes) are favourable and others are unfavourable in all or most of the environments.

2. Non-Linear or Non-Additive Relationship

This type of relation can be grouped in 3 different types.

(i) Type B Interaction

The change in phenotypic values of genotypes may be in the same direction (increase or decrease in phenotypic values) but unequal in magnitude under changed environment (E_2) with a *change in rank order* of two genotypes. This occurs when the animals of a single herd with small differences are tested under macro-environment in order to test the genetic variation in the ability to respond to different environments with large differences *e.g.* interaction between families and date of hatching affecting sexual maturity in poultry, families reared in batteries or on floor, etc., sire – herd interaction, sire – ration (half sib families reared on 2 plane of nutrition), sire – year – season, sire – region interaction, etc. This type of interaction is more important when selection is within a breed under different environments. This interaction indicates that some genes (genotypes) may have effects that differ under different environment.

(ii) Type C Interaction

When the change in phenotypic values of two genotypes under changed environment (E_2) is in the opposite direction but *does not change the rank order* of two genotypes. This involves when animals with large differences (breeds, strains, lines, crosses) are tested under different environments having very less differences (environmental variability within herd). The micro environmental variation cause some genotypes (pure breeds) to vary but without producing any effect on hybrids (heterozygotes), as the hybrids are well buffered to micro-environmental changes. This type of interaction is not important practically.

(iii) Type D Interaction

This occurs when the change in phenotypic values of 2 genotypes under changed environment is in the opposite direction leading to a *change in rank order*. This includes when breed differences are tested under macro-environmental changes. These are important in animal breeding. If this type of interaction exists, it will then decide the relative merits of breeds or lines in different environments and will be required to evaluate the adaptability of different genotypes under different environments. This interaction indicates that some genes may have effects that differ from environment to environment.

Genetic Slippage

From the G-E relationship it can be inferred that some genes (genotypes) will be favourable and others unfavourable in all (or most) of the environments. Some genes may have effect that differ from environment to environment and these will cause the G-E interaction. Such interactions may cause decreased performance when a population selected under one environment moves in a new environment which means a regression in performance to which Dickerson (1962) termed as the "*genetic slippage*" which indicates the reduction in breeding value when population perform in environment other than that in which it was selected.

17.2 Examples of G-E Interaction

The G – E interaction are considered when there is a change in the rank order of genotype under changed environment. The followings are some of the examples of G – E interaction. The change in normal environmental conditions for living to unhealthy and unhappy environment changes the phenotype of the character *viz.* the occurrence of disease, the healthy body (resistance, normal health) become sick (susceptible) in man, animals and plants, and untoward happenings, life turns to end of life (death) through heart attack and suicide in humans, etc.

The resistance and susceptibility to *various diseases* in man, animals and plants are the examples of G – E interaction. This can be understood that a healthy individual has a normal phenotype (normal health, resistance) for the character health. Normal health (resistance) and sickness (susceptibility) are two forms (phenotypes) of health, as a character. The environmental stress due to any type of unhealthy environments (cold and heat stress, hunger, excessive smoking, excessive alcoholic use, food poisoning or a toxin produced by disease causing organism) causes an individual to become sick and finally may lead to death.

Likewise, some people (genotype) remain least affected mentally while others are very much sensitive, responding very much erratically to unhappy environment and ***untoward happening*** (heart felt incidents) like, demotion or termination of their service, harassment/atrocity (physical, mental and sexual), death of their very near and dear, being cheated and looted for their capital, defamation in the society for their honesty and sexual character, etc. The sensitive people become either victim of heart attack or they took very much drastic step like suicide and thus there is end of their life.

17.3 Experimental Evidence of G-E Interaction

The magnitude of G-E interaction can be estimated by growing the experimental material in different environments. Wright (1939) suggested that a population should be bred under different environmental niches to support the non additive G-E relationship. According to Lush (1945), the breeding stock should be selected under such similar environmental conditions where the selected animals are to be used and live to perform. Hammond (1947) put forth a different hypothyeses "the animals should be best selected for a trait under the environment which favours its fullest expression and that once developed can also be used in other environment". Thus there was no GE interaction and one may argue that a favourable environ-ment will allow more rapid progress in a desired character under selection and this improved genotype will attain a higher level of performance on its transfer to less favourable environment than could have been attained by the same amount of selection under the less favourable conditions.

Falconer and Latyszewski (1952) translated the Hammond's hypothesis in genetic terms that this thesis seems to require the following two conditions. The genes determining the expression of the character selected are mainly the same in both good and bad environments which means in other words that there must be an absence of G-E interaction. Secondly, a different sort of interaction between genotype and environment is required, such that the bad environment affects the superior genotype more compared to the inferior genotype and thus the random environmental variation being minimum in a good environment should lower the correlation between genotype and phenotype resulting in higher heritability of a trait in good environment than in the poor. Thus Hammond's thesis supposes that the consequences of a bad environment will be to reduce the genotypic variance alone and consequently also the H^2. The ratio of response would then be less in a bad than a good environment.

Warwick (1951) stated that animals should always be bred in the environment where they are to be used. In the light of these experiments, the choice of environmental conditions under which the selective breeding is to be practiced presented a problem of practical importance for livestock improvement. The problem is that to get good results whether the selection is to be carried out in an environ-ment where the improved genotype will eventually be required to live or whether better results may be attained under another conditions more favourable for the expression of the desired trait. In contrary to the Hammond's thesis, most geneticists are of the opinion that performance in a favourable environment has a different genetic basis from performance in an unfavourable environment. This means that a better genotype in one environment could not be expected to be superior in a different environment. Selection should thus be carried out in an environment where the improved breed is to live.

Experiment on mice: Falconer and Latyszewski (1952) had undertaken the first step as an experimental study of the problem that whether environmental conditions which increase the expression of the desired trait will make selection more successful than unfavourable conditions. They studied body weight of mice on two planes of nutrition *viz.* ad lib and 75 per cent diet for two selection lines from a single population: the selection was being made in exactly the same manner for the same measurement. One line was given full diet (F) and other was given a restricted diet (R) to 7.5 per cent of quantity though the quality of diet was same. A population of about 200 full sibs of single family was obtained and divided into 2 parts *viz.* full diet line and restricted diet line. Twelve animal were selected on individuals own merit out of 100 in each line in the first generation of selection. In general 2 litters were raised from each mated pair in both lines and the number of mice measured per generation in each line averaged 40 of each sex. The plan along with results is as

	Base Population	*Full Diet Line*	*Restricted diet line (75 per cent)*
1)	Rate of gain per generation (gm)	0.33±0.101	0.26±0.061 (1.3 per cent) Non sig. differences (1.5 per cent)
2)	h^2 Non sig. differences	0.197±0.061	0.291±0.127
3)	Total variance in body weight	—	Reduced

4) Conclusion:
Selection was found effective in both line and so the exchange of environments (diet) was made in 5th and 7th generation.

	FF	RF	FR	RR
5)	Higher 6 week weight	Low mean 6 week wt. but with marked improvement	Low rate of gain	High rate of gain
	Difference was slightly sig.		Difference was sig.	

* F = Full diet line
FR = Full diet line shifted on restricted diet
FF = Full diet line remained on full diet
R = Restricted diet line
RF = Restricted diet line shifted on full diet
RR = Restricted diet line remained on restricted diet

The mice of the full diet line raised on restricted diet (FR) were much less heavy than the contemporaneous mice of the restricted diet line (RR). There was no evidence that the increase of weight due to selection on full diet had made any improvement in weight on restricted diet; while mice of the restricted diet line raised on full diet (RF) were nearly equal in weight to the contemporaneous mice of full diet line (FF) and the weights were far above the unselected level for full diet line and this selection for weight on restricted diet was almost equally effective in increasing weight on full diet as was selection on full diet. The data indicated that the full diet line on restricted diet (FR) show lesser rate of response as compared to restricted diet line on restricted diet (RR) and the differences were highly significant whereas when both lines were raised on full diet the differences were small though significant ($p < 0.05$). The mean 6 week weight of restricted diet line on full diet (RF) was low as compared to full diet line on full diet (FF). Conclusively the results were in contrary to Hammond's hypothesis in two ways – h^2 was higher in bad environment than in the good, and the improvement attained by selection under good conditions was not realized when selected strain was transferred to bad condition, instead of being better than the strain selected under bad conditions it was worse.

They also critically evaluated Hammond's hypothesis as well as their own results in terms of variance components, According to Hammond's thesis the σ^2_G alone will be reduced as a consequence of bad environment and so also the h^2 making the response less in a bad environment than in good. But they obtained different results – effect of bad environment was to reduce the σ^2_G by 45 per cent and σ^2_E by 66 per cent, with a consequent increase of h^2 from 20 to 29 per cent and the net result of these changes was that the response in bad environment was reduced by 21 per cent. The response to selection can be increased either by reducing σ^2_E or increasing σ^2_G (and thereby increasing h^2). If the σ^2_G is increased without increasing σ^2_E the h^2 will of course be increased. If the σ^2_E is increased in proportion to σ^2_G, then the h^2 will remains unchanged but the response will be increased. Thus an increase of σ^2_G without changing, the h^2 will increase the response.

Experiment on Pigs

A similar experiment on sows was conducted by Fowler and Ensminger (1957) by giving full diet and 70 per cent as much as the full fed pigs. After 6 generations, half of the pigs in each line were shifted to other plane of nutrition forming 4 lines *viz.* high-high (HH), high-low (HL), low-low (LL) and Low-High (LH). The highest indexed animals were selected for breeding to produce next generation.

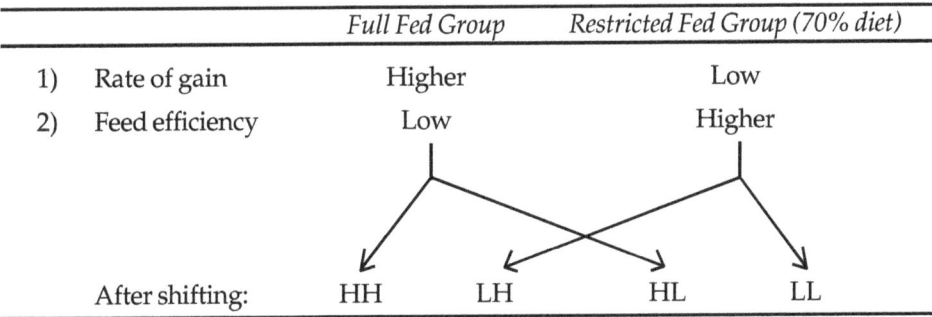

		Full Fed Group	*Restricted Fed Group (70% diet)*
1)	Rate of gain	Higher	Low
2)	Feed efficiency	Low	Higher
	After shifting:	HH LH	HL LL

H group was better than L group up to 6 generation in rate of gain but reverse was true for feed efficiency. After shifting, LH group was better than HH in rate and economy of gain and LL group excelled than HL groups in rate and economy of gain.

17.4 Implications of G-E Interaction

The G-E interaction is of significance when the phenotypic differences of different genotypes in two environments differ significantly. The significance thus depends upon the magnitude of change in the phenotype with a change in environment.

The G-E interaction has the following consequences:

(*i*) The environment differences have greater effect on some of the genotypes. This result in a change in ranking of genotype under changed environment and this is the degree of G-E interaction.

(*ii*) The correlation between phenotype and genotype is reduced.

(*iii*) It leads to an inaccurate/biased estimate of the variance components.

These consequences have the following implications:

1. Choice of Breed and Selection Scheme

A well adapted genotype (breed/variety) shows no or little variation in its performance over a normal range of environment (location). However, no breed is well adapted over locations and each genotype is said to be adapted only under certain set of environmental conditions (local conditions). This implies that each genotype has its certain environmental requirements and any change in that has the adverse effect on the performance of the genotype. The G-E interaction is the cause for the adverse effect. The existence of G-E interaction has an effect that a genotype superior in one environment does not show its superiority in another environment. This creates the problem of the adaptation of genotypes to a wide range of environments. Therefore, there should be a correct choice of breed to be included in the breeding policy for genetic improvement of livestock.

The use of A.I. and frozen semen technology has made extensive use of progeny tested sires throughout the country and world wide. The sires are tested under farm conditions/experimental stations where the environment in terms of rearing and management conditions is better than the field conditions where the progeny of these sires will be raised in future. The note worthy point is to see that how much of the improvement made in one environment will be retained if a breed is shifted in another environment. In the presence of G-E interaction the genetic superiority of sires selected in one environment cannot be fully exhibited under another environment. The G-E interaction exists because the physiological mechanisms for the development and expression of the character in diverse environments are different to some extent and it is likely that separate set of genes express themselves under different environments. This means that the genes required for better performance may be different from the genes that cause poor performance. It is well known that the expression of genes is environment specific. For example, the genes responsible for baldness expresses themselves in old age, and likewise the expression of genes responsible for ill health, milk production, menstruation in women etc are environmental specific. Therefore, when a genotype is shifted to another environment, a single character (milk production) recorded in two different environments may be regarded as two separate characters. The inconsistency in response to selection in different environments will depend upon the magnitude and direction of the genetic correlation (rg) between the performance records of the character in two environments.

Low rg will lead to genetic slippage (reduction in breeding value) in the environment in which selection was not done. Thus it will lead to a disagreement between predicted and observed response to selection and hence the selection made in one environment will not be effective in another environment It will mean that the genotype (breed) is not equally adapted to both the environment. On the other hand, the high *rg* between the records of the same trait in two environments will indicate that the performance recorded in two environments represents the same character controlled by more or less the same genes and that the breed is equally adapted in both the environments.

The problem that under which environment the selection should be made in the presence of G-E interaction was tackled by Falconer (1952) by estimating the r_g between the same traits recorded in two environments. The response in an environment (E_2) to selection done in the other (E_1) can be predicted as correlated response (CR) in environment 2 to selection done in environments 1

$$CR_2 = r_g h_1 h_2 \sigma p_2 i_1$$

Thus if the selection is done in E_1, the CR in E_2 (CR_2) is predicted to test the effectiveness of selection done in E_1.

The answer to the problem of environment and selection can be obtained by taking the ratio of correlated response to direct response in E_2:

$$CR_2 = \frac{(rg\, h_1 h_2\, \sigma p_2 i_1)}{h_2 h_2\, \sigma p_2 i_2} = rg \frac{h_1}{h_2} \quad (taking\ i_1 = i_2)$$

The increase or decrease in genetic gain by selecting parents in an environment (E_1) other than that where the progeny are expected to live (E_2) can be-predicted from the knowledge of the genetic correlation between traits in the two environments and the h^2 estimates. The CR_2 will be less than DR_2 when $r_g h_1$ is less than h_2. In the experiment conducted by Falconer and Latyszwski (1952) for body weight of mice on low and high plane nutrition, it was observed that the improvement made by selection under high plane nutrition (E_1) was not carried forward when the mice were shifted on low plane nutrition (E_2). On the other hand, the improvement made under low plane nutrition (E_2) was retained when the mice were shifted to high plane nutrition (E_1). The gain was well above control levels and nearly as great as was in mice on high plane of nutrition. When high plane mice were shifted to low plane of nutrition, there was no evidence of correlated response to selection. Similar results were obtained by Falconer (1960) in mice for 3 to 6 weeks body weight These results indicated the G-E interaction, The selection in the less favourable environment resulted in genetic improvement of the trait in both favourable and unfavourable environment but selection in favourable environment did not result in genetic improvement of trait in unfavourablé environment. Fowler and Ensminger (1957) had also arrived at the same conclusion for average daily gain in pigs on full feeding and restricted feeding environment that the trait was affected by different genes in the two environments. Thus, the existence of G-E interaction indicated that selection should be made under environmental conditions in which the progeny are expected to live.

2. Heterosis and Environment

The effects of mating systems on the magnitude of inbreeding depression and heterotic effects depend upon the environment in which the population is maintained. The environment conditions change the ranking of lines, strains, breeds or sires within a breed. The selection gain obtained in one environment may not be obtained in other environment if G-E interaction exists. The G – E interaction may decrease the genetic progress. Therefore, the C-E interactions are very important in livestock productivity because they are a potential cause of disagreement between actual and predicted results and hence, lead to disappointment and financial loss to the breeder as the results for genetic manipulation are not obtained according to the expectations.

The mating systems are very important tools of the breeding plans for genetic improvement of livestock. Many traits deteriorate as a consequence of inbreeding and also show heterosis as a consequence of line crossing or crossbreeding. The effects of mating system (inbreeding and cross breeding) depend upon the environmental conditions. The deleterious effects of inbreeding are more under substandard environmental conditions. Thus, when the mating systems (inbreeding vs random mating) x environment interaction are important, it is not possible to predict accurately the inbreeding depression in a herd because the effects of inbreeding depend on the environment. Likewise, the heterotic advantage depends upon environmental conditions under which the comparison is made.

Different amount of heterosis under different systems have been reported by Hohenboken *et al* (1976) in sheep and this indicated the mating system x environment interaction. It is thus not possible to accurately predict the average amount of heterosis in either environ-ment. Thus, interaction of mating system (cross breeding vs random mating) with environment lead to disagreement between expected and actual results obtained. The magnitude of heterosis in relation to environment has been discussed in chapter 16 under section 16.9.

3. Low Accuracy in Predicting B.V.

The correlation between genotype and phenotype is reduced due to the existence of G-E interaction. Therefore it becomes difficult to accurately estimate the genetic worth (breeding value) of a genotype whose ranking may be changed in a changed environment. If a genotype performs better in an environment and if there is no G-E interaction, it can then be predicted and said that it will also prove better in a changed environ-ment. However, such a breed to have high adaptability is generally a low producer or vice versa. There is a negative relationship between adaptability and productivity.

4. Biased Estimate of Variance Components

The G-E interaction can not be estimated in terms of the mean square (σ^2_{GE}) if there is only one environment. In this case the G-E interaction variance is included in the genotypic variance and thus the σ^2_G will be $\sigma^2_G + \sigma^2_{GE}$ which imply that the estimate of σ^2_G is biased upward. Therefore, if the σ^2_G will be used in breeding plan it will have the effect of disagreement between the observed and expected response to selection. Thus it will be the wastage of time, resources and effort, and hence the selection programme will not be effective In view of this it is essential that the G-E interaction should be estimated by testing the genotypes for their performance trait of interest under different environments of years or locations.

17.5 Specification of G-E Interaction

The specification of genetic, environmental and their interaction contribution to the phenotypic values can be given, as the simplest case, for non-segregating genotypes (true breeding lines) differing by only one gene difference (A-a) raised in two environments. The model assumes that additive-dominance effects of genes are adequate to specify the genetic components of phenotypic value. This model can be further extended for many environments and for segregating generations (F_2, B_1 and B_2) also. Mather and Jones (1958) have given the description of genotype-environment interaction in continuous variation whereas the environmental and G-E components of variability of generation means have been discussed by Bucio (1966) for inbred lines, Bucio and Hill (1966) for heterozygotes and Bucio et al (1969) for segregating generations.

17.5.1 Non-Segregating Generations

(i) Two Parental Lines

The two non-segregating genotypes differing for one gene difference (A-a), one is AA and other is aa, are each raised under two environments (E_1 and E_2). Thus there will be four phenotypes (two genotypes each under two environments). The differences among four phenotypes can be specified in terms of gene's effect, environmental effects and the gene-environment interaction effect. The model assumes that the allele A and environment (E_1) have positive/favourable effects on the trait while the allele *a* and E_2 have unfavourable effects. The expression of expected mean performance for any generation can be written in terms of genetic, environmental and interaction components if the genetic components of that generation are known. Here, the generations are two parental lines differing for one gene difference designated as P_1 (larger parent, AA) and P_2 (smaller parent, aa). The differences among four phenotypes will be described by four parameters *viz.* m, a, e and I_{ae} The expected mean performance will be as under

Table 17.1: Expected Mean Performance

Genotype/Environ	E_1	E_1	Mean
G_1 (AA)	$m + a + e + I_{ae}$	$m + a - e - I_{ae}$	$m + a$
G_2 (aa)	$m - a + e - I_{ae}$	$m - a - e + I_{ae}$	$m - a$
Mean	$m + e$	$m - e$	m

where,   m and a are as defined earlier

e = Environmental deviation

= average of the difference between two envi-ronments over two lines.

I_{ae} = Joint effect of a and e components

(ii) F_1 Produced by Two Pure Lines

The above model of two genotypes (parents) – two environments can be further elaborated by including the F_1 (heterozygous genotype, Aa) and its interaction with environment. The genetic effect of heterozygotes is due to the dominance properties of the genes which is denoted by the genetic parameter d. The d represents the deviation in the phenotypic value of the heterozygote from mid parent value of two homozygotes. The d may also interact with the environment (e) which modifies the phenotypic value further. This interaction component of phenotypic value is represented as I_{de} corresponding with I_{ae}. Thus, the expected mean of heterozygous genotype (Aa) raised in two environments will be:

Environments		Expected Mean
Better	–	$m + d + e + I_{de}$
Poor		$m \div d - e - I_{de}$

where,   d = as defined earlier

I_{de} = joint effect of d and e components

Therefore, the estimation of all the parameters (m, a, d, e, I_{ae} and I_{de}) requires to record observations on two homozygotes and their F_1 grown simultaneously in the two environments. There will be six phenotypic classes of 3 genotypes raised in two environments and hence six means from which all these six parameters of interaction model can be estimated.

17.5.2. Segregating Generations

The segregating generations are F_2, B_1 and B_2 etc. The G-E interactions in these generations can be specified by the same parameters used for non-segregating generations. The expected mean performance can be derived for any generation provided the genetic composition of the generation in terms of the proportions of homozygotes and heterozygotes is known for any gene difference.

(i) F_2 Generation

The F_2 generation for single gene difference (A-a) grown in two environments (E_1 and E_2) will have six phenotypic classes and hence six means with their expected composition will be as follows:

Table 17.2: Expected Mean Performance of F$_2$ Generation

Genotypes/ Environment	AA	Aa	aa	Mean
E$_1$	$m + a + e + I_{ae}$	$m + d + e + I_{de}$	$m - a + e - I_{ae}$	$m + \frac{1}{2}d + e + \frac{1}{2}I_{de}$
E$_2$	$m + a - e - I_{ae}$	$m + d - e - I_{de}$	$m - a - e + I_{ae}$	$m + \frac{1}{2}d - e - \frac{1}{2}I_{de}$
Mean	$m + a$	$m + d$	$m - a$	$m + \frac{1}{2}d$

The F$_2$ mean is $m + \frac{1}{2}d$ when the F$_2$ population is grown in two or more environments since $\Sigma e = 0$ and $\Sigma I_{de} = 0$, the environmental effects and its interaction effect with genetic effect are cancelled out for which it is true that environments do not contribute to the mean. However, when the population is grown only in one environment then the *e* component and its interaction with gene's effect contribute to the mean. Therefore, the expected mean of F$_2$ population can be written as:

$$F_2 = m + \frac{1}{2}d + e + \frac{1}{2}I_{de} \quad \text{for better environment}$$

$$= m + \frac{1}{2}d - e - \frac{1}{2}I_{de} \quad \text{for poor environment}$$

$$= m + \frac{1}{2}d \quad \text{averaged over all environments}$$

Thus the F$_2$ mean when averaged over two or more environments gives the genetic contributions to the generation mean.

(ii) First Generation Back Crosses

Similarly, the expression for any generation can be written in terms of the genetic, environmental and their interaction components provided the genetic components of that generation are known. For example, the genetic components of first generation back crosses means are:

$$B_1 = m + \frac{1}{2}a + \frac{1}{2}d \quad \text{over all environments}$$

$$B_2 = m - \frac{1}{2}a + \frac{1}{2}d \quad -\text{do}-$$

The complete specifications of B$_1$ and B$_2$ generations recorded in two environments (E$_1$ and E$_2$) in terms of genetic, environmental and G-E interaction components can be given as:

$$B_1 E_1 = m + \frac{1}{2}a + \frac{1}{2}d + e + \frac{1}{2}I_{ae} + \frac{1}{2}I_{de}$$

$$B_1 E_2 = m + \frac{1}{2}a + \frac{1}{2}d - e - \frac{1}{2}I_{ae} - \frac{1}{2}I_{de}$$

$$B_2 E_1 = m - \frac{1}{2}a + \frac{1}{2}d + e - \frac{1}{2}I_{ae} + \frac{1}{2}I_{de}$$

$$B_2 E_2 = m - \frac{1}{2}a + \frac{1}{2}d - e + \frac{1}{2}I_{ae} - \frac{1}{2}I_{de}$$

17.6 Estimation of G–E Interaction

The presence of G – E interaction to affect a trait can be estimated by applying any of the following methods, depending on the type of population available:

17.6.1 Biometrical Approach

The procedure of estimation of the genetic, environmental and G-E interaction components using the means of non-segregating generations for additive-dominance model has been described as under -

1. Two Genotypes–Two Environments

(i) Mid Parent Value (m)

The mid parent value (m) is the point of origin. It is estimated as the average of both the parents over all the environments as

m = mid parent value

$$= \frac{1}{2}(\overline{P}_1 + \overline{P}_2)$$

$$= \frac{1}{2}[\frac{1}{2}(\overline{P}_{11} + \overline{P}_{12}) + \frac{1}{2}(\overline{P}_{21} + \overline{P}_{22})]$$

Where, $\overline{P}_1$ = Average of P_1 under all environments

$\overline{P}_2$ = Average of P_1 under all environments

$\overline{P}_{11}$ = Average of P_1 under better environment (1)

$\overline{P}_{12}$ = Average of P_1 under poor environment (2)

$\overline{P}_{21}$ = Average of P_2 under better environment (1)

$\overline{P}_{22}$ = Average of P_2 under better environment (2)

(ii) Genetic Component (Additive Genetic)

The additive genetic effect denoted by 'a' measures the difference between means of two homozygotes averaged over both the environments and it is the amount by which the mean phenotypic value of two homozygous genotypes differ from population mean (mid parent value, m) and estimated as half the difference of the means of two genotypes over two (more) environments as:

$\mathbf{a} = \frac{1}{2}(\overline{P}_1 - \overline{P}_2)$ = additive gene effects.

Thus the additive effect of gene (**a**) is the average deviation of two pure lines (for one gene difference) from overall mean (**m**) and measures the average effect of the difference in two genotypes. Thus, **a** is the additive genetic value.

(iii) Environmental Component (e)

The environmental deviation represents the difference between means of two environments averaged over two genotypes (pure lines) and hence measured as:

$\mathbf{e} = \frac{1}{2}(\overline{E}_1 - \overline{E}_2)$ = environmental deviation.

where, E_1 is the average of all genotypes in environment 1 etc.

Thus **e** measures the effect of the difference in environment and it is the amount by which the mean phenotypic value between two environments differs from population mean (u – m). The environmental effect in a particular environment (say j environment) is the deviation of the mid parent value of two genotypes in that environment (say m_1) from the mid parent value over all environments (m). Thus

$$e_j = \tfrac{1}{2}(\overline{P}_{1j} + \overline{P}_{2j})$$

$$= m_j - m$$

= environmental deviation in j^{th} environment

where, m_j = mid parent value in j^{th} environment

(iv) G-E Interaction Component (I_{ae})

This is joint effect of the two *viz.* genetic and environment. This is estimated as the difference between observed phenotypic mean of ith genotype in j^{th} environment and its expected mean obtained by summing the a and e components so that

$$I_{ae} = \overline{P}_{ij} - (m + a + e)$$

for the reason that $\overline{P}_{ij} = m + a + e + I_{ae}$

The I_{ae} component is also obtained as half the difference of mean of two homozygous genotypes under two environments as:

$$I_{ae} = \tfrac{1}{2}(\text{Diff. } \overline{P}_1 - \text{Diff. } \overline{P}_2)$$

where, Diff. P_1 is the difference in mean of P_1 between two environments

or $I_{ae} = a_j - a$

where, a_j is the additive gene effect in j^{th} environment

The scaling test is applied to test the significance of all these genetic parameters after estimating the variance and standard error of each parameter. The absence of G-E interaction is indicated if the I_{ae} component is not significant and confirm that the model $P = G + E$ is adequate.

2. Many Environments–Genotype Interaction

The interaction model can be extended for many environments. The environmental differences are expressed by a series of comparisons equal in number to the degrees of freedom for the environments. Bucio Alains (1966) gave the procedure by illustrating the experimental data of two varieties of Nicotiana rustica and their F_1 along with other generations derived from them growing over 16 years (environments). The different parameters are estimated as under:

m =	mid parent value (average of two homozygotes) over all the environments	
=	$\tfrac{1}{2}(\overline{P}_1 + \overline{P}_2)$	
a =	half the mean difference between two homozygotes over all environments	
=	$\tfrac{1}{2}(\overline{P}_1 - \overline{P}_2)$	

	=	additive genetic value or additive effect of gene
	=	deviation of two lines from overall mid parent value
d	=	average value of deviation of F_1 mean from mid parent value over all the environments.
	=	$\overline{F_1} - m$
	=	dominance effect of gene.
e_j	=	half the difference between the average of two homogyzotes in j^{th} environment minus the average value of this difference overall the environments.
	=	$\frac{1}{2}(\overline{P}_{1j} + \overline{P}_{2j}) - m$
	=	$m_j - m$
	=	environmental effect which is the deviation of the mid parent value of two lines in j^{th} environment from mid parent value over all the environments such that $\Sigma e_j = 0$
$I_{ae\,(j)}$	=	half the difference between two homozygotes in j^{th} environment minus the difference between two homozy-gotes overall environments
	=	$\frac{1}{2}(P_{1j} - P_{2j}) - a$
	=	$a_j - a$
	=	interaction of additive genetic value with j^{th} environment such that $\Sigma\, Iae_{(j)} = 0$
$I_{de(j)}$	=	difference between average value of deviation of F_1 mean from mid parent value for j^{th} environment and the average deviated value of F_1 mean from mid parent value over all the environments.
	=	$\left(\overline{F}_{1j} - m_j\right) - d$
	=	$dj - d$
	=	interaction of dominance effect of gene with j^{th} environment such that $\Sigma\, I_{de(j)} = 0$

It can be seen that the difference between parental means is a linear function of the environments and the deviation of F_1 mean from mid parent is also a linear function of the environments which is larger for good environment than for poor environment. If a is greater than d, the deviation of F_1 mean from mid parent (d, heterosis) is smaller for good environment than for poor environment. Thus, the heterosis is a function of the environment.

17.6.2 Statistical Techniques

The evidence of the presence and estimation of G-E interaction can be obtained by subjecting the breeding data to statistical methods *viz.* Genetic correlation approach, Analysis of variance and Regression analysis

(1) Genetic Correlation as an Evidence of G–E Interaction

The consequence of the presence of G-E interaction is that the correlation between genotype and phenotype is reduced. This makes it difficult to evaluate the genetic worth of a genotype whose ranking in comparison to other genotype may be changed in different environment. This poses the problem of adaptation of a genotype in a range of environments. The adaptation of the genotype (breed/variety) to different environments may be assessed by detecting the genotype environment interaction, This idea of adaptation of breed to different environments in relation to G-E interaction was conceived by Falconer (1952) by considering the performance records of a breed in two environments as two separate characters and to estimate the genetic correlation between them.

Falconer (1952) considered only two different environments and expressed the G-E interaction from an estimate of the genetic correlation between the records of the same character measured in two different environments. The idea was to make the genetic aspect of the situation clear and to obtain a quantitative evaluation of the efficiency of two methods of selection which are the direct and indirect selection by estimating the direct response and correlated response to selection. Such a method will help to solve the problem of environment and selection in the sense whether it is better to make selection for genetic improvement in an environment in which the improved genotype (breed) through selection is required to live or the improvement through selection should be made in some other environment which is more favourable for the better expression of the desired character.

Falconer (1952) regarded the performance of the same charac-ter recorded in two environments as two different characters which should be genetically correlated because the two characters are the two different expressions of the one and the same character recorded in two different environments. This idea is based on the fact that the gene expression is environment specific *viz.* some genes controlling the character express themselves in one environ-ment while others express in other environment. However, the selection of a character in one environment will bring a correlated response (CR) in the same character measured in other environment and this CR may then be compared with that of direct response (DR) to selection for the desired character itself. The answer of the problem of the environment and selection can be obtained by taking the ratio of the CR to the DR as

$$\frac{CR}{DR} = r_g \left(\frac{i h_2 \sigma_{g1}}{h_1 \sigma_{g1}} \right)$$

$$= r_g \left(\frac{h_2}{h_1} \right)$$

Where, the subscripts 1 and 2 refer two environments.

1 is the *primary environment* under which the improved genotype has to live (*e.g.* low plane of nutrition), and

2 is the *secondary environment* under which selection is made (*e.g.* high plane of nutrition) but under which the improved genotype (through selection) is not required to live subsequently.

Thus, the DR is then the improvement in the trait under primary environment (1) and the CR is the improvement in the trail under secondary environment (2).

An advantage of selection in the secondary environment (high plane nuirition = HPN) would accrue only through an increase of h^2 which have to be great enough to offset the loss of efficiency through selection being made for a trait in primary environment (low plane nutrition LPN). When the two environments vary widely like temperature and tropical climate, the genetic correla-tion (r) will be low and thus the difference in h^2 would have to be very great or the CR to be greater than the DR. Therefore, the justification in favour of selection in the secondary environment requires a much high h^2 in the secondary environment.

In the experiment described by Falconer and Latyszewsky (1952) with mice, the two strains were selected for body weight – one on high plane of nutrition and other on a low. After some generation of selection the diet of the two strains were changed and the body weight was measured for each strain on the other diet. With this experiment two main findings were:

(i) Heritability was higher on the low plane (0.29) than on the high (0.19).

(ii) The two correlated response were less than direct response and on comparing with the corresponding direct response, the CR follow-ing selection on the low plane was much greater than CR following selection on the high plane.

The two ratios of CR to DR may be compared taking the r_g as 0.65.

Selection Done at Low Plane

The ratio of correlated to the direct response for weight on high plane of nutrition, where 2 (secondary environment) refer to low plane on which selection was done and 1 (primary environment) to high plane, *i.e.* selection is done at low plane of nutrition (environment 2).

$$\frac{CR_2}{DR_2} = r_g \left(\frac{h_1}{h_2} \right)$$

$$= 0.65 \sqrt{\frac{0.3}{0.2}}$$

$$= 0.8$$

Selection done at High Plane

The other CR which indicates the change of weight on low plane following selection on high plane referring 2 (secondary environment) to high plane and 1 (primary environment) to low plane of nutrition was found. In this case the expected ratio of CR to DR of weight on low plane was found to be about 0.5 as

$$\frac{CR_1}{DR_1} = r_g \left(\frac{h_2}{h_1} \right)$$

$$= 0.65 \sqrt{\frac{0.2}{0.3}}$$

$$= 0.5$$

The values of two estimates of heritability and of two direct and correlated responses would yield two separate estimates of the genetic correlation (Falconer, 1952) which would indicate the effect of environment on the phenotypic expression of the desired trait.

Falconer (1952) first proposed that G-E interaction can be shifted by computing the genetic correlation of the same trait in two separate environments. The idea of considering the same character measured in two different environments as two characters is that the genes controlling the trait in one environment may be different (at least partially) from those which control the trait in the second environ-ments. The low genetic correlation between the same trait of the same genetic group in different environments is indicative that the environ-mental differences have important bearing in influencing the trait which indicates that the G-E interaction is present and that the individuals of the same genetic group are not equally adapted-to the different environment, while the high r_g will indicate less effect of environmental differences and hence very little G-E inter-action and the equal adaptation of individuals of the same genetic group in different environment.

The idea proposed by Falconer to study the G-E interaction was extended to more than two environments by Robertson (1959) by estimating the intra class genetic correlation as a measure of interaction. The genetic correlation of a sire's estimated BV for milk fat production in various herds of different production levels as well as under different housing systems have been reported to be close to unity.

Estimation of Genetic Correlation

The genetic correlation between two records of the same trait measured in two environments is estimated by the procedure outlined in the chapter 22 on association among traits. Thus the genetic correlation may be estimated either from the half sib families or full sib families.

(2) Analysis of Variance Method

This is the most relevant approach to study the genotypic, environmental and G-E interaction effects. This can also be used to estimate the heritability in broad sense since this method estimates the different components of phenotypic variance.

In general, the procedure to estimate the G-E interaction is to test some genotypes (m) under some environments (n). The genotypes may be the different breeds, purelines/isogenic lines, half sib and full sib families etc. The following model is used-

$$Y_{ijk} = u + g_i + e_j + ge_{ij} + e_{ijk}$$

Where, Y_{ijk} is the kth observation of ith genotype recorded in j^{th} macro environment,

    u is the general mean

    g_i is the effect of ith genotype

    e_j is the effect of Jth macro environment

    ge_{ij} is the interaction effect of ith genotype in j^{th} genotype environment.

    e_{ijk} is the random deviation caused by the environmental difference within the ij^{th} genotype environment.

The analysis of variance is conducted to subdivide the phenotypic variance into its components according to the various genotypes (m) and environments (n). The ANOVA takes the following form:

Table 17.3: Analysis of Variance

Sources	D.F.	M.S.	E.M.S.
Genotypes	m − 1	M.S.$_1$	$\sigma^2_{Et} + r\sigma^2_{GEp} + nr\sigma^2_G$
Environment	n − 1	M.S.$_2$	$\sigma^2_{Et} + r\sigma^2_{GEp} + mr\sigma^2_{Ep}$
G − E interaction	(m − 1) (n − 1)	M.S.$_3$	$\sigma^2_{Et} + r\sigma^2_{GEp}$
Residual	m n (r − 1)	M.S.$_4$	σ^2_{Et}

Where, r = r for isogenic lines, r = 0.25 r for Hs and 0.5 r for Fs n = Size of a genotype
        E_p = macro environmenyt, E_t = residual environment

The genotypes may be different breeds, isogenic lines, or half sibs or full sib families.

Solved Examples

Example 17.1

Two genotype – two environments.Find out the different component of phenotypic value from the following information and test the adequacy of the non-interaction model.

Genotypes	Environment	Mean	Model			
			m	a	e	I_{ae}
$G_{1\,(AA)}$	1	153	1	1	1	1
$G_{1\,(AA)}$	2	125	1	1	−1	−1
$G_{2\,(aa)}$	1	127	1	−1	1	−1
$G_{2\,(aa)}$	2	104	1	−1	−1	1

Solution

$$m = ¼(153 + 125 + 127 + 104) = 127.25$$

$$a = ¼[153 + 125) - (127 + 104)] = 11.75$$

or $= ½(\overline{G}_1 - \overline{G}_2) = ½(139 - 115.5) = 11.75$

$$e = ¼[(153 + 127) - (125 + 104)] = 12.75$$

or $= ½(\overline{E}_1 - \overline{E}_2) = ½(140 - 114.5) = 12.75$

$$I ae_1 = ¼(153 + 104) - (125 + 127)] = 1.25$$

or $= ½(153 - 127) - ½[½(153- 127) + ½(125-104)]$

$$= ¼(26 - ½(13 + 10.5)] = 13.0 - 11.75 = 1.25$$

$$Iae_2 = ½(125 - 104) - ½[½(153 - 127) + ½(125 - 104)]$$

$$= 10.5 - 11.75 = -1.25$$

Verification of phenotypic value:

P_{11}	$= m + a + e + 1ae = 127.25 + 11.75 + 12.75 + 1.25$	$= 153$
P_{12}	$= m + a - e - Iae = 127.25 + 11.75 - 12.75 - 1.25$	$= 125$
P_{21}	$= rn - a + e - Iae = 127.25 - 11.75 + 12.75 -1.25$	$= 127$
P_{22}	$= m - a - e + Iae = 127.25 - 11.75 - 12.75 +1.25$	$= 104$

Averaged over two breeds, the phenotypic average was higher in E_1 environment than in E_2 (140 vs 114.5) and the breed average over the two environments was higher for breed G_1 (139) than breed G_2 (115.5). Statistically, the main effects of each environment is the average of both the breeds expressed as deviation from the overall population mean (m = 127.25). The breed main effect of each breed was averaged over both environments and expressed as deviation from the overall population mean (u = 127.25). The sum of the main effects for environments as well as for the main effects for breeds is zero.

When there is no interaction between main effects (genotypes and environments) the phenotypes of the 4 breed x environment subclasses can be predicted accurately from the sum 'of the overall population mean, the main effect for the breed and the main effect of the environment. In example, the phenotype for G_1E_1 subclass is predicted as 127.25 + 11.75 + 12.75 = 151.75 which is lower than the observed average of 153. Thus, there is a difference between the predicted and actual average of the sub class. This indicated that there was an interaction between breeds and environment to produce their effect on phenotype. When G x E interaction exists, the average phenotypic value of some subclass cannot be predicted from the main effects of the corresponding genotype and environment.

Example 17.2: Many Genotypes-Environments

Bucio Alains (1966) reported the data on plant height of N. rustica over 16 years taking 16 years as 16 environments. The data were recorded on two parental varieties (P_1 as better parent and P_2, as inferior parent) and their F_1 below.

Years	P_1	P_2	F_1	F_2	B_1	B_2
1	49.10	39.36	49.74	47.27		
2.	50.14	39.60	50.87	48.14		
3.	48.i6	39.48	49.15	47.45		
4.	41.i7	37.i3	43.33	39.60		
5.	42.94	40.20	45.66	43.21		
6.	37.37	38.34	42.63	38.63		
7.	40.54	38.14	4i.56	41.47		
8.	44.68	41.90	49.78	46.73		
9.	42.50	42.15	47.11	44.64		
10.	32.86	35.84	37.42	39.70		
11.	47.43	44.45	52.40	55.28		
12.	44.62	36.75	46.75	47.42		
13.	60.73	48.70	63.63	60.37		
14.	57.69	47.31	60.11	55.67		
15.	53.47	45.23	55.31	51.44		
16.	60.03	46.36	59.51	57.81		
Mean	47.09	41.31	49.62	47.80	48.23	46.02

Solution

The estimates of m, a and d for 16 environments are:

m = ½ (47.09 + 41.3l) = 44.27 ± 1.008

a = ½ (47.09 – 41.3l) = 2.84 ± 0.993

d = 49.62 – 44.24 = 5.42 ± 0.939

The estimates of e_j and $I_{ae(j)}$ and $I_{de(j)}$ for the different environments have been enlisted below after they are estimated as:

For environment No. 1

e_1 = ½$(P_{11} + P_{21})$ – m = m_1 – m

 = ½ (49.1 + 39.36) – 44.27

 = 44.23 – 44.27 = – 0.04

$I_{ae(1)}$ = a_1 – a

 = ½ (49.1 – 39.36) – 2.84

 = 4.87 – 2.84 = 2.03

$$I_{de(1)} \quad = d_1 - d = [49.74 - \tfrac{1}{2}(49.10 + 39.36)] - 5.82$$
$$= F_{11} - m_1 - d = (49.74 - 44.23) - 5.82$$
$$= 5.51 - 5.82 = -0.31$$

For environment No. 2

Similar procedure to that used for environment no. 1.

Likewise, the different components can be estimated for all the environments. After estimating all the components for all the environments, the results can be presented in the tabular form:

Environ.	e_j	$I_{ae(j)}$	$I_{ae(j)}$	Environ	e_j	$I_{ae(j)}$	$I_{ae(j)}$
1	− 0 04	2.03	− 0.31	9			
2				10			
3				11			
4				12			
5				13			
6				14			
7				15			
8				16			

Mixed population: The procedure to estimate genotypic value, environmental deviation and G – E interaction components of phenotypic value for a character from the means of a number of genotypes (mixed population) kept under a number of environments has been given above under section 15.2 and illustrated with a solved example no. 15.1.

Chapter 18

Phenotypic Variance

The phenotypic value and its causal components along with mean have been discussed in the last chapter. The population mean is used to compare the two or more populations for certain purpose. However, the mean value of a character is not sufficient to describe a population for a quantitative character because the population mean does not give any idea about the variability in phenotypic values of different individuals. The differences in phenotypic values of different individuals of a population are called as variation. The variation may be classified as group variation recorded on individuals of different groups, individual variation recorded on different individuals within a group and within individual variation recorded at different times on the same individuals. The degree or amount of variation is measured by various statistical measures *viz.* range, mean deviation, variance including the standard deviation, standard error and coefficient of variation. The variance is more useful population parameter because it has the properties of additivity and subdivisibility.

The properties of variance are used to partition the total variance in to its causal components analogous to the partitioning of phenotypic value. These various components of phenotypic variance are very useful for their exploitation in bringing genetic improvement of a character.

18.1 Estimation of Variance

The variance is taken as the mean of squares of the deviated values from their mean and referred as the mean of squared values (Mean square, M.S.). Thus, in estimating the variance, the phenotypic value of each individual is taken as its deviation from population mean, the deviated values are then squared and added, and the sum of squared values is divided by the number of individuals (on which the phenotypic values were taken). Thus, it will give the mean of the squared values and hence called as mean square. This mean square is the variance. The variance is calculated by denoting the phenotypic values as X rather than P:

$$V_X = \sum \frac{(X_i - \overline{X})^2}{N} \qquad \text{(i)}$$

$$= \frac{\left[\dfrac{\sum X^2 - (\sum X)^2}{N}\right]}{N} \qquad \text{(ii)}$$

$$= \frac{\sum X^2}{N} - \left[\frac{\sum X}{N}\right]^2$$

$$= \overline{X^2} - (\overline{X})^2 \qquad \text{(iii)}$$

$$= \text{Mean of square values} - \text{Square of Mean Values}$$

The numerator in (i) and (ii) is the sum of squares. This is divided by N – 1 instead of N when the sample variance is estimated.

18.2 Major Components of Phenotypic Variance

The variance has its components corresponding to the components of phenotypic values. The reason is that the phenotypic values are changed as a result of change in either genotype or in environment. Thus the genotype and environment are two major component of variation and form the basis to partition the variance in to corresponding components as the variance has the property of its subdivisibility. Here it is important to note that variation in genotypes causes variation in genotypic values which give rise to the genotypic (genetic) variance and the variation in environment causes the environmental variance. Therefore, the phenotypic variance which is the variance in phenotypic values is partitioned analogous to the partitioning of the phenotypic values as:

$$P = G + E$$
$$(P)^2 = (G + E)^2$$
$$= G^2 + E^2 + 2GE$$
$$V_P = V_G + V_E + 2Cov_{GE}$$

Where, V_P is the phenotypic variance,

V_G is the genotypic variance

V_E is the environmental variance

Cov_{GE} is the interaction variance (genotypic values and environmental deviation).

However, it is assumed that the genotype and environment are independent and hence the G – E interaction is taken as absent or treated as part of environmental variance. For practical purpose, independence is assumed. However, the genotypic and environmental variance components are further partitioned analogous to the partitioning of the genotypic value and environmental deviations, respectively.

18.3 Components of Genotypic Variance

The genotypic variance is composed of the components of genotypic value *viz.* additive gene effects, dominance deviations and interaction deviations. These components of genotypic value create variation in genotypic value of different individuals. Therefore, the variance of genotypic values called as the genotypic or genetic variance is partitioned into variance components associated to these components of genotypic values according to Fisher (1918) as: $V_G = V_A + V_D + V_I$

where,

V_A is the additive genetic variance caused by differences in breeding values of different individuals,

V_D is the dominance variance caused by differences in dominance deviations of different individuals or due to deviation of genotypic value from additive gene action.

V_I is the interaction variance caused by epistasis of genes for two or more loci case.

The sum of $V_D + V_I$ is called the non-additive genetic variance which is due to the gene combination value of the genotypic value. This part is neither fixed nor inherited whereas the additive part of variance (V_A) is fixed and heritable.

Additive-Dominance Variance (Single Locus Variance)

The genotypic value and its variance for a single locus two alleles system ($A_i A_j$ genotype) can be represented as:

$$g_{ij} = a_{ij} + d_{ij}$$
$$(g_{ij})^2 = (a_{ij} + d_{ij})^2$$
$$= a_{ij}^2 + d_{ij}^2 + 2 a_{ij} d_{ij}$$
$$= a_{ij}^2 + d_{ij}^2 \qquad \text{Since, } a_{ij}^2 \text{ and } d_{ij}^2 \text{ are uncorrelated}$$

Thus, $V_G = V_A + V_D$

Interaction Variance (Two or more Loci)

The genotypic value for polygenes taking their interaction effect is:

$$G = A + D + I$$

Therefore, the genotypic variance will be accordingly partitioned as:

$V_G = V_A + V_D + V_I$ since, A, D and I parts are not correlated

The magnitude of V_I is very small and negligible and hence ignored. However, the interaction variance can be divided on two bases, according to the number of loci *viz.* two loci interaction, three loci interaction and so on and according to the interaction involved between breeding values and dominant deviation. Considering two loci interaction, the interaction may be between breeding values of two loci causing additive x additive variance (V_{AA}), interaction between BV of one locus and dominance deviation of other locus producing additive x dominance variance (V_{AD}) and the interaction between dominance deviations of two loci causing dominance x dominance variance (V_{DD}). Hayman and Mather (1955) partitioned the epistatic (interaction) variance as under:

$$I = I_{AA} + I_{AD} + I_{DD}$$
$$V_I = V_{AA} + V_{AD} + V_{DD}$$

Now, the total phenotypic variance (V_P) can be partitioned on the assumption of independence of genotype and environment as:

$$V_P = V_G + V_E$$
$$= V_A + V_D + V_E \qquad \text{for single locus}$$
$$= V_A + V_D + V_I + V_E \qquad \text{for two or more loci.}$$
$$= V_A + V_D + (V_{AA} + V_{AD} + V_{DD}) + V_E$$

18.4 Components of Environmental Variance

The environment surrounding the individual during the course of development and expression of a character form a major part of the phenotypic variance. The environmental factors in this respect can be considered as permanent environmental effects (E_P) and temporary environmental effects (E_T). The corresponding variance caused by these two types of environmental effects is termed as the permanent environmental variance (V_{EP}) and the temporary environmental effects (V_{ET}). The permanent environmental factors affect the phenotypic values in general and hence the variation caused by them is also termed as the general environmental variance (V_{EG}). On the other hand, the temporary environmental factors affect the individual for a specific or temporary period and hence the variation caused by them is also termed as special environmental variance (V_{ES}). Thus, the environmental variance is partitioned as:

$$V_E = V_{EP} + V_{ET}$$
$$= V_{EG} + V_{ES}$$

With this the partitioning of phenotypic variance is complete and can be shown as:

$$V_P = V_G + V_E + V_{GE}$$
$$= (V_A + V_D + V_I) + (V_{EP} + V_{ET}) + V_{GE}$$

Thus, it is clear that the phenotypic variance which is the variance of phenotypic values, can be partitioned corresponding to the components of the phenotypic value. This indicates the differences in phenotypic values attributed to the genes or genotypes of the individuals and the environment received by the individual. The phenotypic variance is partitioned by the statistical technique known as the analysis of variance, more popularly known as Fisher's F-test.

18.5 Importance and Use of Variance Components

The genetics of a quantitative character is the study of the component parts of variance attributed to different causes. The magnitude of the different parts of the variance provide very useful information as given below:

Total Genetic Variance

It is necessary to know the effect of different factors causing variation in a character and to estimate the percent contribution of different causing factors to the total variance. This helps to provide the information about the relative role of heredity and environment to affect a trait and to know the degree of genetic determination expressed in terms of heritability in broad sense which is the ratio of genetic variance to the phenotypic variance as:

$$H^2 = \frac{V_G}{V_P}$$

It is important to know the relative role of heredity (genetic variation) and environment to cause the variation as it is specific to the character, the population and the individual.

Additive Genetic Variance

This part of variance is expressed in terms of heritability in narrow sense (h^2) as:

$$h^2 = \frac{V_A}{V_P}$$

The use and importance of additive genetic variance in terms of heritability in narrow sense (h^2) have been discussed in chapter 17 under section 17.1.2.

Non-additive Genetic Variance

The non-additive genetic variance is not fixed and not inherited. Thus, higher amount of this variance component is not desirable and selection based on this part of variance is not effective. It is thus not desirable to plan for genetic improvement based on the amount of non-additive genetic variance. However, this part of variance can be exploited by special breeding methods.

G-E Interaction Variance

When the expression of genotype (phenotype) becomes dependent on the environment, then different genotypes respond differently to the specific differences of environments and this causes an additional component of variance known as genotype-environmental interaction variance (V_{GE}) which is included with the V_E. The knowledge of the existence of G – E interaction is very useful in a number of ways:

(i) When the VGE exist, a genotype proved to be better in one environment can not be expected to be better in another environment. Therefore, selection should be carried out in an environment where improved genotype has to live. This information is thus helpful to decide the choice of environment for selective breeding and testing of sires. The existence of G-E interaction modifies the gene effects in a different environment while the absence of G-E interaction indicates the same gene effects in all the environments.

(*ii*) The herd comparison is not advisable in the presence of G-E interaction.

(*iii*) The data correction for environmental effects is advisable in the presence of G-E interaction.

Environmental Variance

The environmental variations are also very important for the following reasons:

(*i*) The environmentally determined superiority (environmental variation) is not transmitted to the progeny and hence the parents showing environmental superiority do not produce superior progeny. Thus, the selection based on environmental variance in a trait is not effective.

(*ii*) *The environmental variations overshadow the genetic variation and hence* reduce the correspondence between genotype and phenotype. Thus, the phenotype does not reveal the genotype when environmental effects are more important. The degree of correspondence between genotype and phenotype is increased with the decrease in V_E. The phenotype is produced and completely determined by the genotype when V_E is zero. Thus, the V_E shadows the V_G.

(*iii*) The proper environment is essentially required to an individual for expression of full genetic potential.

(*iv*) However, the uniform and better environment given to a breeding stock reduces environmental variability and is helpful for improvement for livestock production efficiency.

(*v*) The presence of environmental variance suggests the data adjustment for environmental effects.

18.6 Estimation of Components of Phenotypic Variance

The methods used to estimate the variance and its major components are the elimination method and analysis of variance method.

1. Elimination Method

The two major component of variance *viz.* genetic and environmental can be estimated by eliminating the either component in planning the experiment. It is clear that environment is beyond control and hence can not be eliminated. The genotypic variance can be eliminated experimentally by taking the individuals with identical genotype like highly inbred lines or F_1 of a cross between two such lines or clones from a single individual or identical twins (monozygotic). The individuals having identical genotypes will have no genetic variance and hence their phenotypic variance will be entirely the environmental variance. Such a population having no genetic variance is called as the genetically uniform population. The genetically mixed population (random bred population) will have both parts of phenotypic variance (genetic and environmental). The two major components will thus be estimated as:

Mixed population (random bred) $\qquad V_{P\,(M)} = V_G + V_E$

Uniform population $\qquad V_{P\,(U)} = V_E$

Difference $\qquad V_{P\,(M)} - V_{P\,(U)} = V_G$

This method is of very limited use and scope due to non availability of highly inbred lines in large farm animals except identical twins which are very rare. This method is thus limited to plants and small lab animals.

2. Analysis of Variance Method

The data on at least two genotypes (breeds, lines, strains) are collected. The phenotypic value is described by a mathematical model to conduct the statistical analysis of variance. The phenotype is expressed as: $X = \mu + G + E + I_{GE}$

where,

μ is the population mean (all the genotypes),

G is the effect of a particular genotype,

E is the effect of environment,

I_{GE} is the effect of genotype-environment interaction,

Assuming that all the effects except U are random and independent (uncorrelated), the phenotypic variance will be: $\sigma^2_P = \sigma^2_G + \sigma^2_E + \sigma^2_{I(GE)}$

The F test is applied by conducting the analysis of variance as follows-

Sources of Variation	DF	SS	MS	EMS
Genotypes	G-1	SS_G	MS_G	$\sigma^2 e + K\sigma^2_G$
Error	N-G	SS_E	MSe	$\sigma^2 e$
Total	N-1			

where,

K is the number of observations per genotype,

G is number of genotypes,

N is total number of records,

$\sigma^2_G = \dfrac{(MS_G - MS_e)}{K}$, is the genotypic variance due to genetic difference among genotypes,

$\sigma^2 e = MSe,$ $\qquad$ is the environmental variance including I_{GE} component and the error in sampling as well as in recording the data.

3. Generation Analysis Method

The phenotypic variance into its components, in case of large livestock and plants, can be partitioned and estimated from the phenotypic variance of parental lines or breeds (say P_1 an P_2), their F_1 and F_2 generations. The phenotypic variance of P_1, P_2, and F_1 (non-segregating generations) is entirely environmental in nature (V_E) because all the individuals have the same genotype. The F_2 is genetically mixed population whose individuals have different genotypes and hence contains both genetic and environmental parts of phenotypic variance. These informations are used to estimate the two major component of phenotypic components as under:

$$V_E = \frac{\left(V_{P1} + V_{P2} + V_{F1}\right)}{3}$$

$$V_{F2} = V_G + V_E$$

$$V_G = V_{F2} - \frac{\left(V_{P1} + V_{P2} + V_{F1}\right)}{3}$$

18.7 Estimation of Components of Genetic Variance

There are four methods for estimating the various components of genetic variance. These are gene frequency and gene effect method, successive generation data, genetic covariance method estimated from resemblance among relatives and multiple mating methods (diallel analysis).

18.7.1. Theoretical Estimation from Gene Effects and Gene Frequency

The additive genetic values due to additive effect of genes (BV) and the dominance deviation of three genotypes are expressed as deviation from the population mean. The mean BV as well as dominance deviation over the 3 genotypes are both zero, because these are estimated from deviated values. Therefore, no correction for assumed mean is required and the variance is simply the mean of squared values. The variance is thus obtained from sum of cross product of the value of genotypes with their frequency. The variance of breeding values and of dominance variance is obtained as:

Table 18.1: Additive Genetic Variance (V_A)

Genotypes	Frequency	B.V.	Freq x (B.V.)²
AA	p^2	$2q\,\alpha$	$4\,p^2q^2\,\alpha^2$
Aa	$2pq$	$(q-p)\,\alpha$	$2pq\,(q-p)^2\,\alpha^2$
Aa	q^2	$-2p\,\alpha$	$4\,p^2q^2\,\alpha^2$
		Sum =	$2pq\,\alpha^2 = \mathbf{V_A}$
		=	$2pq\,[a + d\,(q-p)]^2$

Table 18.2: Dominance Variance (V_D)

Genotypes	Frequency	Dom. Dev.	Freq. x (Dom. Dev.)²
AA	p^2	$-2q^2d$	$4\,p^2q^2\,d^2$
Aa	$2pq$	$2pqd$	$8\,p^3q^3\,d^2$
Aa	q^2	$-2p^2d$	$4\,p^4q^2\,d^2$
		Sum =	$(2pqd)^2 = \mathbf{V_D}$

Total Genetic Variance

The genetic variance can be obtained from genotypic vales but it being lengthy and hence V_G is estimated as sum of V_A and V_D.

Therefore, $G^2 = (A + D)^2$

$$V_G = V_A + V_D + 2\text{Cov}_{AD}$$
$$= V_A + V_D \text{ (since Cov.}_{AD} = 0)$$
$$= 2pq\,\alpha^2 + (2pqd)^2.$$

The breeding value and dominance deviation are not correlated and their covariance is zero.

Breeding Value and Dominance Deviation are not Correlated

The covariance of breeding values with dominance deviation equals zero. This can be shown as under. The covariance is the sum of the cross product of the breeding value, dominance deviation and frequencies of all the three genotypes.

Table 18.3: Correlation between B.V. and Dominance Deviation

Genotypes	Frequencies	B.V.	Dom. Deviation	Cross Products
AA	p^2	$2q\alpha$	$-2\,q^2\,d$	$-4\,p^2q^3\,d\,\alpha$
Aa	$2\,pq$	$(p-q)\,\alpha$	$2\,pqd$	$4\,p^2q^2\,d\,\alpha\,(q-p)$
Aa	q^2	$-2p\,\alpha$	$-2\,p^2\,d$	$4\,p^3q^2\,d\,\alpha$
			Sum =	$4\,p^2q^2\,d\,\alpha\,(-q+q-p+p)$
				$= 0$

Effect of Gene Frequency and Degree of Dominance on Components of V_G

The above expressions of the two components of the genetic variance (V_A and V_D) indicate that their magnitudes are influenced by the gene frequency and the degree of dominance:

When there is no dominance ($d = 0$), the $V_A = 2pq\,\alpha^2$ and
$$V_D = 0.$$

When there is complete dominance ($d = a$), the $V_A = 8pq^3a^2$ and
$$V_D = (2pqa)^2$$

When the frequencies of all the segregating genes are equal ($p = q = 0.5$) as in F_2 population derived from a cross of two highly inbred lines, the genetic components of variance are then become as:

$$V_A = \tfrac{1}{2}a^2$$
$$= \tfrac{1}{2}V_A$$
$$V_D = \tfrac{1}{4}d^2$$
$$= \tfrac{1}{4}V_D$$
$$V_{G(F2)} = V_A + V_D$$
$$= \tfrac{1}{2}V_A + \tfrac{1}{4}V_D$$

With varying gene frequencies and different degree of dominance, the average effect of gene substitution, the total genetic variance and its additive as well as dominance components will vary as under in Table 18.4.

Table 18.4: Genetic Components in Relation to Gene Frequencies and Degree of Dominance

q	α $= a + d\,(q - p)$	V_A $2pq\,\alpha^2$	V_D $(2pqd)^2$	V_G $= V_A + V_D$
I. Taking a = 4, and d = 2				
0.1	2.4	1.04	0.13	1.17
0.2	2.8	2.51	0.41	2.92
0.3	3.2	4.30	0.71	5.01
0.4	3.6-	6.22	0.92	7.14
0.5	4.0	8.00	1.00	9.00
0.6	4.4	9.29	0.92	10.21
0.7	4.8	9.68	0.71	10.39
0.8	5.2	8.65	0.41	9.39
0.9	5.6	5.64	0.13	5.77
1.0	6.0	0.00	0.00	0.00
II. Taking complete dominance (d = a = 4)				
0.1	0.8	0.12	0.52	0.64
0.2	1.6	0.82	1.64	2.46
0.3	2.4	1.01	2.82	3.83
0.4	3.2	4.92	3.69	8.61
05	4.0	8.00	4.00	12.00
0.6	4.8	11.06	3.69	14.75
0.7	5.6	13.17	2.82	15.99
0.8	6.4	13.11	1.64	14.75
0.9	7.2	9.33	0.52	9.85
1.0	8.0	0.00	0.00	0.00

Contd...

Table 18.4–*Contd...*

q	α $= a + d\,(q - p)$	V_A $2pq\,\alpha^2$	V_D $(2pqd)^2$	V_G $= V_A + V_D$
III. Taking no dominance (d = 0), and a = 4				
0.1	4	2.88	0	2.88
0.2	4	5.12	0	5.12
0.3	4	6.72	0	6.72
0.4	4	7.68	0	7.68
0.5	4	8.00	0	8.00
0.6	4	7.68	0	7.68
0.7	4	6.72	0	6.72
0.8	4	5.12	0	5.12
0.9	4	2.88	0	2.88
1.0	4	0.00	0	0.00

From the figures shown in Table 18.4, the followings are evident:

(1) When the gene frequencies are extreme (q= 0, q = 1), the genetic variance and its both the components are all zero and there is an increase in variance as the gene frequencies move towards the middle. Thus, the contribution of genes is more when at intermediate gene frequencies than when at high or low frequencies. The recessives at low frequency contributes very little variance. At extreme gene frequencies the geno-types are homozygous and hence no genetic difference exists whereas the heterozygosity is increased when the gene frequencies moved towards the middle and maximum heterozygosity is attained at intermediate gene frequencies, with $p = q = 0.5$ the 2pq = 0.50 which is maximum than any values of gene frequencies. Thus, maximum genetic diversity in the population exists at intermediate gene frequencies and this give rise to maximum genetic variance.

(2) When there is no dominance (d = 0) tile genetic variance contained only the additive variance and maximum when $p = q = 0.5$.

(3) In case of complete dominance (d = a), the V_A is maximum when q = 0.75, the V_D is maximum when $p = q = 0.5$, and the V_D is maximum when q = 0.7 ($q^2 = 0.5$). Similar magnitude of genetic variance and its two components are obtained when there is semi dominance.

(4) In case of over dominance (a = 0), the V_D is same as with complete dominance. However, the V_A is zero when $p = q = 0.5$ but V_A is maximum at q = 0.15 and q = 0.85 whereas the V_D is constant over a wide range of gene frequencies.

Multiple Alleles at a Locus

The existence of multiple alleles at a locus complicates the theoretical description of the effect of the locus, though the same principle is followed. The average effect of multiple alleles at a locus contributes to the additive genetic variance and several dominance deviations give rise to the dominance variance.

Interaction Variance

The contributions of genes at different loci affecting a trait to the genetic variation are additive when the genes at different loci are independent in action and in inheritance (no linkage).

The separate effect of all the loci affecting a trait is added to get the variance components, in a random mating population which is in equilibrium. The additive genetic variances attributable to each locus separately are added together and the sum of the contribution of all loci is taken as the additive genetic variance. Likewise, the dominance variance is the sum of the dominance variances contributed by all loci separately.

When a trait is affected by more than one locus, as in case of metric traits, then another component of genetic variance is present due to the epistatic effect of genes (interaction deviation). The interaction deviation, if present, gives rise to the interaction variance. This interaction variance denoted by V_I is the variance of the interaction deviations. The differences in epistatic effects of genes between individuals give rise to the epistatic or interaction variance (V_I).

The interaction between loci affecting a trait occurs frequently. The interaction may be between two loci (digenic interaction) or more loci and it may be between breeding values or dominance deviations at different loci. Thus, $V_I = V_{AA} + V_{AD} + V_{DD}$. Very little is known about the relative importance of interaction variance as a source of the variation. The estimation of the amount of variance generated by the interaction deviations (interaction variance, V_I) is not easy. The interaction variance is included with the dominance component and referred as the non-additive genetic variance. The V_I contributes very little to the resemblance between relatives.

In estimating the coefficients of the interaction variance of different kinds (V_{AA}, V_{AD} and V_{DD}), the products of the coefficients of V_A and V_D are taken. For example, the genetic Variance of F_2 generation will be made of the following component parts –

$$V_{G(F2)} = \tfrac{1}{2} V_A + \tfrac{1}{4} V_D + V_I$$
$$\text{Where,} \quad V_A = (a_A + \tfrac{1}{2} i_A)^2$$
$$V_D = (d_A + \tfrac{1}{2} I_A)^2$$
$$V_I = \tfrac{1}{4} (i)^2 + {}_{1/8} (j)^2 + {}_{1/16}(l)^2$$
$$= \tfrac{1}{4} V_{AA} + {}_{1/8} V_{AD} + {}_{1/16} V_{DD}$$

Disequilibrium Variance

The disequilibrium component of variance arises when the population is not in equilibrium under random mating. The disequilibrium is a situation when the genotypic frequencies are not in accordance to the gamete frequencies for two or more loci considered jointly. This disequilibrium condition gives rise to the variation as explained below:

Assuming two loci which do not interact with each other, the genotypic values of individuals for two loci separately are G_1 and G_2 such that the genotypic value for both loci jointly is $(G = G_1 + G_2)$. The variance due to the two loci will be:

$$V_G = V_{G1} + V_{G2} + 2Cov_{G1G2}.$$

The covariance term is the correlation between the genotypic values at two loci in different individuals. The effect of disequilibrium to increase or decrease the variance depends on the positive or negative correlation. The covariance is zero where there is no disequilibrium.

The disequilibrium is caused by two types of non random mating which is the selection of parents and the assortative mating. These produce two kinds of covariance which represents different correla-tions of gene effects. *e.g.* correlation between genes at different loci in the same gamete (gametic phase or linkage disequilibrium) and the correlation between the genes in uniting pairs of gametes (between the genes the individual receives from its two parents). The selected parents mated at random produces first type of covariance due to gametic phase disequilibrium. The asortative mating creates both types of covariance.

18.7.2 Quantitative Estimation from Successive Generation

(1) Variance of True Breeding Lines and their F_1

A cross is made between two inbred true breeding lines having genetically uniform individuals within the lines, say P_1 line with AA genotype and P_2 line with aa genotype. The F_1 produced by crossing these two lines will have the individuals all with Aa genotype. All these three populations (P_1, P_2, F_1) are genetically uniform and hence there is no genetic variation within line. However there is variation in phenotypic measurements (phenotypic variance) among the individu-als within both the lines $(P_1$ and $P_2)$ and F_1. This variation will be entirely the environmental variance. However, the phenotypic vari-ance of these 3 populations will be of different magnitude. This is because the F_1 individuals are heterozygous and hence less susceptible to environmental conditions than the individuals of P_1 and P_2 lines which are homozygous. As a result the environment will have more effect on the phenotypic values of the individuals of P_1 and P_2 lines than the individuals of F_1 generation. Thus the environmental variance of P_1 and P_2 lines will be more than F_1 generation. Therefore, the mean phenotypic variance of all the three populations is taken as the true estimate of the *environmental variance* as

$$V_E = \frac{(V_{P1} + V_{P2} + V_{F1})}{3}$$

The successive generations produced from parental lines and F_1 generations are the F_2 generation and the two back cross generations.

(2) Genetic Variance of F_2

The F_2 is a segregating generation for genetic differences among its members. The constitution of F_2 population with respect to the frequencies of the individuals of three genotypes will be AA: ½ Aa: aa, and the genotypic values will be a, d, and – a respectively. The mean of F_2 population will be ½d:

The genetic variance of F_2 generation will be obtained as the sum of the squared deviation of each genotype from mean of F_2 multiplying with genotypic frequency as

Genotypes	Freq.	Value	Deviation	Freq.x (Deviation)²
AA	¼	a	a – ½ d	¼ (a – ½d)²
Aa	½	d	d – ½d	½ (½ d)²
aa	¼	– a	– a – ½d	¼ (-a – ½ d)²

The sum of squares of deviations will be:

$$= ¼ (a - ½ d)^2 + ½ (¼ d^2) + ¼ (-a - ½ d)^2$$
$$= ¼ (a^2 + ½ d^2 - ad) + ½ (¼ d^2) + ¼ (a^2 + ¼ d^2 + ad)$$
$$= ¼ a^2 + {}_{1/16} d^2 - ¼ ad + {}_{1/8} d^2 + ¼ a^2 + {}_{1/16} d^2 + ¼ ad$$
$$= ¼ a^2 + ¼ a^2 + {}_{1/16} d^2 + {}_{1/8} d^2 + {}_{1/16} d^2$$
$$= ½ a^2 + ¼ d^2$$

Therefore, the genetic variance of F_2 generation will be:

$$V_{G (F2)} = ½ a^2 + ¼d^2$$
$$= ½ V_A + ¼ V_D$$

The total variance of F_2 generation which also includes the environmental variance will be

$$V_{P(F2)} = ½ V_A + ¼ V_D + V_E$$

Thus the genetic variance of F_2 generation can be partitioned into two components. The first is V_A (additive genetic variance) which depends upon a and measures the difference between homozygotes and this V_A is fixable. The second part is V_D which depends upon d and measures the gene action in heterozygotes and cannot be fixed in selection.

(3) Genetic Variance of Back Crosses

The two back crosses are produced by mating F_1 with two respective parents (P_1 and P_2) as:

$$B_1 = F_1 \times P_1 \text{ and } B_2 = F_1 \times P_2$$

The constitution of both the backcrosses will be that they will have half the offspring homozygotes and another half heterozygotes for each gene pair by which the parent differ. Thus can be shown as under

F_1	x	P_1		F_1	x	P_2
(Aa)	↓	(AA)		(Aa)	↓	(aa)

$$B_1 = ½ \text{ AA}: ½ \text{ Aa} \quad \text{and} \quad B_2 = ½\text{Aa}: ½ \text{ aa}$$

The *population mean of B₁ generation* will be:

Genotype	Freq.	Value	Freq. x Value
AA	½	a	½a
Aa	½	d	½d
	B₁ Mean = ½a + ½d		

The *population mean of B₂ generation* will be

Genotype	Freq.	Value	Freq. x Value
Aa	½	d	½d
aa	½	– a	– ½ a
	B₂ Mean = – ½ a + ½d		

Genetic variance of B₁ generation will be obtained as

Genotype	Freq.	Value	Freq. x (deviation)²
AA	½	a	½ (a – ½a – ½d)²
Aa	½	d	½(d – ½a – ½d)²

Sum $= ½ (½a - ½d)² + ½ (-½a + ½d)²$

   $= ½ (¼a² + ¼d² – ½ ad) + ½ (¼a² + ¼d² - ½ ad)$

   $= ¼ a² + ¼ d²$ (Since ad are zero)

   $= ¼V_A + ¼V_D$

   $= V_{G (B1)}$

Thus, the phenotypic variance of B₁ will be

$V_{P (B1)}$ $= ¼V_A + ¼ V_D + V_E$

Genetic variance of B₂ generation will be obtained as

Genotype	Freq.	Value	Freq. x (Deviation)²
aa	½	– a	½ (-a + ½ a – ½ d)²
Aa	½	d	½ (d + ½a – ½d)²

Sum $= ½ (-½a – ½d)² + ½ (½ a + ½d)²$

   $= ½ (¼ a² + ¼ d² + ½ ad) + ½ (¼a² + ¼ d² + ½ ad)$

   $= ¼ a² + ¼ d²$ (Since ad = 0)

$$= \tfrac{1}{4}V_A + \tfrac{1}{4}V_D$$

$$= V_{G\,(B2)}$$

The phenotypic variance of B_2 is

$$V_{P\,(B2)} = \tfrac{1}{4}\,V_A + \tfrac{1}{4}\,V_D + V_E$$

The above expressions of the phenotypic and genetic variances of B_1 and B_2 generations indicate that these are same for the two generations. –

The phenotypic variances of these 3 segregating generations may now be summarized as:

$$V_{P\,(F2)} = \tfrac{1}{2}\,V_A + \tfrac{1}{4}V_D + V_E$$

$$V_{P\,(B1)} = \tfrac{1}{4}\,V_A + \tfrac{1}{4}\,V_D + V_E$$

$$V_{P\,(B2)} = \tfrac{1}{4}\,V_A + \tfrac{1}{4}\,V_D + V_E$$

The sum of the phenotypic variances of B_1 and B_2 generation will be

$$V_{P\,(B1)} + V_{P\,(B2)} = \tfrac{1}{2}\,V_A + \tfrac{1}{2}\,V_D + 2\,V_E$$

The $V_{G\,(B1)}$ and $V_{G\,(B2)}$ are estimated by substracting the V_E from their phenotypic variances. Thus, sum of the genetic variances of the two back crosses is

$$V_{G\,(B1)} + V_{G\,(B2)} = \tfrac{1}{2}\,V_A + \tfrac{1}{2}\,V_D \text{ and}$$

$$V_{G\,(F2)} = \tfrac{1}{2}\,V_A + \tfrac{1}{4}V_D$$

Therefore, substracting genetic variance of F_2 from the sum of the genetic variances of the two back crosses estimates $\tfrac{1}{4}\,V_D$. The V_D is thus 4 times the difference between the sum of the genetic variance of the two back crosses and the genetic variance of F_2

$$V_A = 4\,[V_{G\,(B1)} + V_{G\,(B2)} - V_{G\,(F2)}]$$

Now substracting the V_D from V_G estimates the V_A as:

$$V_A = V_G - V_D.$$

Evidence of Dominance

The evidence of dominance is indicated in two ways. The first is the deviation of F_1 mean from mid parent value. The direction of deviation of F_1 mean from the mid parent value indicates that which parent (P_1 or P_2) carry the preponderance of dominant alleles. Second evidence comes from the difference between the variance of two back crosses ($V_{B1} - V_{B2}$) which should equal to Σad. Thus, Σad represents the difference between genetic variances of the two back crosses and $\Sigma ad = \sqrt{\dfrac{V_D}{V_A}}$. This difference in genetic variances should be equal to zero ($\Sigma ad = V_{G\,(B1)} - V_{G\,(B2)} = 0$) in case of no dominance. On the contrary, the dominance is indicated when Σad is not equal to zero.

The difference between the genetic variances of the two backcrosses (Σad) must equal to zero under the following conditions:

(i) When F_1 mean equals mid parent value $\left[\overline{F_1} = \dfrac{(\overline{P_1} + \overline{P_2})}{2} \right]$. This indicates no dominance.

(ii) When both the parents are equal in expression of the character.

The degree of dominance is expressed by $\dfrac{d}{a}$. When $\dfrac{d}{a}$ is constant in magnitude for all gene pairs affecting a trait (though not necessarily constant in sign), the additional evidence of dominance is provided by the difference between the variances of two backcrosses which equal Σad. The Σad will equal $\sqrt{V_A V_D}$, then $\dfrac{d}{a} = \sqrt{\dfrac{V_D}{V_A}}$ is a measure of the degree of dominance. This $\sqrt{\dfrac{V_D}{V_A}}$ provides an estimate of the average dominance of the genes.

If the degree of dominance $\left(\dfrac{d}{a} \right)$ differ, it then results Σad small to $\sqrt{V_A V_D}$. The difference between Σad and $\sqrt{V_A V_D}$ will be more, if the variation in d/a is more from one gene pair to another. The degree of dominance differs from one gene pair to another, in case the Σad and $\sqrt{V_A V_D}$ differ too much. A large difference between Σad and $\sqrt{V_A V_D}$ indicate that besides the preponderance of dominant genes in P_1 parent, there are some dominant genes in P_2 parent.

In this case, a and d effects are balanced respectively in the sense that Σad with positive sign will be equal to Σad with negative sign. There is thus the evidence of dominance when Σad is not equal to 0. Therefore, if the two backcrosses differ in their variances, it indicates the evidence of dominance because $V_{B1} - V_{B2}$ should equal to Σad when there is no dominance.

The back cross with low variance indicates the preponderance of dominant alleles carried by that parent of the parental generation from which the backcross is derived. Thus the back cross with parent having preponderance of dominant alleles will have low variance. Therefore, $V_{G(B1)} - V_{G(B2)} = \Sigma ad$ which represents the evidence of dominance. When all d's are of the same sign (all dominant genes are present in one parent) the Σad must equal to $\sqrt{V_A V_D}$. On the other hand, if Σad is not equal to $\sqrt{V_D V_A}$ it then indicates that the dominant genes are present in both the parents (P_1 and P_2), a case of dispersed genes.

The second estimate of the distribution of the dominant genes in two parents is the degree of dominance ($\sqrt{V_D / V_A}$). If the degree of dominance is equal to one it indicates that all dominant genes are present in one parent and when less than one it then indicates that both parents have dominant genes.

The difference between Σ ad and $\sqrt{V_A V_D}$ indicates the followings:

☆ Evidence of dominance,

☆ Degree of dominance differ from one gene pair to another,

☆ Preponderance of dominant genes in one parent

☆ Dominant genes were distributed in both the parental generation with more number of genes in one parent.

18.7.3 Genetic Method (Resemblance among relatives)

The genetic covariance among relatives computed from phenotypic values recorded on relatives is translated into the genetic variance. This procedure is based on resemblance among relatives. The procedure has been detailed in next chapter 15 on resemblance among relatives.

18.7.4 Multiple Matings Method

These include the diallel analysis, triallel and quadrilallel, and other designs (North Carolina Design). These designs are used in plant breeding for the reason that a number of varieties are grown whereas in animal science it is not possible to keep more numbers of breeds.

Solved Examples

Example 18.1

Estimate the genetic variance and its components from the information given below. p=0.6, q=0.4, a=16, d=2

Geno.	Freq.	G	B.V.	Dom. Dev.
AA	0.36	11.84	12.48	– 0.64
Aa	0.48	–2.16	–3.12	0.96
aa	0.16	–20.16	–18.12	– 1.44

Solution

All the values have been expressed as deviations from the population mean and hence the variance is obtained by multiplying the frequency of each genotype by the square of its value and summing over all the three genotypes. The V_G, V_A and V_D are thus estimated as under:

$$V_G = p^2 g^2_{11} + 2pqg^2_{12} + q^2 g^2_{22}$$
$$= 0.36\,(11.84)^2 + 0.48(-2.16)^2 + 0.16(-20.16)^2.$$
$$= 50.4668 + 2.2395 + 65.0281$$
$$= 117.7344$$
$$V_A = p^2 a^2_{11} + 2pqa^2_{12} + q^2 a^2_{22}$$

$$= 0.36 \, (12.48)^2 + 0.48 \, (3.12)^2 + 0.16 \, (-18.72)^2$$

$$= 56.0701 + 4.6725 + 56.0701$$

$$= 116.8127$$

$V_D = p^2 d^2_{11} + 2pq d^2_{12} + q^2 d^2_{22}$

$\quad = 0.36 \, (-0.64)^2 + 0.48 \, (0.96)^2 + 0.16 \, (1.44)^2$

$\quad = 0.1475 + 0.4423 + 0.3318$

$\quad = 0.9216$

The V_G and its two components (V_A and V_D) can also be obtained directly by using their formulae as under:

$V_A = 2pq\alpha^2 = 2pq \, [a + d \, (q - p)]^2$

where, $\quad p = 0.6, q = 0.4,$

$\qquad\qquad a = 16, \text{ and } d = 2$

$\qquad\qquad \alpha = 16 + 2 \, (0.4 - 0.6) = 16 - 0.4$

$\qquad\qquad\quad = 15.6$

$V_A = 2 \times 0.6 \times 0.4 \, (15.6)^2$

$\quad = 116.8128$

$V_D = (2pqd)^2$

$\quad = (2 \times 0.6 \times 0.4 \times 2)^2$

$\quad = 0.9216$

$V_G = V_A + V_D$

$\quad = 116.8128 + 0.9216$

$\quad = 117.7344$

Example 18.2

The relation between genes affecting size and colour in certain species of Nicotiana has been studied by Smith (1937). The results obtained in crosses between tobacco species (Nicotiana) which differed in their flower length are given below -

Generations	No.	Mean	V_p
P_1	47	1292	48
P_2	62	37	32
F_1	38	742	46
F_2	180	684.4	130.5
B_1	56	106.5	85.5
B_2	140	314.5	98.5

Estimate the components of genetic variance and environmental variance. Also interpret the results in terms of the dominance.

Solution

$$m = \frac{(1297 + 37)}{2} = 664.5$$

(i) Variance components:

$$V_E = \frac{(48 + 32 + 46)}{3} = 42$$

$$V_{G(F2)} = V_{P(F2)} - V_E$$
$$= 130.5 - 42.0 = 88.5$$
$$= \tfrac{1}{2} V_A + \tfrac{1}{4} V_D$$

$$V_{G(B1)} = V_{P(B1)} - V_E$$
$$= 85.5 - 42.0 = 43.5$$
$$= \tfrac{1}{4} V_A + \tfrac{1}{4} V_D$$

$$V_{G(B2)} = V_{P(B2)} - V_E$$
$$= 98.5 - 42.0 = 56.5$$
$$= \tfrac{1}{4} V_A + \tfrac{1}{4} V_D$$

$$V_{G(B1)} + V_{G(B2)} = 43.5 + 56.5$$
$$= 100.0$$
$$= \tfrac{1}{2} V_A + \tfrac{1}{2} V_D$$

From above, V_D can be computed as:

$$V_{G(B1)} + V_{G(B2)} - V_{G(F2)} = \tfrac{1}{4} V_D$$
$$43.5 + 56.5 - 88.5 \qquad = 11.5$$
$$= \tfrac{1}{4} V_D$$

Therefore, $V_D = 11.5 \times 4 = 46.0$

Similarly, V_A can be computed as:

$$V_{G(F2)} - \tfrac{1}{4} V_D \qquad\qquad = \tfrac{1}{2} V_A$$
$$88.5 - 11.5 = 77 \qquad\qquad = \tfrac{1}{2} V_A$$

Therefore, $V_A = 77.0 \times 2 \quad = 154$

(ii) Dominance effect:

(a) The F_1 exceeded over mid parent value towards P_1 parent. This indicated dominance effect and that too showing the preponderance of dominance of genes from P_1 parent.

Further, it was observed that B_1 averaged 1065 with average mid parent value as $1017 = [(1292 + 742)/2]$ and B_2 averaged 314.5 with average mid parent value as $389 = [(37 + 742)/2]$ indicated again the preponderance of dominant alleles in P_1 parent because B_1 averaged higher than mid parent value, while B_2 averaged lower than mid parent value. The F_2 mean was lower (648.4) than the F_1 mean (742) which indicated the regression towards P_2 parent and can be explained due to segregation of genes.

The environmental variance (V_E) was the only source of variance in parental and F_1 generations and it varied from 32 to 48 with an average $(48+32+46)/3 = 42$.

The degree of dominance (d/a) is:

$$\frac{d}{a} = \sqrt{\frac{V_D}{V_A}}$$

$$= \sqrt{\frac{46}{154}}$$

$$= 0.55$$

This provides an estimate of the average dominance of the genes.

(b) The additional evidence of dominance is provided by the difference between the variances of the two back crosses, if the measure of dominance (d/a) is constant in magnitude for all gene pairs. This difference $(V_{B1} - V_{B2})$ equals Σad. The Σad will equal to $\sqrt{V_A V_D}$ in case of no dominance.

Thus $\Sigma ad = V_{B1} - V_{B2} = \sqrt{V_A V_D}$

$$= 98.5 - 85.5 = 13 \text{ and}$$

$$\sqrt{V_A V_D} = \sqrt{46 \times 154} = 84$$

Therefore, in this case Σad is not equal to $\sqrt{V_A V_D}$ and hence it indicated dominance.

If the degree of dominance (d/a) differ, it then results Σad small to $\sqrt{V_A V_D}$. The difference between Σad and $\sqrt{V_A V_D}$ will be more, if the variation in d/a is more from one gene pair to another. In the above case the Σad and $\sqrt{V_A V_D}$ differ too much and thus it indicated that the degree of dominance differ from one gene pair to another. And also such a large difference between Σad and $\sqrt{V_A V_D}$ indicate that besides the preponderance of dominant genes in P_1 parent, there are some dominant genes in P_2 parent, which was also evident from degree of dominance being 0.55 and thus the dominants genes were distributed in both the parental generation (P_1 and P_2) with more number of them in P_1 parent.

Example 18.3

Find out the components of variance, degree of dominance and heritability for flowering time in wheat from following data:

	Varieties and their Crosses	Mean	Variance $_{(P)}$
P_1	Early flowering	12.99	11.04
P_2	Late flowering	27.61	10.32
F_1		18.45	5.24
F_2		21.20	40.35
B_1		15.63	17.35
B_2		22.88	34.29

Solution

(i) *Variance components:*

Average $V_E = (11.04 + 10.32 + 5.24)/3 = 8.87$

$V_{G\,(F2)} = \frac{1}{2} V_A + \frac{1}{2} V_D = 40.35 - 8.87 = 31.48$

$V_{G\,(B1)} = \frac{1}{4} V_A + \frac{1}{4} V_A = 17.35 - 8.87 = 8.48$

$V_{B\,(B2)} = \frac{1}{4} V_A + \frac{1}{4} V_A = 34.29 - 8.87 = 25.42$

$V_{G\,(B1)} + V_{G\,(B2)} = \frac{1}{2} V_A + \frac{1}{2} V_D = 38.90$

Now, $\frac{1}{4} V_D = 33.9 - 31.48 = 2.40$ and

$V_D = 2.40 \times 4 = 9.6$

$\frac{1}{2} V_A = 31.48 - 2.40$

$= 29.08$ and

$V_A = 29.08 \times 2 = 58.16$

The variance components are as:

$V_P = V_A + V_D + V_E$

$= 58.16 + 9.6 + 8.87$

$= 76.63$

(ii) *Evidence of dominance*: This can be obtained in two ways as under:

$$\text{Degree of dominance} = \frac{d}{a} = \sqrt{\frac{V_D}{V_A}}$$

$$= \sqrt{\frac{9.6}{58.16}} = 0.406$$

(a) Σ ad $= V_{G(B1)} - V_{G(B2)}$

$\qquad = 25.42 - 8.48 = 16.94$

$$\sqrt{V_A V_D} = \sqrt{58.16 \times 9.6} = 23.63$$

The Σ ad and $\sqrt{V_A V_D}$ differed and this difference indicates the followings:

— Evidence of dominance,

— Degree of dominance differ from one gene pair to another,

— Preponderance of dominant genes in one parent and

— Dominant genes were distributed in both the parental generation with more number of genes in one parent.

(b) Mid parent value $= \dfrac{(12.99 + 27.61)}{2} = 20.30$

$\qquad$ F$_1$ mean $= 18.45$

$\qquad$ F$_1 - $m $= 20.3 - 18.45 = 1.85$

Thus, F$_1$ mean deviates from **m** towards P$_1$ and hence it indicated the preponderance of dominant genes in P$_1$ parent.

$\qquad$ B$_1$ mean $= 15.63$ and

$\qquad$ m between F$_1$ and P$_1 = \dfrac{(18.45 + 12.99)}{2} = 15.72$

$\qquad$ B$_2$ mean $= 22.80$ and

$\qquad$ m between F$_1$ and P$_2 = \dfrac{(18.45 + 27.61)}{2} = 23.03$

Thus, the mean values of F$_1$, B$_1$ and B$_2$ deviated towards P$_1$ parent.

(iii) Heritability $= \dfrac{V_A}{V_P}$

$\qquad = \dfrac{58.16}{76.63} = 0.759$

This indicated that 75.9 percent of the total variation in flowering time is due to additive genetic differences.

Chapter 19
Resemblance among Relatives

The relatives are more alike genetically than unrelatives. Thus, the relatives will tend to look more alike for a given trait (similar performance) than unrelatives. This is called as resemblance among relatives. The resemblance among relatives for metric traits is measured from observations recorded on individuals of a population, is basic to the study of the genetics of quantitative characters, is the property of the character, and used to estimate the amount of additive genetic variance which forms the basis of estimating heritability. The additive genetic variance is heritable and fixed component of genotypic variance, and used to determine the best breeding method for genetic improvement.

19.1 Causes of Resemblance

A group of related individuals have similar performance (look alike) for any metric character because they have common genes and also share common environment. The similarity in performance (resemblance) is increased with increase in number of common genes. The more close relatives have more number of common genes and hence show more resemblance (similarity). Therefore, the relatives will have similar performance in metric traits, if they share more common genes and also they will inherit more number of common genes to their progeny. On the contrary, the relatives will have less similarity in performance if they share less common genes and hence they will inherit less common genes to their progeny.

The common environment shared by relatives has also the similar effect to cause similarity in performance among relatives. The resemblance among relatives is increased with increase of common genes and common environment or vice versa.

Therefore, the common genes and the common environment shared by the relatives are the determinants of resemblance among relatives.

The extent of resemblance between relatives thus depends on the extent to which the relatives have

☆ Genes in common

☆ Genotypes in common

☆ Common environment

19.2 Measurement of Resemblance

The resemblance (similarity) in performance of relatives shows that they (relatives) are correlated genetically as well as environmentally to some degree with each other. The correlation among relatives for a trait can be estimated as a measure of resemblance among them. The different kinds of relatives are parent – offspring, half sibs, and full sibs that are easily available in farm animals.

The correlation among relatives is measured by the covariance among them. The covariance among relatives is thus used to measure the resemblance among them (relatives). Therefore, it requires the estimation of the amount of covariance (co-variation) that exists among the individuals of a group.

The covariance is a part of the total phenotypic variance and hence the *covariance is taken as a proportion of the total variance.* The covariance between relatives expresses the amount of variation common to the members of a group and is equivalent to the corresponding variance components between that group of relatives attributed to the cause and the extent of genetic relationship (Table 19.1). The degree of resemblance among relatives, in terms of the covariance, is thus measured by partitioning the phenotypic variance into its components corresponding to the grouping of individuals. Therefore, a population is divided in a number of groups depending on the genetic relationship between relative *viz.* parent-offspring groups, half sib groups and full sib groups.

Covariance among Relatives Equals to the Variance Component Corresponding to Group of Relatives

The covariance measures the resemblance and equals the variance (which measures the differences among the groups of relatives). For example, the covariance between half sib is equal to the sire variance because the half sibs are related by sharing common genes of the same sire and hence common sire is the cause of relation. Further, the genetic relationship between half sibs is 25 per cent which is due to their common breeding values. Thus, $\text{Cov}_{(HS)}$ = sire variance = $\frac{1}{4} V_A$. Likewise, the covariance between full sibs is equivalent to sire plus dam variance because they are the progenies of same sire and same dam and they have 50 per cent genetic relationship due to their common breeding values. Therefore, $\text{Cov}_{(FS)} = \sigma^2_s + \sigma^2_d = \frac{1}{2} V_A + \frac{1}{4} V_D$. Mathematically, this has been shown in estimating the genetic covariance among relatives.

It is therefore that the covariance measures the degree of resemblance between relatives based on the grouping of individuals into families *viz.* sire families or dam families (half-sibs), sire-dam families (full sibs), parent-offspring (sire-daughter groups) etc. and used to partition the phenotypic variance into variance components corresponding to the group of relatives.

Table 19.1: Relation of Covariance (Resemblance) among Relatives with Variance Components

Relatives	Covar. = Variance Comp.	Regression (b) or Correlation (r)
Offspring-one parent	$Cov_{Op} = \frac{1}{2} V_A + \frac{1}{4} V_I$	$b = \frac{1}{2} \dfrac{V_A}{V_P}$
Offspring-mid parent	$Cov_{OP} = \frac{1}{2} V_A$	$b = \dfrac{V_A}{V_P}$
Half-sibs	$Cov_{HS} = \frac{1}{4} V_A + \frac{1}{16} V_I$	$r = \frac{1}{4} \dfrac{V_A}{V_P}$
Full sibs	$Cov_{FS} = \frac{1}{2} V_A + \frac{1}{4} V_D + V_{Ec}$	$r = \frac{1}{2} V_A + \frac{1}{4} \dfrac{V_D}{V_P}$

where, $\quad V_P = \frac{1}{2} V_P$ but $V_P = \sigma^2_P$;

$\qquad\qquad V_P = V_O$ and hence $V_P/V_O = \sigma^2_P$

$\qquad\qquad h^2 = 2 b_{OS} = 2b_{OD} = b_{OP} = 2 r_{OP}$

The analysis of variance is conducted to partition the total observed variance of a character into the following two components:

Between group variance (σ^2_B), is variance of means of groups about the population mean,

Within group variance ($\sigma^2_W = \sigma^2 e$), is variance of individuals of a group about their group mean.

The between group component of variance (sire variance, etc.) as a proportion of the total variance expresses the amount of variation common to members of the same group and called as the intra – class correlation. This amount of variance is equally referred to as the covariance of members of the same group.

Similarity within Group vs Variance between Groups

The resemblance (similarity) between relatives can be taken either as similarity of individuals of a group or as the differences between individuals of different groups. It is proper to think that more is the similarity within a group of relatives more will be the differences between groups. Therefore, the amount of similarity (degree of resemblance) can be expressed as a proportion of between group components to the total variance, expressed by intra class correlation (t) as: $t = \dfrac{\sigma^2_B}{\left(\sigma^2_B + \sigma^2_W\right)}$

The variance among groups is a measure of the similarity within group. This can be understood by two situations of large and small variation between groups.

(i) Large Variation between Groups

When there will be large variance between groups, the variance within group will be small. This indicates that individuals belonging to a group (*e.g.* half sibs or full sibs) are more similar (resemble) in their performance and hence they will have their phenotypic values closer to the mean phenotypic value of their group and so variance within group will be small but the variance among group means will be large which will result into large intra class correlation.

(ii) Small Variation within Group

On the contrary, when variation between groups is small but within group variation is large, this will indicate that individuals of a group are not similar in their performance (phenotypic values) but have their phenotypic values widely spread about their group mean. This will result small variance among means of the groups compared to the variance among individuals within group and thus intra class correlation will be small. Therefore, the magnitude of intra class correlation is an indication of the amount to which the means of the different groups differ from each other.

Extent of Common Genes:

The factor of having genes in common by the relatives causes the additive genetic relationship between them, denoted by '*a*' and this means that they have the same B.V. because the additive genetic relationship (*a*) is due to the additive effect of genes. The resemblance between relatives is also affected by the differences in B.V. of the individuals of a population. This can be understood by taking the similarity and differences in the B.V. of the members of a population.

(i) Similarity in B.V.

When all members of a population, whether relatives or not, have exactly the same set of genes. This indicates that they have the same B.V. and hence $V_A = 0.0$. In this case, there will be no contribution of having genes in common by the relatives to the resemblance between relatives.

(ii) Differences in B.V.

The variation in B.V. means that there exists the V_A in the population. Thus, different genes exist in unrelated individuals within a population. In this situation, the resemblance between relatives will increase along the extent to which the relatives have genes in common compared with unrelated individuals of the population. In this way, the importance of having genes in common depends on the extent of V_A in the population. The maximum value of V_A equals V_P ($V_A = V_P$) and hence the relative importance of having genes in common equal $\dfrac{V_A}{V_P}$ which is the heritability. Therefore, the resemblance between relatives increases with the increase in additive genetic relationship ((a) and h^2. The resemblance due to having genes in common equals ah^2 when the relatives are not inbred. This is the basis of estimating heritability. Therefore,

Resemblance = ah^2

$$h^2 = \frac{\text{Resemblance}}{a}$$

where, a is the additive genetic relationship

In a similar way, the contribution of having genotypes in common to the resemblance between relatives depends on the values of $\frac{V_D}{V_P}$ and $\frac{V_I}{V_P}$ whereas the contribution of having environment in common depends on $\frac{V_{EC}}{V_P}$.

Now, taking the effect of all the factors causing resemblance between relatives, the total resemblance will be as –

$$\text{Resemblance} = ah^2 + d\left(\frac{V_D}{V_P}\right) + \frac{V_{EC}}{V_P}$$

where, d is the probability of relatives having same genotype

(dominance relationship)

V_I is ignored for relatively unimportant

The heritability is thus estimated as:

$$h^2 = \frac{\text{Resemblance}}{a} = \frac{ah^2}{a} + \frac{d\,V_D}{a\,V_P} + \frac{a\,V_{EC}}{a\,V_P}$$

$$= h^2 + \frac{d\,V_D}{a\,V_P} + \frac{V_{EC}}{V_P}$$

It is thus clear that h^2 estimate becomes biased upward if the relatives have genotypes or environment in common. However, this biasness can be eliminated.

Observational vs Causal Components

The variance components estimated directly from observations (phenotypic values) based on the degree of resemblance between relatives are called as observational components, denoted as σ^2 like sire variance (σ^2_S) which is Cov $_{HS}$ or dam variance (σ^2_D) which equals Cov $_{FS}$ – Cov $_{HS}$. The Cov $_{FS}$ = $\sigma^2_S + \sigma^2_D$.

The causal components are the components of phenotypic variance attributable to different genetic and environmental causes (estimated in preceding chapter), denoted by the symbol V, like additive genetic variance (V_A), dominance variance (V_D), interaction variance (V_I).

19.3 Phenotypic Resemblance

The significance of estimating the degree of resemblance between relatives is to estimate the proportionate amount of additive genetic variance to the total phenotypic variance, $\dfrac{V_A}{V_P}$. The degree of resemblance is observed from measurements of phenotypic values of relatives and expressed as a regression or correlation by dividing the covariance among relatives with the appropriate variance.

(1) Correlation and Regression Analysis

The degree of resemblance between offspring and parent is expressed as the regression of offspring on parent. The offspring receives only ½ its inheritance from either parent. Therefore, the regression of progeny on one parent measures only ½ the genetic variation.

$$b_{OP} = \frac{1}{2}\frac{\sigma^2_A}{\sigma^2_P} \qquad \text{for single parent}$$

where, σ^2_P is the phenotypic variance of parent.

In case of mid parent value, the covariance is to be divided by the variance of mid parent value which is half the phenotypic variance giving the regression as:

$$b_{OP} = \frac{\sigma^2_A}{\sigma^2_P}$$

The regression coefficient of one sib on another can also be determined. The correlation between two variables is about equal to the regression of one variable on the other, in case of equal variances of two samples. The degree of resemblance is also thus taken as a correlation between sibs.

(2) Analysis of Variance

The full sibs are the members of the same family and likewise are the half sibs. Thus, the FS and HS are genetically more alike among themselves than individuals from different families. Therefore, analysis of variance can be used to compare variation within families to the variation among families. The families are of full sibs as well as of half sibs.

$$r_{HS} = \frac{1}{4}\left(\frac{\sigma^2_A}{\sigma^2_P}\right)$$

$$r_{FS} = \frac{1}{2}\left(\sigma^2_A + \frac{1}{2}\sigma^2_D + \frac{\sigma^2_{EC}}{\sigma^2_P}\right)$$

19.3.1. Genetic Resemblance (Covariance)

The common genes shared by the relatives cause the genetic covariance between relatives and hence it is estimated depending on the type of relatives. The genetic covariance between relatives can be obtained either using the concept of the coefficient of parentage (Malecot, 1948) or from observations made on relatives.

I. Genetic Covariance from Observations

The genetic covariance can be estimated directly from observations (phenotypic values) recorded on relatives and this comes equal to the genetic covariance obtained using the concept of the coefficient of parentage based on the probability of genes, identical by descent, possessed by two related individuals.

(i) Covariance between Offspring and One Parent

This is equal to the cross product of the genotypic value of parent and its offspring. Expressing the value as deviation from population mean, the mean genotypic value of offspring is half of the breeding value of the parent. Thus the covariance of parent offspring (Cov_{OP}) is:

$$\text{Cov}_{OP} = \text{Parent value} \times \text{Mean of offspring}$$
$$= G\,(\tfrac{1}{2}A) = [(A+D)\,\tfrac{1}{2}A]$$
$$= \tfrac{1}{2}A^2 + \tfrac{1}{2}AD$$
$$= \tfrac{1}{2}V_A \text{ since, A and D are uncorrelated}$$

where,   G is the genotypic value of parent and equals to A + D

A^2 is the sum of squares of breeding values

The regression coefficient as an expression of degree of resemblance is obtained by dividing the Cov_{OP} with the total phenotypic variance of parent (V_P). Thus

$$b_{OP} = \frac{\text{Cov}_{OP}}{V_P}$$

$$= \frac{1}{2}\frac{V_A}{V_P}$$

$$r_{OP} = \frac{\text{Cov}_{OP}}{V_P\,V_O}$$

$$= \frac{\text{Cov}_{PO}}{V_P} \quad \text{Since } V_P = V_O$$

$$= \frac{1}{2}\frac{V_A}{V_P}$$

(ii) Genetic Covariance between Offspring and Mid Parent

This covariance (Cov_{OP}) is obtained as:

$$\text{Cov}_{O\overline{P}} = \text{Offspring with } \tfrac{1}{2}\,(P_1 + P_2)$$
$$= (\text{Cov}_{OP1} + \text{Cov}_{OP2})$$

Now taking that both parents have equal variance

$$\text{Cov}_{OP1} = \text{Cov}_{OP2} \text{ and Cov}_{O\bar{P}} = \text{Cov}_{OP}$$

Since, $\text{Cov}_{OP} = \frac{1}{2} V_A$ so $\text{Cov}_{O\bar{P}} = \frac{1}{2} V_A$

The regression of offspring on mid parent as a measure of degree of resemblance between them will be:

$$b_{O\bar{P}} = \frac{\text{Cov}_{O\bar{P}}}{V_P}$$

$$= \frac{\frac{1}{2} V_A}{\frac{1}{2} V_P}$$

$$= \frac{V_A}{V_P}$$

The variance of mid parent value (V_P) is half the phenotypic variance ($\frac{1}{2} V_P$).

(iii) Genetic Covariance between Half Sibs

Suppose there are **m** numbers of sires or sire families (1, 2, …, i,., m) and each sire or sire family have n individuals (1, 2,., j,.,n). The measurement recorded on j th progeny of i th sire (X_{ij}) can be written as:

$$X_{ij} = \mu + S_i + e_{ij}$$

where, μ = Overall mean of the population

S_i = effect of ith sire common to all members of ith family *i.e.* true mean of ith sire about the population mean

e_{ij} = random error with the jth progeny of ith sire family

The covariance between half sibs, Cov (X_{ij}, X_{ik}), will be the covariance between the measurements of two members of the family:

$$\begin{aligned}
\text{Cov}_{HS} &= \text{Cov} (X_{ij}, X_{ik}) \\
&= E[(S_i + e_{ij})(S_i + e_{ik})] \\
&= E S_i^2 + E(S_i e_{ij}) + E(S_i e_{ik}) + E(e_{ij} e_{ik}) \\
&= \sigma^2_S \text{ Since other products are not correlated} \\
&= \frac{1}{4} V_A \text{ Since half sibs are 25 per cent genetically correlated.}
\end{aligned}$$

Thus, the covariance between half sibs is equal to the variance between half sib family means (σ^2_S) which is equal to $\frac{1}{4} V_A$. The covariance is thus the variance of the means of the half sib groups as: ($\frac{1}{2}$ A) ($\frac{1}{2}$ A) = $\frac{1}{4} \sigma^2_A$.

Therefore, the variance of half the B.V. of parent is equal to the covariance between half sibs which is a quarter of the additive genetic variance.

The variance of phenotypic values (σ^2_X) or (σ^2_P) is:

$$\sigma^2_P = \sigma^2_S + \sigma^2_W$$
$$= Cov_{HS} + \sigma^2_W$$

Therefore, $\sigma^2_W = \sigma^2_P - Cov_{HS}$

$$= \sigma^2_P - \sigma^2_S$$

The two variance components of phenotypic values estimate the followings:

$$\sigma^2_S = Cov_{HS}$$
$$= \tfrac{1}{4} V_A + 1/16 V_{AA} + {}_{1/64} V_{AAA}$$

$$\sigma^2 e = \sigma^2_P - Cov_{HS}$$
$$= \tfrac{3}{4} V_A + {}_{15/16} V_{AA} + {}_{63/64} V_{AAA} + V_D + V_{AD} + V_{DD} + \ldots + V_E$$

Thus the σ^2_W or $\sigma^2 e$ estimates the remainder of the genetic variance plus all the environmental variance.

The correlation between two half sib is:

$$r_{(x_{ij}, x_{ik})} = \frac{Cov_{(x_{ij}, x_{ik})}}{\sigma^2_S + \sigma^2_W}$$

$$= \frac{\sigma^2_S}{\sigma^2_S + \sigma^2_W}$$

Thus, $\quad r_{(HS)} = \dfrac{\sigma^2_S}{\sigma^2_P}$

$$= \frac{1}{4} \frac{\sigma^2_A}{\sigma^2_P}$$

This correlation measures the degree of relationship (resemblance) expressed as the between group component of variance as a proportion of total variance and known as intra class correlation. Here, σ^2_S is the between group component of variance and σ^2_W is the within group component of variance. It is thus the between group component of variance (covariance between group) which expresses the amount of variation common to members of the same group. The components of variance (between groups, σ^2_S and within group, σ^2_W) are estimated by analysis of variance.

(iv) Genetic Covariance between Full Sibs

A number of sires are each mated to many dams and a number of progenies from each dam are born which are measured for metric trait. The measurement recorded on k^{th} progeny of jth dam mated to i^{th} sire (X_{ijk}) is described by the following mathematical model:

$$X_{ijk} = \mu + s_i + d_{ij} + e_{ijk}$$

where, $\quad \mu =$ Overall mean of the population

s_i = Sire effect (deviation) common to members of i th sire family

d_{ij} = Dam effect (deviation) common to members of j th dam family mated to i th sire

e^{ijk} = error component associated with k th progeny of j th dam family of ith sire.

So that the phenotypic variance $(\sigma^2_x = \sigma^2_p)$ is

$$\sigma^2_x = \sigma^2_p = \sigma^2 s + \sigma^2 d + \sigma^2 w$$

Now, the covariance between two members (full sibs) for their measurements (X_{ijk1} and X_{ijk2})

$$\begin{aligned} \text{Cov}_{FS} \quad &= \text{Cov} (X_{ijk1}, X_{ijk2}) \\ &= E(s_i + d_{ij} + e_{ijk1}) (s_i + d_{ij} + e_{ijk2}) \\ &= E(\sigma^2 s_i) + E(\sigma^2 d_{ij}) \text{ since other products are zero being uncorrelated.} \end{aligned}$$

The sire and dam progenies having both parents in common also contains the half sibs, so the covariance between half sibs for their measurement X_{ijk1} and X_{ijk2} is:

$$\begin{aligned} \text{Cov}_{HS} \quad &= \sigma^2 s = \tfrac{1}{4} V_A + 1/16\, V_{AA} \text{ as obtained earlier} \\ \sigma^2 d &= \text{Cov}_{FS} - \text{Cov}_{HS} \\ &= (\sigma^2 s + \sigma^2 d) - \sigma^2 s \\ \sigma^2 w &= \sigma^2_p - \text{Cov}_{FS} \end{aligned}$$

The phenotypic variance of a trait $\left(\sigma_x^2\right)$ is partitioned in to observational components attributable to the followings-

(i $\sigma^2 s = \text{Cov}_{HS}$ = variance between the means of half sib families (sire families) which represents the difference between the progeny of different sires (known as sire component of variance) and estimates the covariance of half sibs (Cov_{HS}). Thus,

$$\sigma^2_s = \text{cov}_{HS} = \tfrac{1}{4} V_A.$$

(ii) $\sigma^2 d = \text{Cov}_{HS}$ = variance between the means of half sib families (dam families) which represents the difference between the progeny of dams mated to same sire (known as between dam within sire component), obtained as:

$$\begin{aligned} \sigma^2 d &= \text{Cov}_{FS} - \text{Cov}_{HS} \\ &= \sigma^2_T - \sigma^2 w - \sigma^2 s \\ &= \tfrac{1}{4} V_A + \tfrac{1}{4} V_D. \end{aligned}$$

(iii) $\sigma^2 w$ = error variance = variance within progeny component which represents the differences between individual progeny of the same dam (known as within progeny component) and obtained as: $V_p - \text{Cov}_{FS} = \tfrac{1}{2} V_A + \tfrac{3}{4} V_D$. This is because the progenies of dams are full sib families and the within group component is obtained by substracting the covariance of members of the groups from total variance. Thus,

$$\sigma^2_w = \tfrac{1}{2} V_A + \tfrac{3}{4} V_D.$$

(iv) $\sigma^2 s + \sigma^2 d = \text{Cov FS} =$ variance of the means of full sib families and equals the sum of between sire and between dam components of variance. Thus,

$$\text{Cov}_{FS} = \sigma^2 s + \sigma^2 d$$
$$= \tfrac{1}{2} V_A + \tfrac{1}{4} V_{D'} + \tfrac{1}{4} V_{AA} + 1/8\, V_{AD} + 1/16\, V_{DD}$$

The correlation (two full sibs) is:

$$r_{(x_{jki1}, x_{ijk2})} = \frac{\text{Cov}_{(x_{ijk1}, x_{ijk2})}}{\sigma^2_P}$$

$$= \frac{\left(\sigma^2_s + \sigma^2_d\right)}{\left(\sigma^2_s + \sigma^2_d + \sigma^2_w\right)}$$

II. Coefficient of Parentage Method

This is based on the probability of genes identical by descent, possessed by two relatives (X and Y). The probability is calculated from the fact that each offspring receives half its genes from each parent.

Consider that X and Y individuals have X_1 and Y_1 genes from paternal side while X_2 and Y_2 from maternal side, then according to Malecot (1948):

1. The probability that the paternal allele in one relative (X_1) is identical to an allele in other relative (Y_1) = $\tfrac{1}{2}$ = O
2. The probability that the maternal allele in one relative (X_2) is identical to an allele in other relative (Y_2) = $\tfrac{1}{2}$ = O'

The covariance between two relatives (X and Y) is obtained as:

$$\text{Cov}(X,Y) = \tfrac{1}{2}(O + O')\, \sigma^2_A + OO' \sigma^2_D$$

where, $\tfrac{1}{2}(O + O')\, \sigma^2_A$ = Coancestry between additive gene effects

or covariance due to additive effect of genes

$OO' \sigma^2_D$ = Coancestry between dominance effects

or covariance due to dominance effects.

According to Malecot (1948), the coefficients for additive gene effects (A) and for dominance effects (D) are:

$$A = \tfrac{1}{2}(O + O')$$

$$D = OO'$$

Therefore, the covariance $(X,Y) = A\, \sigma^2_A + D\, \sigma^2_D$

The coefficient of dominance effect (A = OO') is zero if either O or O' is zero. The covariance due to dominance effects appears only when both genes which cause the dominance are identical by descent in both individuals (Full sibs or double first cousins) which are related to each other on both sides by the pedigree. The coefficient of dominance variance represents the probability of relatives having the same genotype through identity by descent.

The *epistatic effects* also cause to the covariance between relatives and estimated as -

1. $V_{I(AA)} = \frac{1}{2}(O+O')^2 \sigma^2_{AA}$
   = Interaction variance between additive effects of two genes at different loci.

2. $V_{I(DD)} = (O+O')^2 \sigma^2_{DD}$
   = Interaction variance between dominance effects of two genes at different loci.

3. $V_{I(AD)} = \frac{1}{2}(O+O')(OO')\sigma^2_{AD}$
   = Interaction variance between additive effects of one locus and dominance effect of other locus.

The interaction covariance between dominance effects of two loci becomes zero when the individuals are related only through one parent. However, the interactions are not important cause of variation their coefficients are exponential ratios contributing smaller part.

The genetic covariance between different sort of relatives are as -

(i) Half sibs:

$A = \frac{1}{2}(O+O') = \frac{1}{2}(\frac{1}{2}+0) = \frac{1}{4}$

$D = OO' = \frac{1}{2}(0) = 0$

$Cov_{HS} = A\sigma^2_A + D\sigma^2_D + A^2\sigma^2_{AA}$
$= \frac{1}{4}\sigma^2_A + 1/16\,\sigma^2_{AA}$

(ii) Full sibs:

$A = \frac{1}{2}(O+O') = \frac{1}{2}(\frac{1}{2}+\frac{1}{2}) = \frac{1}{2}$

$D = OO' = \frac{1}{2} \times \frac{1}{2} = \frac{1}{4}$

$Cov_{FS} = A\sigma^2_A + D\sigma^2_D + A^2\sigma^2_{AA} + AD\sigma^2_{AD} + D^2\sigma^2_{DD}$
$= \frac{1}{2}\sigma^2_A + \frac{1}{4}\sigma^2_D + \frac{1}{4}\sigma^2_{AA} + 1/8\,\sigma^2_{AD} + 1/16\sigma^2_{DD}$

(iii) Parent – offspring:

$A = \frac{1}{2}(O+O') = \frac{1}{2}(1+0) = \frac{1}{2}$

$D = OO' = 1 \times 0 = 0$

$Cov_{OP} = A\sigma^2_A + D\sigma^2_D + A^2\sigma^2_{AA}$
$= \frac{1}{2}\sigma^2_A + \frac{1}{4}\sigma^2_{AA}$

(iv) Mid parent offspring: This is same as Cov_{OP}.

Interaction Component of Covariance

The genetic covariance among different sort of relatives also contains the interaction component of variance besides additive and dominance components. The interaction is not considered an important part of genetic variance but neglected for two reasons. The first is that it has very small contribution to the covariance because of their coefficients in exponential ratios and hence it contributes very less to the resemblance between relatives. Secondly, the separation of interaction variance from other components is not easy but requires special experimental techniques, like use of inbred lines which partition the V_P into V_A and the rest $(V_D + V_I + V_E)$.

Genetic Explanation

The genetic explanation of the expected composition of the variance components of different types of relatives has been given here as under –

(i) Half Sibs

Half sibs inherit the identical genes at a locus from their sire or dam and this causes resemblance between them. The probability of the gene to be transmitted to one sib is 0.50 and the probability of transmitting the same gene to another sib is also 0.50. The combined probability that two half sibs will inherit from their sire the identical genes (copies of the exact same gene) at a locus, according to the multiplication law of independent events (here, the independent events are separate meiosis and crossing over, mating and fertilization) is $0.5 \times 0.5 = 0.25$. Thus, these identical genes will cause similarity between half sibs to the extent of 25 per cent of the observed resemblance.

Likewise, the probability that half sibs inherit exactly the same genes at two unlinked loci is $0.25 \times 0.25 = 0.0625 = 1/16$ which causes the additive x additive epistatic interaction. This is an additional cause of resemblance between half sibs.

The half sibs can not have identical genotypes at a locus because they get the common genes either from their sire or dam and hence there will be no portion of dominance genetic variance. Therefore, the resemblance between half sibs measured as covariance between them (Cov_{HS})

$$Cov_{HS} = \sigma^2 s$$
$$= \tfrac{1}{4} V_A + 1/16 V_{(AA)}$$

This means that between sire components of variance estimates $\tfrac{1}{4}$ of the additive genetic variance (V_A) plus $1/16$ of the additive x additive epistatic interaction genetic variance. This is the expected composition of the variance component between sires $(\sigma^2 s)$.

(ii) Full Sibs

The full sibs receive 25 per cent genes in common from sire and additional 25 per cent genes in common from dam. Thus, the total genes in common among full sibs will be $25 + 25 = 50$ per cent which is the amount of resemblance among full sibs due to common genes causing the additive genetic variance $(\tfrac{1}{2} V_A)$.

Secondly, the *dominance deviation* to the extent of 25 per cent of the variance $(\tfrac{1}{4} V_D)$ will contribute to the phenotypic resemblance. This means that 25 per cent of similarity of one full sib with another full sib is expected from dominance effects of genes. This is because full sibs have a 25 per cent chance of having exactly the same genotype at a particular locus (both alleles identical by descent from the same sire and dam). This is explained as under –

Consider one locus (A) on which sire has A_1A_2 genotype and the dam has A_3A_4 genotype. The probability of receiving A_1 gene from sire by an offspring is $\tfrac{1}{2}$ and of receiving A_3 gene from dam is also ½. Thus, the probability of the combination $A_1 A_3$ = ½ x ½ = ¼. Likewise, the probability is also ¼ for another sib. Therefore, the probability of the two full sibs to get the combination $A_1 A_3$ from the same sire and dam is ¼ x ¼ = 1/16, because all these events are independent. There will be 3 more combinations of $A_1 A_4$, $A_2 A_3$ and $A_2 A_4$ whose probability will also be ¼ for each combination. Thus, the combined probability of full sibs having identical genotypes at locus **A** is 4 x 1/16 = ¼ being mutually exclusive events. This proportion will be applicable for all loci for which the full sibs are expected to have identical genotype.

The *epistatic interaction variance* also causes the observed resemblance to the extent of 25 per cent [$V_{I(AA)}$]. This is because the full sibs have a probability of 25 per cent to inherit genes at two unlinked loci causing epistatic interaction among average effect of genes. In addition to $V_{I(AA)}$, the epistatic genetic variance caused by interaction between dominance gene effect at two loci (V_{DD}), and by interaction between average effect at one locus and dominance effect at another locus (V_{AD}) will add in smaller proportion to the extent of $1/16 V_{DD}$ and $1/8 V_{AD}$ towards the observed resemblance.

In addition to the genetic resemblance, the full sibs also share common environment. These are similar uterine and post-natal maternal environment like nursing, protection and learning by same dam at the same time, and sharing the similar weather, management etc for litter mates. These similar environmental factors shared by full sibs also cause the resemblance among them, denoted as V_M.

The above causes of resemblance measured as covariance among full sibs (Cov.$_{FS}$) can be collectively written as –

$$\text{Cov.}_{FS} = \sigma^2 s + \sigma^2 d + V_M$$
$$= ½ V_A + ¼ V_D + ¼ V_{I(AA)} + 1/8 V_{I(AD)} + 1/16 V_{I(DD)} + V_M$$

Effect of Linkage on Covariance between Relatives

In derivation of the covariance between relatives it was assumed that the concerned loci affecting the character are not linked (linkage equilibrium). In a random mating population with genotypic frequencies in linkage equilibrium, the covariance between relatives is not affected by linkage. Thus linkage does not affect the covariance of direct relatives (offspring and parent) while the covariance of collateral relatives (sibs, cousins, uncle and nephew) is affected by linkage.

The linkage increases the covariance of sib families depending on the strength of linkage recombination frequencies in a way that closer is the linkage the greater will be the increase in covariance. This increase appears only with the interaction component. The amount of bias due to linkage decreases with increase in number of generations from one relative to the other through common ancestor. Thus, the bias in covariances between relatives due to linkage depends on the type of relatives, closeness of relatives and strength of linkage.

19.3.2 Environmental Resemblance (Covariance)

In addition to the genetic causes, there are environmental circumstances which cause the relatives to resemble each other. All sort of relatives are subject to environmental source of resemblance due to sharing common environment. The members of a family born in the same gestation in litter bearing animals (mice and pigs) or reared together (half sibs and full sibs, particularly in human and farm animals) share a common environment. The cultural influences in humans, nutrition and climatic factors etc are also the sources of common environment. The common environment shared by relatives tends to make the relatives more resemble with each other and hence contribute to the resemblance (covariance) between relatives. On the other hand, the common environment causes differences between groups of unrelated individuals and hence contributes to the variance between means of different families.

Considering the resemblance (covariance) between relatives due to sharing common environment, the environmental variance (V_E) can be partitioned into the following two components:

$$V_E = V_{EC} + V_{EW}$$

Where, V_{EC} represents the environmental component of variance between means of groups arises due to sharing common environment by relatives. Thus it represents the environmental causes of similarity between relatives. This contributes to the variance between the members of the families and hence contributes to the covariance of the related individuals.

The V_{EC} component of environmental variance contributes more to the covariance of full sibs than any other types of relatives because they have also a common maternal environment which is most difficult to remove by experimental design. The V_{EC} component can be reduced or eliminated by proper designing the experiment to distribute the relatives over a range of environment but the component due to maternal effect (a source of common environment) is not possible to eliminate. The V_{EC} can be measured by replication.

V_{EW} is the remainder of environmental variance and known as within group component of variance, arises from causes of differences not connected with the relationship among individuals and it does not contribute to the variance of the true means of the group (between group component).

The environmental effects that are same (common) to all members of the family, are called as the *common environmental effects*. There are two types of the common environments. The first is the common maternal environment called as **maternal effect** and second is the **contemporary environment effect.**

Maternal Effects

The *maternal environment* which causes *maternal effects* includes prenatal and post natal common maternal environment shared by litter mates in pigs and mice. The litter mates share common maternal environment mainly through the nutritional effect of the mother on the foetus and the young, common intra uterine environment, milk yield and mothering ability in mammals (pigs and sheep). This maternal environment during early stages in the life of the young results the offspring of the same dam to show resemblance to each other more than others which differentiate the members of different dams or families. Thus, maternal effects influence the resemblance of maternally related individuals like full sibs, maternal half sibs and dam-daughter groups and thereby contribute to their covariance.

The maternal effects can be studied in two ways. The first is that the phenotypic value of the mother may have its effect on the phenotypic value of the offspring *e.g.* large mothers provide better nutrition to their foetus and young ones during early ages compared to small mothers, causing to produce heavier progeny with faster growth rate in early ages. This causes a resemblance between parents – offspring as well as among the offspring themselves (full sibs and maternal half sibs) particularly for body size in mammals. Secondly, the maternal effect causes the resemblance among the offspring of the same dam but not between the mother and offspring. The maternal effect thus increases the covariance (resemblance) between relatives. The maternal effects have more impact on juvenile (young hood) characters and are reduced in later ages.

Baker *et al* (1943) have worked out that the variance caused by litter environment for 3 week weight in piglets had 50 per cent while the genetic variance was only 5 per cent of the total whereas at 6 months of age each effect caused 25 per cent of the total variance. The compensatory growth counter balances the maternal effects as evidenced by the negative correlation between growth in early and in post puberal stages.

The phenotype of a metric trait affected by maternal effects is influenced by two genetic components *viz.* direct genetic effects which are due to individuals own genotype plus maternal genetic effects which are due to genotypic differences among dams for maternal effects, and by the maternal environmental effects (non-genetic) which the dam induces in her offspring through cytoplasmic factors, intrauterine environment and early postnatal nutrition.

C-Effect

The *contemporary environmental conditions* to a group of individuals provide similar environment to contemporary individuals, thereby increasing the similarity (resemblance) within members of the same group born and grow together. The *contemporary environment* includes the same period of birth and rearing (members of a family like half sibs in animals are more likely to be born and reared during the same period), the same conditions of culture media in Drosophila, same cultural and soil conditions for plants. The similar environmental effects reduce the differences within family members reared/grown together and cause the families more alike than if the only source of similarity would have been the genetic relationship. This causes a group of relatives to be more similar and hence contributes to the resemblance within family members. Such common environmental effects which differ from one group of relatives to another due to be contemporaneous cause the members of the same family alike (similar) were called C – effects by Lerner (1950). The c – effects create differences between families not receiving contemporary environment, are difficult to separate and create complication to estimate correctly the covariance (resemblance) between relatives due to genetic effects only. The increase in size of families also does not decrease the c- effects. The c- effects among full sib families are larger than half sib families. The portion of total variation caused by c – effects is increased.

The within family selection eliminates the non genetic familial effects, because within family selection is made among the individuals having C-effects. Therefore, the familial effects being held in common to all members of the family, individuals deviating from family mean is supposed to be genetically superior and deserve to be selected. The within family selection is used when the environmental effects are large (low h^2) but common for all family members.

It is important to remove the environmental likeness before estimating genetic covariance. This can be done by comparing the animals within the same environment or to adjust the data for the environmental effects.

Chapter 20
Heritability

Selective breeding primarily aims the genetic improvement of progeny generation. The genetic progress in performance is estimated by genetic parameters which are heritability, repeatability and genetic correlation among characters. The heritability estimates the progress in terms of response to selection in a trait whereas the heritability along with genetic correlation estimates the progress in terms of correlated response in a correlated character. The repeatability is used to estimate the increase in mean performance at subsequent age whereas the repeatability along with phenotypic correlation estimates the improvement in correlated trait at subsequent age of the animal. The use and importance of all these three genetic parameters have been discussed in subsequent chapters along with their definition and methods of estimation.

20.1 Definition of Heritability

The term heritability was coined by Lush (1948) to indicate the relative importance of heredity in determining the phenotypic value of a character. The heritability can be defined in a number of ways *viz.* mathematically, statistically and genetically. However, it expresses the genetic part of the phenotypic variance. It is taken in two sense *viz.* broad sense and narrow sense heritability according to that which genetic part (genotypic or additive) is to be expressed as a ratio to the total phenotypic variance. When only additive genetic part is taken, it is then said as the heritability in narrow sense and denoted as h². Thus, $h^2 = \dfrac{\sigma^2_A}{\sigma^2_P}$. Whereas when the complete genetic part is taken, it is then said as the heritability in broad sense denoted $H^2 = \dfrac{\sigma^2_G}{\sigma^2_P}$. The heritability is taken in narrow sense unless other wise mentioned.

Mathematically, the heritability is the portion of differences in phenotypic values of a character attributable to the differences in breeding values for that character. In other words, the heritability is the ratio of additive genetic variance to the phenotypic variance as:

$$h^2 = \frac{\sigma^2_A}{\sigma^2_P}$$

Statistically, the heritability is defined in terms of the relationship between breeding value and phenotypic value of a character in a population taken as a measure of the strength (reliability or correspondence or consistency) of relationship between the two values. Heritability in term of the correlation between the two values is taken as square of the correlation between phenotypic value and breeding value. Therefore, $h^2 = (r_{AP})^2$.

The heritability, also in statistical term, is the regression of breeding value (A) on the phenotypic value (P) and hence, $h^2 = b_{AP}$.

Genetically, the heritability measures the degree to which the offspring resemble their parents in performance traits. Thus, it indicates the resemblance between parent and offspring. It is also taken as the portion of genetic superiority of parents inherited and expressed by the offspring.

20.2 Limits of Heritability

The variance can not be negative and it may be close to zero or completely zero in some particular cases (completely pure line). Therefore, the heritability can not be greater than one or less than zero. The values of heritability range between zero to one depending on the magnitude of phenotypic variability attributed to genetic effects. However, heritability is estimated from resemblance among relatives based on certain assumptions which may not always be fulfilled. Thus, heritability may exceed the mathematical and biological bounds.

Interpretation of Heritability Values

In a random mating population of farm animals, the phenotypic value of a quantitative trait is the joint product of the genotype and the environment. Therefore, the phenotypic variability in quantitative traits of farm animals is neither completely due to genetic differences nor completely due to the environment differences but partly assigned to both the effects. The proportion of genetic variance among phenotypic values is expressed by heritability in broad sense while the contribution of environmental variance to the phenotypic variance is obtained by substracting heritability value from 1.

H^2 = proportion of genetic variance

$1-H^2$ = proportion of environmental variance

h^2 = proportion of additive genetic variance

$1-h^2$ = proportion of non-additive genetic variance plus environmental variance.

Thus, the heritability of a quantitative trait may range between any value from zero to 1 depending upon the contribution of genes effect and the environmental effects in final expression of the phenotypic values of a trait.

(a) Complete Heritability

If the differences in the phenotypic values are entirely due to the genes effects then the heritability is 1. This is because $\sigma^2 e = 0$ and $\sigma^2_G = \sigma^2_P$ in this case and so $H^2 = \sigma^2_G = \sigma^2_P = 1.0$. The complete heritability or the heritability value as 1 indicates that:

☆ The phenotype is completely and exclusively determined by genes,

☆ The phenotypic variability is caused entirely due to the gene effects with no role of the environment in modifying the phenotypic values,

☆ The offspring of the selected parents inherit in full the excess value of the character over the population average,

☆ The genetic gain equals in size to the selection differential,

☆ Further the phenotype of progeny will equal to the average phenotype of the mid-parent.

(b) Zero Heritability

If the phenotypic values differ entirely due to environmental factors, then the heritability is equal to zero. This is because the $\sigma^2_P = \sigma^2_E$ in this case and hence $\sigma^2_G = 0$. This is the case in pure lines and in identical twins which are completely homozygous (have the same genotypes) and hence have no genetic differences. This makes the σ^2_G equal to zero. In this case, the variation in phenotypic values is entirely environmental in nature and the genetic variation is absent. The consequences are that there will be no genetic gain through selection and thus the genetic improvement will be zero. This is because selection acts on genetic variability. Thus, the selection will not be effective and hence the offspring are not expected to have any superiority over the population average. The mean value of the progeny fully regresses on the mean value of the selected parents. This implies that the average for the offspring generation is the same as that for the parents.

In case of identical twins or highly inbred lines the heritability is zero, it does not mean that the trait is not heritable or not affected by genes but it indicates that there is no genetic difference in the phenotypic values of different individuals of the population.

20.3 Misconceptions about Heritability

1. *Inherited Vs Heritable Traits*: A genetically determined trait is called inherited trait which is coded for somewhere in everyones' DNA. But every inherited trait (genetically determined) is not said to be heritable. The term heritable trait implies that a genetically determined trait (inherited trait) should have differences in performance among individuals of a population. Therefore, a genetically determined trait is said to be heritable only when there exist differences in performance for the trait. Some traits are completely determined genetically but do not show differences and hence not said to be heritable *e.g.* number of legs, hands and eyes etc. An individual of any

species is born with fixed number of legs *e.g.* cows, buffaloes, sheep, goat, pigs, dogs have four legs provided there are congenital deformities. The number of legs is a trait and certainly genetically determined but this trait is not said to be heritable because differences in number of legs do not exist. Therefore, a trait is said to be highly heritable in terms of heritability.

2. The heritability indicates the relationship between breeding value and phenotypic value. In view of this, it is wrongly interpreted that if a trait has high heritability, then the breeding values for the trait will also be high.

3. *Heritability is a Population measure:* It is a population and not of an individual. Thus an individual can not have a low or high heritability of a trait.

4. *Heritability is the property of the trait, the population and environmental conditions:* The h^2 estimates vary for a trait for different populations because of differences among individuals of the population attributed to additive gene effects and under different environmental conditions, it changes over time (generations) and have different values for different traits. Thus, the h^2 estimate is valid only for the population for which it has been estimated.

   (i) *Property of a trait:* The $V_A = 2pq [a + d (q - p)]$ and thus depends upon the genetic properties *viz.* type of gene action, number of loci affecting a trait, their frequencies and the magnitude of effects. These are all specific to the trait and to the population. Thus, any change in gene frequencies leads to a change in the amount of V_A and hence h^2.

   (ii) *Property of population:* The genetic structure of the population and its size affect the h^2. Genetically uniform population has low h^2 because of having similar genes and genotypes. Low population has low h^2 because of sampling effect and unavoidable inbreeding.

   (iii) *Environmental conditions:* Population with uniform environmental conditions has low h^2 of a trait because uniform environment to all individuals of a population reduces the environmental differences among individuals, thereby reducing the total phenotypic variance which is denominator term used to estimate h^2. Therefore, h^2 is higher under uniform environment.

The different h^2 values are obtained under different feeding regimes. The animals which are not well fed and conditioned, can not fully exploit their genetic potential and hence the genetic differences are reduced among animals.

The herd performance for milk production also influences the h^2. The h^2 of milk production is low in a herd with low average compared to medium and high average herd. The G – E interaction seems to be important in this respect. The environmental factors are not expected to be moderate/optimum in a herd with low average and this affect the expression of genetic variation in animals. The genetically superior animals under poor environmental conditions may not fully exhibit their superiority whereas the expression of genetic variation in animals under moderate environmental factors is not affected to the extent that genetically superior animals may fail to exhibit their superiority. The genetic differences are thus reduced in a herd which is not well fed and conditioned (low herd average) because the animals can not fully exploit their genetic potential.

The age of the animals has also influence on h^2 of the character. Certain age groups (young age) are more sensitive to environmental conditions which increases the environmental variance and thereby reducing the h^2. For example, the h^2 of mortality in calves upto 3 months of age is low than at subsequent ages.

The h^2 of first lactation milk yield is higher than in second lactation. This may be due to the reason that cows in first lactation are well conditioned to exploit their genetic potential better than in second lactation. Secondly, the high producers are exhausted and depleted in first lactation and hence can not display their genetic potential fully subsequently. Thirdly, there is some selection of cows after first lactation.

Age differences among animals also reduce the h^2 of the character because variation in age increases the error variance which increases the phenotypic variance leading to a decrease in h^2. Therefore, it is advocated that h^2 should be estimated based on the records of animals of the same age.

20.4 Limitations of Heritability

The h^2 estimates have great role in animal breeding. However, there are certain limitations in its use.

(i) There are certain assumptions in h^2 estimation (see section 17.5) below. In real situations, these assumptions may not fulfill and hence the h^2 estimate may not be accurate.

(ii) The h^2 of a trait is the property of a particular population at a particular time in a range og environments. Therefore, the once estimated for one population at one time can not be used for the same population in future or for other population or for other environmental conditions.

(iii) The change in environment has two fold effects on h^2 estimate. The first is that an increase in environmental variance reduces the h^2 estimate. Secondly, the values of genetic parameters (*a* and *d*) which affect V_A depend on the environment (See section 16.8).

(iv) The h^2 is a single value affected by gene frequency, gene action and environmental effects as well as represents the combined effect of all the polygenes affecting a trait without indicating about any of the polygene. Thus, it is not easy to interpret the h^2 in simple genetic terms. The gene frequency and the gene effects may be different for different polygenes. These values can not be integrated and said to be statistically confounded. The h^2, being representing the cumulative effect of polygenes affecting a trait, does not tell about the actual mode of inheritance of a trait.

(v) The gene frequencies undergo changes during selection which leads to a change in h^2 estimate. However, the change in h^2 is sufficiently slow over a few generations of selection and it can not be regarded as constant. The constancy in gene frequency is for two reasons. The first is that a gene may have small effect on the phenotypic variance of a trait. Secondly, the change in environment influence the values of gene effects and thus if the environment does not change over generations, there will be no change in the values of **a** and **d**. Therefore, the h^2 usually remains approximately constant for the first 10 generations or so under selection. However, under long term selection, the h^2 is expected to be decreased. It is known that the additive genetic variance is completely exhausted at selection limit because either of the two alleles at a locus is fixed, resulting either $p = 0$ or $q = 0$. In case of overdominance, under selection equilibrium, the gene does not contribute to V_A.

20.5 Assumptions in Heritability Estimation

The heritability is based on the partitioning of the total phenotypic variance into different genetic and environmental components. The partitioning of variance has certain complications and is valid under certain assumptions given as under:

1. *There is No Inbreeding*: The h^2 is expected to decline with the inbreeding in a small popuulation. The inbreeding results in increased homozygosity and reduces the genetic variance. Secondly, it increases the environmental variance ($\sigma^2 e$) because inbred animals are more sensitive to environment or less well buffered. Certain characters show more environmental variance among inbred individuals than among outbreds. With inbreeding the gene frequencies in separate lines tend towards the extreme values and thus the lines become differentiated in gene frequency. This will affect mean genotypic value because it depends on gene frequency. This will decrease the genetic variance within the lines because the genetic variance is reduced as the gene frequencies tend towards the extreme values. Thus, inbreeding leads to genetic differentiation between lines and genetic similarity within line. Thus, h^2 within line will be low due to low genetic variance within line.

   The environmental component of variance may differ according to the genotype, and the inbred animals often have great environmental variance than outbreds. Though the cause is not fully understood but it has been explained by Robertson and Reeve (1952) that possession of different alleles at specific loci provides the hybreds with greater biochemi-cally versatility which makes the outbreds more buffered to the circum-stances of the environment. The fact that inbreds are more susceptible to environmental sources of variation has been observed for many characters and in many organisms. Thus, environmental variance is dependent on genotype. One genotype may be more or less susceptible to environmental influence than other line and thus have more or less h^2. The continuous inbreeding increases the homozygosity appreciably and then the estimation of BV is vague and doubtful. In partitioning the components of variance it is assumed that the environment is same for all genotypes.

2. *There should be no selection of data*, and all the available values or their random sample is included in the assessment of breeding value. Thus, the

information (observations) should be representative. For example, when a bull is assessed on collateral relatives or on progeny performance, then all the collaterals and offspring with known performance must be included. Likewise a selection criterion must be fixed in case of selection of cows for milk production. The cows may either be selected on the basis of first lactation record or on the average of first 2 or 3 lactation records and there should not be selection of data like to that selection based on best lactation performance.

3. *There is no genotype-environmental correlation* and the trait is inherited additively. In assessing the breeding value (partitioning of variance components) it is assumed that genotypic value and environmental deviation are independent of each other which means that these are not correlated with each other. The correlation between them is not important complication because of randomly distribution of environmental influences within the population and more over the observations are corrected. Under certain conditions the correlation exists or a correlation is introduced between genotype and environment. For example, milk yield in dairy animals. The dairy animals are fed according to their milk production. The presumptive dams of bulls are fed and managed better to enhance their production than their contemporaries. Thus, the cows with better genotypes are given better environment and they appear better than actually they are. The mothering ability and suckling capacity of the dams in pigs give rise to systematic differences between contemporary litters. Similarly, different time of hatching also produce environmental differences between groups of chicks. Human intelligence is another example. The environment given to the children at home by the parents during their development stage influence the intelligence of the children. In other words, the family status, education, facilities and guidance affect the environment in which the children grow up and this environment has its impact on the intelligence of the children. This creates a correlation between genotype and environment of the children. The intelligent parents provide better environment to the extent that their children become intelligent and it is then said that intelligence is inherited. The environmental effects given by the parents are not the consequence of the children's genotype but are of their parent's genotype. Under such situation the phenotypic values are influenced by environmental deviations and because genotypic and phenotypic values are correlated, therefore, it introduces a correlation between phenotypic and environmental deviations. This means that the genotype environment correlation is produced. This leads to the phenotypic variance to be composed as:

$V_P = V_G + V_E + 2Cov_{(GE)}$ instead of $V_P = V_G + V_E$ which is valid when there is no correlation between genotypic value and environmental deviation.

The special environment (feeding level etc.) is regarded as part of the genotype to overcome the complication of genotype environment correlation. This is because non-random environment is the consequence of the genotypic value and hence the environment given to an individual is taken as part of its genotype. The genotypic variance in this case also includes twice the covariance of the genotypic values and environmental deviations. Thus considering any such covariance as part of the genetic variance is convenient theoretically but in practice it is unavoidable. This type of errors has a misleading effect in selection. Therefore, it is assumed that all environmental influences are randomly distributed, without any G-E correlation.

4. *There should be no genotype – environment interaction –* It is assumed in partitioning the phenotypic variance into its components that the genotypic values and environmental deviations are uncorrelated. This means that specific difference in environment should have the same effect on different genotypes. When a specific difference in environment has different effects on the different genotypes, an interaction between genotypes and environments is introduced, and thus the effects of genotype and environment are not independent. The interaction may be of several forms. It may be that a specific difference of environment may have more effect on one genotype than on other genotypes. This results sometimes the change of ranking of different genotypes in two or more environments. This type of observation of genotype and environment on each other creates the G-E interaction. For example, genotype X may perform better than genotype Y in one environment (say good feeding) but with a change of environment (say poor feeding) the genotype Y may perform better than genotype X. This gives rise to an additional compo-nent of phenotypic value of an individual and the equation becomes as $P = G + E + I_{GE}$ instead of $P = G + E$. This interaction component of phenotypic value (I_{GE}) gives rise to an additional source of variation known as interaction variance and the phenotypic variance becomes as:

$V_P = V_G + V_E + V_{GE}$ instead of $V_P = V_G + V_E$ which is valid when there is no interaction between genotype and environment.

The interaction variance is included with the environmental variance. This is based on the fact that phenotypic variance of a genetically uniform group (being treated as single genotype) is entirely the environmental variance because the differences in phenotypic values are entirely due to environmental differences among individuals. Moreover, the environmental variance depends on the extent to which a particular genotype responds to environmental differences as some genotypes are more sensitive to environmental effect than other genotypes. Thus, the environmental variance is a property of the genotype, to some extent but the source of variation is environmental and genetic in nature. Therefore, the interaction variance (V_{GE}) is regarded as part of the environmental variance.

This G-E interaction is quite important because the genes besides interacting among themselves also interact with the environment under which the organism is reared. But when a specific difference in environment has same effect on different genotypes, it does not affect the result and a certain environmental deviation can be associated with a specific difference of environment irrespective of genotype. The G-E interaction may be avoided by distributing the genotypes at random over a common range of environments.

The importance of G-E interaction is more in view of the fact that the individuals of a breed are reared under different environmental conditions of feeding, housing and management, etc. The different environmental conditions (farms or locations etc.) are specific environ-ments. Rearing of individuals under specific environmental conditions of nutrition, location, temperature, etc. is helpful to study the genotype environment interaction by analysis of variance. The presence of G-E interaction is helpful to recommend the specific environment to a particular genotype while in the absence of interaction any genotype can be kept under all available environments.

20.6 Ways to Improve Heritability

The best way to increase the h^2 is to reduce the environmental variations among the individuals of a population. The $\sigma^2 e$ can be reduced by managing the animals under uniform environment, to measure accurately the performance of the animals for a trait, mathematical adjustment of environmental effects, use of multiple records per animal and expressing the performance of an animal (i^{th} animal) for a trait from contemporary group mean either as a deviation or as a trait ratio.

1. *Providing Uniform Environment*: The animals should be raised and managed under similar environmental conditions. This makes the environmental effects smaller and hence the variation in phenotypic values due to environmental effects is reduced. The performance be-comes a better indicator of breeding value which, in other words, means that h^2 is increased. The environmental differences lead to biasness in performance records and the relationship between phenotypic value and breeding value is poor.

   Suppose a herd of dairy cows is divided in two groups. Half of them are chosen at random and given good environment (say high feeding level or calved in a favourable season) whereas the other half could not get better environment. Now the milk production of all the cows of both the groups is recorded. There are chances that the cows getting better environment will produce more than those cows which received poor environment. However, some of the cows of group II (poor environment) may have high breeding value for milk production but their milk production may be low due to poor environment. On the other hand, some cows of group I (better environment) may have average breeding value but even though they produce more milk only because of getting good environment. Therefore, in this case of milk production example, the milk yield (phenotype) is not a good indicator of the breeding value because of differences in environment and hence the h^2 of milk production is low. Now think that all the cows of the herd get similar environment. In this case, the cows with better breeding values are likely to yield more than those with poor breeding values. In other words, the relationship between milk production and its breeding value is high than the previous case of dividing the cows in two groups of better and poor environment. Heritability is increased due to the uniform environment to all the cows.

2. *Use of Multiple Measurements*: The h^2 based on more records (h^2_n) is higher than based on single record per animal. An animal experiences different environments at different ages (poor as well as better environment) which are of temporary in nature. Thus the positive and negative effects of these temporary environmental factors are cancelled in taking the average of more records per animal and hence the temporary environmental variation is reduced which in turn reduces the total phenotypic variance. The h^2 based on n records (h^2_n) is:

$$h^2_n = \frac{nh^2}{1+(n-1)r}$$

where, r = repeatability of the trait

n = no. of records per animal

h^2 = heritability based on one record.

and hence h^2 is increased by increase in number of records per animal.

3. *Adjustment of records*: There are many known environmental factors which modify the gene's expression and hence mask the animal's true breeding value. The performance records are adjusted (corrected) to a common basis for the significant environmental effects to minimise the environmental variations.

To remove the environmental effects from the performance data the correction factors (C.F.) for each source of variation are estimated by using all the least squares constants irrespective of their significance. The C.F. is added to the original record of each animal with sign changed and the resultant quantity is the adjusted record. Gacula *et al* (1948) described the following adjustment formula:

$Y = y_i - C.F.$

where, Y = adjusted record

y_i = unadjusted or original record

C.F. = sum of all constants

The other methods for adjustment of data are:

Ratio factor, paired comparison, difference method and Regression method.

4. *Accurate measurement of Data*: A bias is introduced when there is no accurate measurement of performance record. This is called the error of measurement and introduces one sort of environmental effect. The example can be cited in this context of the body weight recorded at different ages viz, birth weight, weaning weight and body weight at calving. It is a general practice to record the birth weight within 8 hours of calving but sometimes the interval

for recording the birth weight is increased from two hours to twenty four hours. Likewise, the body weights at subsequent ages (weaning weight) of some calves/lambs/kids are recorded when the water and feed in their digestive tract is not equal _i.e._ some ones are recorded after watering and feeding while others are recorded without providing feed and water. Thirdly, a particular date is fixed to record the weights irrespective of the age of the animal with ± 10 days or more. Moreover, the scale used to record the body weight may read the increment of 10Kg or 5Kg. or 1Kg. The more precise and accurate measurement of body weight will be on the scale having the minimum increment or graduation. Thus the scale of measurement should be a sensitive scale. The body weight recorded with equal accuracy is more heritable because they do not have the error of measurement and hence the environmental variance is less in such records. Likewise, there should not be any error in recording the milk yield of different cow _viz._ use of faulty scale, stealing of milk of some cows and any other kind of error in recording the milk yield.

5. _Analysis of data based on contemporary group mean_: The animal performance data should not be analyzed in absolute unit but in relation to the contemporary group either as the deviation or as a ratio. This is one way to reduce the environmental variation in case when all the animals are not managed under similar conditions.

(i) One way to express the phenotypic value of an individual (P_i) is to take its deviation from a contemporary group mean (Pcg) as: $(P_i - P_{cg})$.

When phenotypic value is taken as a deviation from contemporary group mean, it is advantageous when groups of animals experience different environments. This increases the heritability. The presence of environmental differences between groups of animals reduces the relationship between breeding values and absolute phenotypic values. The reason is that some animals with low breeding values may have high phenotypic value under favourable environment while some animals with high breeding values may have low phenotypic values due to poor environ-ment. The environmental differences are accounted for when the pheno-typic value is expressed as a deviation from contemporary group mean and this increases the relationship between animal's breeding values and deviated phenotypic value which can be expressed as:

$$r_{A(Pi - Pcg)} > r_{AP}$$

The deviated phenotypic value is an alternate way for adjustment of data for significant environmental effects. Thus, the contemporary groups are used to account for environmental differences between groups of animals. The reason of using contemporary groups is to account for the contemporary group effects which are the environmental effects common to all members of a contemporary group. However, it should be kept in mind that the contemporary groups should not be genetically different _e.g._ animals from different herds or flocks.

(ii) Another way to express the performance as a deviation from contemporary group mean is the trait ratio which is an expression of relative performance. The trait ratio is taken as a ratio of an animal's performance to the average performance of all animals of contemporary group. However, the trait ratio is calculated after adjusting the data for environmental effects.

Trait ratio = Pi/Pcg x 100

20.7 Sources of Error in Heritability

There are certain factors which affect the accuracy in estimating heritability and create error or pitfalls in estimation of heritability.

1. Scale Effect

The trait showing skewed distribution posed problem and error in estimating h^2 on untransformed data. The scale effect is a phenomenon which arises when the variance changes with mean. When the variance is not independent of mean, then the change of variance can be attributed to the scale of measurement to some extent. It should not be taken that each character has its natural scale of measurement. For example, growth is measured in arithmetic units but actually it is a geometrical process, and therefore, a geometric scale is the most natural and appropriate for expressing growth. The criteria to an appropriate scale are: that the distribution of phenotypic values should follow a normal curve, and that the variance should be independent of mean. A skewed distribution indicates that the data should be transformed before analysis. The relationship between the amount of variance and the mean determines the degree of departure from normality, and it is expressed in terms of coefficient of variation. Transformation of data is less needed when the coefficient of variation is low than when it is high. When the variance changes following a change of the population mean, it requires transformation of data but if the transformation in not done certain phenomenon arise called scale effect. Transformation of measurements to an appropriate scale makes the variance independent of mean. Thus, the scale effects disappear on changing the scale of measurement of the character. The scale effect in relation to variance and mean complicated the comparison of variances of two populations with different mean, *e.g.*, inbreds and hybrids. The coefficient of variation provides a test for the appropriateness of transformation of data. When two populations differ in their variance but the coefficient of variation are nearly alike it then indicates that the variance is dependent of mean. This shows that there is a change of variance following a change in mean. Therefore, the coefficient of variation should vary if the variance is independent of mean. The realized heritability which is the ratio of response to selection differential is very little influenced by scale effects and is a convenient way of eliminating scale effects. Both the dominance and epistatic interaction between different loci are affected by the scale. The scale transformation may reduce the variance attributed to epistatic interaction.

2. Unadjustment of Data

It is necessary to adjust the data for significant environmental effects. This reduces the environmental vari-ance and error in h2 estimation. If per chance the progeny of a sire get better environment, it is most likely that they will have better performance compared to the performance of the progeny of another sire under poor environment if the environment has significant effect on the trait. Under such a condition the bull's genotype is not responsible for better or poor performance but the same is attributed to the environment. These environmental variations are combined with genes effect. Thus, the differences between sires will not be real but erroneous due to environmental effects. Therefore, it is required to adjust the data for environmental effects before genetic analysis.

3. Method of Estimation of h^2

This also influences the size of h^2. The h^2 obtained by different methods gives biased estimated for the reason discussed in chapter 15.

4. Violation of the Assumptions in h^2 Estimation

(i) G x E Interaction

This component of phenotypic value influences the h^2 estimate. There should be no G x E interaction. All the genotypes should react in an identical manner to environmental changes. In the presence of G x E interaction the different genotypes respond differently to environment changes and it affects the variance. The $V_{I(GE)}$ is increased and included with V_E. The different change in phenotypic value of different genotypes indicate that a change in environment do not have the same effect on all the genotypes to produce a change in phenotypic values. This reflects the presence of I_{GE}. On the other hand, equal change in phenotypic values of all the genotypes due to a change in environment does not change the variance. This reflects absence of I_{GE} and had no effect on h^2 estimate.

(ii) G x E Correlation

In partitioning the variance it is assumed that genotypic values and environmental deviations are independent of each other. Thus, they have no correlation among themselves. The correlation between the two arises when better genotypes are given better environment. Under some situation the correlation exists *e.g.* when dairy cows are fed according to their milk yield, the high yielding cows are given more food. The correlation increases the phenotypic variance by the amount equal to twice the covariance of genotypic values and environmental deviation (2 Cov $_{GE}$). This covariance part is regarded as part of genetic variance because the non-random aspect of environment is a consequence of genotypic values and, therefore, an individual's environment is thought of the part of its genotype.

(iii) Selection of Parents

Random mating is another assumption in estimating the resemblance among relatives. When the parents are a selected group it reduces the phenotypic variance among parents compared to unselected group and consequently, the covariance of sibs is reduced. Therefore, the h^2 estimated from intra-class correlation is reduced. However, the selection does not affect the regression of offspring on parent because the covariance between parent and offspring is reduced to same extent as the variance of parents. However, the covariance is not a valid measure of additive genetic variance and similarly the variance of parents is not a valid measure of the phenotypic variance. The selection of parents affects the h^2 estimates obtained from correlation of parent and offspring.

(iv) Assortative Mating

When the parents are mated according to phenotypic resemblance, then a correlation exists between the pheno-typic values of the mated pairs. This correlation changes the frequencies of the different types of mating which increase the variance of mid parent value as well as the Cov_{FS}. The h^2 estimate is increased due to assortative mating. The increased variance of mid parent value due to assortative mating reduces the sampling error of the regression coefficient and thus to the h^2. Thus the precision of estimate is increased.

(v) Inbreeding

The h^2 is reduced with inbreeding in a small population provided there is no selection. The inbreeding reduces the genetic variance. Secondly, the inbreds are more sensitive to environ-mental changes. This increases the environmental variance. However, the natural selection operates which results in less reduction of heritability than the expectation. It is possible to find out the h^2 value corrected to base population (h^2_B) as:

$$h^2_B = \frac{h^2_1}{\left[1 + \left(h^2_1 - 1\right)\right]}$$

where, h^2_1 = Heritability within lines

$$\frac{(1-F)\sigma^2_G}{(1-F)\sigma^2_G + \sigma^2_E} = \frac{h^2_B(1-F)}{1 - h^2_B F}$$

where, F is the inbreeding coefficient

$(1-F)\,\sigma^2_G$ is the within line valance

The genetic and environmental components of the phenotypic variance may show unequal changes. This leads to a change in heritability. The environmental part is not constant but depends on a number of factors which may or may not be controlled by the breeder.

20.8 Importance and Use of Heritability

The heritability is the most useful genetic parameter in providing a number of useful information, predicting the possibility and amount of change in the genetic improvement of population as result of selection, and deciding the proper selection and mating systems.

1. The heritability of a character provides the following useful information:

   (i) The heritability is a *measure of the genetic variability* in phenotypic values of a character among the individuals of the population. Heritability is expressed in two ways *viz.* the amount of total variability attributed to differences in genotypic values (H^2) and secondly to those attributed to differences in the breeding values (h^2) of the individuals of a population.

   (a) *Heritability in broad sense* (H^2) – The proportion of total variation in a trait among the individuals of a population attributed to the genetic differences is called as the heritability in broad sense (Lush, 1937)

   and denoted as: $H^2 = \dfrac{\sigma^2_G}{\sigma^2_P}$.

   This estimate of heritability is used to know the relative contribution of genotype and environment to create the differences in phenotypic values among the individuals of a population for a trait. The H^2 is thus called as the degree of genetic determination. The H^2 indicates the proportion of total phenotypic variance attributed to the genes effect of all types *viz.* additive, dominance and interaction (epistatic)

   effects which are combined denoted by $H^2 = \dfrac{\sigma^2_G}{\sigma^2_P}$.

   (b) *Heritability in narrow sense* (h^2) – Among the genetic effects of all kinds, the additive genetic effect is more important in causing the variation Secondly, the differences (variance) caused by additive gene effects (denoted by σ^2_A) are only transmitted to the progeny as such and hence of the total variance caused by additive gene effects is fixed whereas the differences among individuals caused by non-additive gene effects are not transmitted as such for the reason that new gene combinations are formed in each subsequent generation. Thus, the heritability is expressed as the proportion of additive genetic variance to the total phenotypic variance. This is called as the heritability in narrow sense, denoted as h^2, and expressed or measured as:

   $h^2 = \dfrac{\sigma^2_A}{\sigma^2_P}$

   Therefore, the heritability provides a measure of genetic variability in a trait among the phenotypic values of the individuals of a population and expressed as the amount of total variability attributed to differences in genotypic values (H^2) or to differences in the breeding value (h^2) of the individuals of a population. Thus, the heritability indicates the relative role of heredity and environment in affecting the phenotypic values of different individuals (in controlling a trait) and hence in contributing the variability among individuals. Therefore, heritability indicates the extent to which the trait is by genotype (from the value of

H²) or by the breeding value of the individual (indicated from the value of h²)

(ii) The heritability is a *measure of the portion of phenotypic superiority of parents passed on to the progeny*. This is because the heritability expresses the amount of phenotypic superiority of parents (the phenotypic differences between the selected and rejected parents), attributed to additive effect of genes which is transmitted (inherited) by the parents and hence passed on to their progeny.

(iii) The heritability is a *measure of the degree of correspondence (agreement) between the phenotypic value and breeding value*. This is because the square root of heritability (h) is equal to the correlation between breeding value and phenotypic value (h = r_{AP}) which indicates the association between the two values.

(iv) The heritability is a *measure of accuracy of selection* based on phenotype. This is because if the heritability is higher, the r_{AP} will also be higher, the higher proportion of superiority will be transmitted and hence the selection will be more accurate.

(v) The heritability is an *indication of type of gene action*. This is because the heritability indicates about the amount of additive genetic variance arising due to additive gene action. Thus, the magnitude of heritability indicates the type of gene action and hence the heritability is an indicator of the extent to which the trait is affected by additive gene action. This is because the heritability estimate is a measure of the proportion of the total variation in a trait due to additive genetic variance arises due to additive gene action.

(vi) The heritability indicates about the *basic genetic phenomenon* of metric traits which are resemblance between relatives and the inbreeding depression with its converse hybrid vigour (heterosis). The resemblance between relatives is due to the effect of genes commonly shared by them. The heritability is a measure of the additive genetic variance which arises due to additive gene effect that are measured in terms of the breeding value. The relatives sharing common genes will have similar additive gene effects and hence similar breeding values. This similarity in breeding values causes resemblance between relatives which forms the basis to estimate the heritability (additive genetic variance arising due to additive gene effects). Secondly, the inbreeding depression or its converse heterosis depends on the type of gene action. Both these phenomenon (I.D. and heterosis) depend on the occurrence of dominance and epistasis. The loci with additive gene action cause neither inbreeding depression nor heterosis. Therefore, the magnitude of heritability which is a measure of gene action gives an indication of the inbreeding depression or heterosis likely to occur or not.

2. The heritability has its ***predicting role*** to predict the breeding value of an individual and the genetic gain in a population through selection.

(i) The heritability is used to predict the *breeding value* of an individual. The heritability is regression of breeding value on phenotypic value ($h^2 = b_{AP}$). The regression is used to predict the unknown variable based on the value of a known variable as: $Y = b_{YX}(X_i - X)$. The animal breeder is interested to know the breeding value (A) which is unknown for an individual based on its phenotypic value which is known. Thus, the estimate of an individual's breeding value for a trait is obtained by multiplying its phenotypic value (P) with heritability (h^2) of the trait as: $A = h^2 P$ by taking both the values as deviation from population mean Thus, the best estimate of the absolute B.V. from phenotypic value for each individual in a population can be obtained as: $B.V. = \mu + h^2(P_i - \mu)$. Where, μ is population mean and P_i is the phenotypic value of ith individual.

(ii) The heritability is used to predict the *genetic gain* (ΔG). The genetic gain or genetic improvement or response to selection is the average superiority of the progeny over their parental generation mean before selection ($X_O - X_P$). The mean of progeny generation is estimated as:

$$X_O \quad = \mu + h^2(X_S - \mu)$$
$$X_O - \mu \quad = h^2(Xs - \mu)$$
$$\Delta G \quad = h^2(Xs - \mu)$$

where,

μ = Population mean before selection;

X_S = Mean of selected parents;

X_O = Mean of offspring.

$X_S - \mu$ = Phenotypic superiority of selected parents known as selection differential

$X_O - \mu$ = Response to selection or genetic gain per generation

ΔG = Av. superiority of progeny.

3. The heritability plays very important role in *decision on the criteria of selection and the mating system*. The uses of heritability in designing the breeding programmes are as under:

(i) **Selection of traits**: In a breeding programme, multiple trait selection is preferred rather than single trait selection. The heritability is one of the most important aspects to decide that which traits should be included in construction of selection index for multi trait selection. The traits with high heritability are included.

(ii) **Optimum family size**: The sib selection is applied for selection of sex limited traits *viz.* milk yield etc. The efficiency of sib selection depends on family size (no. of sibs to be recorded) because larger is the family size larger will be the response. However, it is not so in practice because of the involvement of intensity of selection as a factor affecting response. There is a limitation of breeding space or facilities to evaluate so many families with larger number of individuals. This impose restriction either to maintain smaller families (having lesser number of individuals per family) or to maintain larger families (having more number of individuals per family). The larger families (having more number of individuals per family but with few numbers of families) result in low intensity of selection. Thus, family size and family number has a conflict and a compromise has to be made. Taking into consideration the intensity of selection, there should be optimal family size to give maximum expected response. The optimal family size (n) depends on the magnitude of heritability as:

$$n = 0.56 \sqrt{\left(\frac{T}{N h^2} \right)}$$

where, N = no. of families to be selected;

T = Family size (total number of individuals to be measured)

(iii) **Selection criterion:** The selection criterion may be the phenotypic value or the combining ability of the trait. The selection based on phenotypic value rests on the breeding value of the individuals estimated either from individuals' own record (individual selection) or from the records of its relatives (sib selection, within family selection). The selection criterion based on phenotypic value are often used to improve the performance of a single purebred population whereas the selection criterion based on individuals' combining ability for the trait is used in commercial application involving crossbreeding.

(a) *Pure breeding programme*- The choice of selection criterion based on phenotypic value depends on the magnitude of heritability of the trait. The individual selection based on individuals' own performance is advocated for traits with high heritability whereas family selection is used to improve the traits with low heritability. In family selection, either whole family is selected or few individuals with phenotypic values above family mean are selected.

When the selection criterion is the family mean and whole family is selected and it is called as family selection. This family selection is used when environmental effects are large (low h^2) but different for different individuals so that the environmental effects are cancelled by taking the mean. On the contrary, when one or few individuals of a family are selected it is known as within family selection. The few individuals within a family are selected on the basis of the deviation of their phenotypic values from the family mean. This within family selection is also used when the environmental effects are large (low h^2) but these environmental effects should be same (common) to all the family members (C-effects). The C-effects are eliminated in within family selection because the selection is made among the individuals having C-effects. Therefore, individuals deviating from family mean are supposed to be genetically superior and should be selected.

(b) Crossbreeding programme: The individuals combining ability for a trait is measured as the average phenotypic value of the progeny produced by crossbreeding the individuals of two populations. The combining ability is of two types *viz.* general (G.C.A.) and special (S.C.A.). The selection is done for utilizing both types of combining ability using two selection procedures *viz.* recurrent selection (RS) and reciprocal recurrent selection (RSS). Both these selection procedures are useful for improvement in traits affected by non additive gene action like over dominance *i.e.* traits with low heritability.

20.9 Methods of Estimating Heritability

The method of estimation of heritability depends on the resemblance among relatives. This is because the relatives tend to look more alike for a trait due to the reason of having similar genes and genotypes than unrelatives. Thus the type of data available *viz.* parent offspring performance or sib performance (half sibs or full sibs) determines the method of estimation of heritability. The heritability can also be estimated from analysis of twin data as well as from the data collected on selection experiment by comparing the performance of parental and progeny generation.

20.9.1 Regression of Offspring on Dam

This method is used when the mating is random, all groups are raised together and each dam (X) has one offspring (Y).

Statistical Model

The observation of progeny (Y_i) is taken as:

$$Y_i = b\, X_i + e_i.$$

Where,   Yi = observation of the ith dam

            b = regression of Y on X

            e_j = random error associated with Y's

Genetic Model

$$\text{Cov}_{OP} = \tfrac{1}{2} V_A + \tfrac{1}{4} V_{AA} + V_M.$$

The heritability is estimated as:

$$h^2 = 2\, b_{OP}$$

Where, b_{OP}
$$= \frac{\text{Cov}_{XY}}{V_X}$$

$$= \frac{\sum xy}{\sigma^2 x}$$

$$\sum xy = \frac{\sum XY - \left(\sum X \sum Y\right)^2}{N}$$

$$\sigma^2 x = \sum x^2 - \frac{\left(\sum x\right)^2}{N}$$

N   = No. of dam – daughter pairs

$$\text{S.E. (b)} = \sqrt{\frac{\left(\sigma^2_b\right)}{\sum x^2}}$$

where, $\qquad \sigma^2_b = \sum y^2 - \frac{\left(\sum xy\right)^2}{\sum x^2}$

$$\text{S.E. } (h^2) = 2 \text{ S. E.(b)}$$

Merits of the Method

The estimate does not contain dominance variation but only a little amount of epistatic variation (Cov $_{OD}$ = ½ V_A + ¼ V_I + V_M).

It is free from environmental covariance because parent and offspring are measured at different times.

Selection of parents does not affect the estimate because selection has same effect to reduce the V_p and Cov $_{OP.}$

The estimate is least affected by mating system. It provides a more precise estimate of heritability.

The b_{OP} has less sampling variance and provides a more precise estimate of h^2.

Demerits and Limitations

It requires the records on two generations. The information on two generations are rarely available for certain traits like slaughter traits.

The method of regression of offspring on mid parent value can not be used for sex limited traits.

The regression of offspring on dam (b $_{OD}$) and on mid parent value for traits particularly measured early in life (birth weight, litter weight etc.) are affected by maternal effects, though regression of offspring on sire(b $_{OS}$) does not contain maternal effect but its application is limited due to lesser degree of freedom and for sex-limited traits.

20.9.2 Intra-sire Regression of Offspring on Dam (ISRD)

This method is used when a number of sires are mated to several dams and each mating produces one offspring. It is estimated as the average regression of daughter on dam within sire. The regression of daughter on dam is calculated separately for each dam group mated to one sire and then the regression from each sire is pooled in a weighted average. This removes the sire effect.

Statistical Model

The observation of progeny (Y_{ij}) born to j^{th} dam mated to i^{th} sire is taken as:

$Y_{ij} = \mu + S_i + b(X_{ij} - X.) + e_{ij}$.

Where, Y_{ij} = record of daughter of ith sire mated to j^{th} dam

μ = overall mean

S_i = effect of ith sire

b = regression of coefficient of Y on X

X = mean of dams

e_{ij} = random error

Genetic Model

$\text{Cov}_{OP} = \frac{1}{2} V_A + \frac{1}{4} V_{AA} + \frac{1}{2} V_M$.

The heritability is estimated by conducting the analysis of variance and covariance as:

Table 20.1: ANOVA and Covariance

S.V.	D.F.	Dam (X)	Daughter (Y)	Cross Product
Sires	S-1	$SS_{S(X)}$	$SS_{S(Y)}$	$SCP_{S(XY)}$
Dams/sire	D-S	$SS_{DS(X)}$	$SS_{DS(Y)}$	$SCP_{DS(XY)}$
Total	D-1	$SS_{T(X)}$	$SS_{T(Y)}$	$SCP_{T(XY)}$

The procedure to calculate sum of squares for sires (SS_S), dams within sire (SS_{DS}) and total sum of squares (SS_T) on both dams (X) and daughter (Y) observations, and the sum of cross products (SCP_{XY}) is given as under:

Sum of Squares for Dams

$$\text{Correction Factor (C.F.)} = \frac{\left(\sum X_{ij}\right)^2}{D};$$

$$S.S._{T(X)} = \sum X^2_{ij} - C.F.;$$

$$S.S._{S(X)} = \left[\frac{\sum X^2_{i.}}{n_i}\right] - C.F.$$

$$S.S._{DS(X)} = S.S._{T(X)} - S.S._{S(X)}$$

$$= \sum X^2_{ij} - \frac{\sum X^2_{i.}}{n_i}$$

Sum of Cross Product (C.S.P. $_{XY}$):

Correction Factor $= \dfrac{\left[\left(\sum X_{ij}\right)\left(\sum Y_{ij}\right)\right]}{D}$

S.C.P. $_{T(XY)}$ $= \Sigma X_{ij} Y_{ij} - C.F.$;

S.C.P. $_{S(XY)}$ $= \dfrac{\sum \left(X_{i.} Y_{i.}\right)}{n_{i.}} - C.F.$

S.C.P. $_{DS(XY)}$ $= $ S.C.P. $_{T(XY)} - $ S.C.P. $_{S(XY)}$

$$= \sum X_{ij} Y_{ij} - \left[\dfrac{\left(\sum X_i Y_i\right)}{n_i}\right]$$

Where, $D = $ number of total dams $= \Sigma n_{i.}$

$n_{i.} = $ number of dams mated to i^{th} sire

$X_{i.} = $ Sum of phenotypic values of all the dams mated to i^{th} sire

$Y_{i.} = $ Sum of phenotypic values of all the daughters born to i^{th} sire

$X_{ij} = $ phenotypic value of jth dam mated to i^{th} sire

$Y_{ij} = $ phenotypic value of jth daughter born to i^{th} sire

$b_{YX} = $ Intra-sire regression of daughter on dam

$$= \dfrac{\text{S.C.P.}_{DS(XY)}}{\text{S.S.}_{DS(X)}}$$

h^2 $= 2 b_{YX}$

S.E. (h^2) $= 2\,SE\,(b)$

$$= 2 \sqrt{\dfrac{\sigma^2_b}{SS_{dS(x)}}}$$

where, $\sigma^2_b = \dfrac{\left\{ SS\,ds(y) - \dfrac{\left[SCP_{dS(XY)}\right]^2}{SS_{dS(x)}} \right\}}{D - S - 1}$

Merit of Method

The ISRD method is best because of the followings:

☆ No correction is required for mating system because progeny within group are produced from the same sire.

☆ Environmental component is much reduced by similar environment within group.

☆ This provides useful estimate of h² when there is no selection in progeny generation and when the maternal effects are absent.

☆ This method is most suited for sex – limited traits.

☆ This method is more appropriate and suitable than other regression estimate.

Limitation

This method has the *limitation* that it does not eliminate the environmental differences among dams within sires. Secondly, the characters measured in early life may have some maternal effect which may increase the estimate.

20.9.3 Weighted Regression Method

This method is used when the numbers of progeny per dam are more than one. The estimate may be obtained in any of the three possible ways:

(i) Regression of individual progeny on parent by repeating the parent value with its each progeny

(ii) Regression of mean value of all the progeny of a parent on parent value

(iii) Weighted regression is obtained based on the phenotypic correlation between progeny with parent and number of progeny per parent. This method was devised by Kempthorne and Tandon (1953). The weighted regression is obtained as:

$$b = \frac{\sum W_i (X_i - \overline{X})(Y_i - \overline{Y})}{\sum W_i (X_i - \overline{X})^2}$$

$$where, \quad W_i = \frac{n_i}{(1 + n_i t)}$$

t = intra – class correlation between sibs within parent

n_i = no. of progeny for i^{th} sire

20.9.4 Correlation between Offspring and Parent

The heritability is estimated as twice the correlation between offspring and parent as:

$$h^2 = 2 \, r_{OP}$$

The intra sire correlation between parent and offspring can also be used to estimate the h² like regression. However, the correlation method gives biased estimate, if dams are selected. The Cov_{OP} and V_P are both affected by selection of dams whereas V_O is not affected. The V_P is reduced due to dam selection and is less than V_O. Thus, correlation is biased but the regression is not biased till the b_{OP} is linear.

20.9.5 Paternal Half Sib Correlation Method

The half sibs are of two types *viz.* paternal and maternal. The intra class correlation between paternal half sibs is more commonly used to estimate heritability for the reason that these are available more in numbers than maternal half sibs. The correlation compares the resemblance among HS to the resemblance among individuals related by an average amount for the population. This is the ratio of variance component among the means of HS group to the total phenotypic variance. The variance among groups is a measure of similarity within group.

This method is used when a number of females (dams) are mated to a number of sires and each dam produces one offspring.

Statistical Model

The observation (phenotypic value, X_{ij}) on a progeny (X_j) of ith sire is taken as:

$X_{ij} = \mu + S_i + e_{ij}$.

Where, μ = overall mean

S_i = Effect of i th sire

e_{ij} = random error attributed to individuals within sire group

Genetic Model

$\sigma^2_P = \sigma^2_S + \sigma^2_e$

$Cov_{HS} = \sigma^2_S$ (Sire variance)

$\qquad = \frac{1}{4} V_A + 1/16 V_{I(AA)}$.

$\sigma^2_P - Cov_{HS} = \sigma^2_P - \sigma^2_S$

$\qquad\qquad = \sigma^2 e$

$\qquad\qquad = \frac{3}{4} V_A + V_D + 15/16 V_{AA} + V_{AD} + V_{DD} + V_E$.

The analysis of variance is conducted to partition the phenotypic variance (σ^2_P) into σ^2_S and $\sigma^2 e$ after estimating the sum of squares.

The mean square between sire groups (MSs) is an estimate of variance component within HS group ($\sigma^2 e$) plus K times the σ^2_S. Thus, MSs = $\sigma^2 e$ + K σ^2_S.

The σ^2_S is the variance of sire group means about the population mean or the component of variance among HS group means. The size of variance component (σ^2_S) is due to the fact that the sire groups differ and thus indicates the differences between the progenies of different sires.

This ($\sigma^2 e$) indicates the difference between the progenies of the same sire (within sire component) and is the variance of individual observations about their group mean.

The procedure to calculate the sum of squares and different component of variance is as under-

$$\text{Correction Factor (C.F.)} = \frac{\left(\sum x\right)^2}{N} = \frac{\sum x^2.}{n.}$$

Total sum of squares (T.S.S.) = $\sum X^2_{ij} - \text{C.F.}$

Sire Sum of square $= \Sigma X^2_{i.} - C.F.$

Progeny within sire S.S. (Error S.S.) = T.S.S. – Sire S.S.

Table 20.2: Analysis of Variance for Half Sib Groups

S.V.	D.F.	Sum of Square	Mean Square	Expected Mean Square
Sires	S – 1	Sire S.S.	$M.S._s$ = Sire S.S./S-1	$\sigma^2_e + K\sigma^2_s$
Progeny/Sire or Error	N – S	Error S.S.	$M.S._e$ = Error S.S./N – S	σ^2_e

Where, K = Average number of daughters per sire $= [1/S-1][n. - \Sigma n_i^2/n.]$

n_i = number of daughters of ith sire and

n. $= \Sigma n_i$

$$\sigma^2_s = \frac{(M.S._s - M.S._e)}{K};$$

$\sigma^2 e = M.S.\, e;$

$\sigma^2_p = \sigma^2_s + \sigma^2_e$

$$t = \frac{\sigma^2_s}{\sigma^2_p}$$

$h^2 = 4\,t.$

Merits of Half Sib Method

☆ Half sib correlation does not contain variance due to dominance or maternal effect or common environment and hence free from bias. The records of all daughters are recorded at the same time.

☆ The method can be used for sex limited traits and for the traits expressed after death of animals.

☆ It does not require records of parents.

The heritability estimated from maternal HS correlation contains epistatic effect, maternal effect and some common environmental effect. The paternal Hs method is more commonly used than maternal HS because the maternal HS are not available in dairy animals, measured in different years and contain maternal effect as well as common environmental effect. This inflates the heritability. The maternal component of variance can be obtained as a difference in the intra class correlation between maternal HS and paternal HS.

Maternal component $(V_M) = Cov_{MHS} - Cov_{PHS}$

Limitations of Half Sib Method

☆ Half sib correlation contains some interaction component equal to $1/16\, V_{I(AA)}.$

☆ The heritability is obtained by multiplying the intra class correlation with 4, the environmental correlation (if exist) are also quadrupled. The environmental correlation exists in the presence of genotype–environment correlation when the daughters of one bull get better environment than others. This increases the genetic differences. The common environment increases the likeness in records of the same sire and hence inflates the h^2.

☆ It is valid in random mating population because the estimate is affected by selection.

☆ The heritability estimated based on small numbers of sire increases the chance of large error.

20.9.6 Full Sib Correlation Method

This method is used in species with larger full sib families like pigs, poultry, mice, goat when each male is mated to several females and each mating produces several offspring (multiple births) or when repeated mating are common. The progenies are arranged as full sib families according to sires taking that i^{th} sire is mated to a set of d_i dams producing n_{ij} progeny. The observation (X_{ijk}) on the kth progeny born from j^{th} dam mated to i^{th} sire can be described from the following mathematical model as:

Mathematical Model

$$X_{ijk} = \mu + S_i + d_{ij} + e_{ijk}$$

μ = overall mean

S_i = Effect of ith sire (deviation common to all the progeny of ith sire from μ.

d_{ij} = Effect of jth dam mated to i^{th} sire (deviation common to the progeny of jth dam and i^{th} sire).

e_{ijk} = Random error or deviation attributed to the individual due to uncontrolled environmental and genetic factors.

All these effects are assumed random and independent with mean.

Genetic Model

$$\sigma^2_P = \sigma^2_S + \sigma^2_D + \sigma^2_{EC} + \sigma^2_e$$

$$\sigma^2_S = Cov_{HS} = \tfrac{1}{4}\sigma^2_A$$

$$\sigma^2_D = Cov_{FS} - Cov_{HS} = \tfrac{1}{4}\sigma^2_A + \tfrac{1}{4}\sigma^2_D + \sigma^2_{EC} + \sigma^2_M$$

$$\sigma^2_S + \sigma^2_D = Cov_{FS} = \tfrac{1}{2}\sigma^2_S + \tfrac{1}{4}\sigma^2_D + \sigma^2_{EC} + \sigma^2_M$$

$$\sigma^2_e = \sigma^2_P - Cov_{FS} = \tfrac{1}{2}\sigma^2_A + \tfrac{3}{4}\sigma^2_D + \sigma^2_{EW}$$

The analysis of variance is conducted to partition the phenotypic variance into observational components attributable to;

(i) Differences between the progenies of different sires (σ^2_S) which is the variance among means of HS families about overall mean. This is between sire component arises due to the sire groups being different. Thus $\sigma^2_S = Cov_{HS}$;

(ii) Differences between the progenies of different dams (σ^2_D) mated to same sire (between dam within sire component, MS_D or between full sibs within half sib groups). The σ^2_D arises due to differences between dam groups. The $\sigma^2_D = Cov_{FS} - Cov_{HS}$ of sires.

(iii) Differences between the progenies of same female ($\sigma^2 e$) which is within progeny component.

Sources	D.F.	S.S.	M.S.	E. M. S.
Sire	S-1	Sire S.S.	$M.S._S$	$\sigma^2_e + K_2 \sigma^2_D + K_3 \sigma^2_S$
Dam/sire	D-s	Dam S.S.	$M.S._D$	$\sigma^2_e + K_1 \sigma^2_D$
Progeny/dam (full sibs within dam)	N-D	Error S.S.	$M.S._e$	σ^2_e

Where,

$$K_1 = \text{Average no. of dams per sire} = \frac{n. - \left(\sum \dfrac{n^2_{ij}}{n_i} \right)}{D-S}$$

$$K_2 = \text{Average no. of progeny per dam} = \frac{\sum \dfrac{n^2_{ij}}{n_{i.}} - \sum \dfrac{n^2_{ij}}{n_.}}{S-1}$$

$$K_3 = \text{Average no. of progeny per sire} = \frac{n - \sum \dfrac{n^2_{i.}}{n_.}}{S-1}$$

N = n. = Total no. of progeny;

$n_{i.}$ = No. of progeny per sire;

n_{ij} = No. of progeny per dam;

S = No. of sires; D = No. of dams

The different components of variance are computed as:

$$\sigma^2_s = \frac{MS_S - MS_e - K_2 \sigma^2_D}{K_3}$$

$$= \frac{MS_S - MS_D}{K_3}$$

$$\sigma^2_D = \frac{MS_D - MS_e}{K_1} ;$$

$$\sigma^2_e = MS_e$$

$$\sigma^2_P = \sigma^2_S + \sigma^2_D + \sigma^2_e$$

The heritability is estimated from half sib correlation based on σ^2_S and σ^2_D as well as from full sib correlation based on $\sigma^2_S + \sigma^2_D$.

$$h^2_S = 4\left(\frac{\sigma^2_S}{\sigma^2_P}\right);$$

$$h^2_D = 4\left(\frac{\sigma^2_D}{\sigma^2_P}\right);$$

$$h^2_{(S+D)} = 2\left(\frac{\sigma^2_S + \sigma^2_D}{\sigma^2_P}\right)$$

Standard Error

The S.E. of h^2 from 3 components is estimated as:

$$SE\,(h^2_S) = 4\sqrt{\frac{\left[Var\left(\sigma^2_S\right)\right]}{\sigma^2_P}}$$

$$SE\,(h^2_D) = 4\sqrt{\frac{\left[Var\left(\sigma^2_D\right)\right]}{\sigma^2_P}}$$

$$SE\,(h^2_{S+D}) = 2\sqrt{\frac{\left[Var\left(\sigma^2_S\right) + Var\left(\sigma^2_D\right) + 2\,Cov\left(\sigma^2_S\,\sigma^2_D\right)\right]}{\sigma^2_P}}$$

Where,

$$Var.\left(\sigma^2_S\right) = \frac{2}{K_3^2}\left[\frac{MS_S^2}{S+1} + \frac{MS_D^2}{D-S+2}\right]$$

$$Var.\left(\sigma^2_D\right) = \frac{2}{K_2^2}\left[\frac{MS_D^2}{D-S+2} + \frac{MS_e^2}{N-D+2}\right]$$

$$Cov\left(\sigma^2_S\,\sigma^2_D\right) = \frac{K_2}{K_3}\left[Var\left(\sigma^2_D\right) - \frac{2\,MS_e^2}{K_1^2(n.....-D+2)}\right]$$

The heritability estimated from full sib component [$h^2_{(S+D)}$] contains twice the maternal effects and ½ V_D

The heritability from dam component (h^2_D) contains four times the maternal effects plus all the dominance effect. The σ^2_D contains variance due to the maternal effect (V_M) during early life of an individual.

Merits and Limitations of Full Sib Method

(i) The h^2_{FS} contains dominance deviations, epistatic variance, maternal effects and common environment in addition to the additive gene effects. Maternal effects strongly bias the covariance in full sibs. Thus the estimate is subject to bias and is least reliable to other methods. Therefore, this method is not valid for traits affected by maternal effects.

(ii) This method gives larger standard error than other estimates.

(iii) This method requires larger full sib families which are, in general, not available particularly for large farm animals.

(iv) The difference between dam and sire component of variance from FS analysis indicates the importance of dominance, interaction and maternal effects. The h^2_S is relatively unbiased, whereas h^2_D is biased in comparison to h^2_S and $h^2_{(S+D)}$. The combined estimate of non-additive and maternal effects can be known from three estimates of heritability.

Comparison between Sib Correlation and Parent Offspring Relation

The sib correlation requires the measurement on progeny generation whereas the parent offspring regression requires the measurements on parent and offspring generation. Thus the data utilized in sib correlation are more contemporaneous and more comparable than data on parent offspring collected over years. The techniques of measurement may differ in collecting data on two generations and this creates the error of measurement. The heritability of slaughter traits or traits of animals which do not yet have progeny can only be estimated by sib correlations. The sib correlation estimates can easily be obtained from test station/field data and it is difficult to get data on parent and offspring in test station and under field conditions. The regression method is preferred to estimate heritability with moderate value and the sib correlation method is preferred for traits of low heritability. This is based on the sampling variance of h^2 by two methods. The regression method has low sampling variance for high h^2 while the sib correlations have low sampling variance at low h^2. When common environment makes the full sib correlation unsuitable, the heritability is estimated based on the between sire component (half sibs correlation).

The comparison of co-variances of paternal and maternal half sisters and half brothers are used to study the sex linked inheritance. The sire covariance for sex-linked inheritance in female also contains $\frac{1}{2} \sigma^2 A$ in addition to $\frac{1}{4} \sigma^2 A$. The $\sigma^2 A_{SL}$ is the additive genetic sex linked variance. The sire covariance for sex linked traits in males is equal to $\frac{1}{4} \sigma^2_A$. Thus

$$\sigma^2_S \text{ in males} = \frac{1}{4} \sigma^2_A$$

$$\sigma^2_S \text{ in females} = \frac{1}{4} \sigma^2_A + \frac{1}{2} \sigma^2_{A\,(SL)}$$

Thus the additive genetic variance for male offspring is obtained by multiplying it by four while for female offspring the multiplication by four overestimates the sex linked additive variance by two. The covariance among maternal half sibs of the two sexes is:

$$\sigma^2_D \text{ in males} = \frac{1}{4} \sigma^2_A + \frac{1}{2} \sigma^2_{A\,(SL)}.$$

$$\sigma^2_D \text{ in males} = \frac{1}{4} \sigma^2_A + \frac{1}{4} \sigma^2_{A\,(SL)}.$$

Thus twice the difference of σ^2_S in males and in females estimate the sex linked additive genetic variance in males $\sigma^2_{A\ (SL)} = 2(\sigma^2_S\ \text{females} - \sigma^2_S\ \text{males})$, whereas in females it is obtained as four times the difference of $\sigma^2 D$ in males and females. Thus $\sigma^2_{A(sL)} = 4(\sigma^2_{SD}\ \text{males} - \sigma^2_D\ \text{females})$.

Equal variance in two sexes is assured. Thus the importance of sex linked inheritance is considered negligible. This assumption is more valid and reasonable in species having many chromosomes and too of small size chromosomes like cattle, buffalo, sheep and goat. But some sex linked inheritance is expected in species that contained fewer pairs of chromosomes and the largest sex chromosomes like domestic fowl. Thus the variability in a trait due to sex linked inheritance is indicated when variance component are quite different in the two sexes.'

20.9.7 Twin Data Analysis

A group of individuals having similar genotypes are called as the isogenic lines, like identical twins and multiplets.

Isogenic lines also include the highly inbred lines with more than 0.9 inbreeding co-efficient as well as the clones in plants. The twins are of two types *viz.* one – egg and two – egg twins which are called as monozygotic twins (identical twins) and dizygotic twins respectively. The dizygotic twins are equivalent to the litter mates or full sibs. The one egg twins contains the same genotype and therefore, the variation between them is purely of environmental nature, but the variation between two egg twins (fraternal twins) is due to both heredity and environment because they are no more alike genetically than FS that are not twins. Therefore, the comparison of these two types of twins provides an estimate of the relative influence of heredity and environment. The composition of the observational components of variance can be as:

Types of Twins	*Between Twin Pairs*	*Within Twin Pairs*
Monozygotic (identical)	$\sigma^2_A + \sigma^2_D + \sigma^2_{EC}$	σ^2_{EW}
Dizygotic (fraternal)	$\frac{1}{2}\sigma^2_A + \frac{1}{4}\sigma^2_D + \sigma^2_{EC}$	$\frac{1}{2}\sigma^2_A + \frac{3}{4}\sigma^2_D + \sigma^2_{EW}$
Difference	$\frac{1}{2}\sigma^2_A + \frac{3}{4}\sigma^2_D$	$\frac{1}{2}\sigma^2_A + \frac{1}{4}\sigma^2_D$

Thus, if the NAGV is not present, then twice the difference between the correlation coefficients of identical and fraternal twins estimates the heritability. The correlation between monozygotic twins estimates herita-bility in broad sense but in narrow sense if σ^2_D and σ^2_I are negligible. The expected covariance between the two types of twins is: -

$$\text{Cov}_{MZ} = \sigma^2_A + \sigma^2_D + \sigma^2_I + \sigma^2_M$$

$$\text{Cov}_{DZ} = \frac{1}{2}\sigma^2_A + \frac{1}{4}\sigma^2_D + \text{some }\sigma^2_I + \sigma^2_M$$

Twice the difference between Cov_{MZ} and Cov_{DZ} is suggested to estimate heritability in broad sense. The h^2 is larger due to the fact that maternal environment makes the twins more alike The resemblance is increased in addition to having by them the common genes. Secondly, one egg twin contains the genetic variance due to the dominance and epistatic effects in addition to the additive genetic variance.

The estimation of heritability will take the following form of analysis of variance based on identical twins, clones or highly inbred lines, taking l isogenic lines, each line having n_i individuals. The phenotypic measurement (X_{ij}) of the jth individual of the ith line can be represented as:

$$X_{ij} = G_i \pm E_{ij}$$

Where, G_i is the genotypic value

E_{ij} is the environmental deviation

The σ^2_X can be partitioned into two components as follows:

S.V.	DF	E(MS)
Between lines	$l-1$	$\sigma^2_d + k\,\sigma^2_G$
Within	$n-I$	σ^2_e

$$where, \quad K = \frac{1}{\ell-1}\left(N - \frac{\sum N^2_i}{N}\right)$$

The h^2 is estimated as intraclass correlation assuming no common environment between the members of a line.

$$H^2 = \frac{\sigma^2_G}{\sigma^2_G + \sigma^2_E}$$

Newman (1941) estimated the heritability for certain human traits using the following formula

$$H^2 = \frac{(Ir - Fr)}{1 - Fr}$$

Where, Ir = intrapair coefficient of correlation of identical twins,

Fr = intrapair correlation of fraternal twins

20.9.8 Heritability Estimation from Selection Experiments

The heritability is also measured by comparing the performance of parental generation with progeny generation. The followings are two procedures:

(a) Apparent Heritability

Lush and Stratus (1942) outlined the way to estimate h^2 by dividing the dams mated to a sire in two groups $viz.$ better and inferior. The performance of the progeny of the two groups of dams is recorded and h^2 is obtained as:

$$h^2 = 2 \left(\frac{\text{difference in daughters of two groups}}{\text{difference in dam's records of two groups}} \right)$$

$$= 2 \left[\frac{(P_H - P_L)}{(M_H - M_L)} \right]$$

Therefore, the heritability of differences is estimated by twice the ratio of the differences in two generations. This example illustrates the concept of regression (Galton) with the regression of the average of the dam's records and the average of the daughters towards the mean. In this example, low producing group is represented by cows with lower inherent ability and poorer than average environmental circumstances. But in progeny generation, a new herd circumstances may be representative for both low and high group. Thus environmental effects are removed and the existing differences in daughter's performance of two groups represented half the genetic differences, while the existing differences in darns groups included both genetic plus the environmental differences. Thus twice the ratio of differences estimates heritability.

When the daughters of many sires are available, the sire effect may be removed by appropriate weighting factor. The mates of each sire are divided into two groups *viz.* high and low producing (M_{iH} and M_{iL}) and the differences between their daughters is computed as D_{iH} and D_{iL} for each (i^{th}) sire separately. Now the difference between the two groups of mates and of daughters of each sire are weighted and summation being taken over all sire. The heritability is then taken as

$$h^2 = 2 \left(\frac{Wi(P_{iH} - P_{iL})}{Wi(M_{iH} - M_{iL})} \right)$$

Where, P_{iH} and M_{iH} indicate the average of high group of progeny and dams sired by sire i, and

P_{iL} and M_{iL} indicate the average of low groups of progeny and dams respectively sired by the sire i,

W_i is the weighting factor of the difference between the animals of sire i.

(b) Realised or effective Heritability

The direct comparison of response to selection and selection differential in the selection experiment estimates the heritability which is called as the realized heritability as:

$R = h^2 S$

Therefore, $h^2 = \dfrac{R}{S}$

$$= \frac{\left(\overline{X}_0 - \overline{X}\right)}{\left(\overline{X}_s - \overline{X}\right)}$$

$$= \frac{\text{Superiority of progeny}}{\text{Superiority of parents}}$$

Falconer (1955) called this estimate as effective heritability, because this represents the actual breeding gain.

The realized h^2 is estimated by plotting the generation means against the cumulative selection differential. A regression line is fitted to the points and the slope of this line is the realized heritability.

Limitations of Realized h^2

This method is an indirect approach. There are certain important conditions for the valid estimation of h^2 by this method *viz.* absence of maternal effects, no dominance, and panmixia. The observed response should not be confounded with systematic changes of generation means due to the environment or the effect of inbreeding. Thus, the number of parents should be large enough to avoid inbreeding. This method is mostly applied in lab animals.

1. The realized h^2 can only be estimated after the selection results are made available.

2. This method cannot be applied in animals having long generation interval and having low reproduction rate.

3. It requires proper monitoring on environmental changes between the periods the parents and progeny measurements are taken. This can be solved by maintaining a control population or by use of repeat mating or to conduct the two way selection experiment which is expensive and not justified to select for poor performance in large livestock species,

In case of small size of selection lines, inbreeding will occur and hence inbreeding depression will occur in the selected trait. It may then be difficult to separate the effect of selection from the effect of inbreeding in the population Therefore, the number of parents should be large enough and inbreeding should be avoided.

This method of estimating heritability seems to be optional. But it may over estimate. The heritability estimated by this method should correspond to that estimated by offspring-parent regression method. The maternal effects can influence the genetic gain in both direction (positive and negative) and consequently the heritability will be influenced. When interaction effects (dominance and epistasis) are not important, the heritability obtained by sib correlation should be similar to realized heritability. But when interaction effects are important the selection gain will be larger in early than in later generations of selection. However, the epistatic gene combinations are not permanent but disintegrate when selection ceases, and consequently the selection gain disappear. Thus the realized heritability may be larger in the first few generations with direct proportion to the transmitted additive interaction effects.

Falconer (1955) gave the concept of realized heritability and this is applied mostly to laboratory animals in which the generation interval is short and control population can be kept or selection in opposite direction can be applied.

Procedure

The realized heritability is estimated by plotting the generation means against the cumulated selection differential. The cumulated S is the selection differential summed over successive generations which means the total selection applied up to that generation. Now a regression line is fitted to the points and the slope of this line is the realized heritability $\left(h^2 = \dfrac{R}{S} \right)$. Thus, the method computes the ratio of final response (cumulative selection gain, R) to the total selection differential (cumulative selection differential, S) as:

$$h^2 = \frac{\sum R_i S_i}{\sum S_i}$$

Where, i is the generation.

The selection differential and response of individual generation can also be taken to estimate the heritability.

The difficulty in using this method particularly for cattle, buffalo and sheep is that generation interval is long and also the reproductive rate is too low making the replacement low. Low reproductive rate makes the generations to overlap and requires the biometrical skill for statistical analysis, whereas the first problem of long generation interval posses financial problem. Thirdly, the parents and offspring are measured at different time particularly in large mammals and by the time the environmental conditions as well as the management practices may be changed. The parents and offspring must be measured under similar conditions to get a valid estimate of realized heritability. The reason for this is that changes in environmental conditions will change the h² estimate. The better environment will improve the response to selection in offspring generation and hence the h² will be biased towards higher side, whereas the poor environment of progeny generation will result low response to selection and hence the h² will be an under estimate. Therefore, it is required to have a proper monitoring on environmental effects, if any. There are three other alternatives to overcome the difficulty of changes in environment. The first is to maintain a control population without selection as a contemporary to the selected population. The change in the average phenotype in control population over years will represent the effect of change in environment. The second is the use of repeat mating to obtain full sibs which will be genetically identical. Therefore, the differences in means of full sibs in subsequent years will represent the effect of change in environment. The third means to estimate the environmental change is to conduct two way selection experiments for the trait (upward and downward selection). The response in the two lines is assumed to be symmetrical though it is not in practical. Thus, this method does not measure the environmental change in real sense. The more important point to use the two way selection experiment as a measure of change in environment is that this method is expensive and not advocated for selection for poor performance.

20.10 Precision of Heritability Estimate

The precision (reliability) of h^2 estimate depends on a number of factors given below:

1. Data recording is correct or inaccurate
2. Similar or different environmental conditions for different animals
3. Scale effect
4. Unadjustment of data
5. Violation of assumptions in h^2 estimation
6. Methods of h^2 estimation

The precision (reliability) of an estimate is indicated by its standard error. Low standard error indicates that the estimate is more precise. The h^2 is estimated from the degree of resemblance between relatives by estimating either correlation or regression. The standard error of h^2 is obtained from the variance of the correlation or regression.

The magnitude of the S.E. of h^2 depends on the closeness of relatives and the sample size used to estimate h^2. In general, the estimate is more precise if the relatives have close relationship. The reason is that to get the h^2 the correlation or regression is multiplied by the factor $1/r$ where r is the genetic relationship between relatives and the S.E. of correlation or regression is also multiplied by the same factor $(1/r)$. Secondly, the S.E. of h^2 is large when the correlation or regression is estimated on small sample size. The reason is that the S.E. of an estimate depends on the sample size. Therefore, the r or b used to estimate h^2 should be based on large numbers to minimise the standard error. However, the available facilities (space, labour, and cost) limit the sample size. In estimating the h^2 the sample size depends on the number and size of families. The h^2 with high precision requires a large number of families and more number of individuals per family. Keeping large number of families reduces the family size and an increase in family size limits the number of families due to the available facilities. Thus the design of experiment (number and size of families) is an important aspect and a compromise has to be made between the number and size of the families.

1. Sib Analysis

The intra-class correlation (t) is estimated either from half sib or full sib families to get an estimate of h^2. The variance of intra-class correlation (t) is:

$$\sigma_t^2 = \frac{2[1 + (n - 1)t]^2}{n(n - 1)(N - 1)}$$

where,   n = no. of individuals per family (family size)

N = no. of families

nN = Total no. of individuals to be measured.

The σ_t^2 is low when $n = 1/t$. Thus, optimum family size $(n) = 2/h^2$ for full sibs and $n = 4/h^2$ for half sib families because $t = h^2/2$ or $h^2/4$ for FS and HS families, respectively. Therefore, the optimum family size (n) depends on the correlation (t) and hence on the h².

Now, the variance of intra-class correlation is:

$\sigma^2_t = 8t/nN$ approx. by putting the value of $n = 1/t$,

and hence the variance of h², after replacing $t = h^2/2$ for FS and $t = h^2/4$ for HS, becomes as:

$$\sigma^2\left(h^2_{FS}\right) = 4\sigma^2_t = \frac{4\left(\dfrac{8h^2}{4}\right)}{nN} = \frac{16h^2}{nN} \text{ approx.}$$

$$\sigma^2\left(h^2_{HS}\right) = 16\sigma^2_t = \frac{16\left(\dfrac{8h^2}{4}\right)}{nN} = \frac{32h^2}{nN} \text{ approx.}$$

Thus, the h^2_{FS} is more precise (twice) than h^2_{HS}.

Robertson (1959) suggested the following formula of optimal family size with half sib families:

$$n = 0.56\sqrt{\frac{T}{Nh^2}}$$

where, $T = nN$

and he further suggested that if h² estimate is not known then n should range between 20 to 30.

2. Parent-Offspring Regression

The variance of regression coefficient (σ^2_b) is:

$$\sigma^2_b = \frac{1}{(N-2)}\frac{\left[\sigma^2_Y - \left(\sum xy\right)^2\right]}{\sigma^2_x}$$

$$= \frac{1}{N-2}\left[\frac{\sigma^2_Y}{\sigma^2_x} - b^2\right] \text{ after rearrangement}$$

$$= \frac{1}{N}\left(\frac{\sigma^2_Y}{\sigma^2_x}\right) \text{ approx}$$

Where,   X = Parent's record

Y = Offspring record

N = No. of families paired records of x and y.

Now, taking the σ^2_x and σ^2_y in terms of numbers

$$\sigma^2_x = \frac{1}{K}V_P \quad ; \quad \sigma^2_y = \frac{1+(n-1)t}{n}V_P$$

Where,   n = No. of offspring per family (family size)

K = No. of parents = 1 or 2

T = phenotypic correlation between family members

The variance of regression becomes as:

$$\sigma^2_b = \frac{K[1+(n-1)t]}{nN}$$

where, nN = T = Total no. of offspring measured.

3. Regression on Single Parent

If the denominator (nN) of variance of regression is the limiting factor of the design of experiment, then nN is fixed and the σ^2_b is minimum when n = 1 which makes (n-1) t = 0. Therefore, more number of families should be measured with only one offspring per family. This will make the standard error of heritability estimate as:

S.E. (h^2) $= \sqrt{\sigma^2_b}$

$= 2/\sqrt{N}$ approx.

This indicates that large number of families are required (say about 400) to get precise estimate of about 0.1 and about 100 families should be measured to get standard error of about 0.2 which implies that an estimate of h^2 below 0.4 will not be significantly different from zero. The precision will be increased by increasing n without reducing N (number of families). Further the precision depends on the correlation between family members (t). When t is low the additional offspring gives more information about family mean.

4. Regression on Mid-Parent Value

In this case both parents are measured (K=2) and if only one offspring per family (n = 1) is measured, the standard error of h^2 is:

SE. (h^2) = $\sqrt{\sigma^2_b}$ = $\sqrt{2}/N$ approx.

Now, if K = 2 and n = 2, the S.E. of estimate is $\dfrac{\sqrt{(1+t)}}{N}$

where t = full sib correlation.

The regression on mid parent results more precise estimate than the regression on one parent.

Effect of Assortative Mating and Selection of Parents

The assortative mating of parents increases the precision for the regression on mid-parent value. The reason is that the assortative mating increases the variance of mid parent value and this increase is more than increase in the variance of offspring. The variance of mid-parent value under assortative mating is:

$\sigma^2_X = \frac{1}{2}(1+r)\,Vp$

where, r = correlation between mates

Now substituting the value of $\sigma^2_X = \frac{1}{2}(1+r)\,Vp$ and $\sigma^2_Y = [1+(n-1)\,t/n]\,Vp$ in the equation of $\sigma^2_b = 1/N\,(\sigma^2_Y/\sigma^2_X)$, the variance of regression with assortative mating becomes approx. as:

$\sigma^2_b = 1/(1+r)$ times the σ^2_b under random mating.

$$= \frac{1}{1+r}\,\frac{K[1+(n-1)t]}{nN}$$

Therefore, the precision is increased by (1+r) or by $\sqrt{2}$ if r = 1 (complete assortative mating).

The selection of parents, though does not affect the regression estimate on parent (single parent or mid-parent), reduces the precision by reducing the variance of parents (σ^2_X). An under estimate of h^2 is obtained from intra-class correlation if the parents are selected. The selection results the variance between parents to be reduced which in turn reduces the covariance of sibs.

Solved Examples and Exercises

Example 20.1

Six sires were mated to 21 dams which produced different number of progenies. Estimate the heritability of the character (birth weight) from half sib (paternal and maternal) and full sib components.

Sires	Dams	Progeny Records (X_{ij})				Totals		
		1	2	3	4	n_{ij}	X_{ij}	X_i
1	1	21	24	–	–	2	45	
	2	16	18	20	–	3	54	
	3	16	17	19	20	4	72	171
2	4	18	20	19	–	3	57	
	5	17	21	23	–	3	61	
	6	23	21	–	–	2	44	
	7	19	19	–	–	2	38	200
3	8	17	20	20	–	3	57	
	9	18	19	22	23	4	82	139

Contd...

Sires	Dams	Progeny Records (X_{ij})				Totals		
		1	2	3	4	n_{ij}	X_{ij}	X_i
4	10	16	19	20	21	4	76	
	11	20	20	24	–	3	64	
	12	22	22	–	–	2	44	
	13	19	20	21	–	3	60	
	14	19	20	22	23	4	84	328
5	15	19	20	19	–	3	58	
	16	22	23	23	–	3	68	
	17	20	22	–	–	2	42	168
6	18	22	23	21	20	4	86	
	19	20	22	23	–	3	65	
	20	21	22	24	–	3	67	
	21	20	21	22	22	4	85	303
Total						64	1309	

Solution

The first step is to calculate the values of K_1, K_2 and K_3.

Sires	Dams/Sire	Progeny/Dam (n_{ij})	Progeny/Sire (n_i)
1	3	2, 3, 4	9
2	4	3, 3, 2, 2	10
3	2	3, 4	7
4	5	4, 3, 2, 3, 4	16
5	3	3, 3, 2	8
6	4	4, 3, 3, 4	14

K_1 = Average no. of dams per sire

$$= \frac{64 - \left[\dfrac{\left(2^2 + 3^2 + 4^2\right)}{9} + \dfrac{\left(3^2 + 3^2 + 2^2 + 2^2\right)}{10} .... + \dfrac{\left(4^2 + 3^2 + 3^2 + 4^2\right)}{14}\right]}{(21 - 6)}$$

$$= \frac{(64 - 19.09)}{15}$$

$$= 2.99$$

K_2 = Average no. of progeny per dam

$$= \frac{\left[\dfrac{19.09 - \left(2^2 + 3^2 + 4^2 + 3^2 + 3^2 + 2^2 + \ldots + 3^2 + 3^2 + 4^2\right)}{64}\right]}{(6-1)}$$

$$= \frac{(19.09 - 3.22)}{5}$$

$$= 3.17$$

K_3 = Average no. of progeny per sire

$$= \frac{\left[64 - \dfrac{\left(9^2 + 10^2 + 7^2 + 16^2 + 8^2 + 14^2\right)}{64}\right]}{(6-1)}$$

$$= \frac{(64 - 11.66)}{5}$$

$$= 10.47$$

Correction Factor $\quad = \dfrac{(1309)^2}{64} = 26773.14$

T. S. S. $\quad = X^2_{ijk} - \text{C.F.}$

$\quad = 27029 - 26773.14$

$\quad = 255.86$

Sire S.S. $\quad = \dfrac{(171)^2}{9} + \ldots\ldots + \dfrac{(303)^2}{14} - \text{C.F.}$

$\quad = 26818.93 - \text{C.F.} = 45.78$

Dam within sire S.S. $\quad = \left[\dfrac{45^2}{2} + \dfrac{54^2}{3} + \ldots\ldots\ldots + \dfrac{67^2}{3} + \dfrac{85^2}{4}\right] - \text{Sire S.S. (crude)}$

$\quad = 26903.75 - 26818.93 = 84.82$

Progeny within dam S.S. = T.S.S. (crude) – Dams within sire S.S. (Crude)

$\quad = 27029 - 26903.75 = 125.25$

ANOVA table for HS and FS for computing different components of variance:

Sources of Variation	D.F.	S.S.	M.S.
Sires	5	45.787	9.157
Dams/sire	15	84.821	5.654
Progenies/dams	43	125.25	2.912

$$\sigma^2_s = \frac{(9.157 - 2.912)}{10.47} = 0.596$$

$$\sigma^2_D = \frac{(5.654 - 2.912)}{2.99} = 0.917$$

$$\sigma^2 e = 2.912$$

$$\sigma^2 P = \sigma^2_s + \sigma^2_D + \sigma^2 e = 4.425$$

The heritability can be estimated from sire, dam and full sib component of variance as:

$$h^2_s = 4\frac{\sigma^2_s}{\sigma^2_P} = \frac{(4 \times 0.596)}{4.425} = 0.539 \ ;$$

$$h^2_D = 4\frac{\sigma^2_D}{\sigma^2_P} = \frac{(4 \times 0.917)}{4.425} = 0.828$$

$$h^2_{(S+D)} = 2\frac{(\sigma^2_s + \sigma^2_D)}{\sigma^2_P} = \frac{2(0.596 + 0.917)}{4.425} = 0.684$$

Example 20.2

Find out the heritability of the character based on paternal half sib correlation from the data given above in example 20.1 considering that the information on dam number's of progenies (Dam's identity) were not available, for which full sib pairs can not be sorted out.

Solution

In this case, the C.F., T.S.S. and sire S.S. will remain the same but the error sum of squares and error variance will be higher and it will be calculated as:

Error S.S. = T.S.S. – Sire S.S. (crude)

$$= 27029 - 26818.93 = 210.07$$

ANOVA table for paternal HS

Sources of Variation	D.F.	S.S.	M.S.
Sire	5	45.78	9.157
Progeny/sire	58	210.07	3.62

$$\sigma^2_s = \frac{(9.157 - 3.63)}{10.66}$$

$$= \frac{5.527}{10.66} = 0.58$$

$$\sigma^2 e = 3.62$$

$$h^2_s = 4\left(\frac{\sigma^2_s}{\sigma^2_P}\right)$$

$$= \frac{(4 \times 0.518)}{3.62}$$

$$= \frac{2.072}{3.62} = 0.572$$

Example 20.3

Lactation length of 22 dams and their daughters sired by 6 sires were recorded Find out the heritability of the character based on regression of daughter on dam method and also from intra sire regression of daughter on dam method.

Sire No.	Pairs	Lactation Length				Sire No.	Pairs	Lactation Length			
		Dams		Daughters				Dams		Daughters	
		(X_{ij})	X_I	(Yij)	Y_i			(X_{ij})	X_I	(Yij)	Y_i
1	1	308		300		4	12	282		295	
	2	290		295			13	280		285	
	3	288		302			14	300	862	295	875
	4	307	1193	285	1182	5	15	270		260	
2	5	290		297			16	282		298	
	6	305		295			17	310		304	
	7	310	905	315	907		18	292	1154	297	1159
3	8	277		291		6	19	267		270	
	9	280		295			20	280		285	
	10	397		305			21	301		310	
	11	310	1264	295	1206		22	290	1138	300	1165
Total									6516		6494

Solution

S.S. (Dams)

C.F. $= \dfrac{(6516)^2}{22} = 1929920.7$

T.S.S. $= (308)^2 + \ldots + (290)^2 - \text{C.F.}$

                                  $= 1944322 - \text{C.F.} = 14401.27$

Sire S.S. $= \dfrac{(1193)^2}{4} + \ldots + \dfrac{(1138)^2}{4}$

                                  $= 1932615.9 - \text{C.F.} = 2695.2$

Dams/sire S.S. $= \text{T.S.S.} - \text{Sire S.S.}$

                                  $= 14401.27 - 2695.2 = 11706.07$

Sum of Cross Products:

C.F. $= \dfrac{[6516 \times 6494]}{22} = 1923404.7$

Total S.C.P. $= (308 \times 300) + \ldots + (290 \times 300) - \text{C.F.}$

                                  $= 1927008 - 1923404.7 = 3603.3$

Sire S.C.P. $= \dfrac{(1193 \times 1182)}{4} + \ldots + \dfrac{(1138 \times 1165)}{4} - \text{C.F.}$

                                  $= 1924469.9 - 1923404.7 = 1065.2$

Dams within sire S.S $= \text{Total S.C.P} - \text{Sire S.C.P.}$

                                  $= 3603.3 - 1065.2 = 2538.1$

ANOVA table

S.V.	D.F.	S.S. Dams	S.C.P.
Sires	5	2695.2	1965.2
Dams/sire	16	11706.07	2538.1
Total	21	14401.27	3603.3

Answer: Intra-sire regression of daughter on dam method:

$$b_{OD} = \dfrac{2538.1}{11706.07} = 0.2168$$

$$h^2 = 2b_{OD} = 2 \times 0.2168 = 0.4336$$

Regression of daughters on dam method:

$$b_{OD} = \frac{3603.3}{14401.27} = 0.25$$

$$h^2 = 2 b_{OD} = 2 \times 0.25 = 0.50$$

Example 20.4

Find out the heritability of first lactation length from the following data by sire, dam and full sib component.

Sire	Dam	Daughter			Dam Total	Sire Total
		1	2	3		
1	1	341	303	291	935	
	2	301	260	278	839	
	3	261	288	276	825	2599
2	4	285	299	335	919	
	5	275	312	327	914	
	6	327	300	313	940	2773
3	7	274	302	300	876	
	8	288	316	285	889	
	9	272	308	299	879	2644
4	10	345	300	297	942	
	11	326	320	293	939	
	12	300	280	291	871	2752
5	13	302	289	294	885	
	14	322	334	334	990	
	15	318	303	331	952	2827
	Total					13595

Solution: (Hint)

S.V.	D.F.	S.S.
Sires	4	3965.955
Dams/sire	10	5507.066
Prog./dam	30	10315.3

Example 20.5

Find out the heritability from the information given below:

$S = 5$; $D = 15$; $K_1 = 3$; $K_2 = 3$; $K_3 = 9$;

$\Sigma X_{ijk}^2 = 4126989$

Dam's Total $(\Sigma X_{ij}) = 93, 84, 83, 93, 92, 94, 87, 90, 88, 95, 94, 87, 88, 98, 95$

Sire's Total $(\Sigma X_{i.}) = 260, 279, 265, 276, 281$

G. Total $(X) = 1361$

Solution: Hint

$MS_S = 9.41$; $MS_D = 5.266$ $MSe = 3.733$

$h^2_S = 0.39$ $h^2_D = 0.434$ $h^2_{(S+D)} = 0.4129$

Example 20.6

A sire is mated to two groups of cows. The high yielding groups produced 2650 kg. milk and the low producing group yielded 2500 kg. The daughters of these two groups of dams averaged 2585 and 2570 kg., respectively. Estimate the apparent h^2 of milk yield.

Groups	Dams	Daughters
1.	High producing	High producing
	$X_1 = 2650$	$Z_1 = 2585$
2.	Low producing	Low producing
	$X_2 = 2500$kg	$Z_2 = 2570$kg
Difference	$= 150$ kg	$= 15$ kg

$$h^2 = \frac{2\,DPR}{DDR} = \frac{(Z_1 - Z_2)}{(X_1 - X_2)}$$

$$= \frac{2 \times 15}{150} = 0.20$$

Where,   DPR = Difference in progeny records

          DDR = Difference in dams records

The daughter's records of these two groups of cows indicated that of the 150 kg difference in the cows, one half of the average difference in breeding value among these cows was 15 kg.

Example 20.7

Mackay (1948) conducted an experiment on the number of sternital bristles in two consecutive generations (G_1 and G_2) for increased bristle number. In G_1 the bristle number were observed to vary from 16 to 25. The individuals having 22 or more number were selected and mated at random to produce G_2 generation. Estimate the realized heritability of the sternital bristle numbers from the data given below:

Bristle Number (X)	15	16	17	18	19	20	21	22	23	24	25	26	27	28	
No. of G_1	–	21	5	18	17	20	12	13	3	5	1	–	–	–	= 115
Individ. G_2 (n)	2	4	7	16	17	13	14	12	6	3	3	2	–	2	= 101

Solution

ΣXn_1 = $(16 \times 21) + (17 \times 5) + \ldots\ldots + (24 \times 5) + (25 \times 1) = 2220$;

ΣXn_2 = $(15 \times 2) + (16 \times 4) + \ldots\ldots\ldots + (26 \times 2) + 28 \times 2) = 2035$

Σn_1 = No. of individuals in G_1 generation =115;

Σn_2 = No. of individuals in G_2 generation = 101;

Σn_3 = No. of individuals of G_1 generation, selected

$\quad = 13 + 3 + 5 + 1 = 22$

ΣXn_1 = $(22 \times 13) + (23 \times 3) + (24 \times 5) + (25 \times 1) = 500$, where 1 = 22 to 25

$X = \mu$ = Mean of G_1 generation (before selection)

$$= \frac{\sum Xn_1}{\sum n_1} = \frac{2220}{115} = 19.3 \; ;$$

Xs = Mean of selected individuals of G_1 generation

$$= \frac{\sum Xn_1}{\sum n_3} = \frac{500}{22} = 22.7 \; ;$$

$Xp_{(G2)}$ = Average of next generation (G_2) obtained after selection and mating

$$= \frac{\sum Xn_2}{\sum n_2} = \frac{2035}{101} = 20.1$$

$S \quad = X_s - \mu$

$\quad = 22.7 - 19.3 = 3.4;$

$R \quad = X_p - \mu$

$\quad = 20.1 - 19.3 = 0.8$

$h^2 \quad = R/S$

$\quad = 0.8/3.4 = 0.235$

Exercise 20.8

Clayton *et al* (1956) established 5 populations and practiced selection for increased number of sternital bristles. The data after one generation of selection showed as under:

Populations	1	2	3	4	5
$\mu_{(G1)}$	35.3	35.3	33.5	33.0	34.0
Xs	40.0	40.0	38.2	37.7	38.7
$X_{Progeny\ (G2)}$	37.9	37.2	35.8	36.3	36.7

Calculate the realized heritability in all 5 populations and the overall mean heritability.

Hint: $S = Xs - \mu$; $R = X_{P\,(G2)} - \mu$

Realized $h^2 = R/S$

Exercise 20.9

Dudley (1977) reported in a long term selection experiment for oil content in maize that it increased linearly for 76 generations from 4.8 to 18.8 per cent, whereas the cumulative selection differential increased at an approx. constant rate of 1.1 per generation. Estimate the h^2 for oil content.

Solution

Total response $= \mu.^{76} - \mu.^{0} = 18.8 - 4.8 = 14$

Cumulative Selection differential for 76 generations $= 1.1 \times 76 = 83.6$

Realized heritability $= \dfrac{R}{S} = \dfrac{14}{83.6} = 0.167$

Exercise 20.10

The following values were calculated from a given data:

$\sigma^2_A = 500$, $\sigma^2_{(D+I)} = 100$, $\sigma^2_{EP} = 200$, $\sigma^2_{Et} = 1200$

Calculate h^2, H^2, t (repeatability), σ^2_G and σ^2_P

Exercise 20.11

A herd of cattle has an average body weight of 395 Kg. The owner selects for breeding purpose cows weighing 405 Kg. and sires that average 425 Kg. The progeny produced had an average adult body weight of 405 Kg. Estimate the heritability.

Exercise 20.12

Find out the h^2 of birth weight from the given data on 26 dams-daughter pairs sired by 4 sires, wherein X is the dam's and Y is the daughter's birth weight.

Pairs No.	S_1		S_2		S_3		S_4	
	X	Y	X	Y	X	Y	X	Y
1.	24	26	36	28	34	30	20	22
2.	28	26	26	24	16	20	32	28
3.	20	24	28	26	22	24	18	24
4.	24	26	30	26	20	24	26	16
5.	20	24	20	24	28	26	30	28
6.	26	26	24	26	32	28	20	24
7.	28	26	22	26	—	—	26	26

Exercise 20.13

A herd of 225 cows was sired by 25 sires with an average of 16 daughters per sire and 5 cows per sire. From the data given below estimate the h^2 and interpret the differences in h^2 estimates from different components.

S.V.	D.F.	MS	
Sires	24	734	$\sigma^2_e + K_2\sigma^2_D + K_3\sigma^2_S$
Dam/sire	200	514	$\sigma^2_e + K_1\sigma^2_D$
Full sibs/dams	175	293	σ^2_e
	$K_1 = K_2 = 5; K_3 = 16$		

Exercise 20.14

Nine months body weight of Murrah buffaloes were recorded on108 progenies of 4 sires which were each mated to 3 dams and hence each dam produced 9 progenies, The statistical analysis of data indicated that MS(sire) was 902.0, MS (among dams/sire) was 220.0 and MS among progeny was 152.5. Estimate the h2 from sire, dam and full sib component

Hint: $K_1 = 3; K_2 = 9; K_3 = 27$

Chapter 21
Repeatability

There are many economic characters of farm animals which occur (repeated) more than once in the life time of an animal and take different phenotypic values at different times (ages of animal). Such characters are milk yield, lactation length, service period, calving interval in dairy animals; fleece (wool) production and wool quality traits in sheep; egg production and quality traits in poultry etc. These characters are called as repeated or repeatable characters and the measurements on these characters are called multiple measurements. These characters recorded at different times (at different ages of the animals) take different phenotypic values inspite of the fact that genotype of an individual is fixed at fertilization and do not change throughout the life. In view of no change in genotype, the only source of differences in phenotypic values of the same individual at different age is the variation in environment to which the individual is exposed.

21.1 Causes of Variation in Repeated Measurements

These environmental sources of variation in repeated characters are of two types *viz.* permanent and temporary. Accordingly, the environmental variance can be partitioned into its two components.

The first category includes the permanent environment effects denoted, as V_{EP}. These effects cause permanent environment variance and these are general environmental effects. The V_{EP}, the variation due to permanent environmental effects, are the between individual component of variance and are the persistent effect over repeated records of the same animal like udder damage has persistent effect on milk production in subsequent lactations, nutrition during calf hood age, and training of horses, etc.

The second category comprises the temporary environment effects, denoted as V_{ET}. These effects cause temporary environment variance and these effects are for a specific time and not always, for which it is called as special environmental variance. These environmental factors vary from time to time. The V_{ET} are caused by differences between the different records of one individual at different time due to temporary environmental effects (which vary from record to record taken at different times) indicates the within individual variation. These are thus the within individual variation and remain for a specific time. Theses temporary factors are climatic factors (temperature, humidity, season of a year), feeding regime, age, management practices which vary from year to year and their effects are likely to have positive and negative effects on the phenotypic values and hence their effects tend to average zero over several periods.

Inspite of the different phenotypic values of repeated character at different ages, there exist a correlation between any two records of the individual and the magnitude of correlation between two records depends on the adjacency of the two records as well as the extent of genetic and permanent environment effects affecting the repeated records. More adjacent are the two records and more is the variability due to genetic and permanent environment effects between two records, higher will be the correlation between the two records. The magnitude of correlation between two records will indicate the reliability of the previous record in predicting the future record. When the correlation is higher, the reliability of previous record will be higher in predicting the future record or vice versa. The correlation between two repeated records will be higher if these records are less affected by temporary environmental effects existing for a specific time. Therefore, it is required to measure the extent to which the observed variations among the repeated records are affected by permanent (both genetic and environmental) and temporary environmental effects.

The ratio of the between individual component of variance comprising $\sigma^2_G + \sigma^2_{EP}$ to the total phenotypic variance (σ^2_p) measures the correlation (r) between repeated records of the same individual and called as the **repeatability** coined by Lush (1937) and denoted by either t or r.

21.2 Producing Ability

The producing ability (PA) is important for repeated traits. The PA refers to the performance potential of an animal for a repeated trait which means the potential of an animal to produce the trait in future. It is a function of all those factors that permanently affect an individual's performance potential. The genotypic value (Breeding value – B.V. and gene combination value – G.C.V.) is determined at conception and hence called permanent genetic effects. Besides these, there are some environmental effects which are also permanent and known as permanent environmental effects. Therefore, the genetic model for producing ability can be written as:

$$PA = G + E_p$$
$$= B.V. + GCV + E_p$$

Thus, the producing ability is neither a purely genetic value nor a purely environmental one, but it is a combination.

The prediction of producing ability is called the most probable producing ability (MPPA) which is very useful in dairy animals and calculated from the data. The MPPA is a prediction of the animal's future record and mathematically,

PA = μ + MPPA.

The producing ability is more important to commercial producers rather than to the seed stock breeders.

21.3 Definition of Repeatability

The repeatability is a measure of the similarity between two or more records of the same trait taken at different times on the same individual of a population. Thus, repeatability indicates the correlation between repeated records of the same trait on the individuals of a population. The repeatability is denoted by t or R. Now take X_1 and X_2 as the two records of the same trait recorded at different ages on the same individual. Thus, $t = r_{X1X2}$. The repeatability has its meaning and use depending on the manner the repeatability is measured.

First, the repeatability is the correlation between two and more records taken at different times on the same individual. Therefore, the first record on an individual (X_1) is an indicator of the consistency and reliability of the second record of the same individual (X_2).

Secondly, the repeatability is also taken as the regression of second record on the first record. The repeatability as regression will indicate the change in future record per unit change in first record. Thus, $t = b_{x2x1}$. In this way the repeatability is useful in predicting the future performance (record) from early record. Thus the repeatability is the fraction of differences between single records of individuals that are likely to occur in future record.

Thirdly, the repeatability is also expressed as a ratio of variances of records that are due to the permanent effects (genetic and environmental) *viz.* proportion of differences in first record that are attributable to the differences in future record due to permanent effects. Thus, $t = \dfrac{\left(\sigma^2_G + \sigma^2_{EP}\right)}{\sigma^2_P}$. Therefore, the repeatability indicates the fraction of the observed differences among individuals due to permanent effects and the remaining portion of the differences (1-t) caused by temporary environmental effects. Thus, the repeatability provides information on the relative importance of permanent effects and temporary environmental effects.

Like heritability, the repeatability is also a population parameter. It is the property of a trait, population and the environmental effects. It is also affected by same factors which affect the heritability and thus the repeatability can be increased by the same ways that are used to increase the heritability.

21.2 Importance and Use of Repeatability

1. The main property of repeatability is that its *determination is much easier* than heritability in either sense. The repeatability can be estimated without

information on groups of relatives (parentage information) and hence the repeatability can be used as the preliminary genetic information.

2. The repeatability sets *upper limit of heritability* in broad sense because the repeatability includes all the genetic (additive and non additive components) plus permanent environmental influences which contribute to the real differences among animals whereas the heritability in broad sense includes only the genetic differences. The repeatability is:

$$r = \frac{\sigma^2_G + \sigma^2_{EP}}{\sigma^2_P}$$

whereas the heritability in broad sence (H^2) is :

$$H^2 = \frac{\sigma^2_G}{\sigma^2_P}$$

3. *Prediction of future record:*

   (i) *Based on single record* on the individuals. The future record (X_2) may be estimated as;

   $X_2 = \mu + r(X_S - \mu)$

   $X_2 - \mu = r(Xs - \mu) = \Delta S$

   where, μ = Population mean before selection;

   Xs = Mean of selected individuals;

   X = Mean of 2nd record.

   $Xs - \mu$ = Phenotypic superiority of selected individuals known as selection differential

   $X_2 - \mu$ = ΔS Gain in future record by selection

   = Av. superiority of future record (X_2).

   This indicates the change in population mean for a future record due to selection based on previous record and hence it is the portion of superiority or inferiority of a given record on an individual as compared to the herd average. Thus it is used to estimate the performance potential or real producing ability of an animal and to compare different individuals in the same herd/flock.

   (ii) *Based on more records:* More than one record of the same trait on the same individual taken at different times are known as multiple records. The repeatability is useful to know the relative efficiency of using single or more records. The repeatability estimate gives an indication that how many records on an individual should be taken before it is culled. The *repeatability of multiple records* (R) *is estimated* as:

   $$R = \frac{nr}{1 + (n-1)r}$$

where, n = number of records;

r = repeatability based on one record.

The estimate R increases with increase in number of repeated records. When repeatability is high, single record is enough to predict the real producing ability (future performance) than considering several records of a trait on an individual with low repeatability will do. This means that when temporary environmental effects are less important (high repeatability) the use of repeated records is of no use, hence the repeated records do not add to the accuracy and the culling on the basis of single record will be effective. On the other hand, the repeated records add to the accuracy when repeatability is low. This is because increase in multiple records cancelled out the temporary environmental effects. The change in later record based on repeatability of multiple records (R) can be predicted by replacing the value of **r** with R in the above equation of predicting of future record (performance) based on single record. The gain due to selection (mean change) at subsequent age based on **n** records is estimated as:

$$\Delta S = \frac{nr}{1+(n-1)r}(X_s - \mu)$$

Lush (1945) used the above relationship to predict the *most probable producing ability* (MPPA) for dairy cows with varying number of records per cow to adjust the records of cows to the same basis for comparing the different cows in the same herd. The MPPA is estimated as:

$$\textbf{MPPA} = \mu + \frac{nr}{1+(n-1)r}(C - \mu)$$

where, C is the cow's own average = X_i

μ is the herd average *i.e.* average before selection.

The temporary environmental effects vary from time to time and are likely to have positive and negative effects at different times and thus cancelled. The permanent environmental effects together with genotypic effects decide an individual's performance potential for its whole life. This performance potential is called as the *'real producing ability".*

4. *Relative efficiency of using different records:* The efficiency of different records can be tested for predicting life time production by estimating the correlation between total and individual record (r_{Ti}) as: $r_{Ti} = \sqrt{\frac{1}{n}[1+(n-1)r]}$

where, n =Number of records used to calculate total of all the records (T).

The relative efficiency of ith record to predict the total production is estimated as:

$$Q = \frac{r_{Ti}}{r_{Tj}}$$

This relationship (Q) is used to determine that which record is more useful in selection.

5. *Culling decision:* The animals with low performance based on first record can be culled when repeatability of the trait is high but when repeatability is low the poor performing animals based on first record should not be culled because the first record is not reliable of the producing ability of the animal in case of low repeatability. Thus when repeatability is low the additional future record has its importance. On the other hand, the additional future record is not important when repeatability is high to take the culling decision.

6. The repeatability estimate can be used in *feed lot experiment*. In case of high repeatability, it requires to distribute equally the different progeny of a sire or dam in different lots. This is because in case of high repeatability the lot differences will largely be due to the genetic differences rather than actually to the lot differences ascribed to treatments.

21.3 Methods of Estimation of Repeatability

The estimation of repeatability requires multiple/repeated records of the same character on the same animal. The number of records per animal may vary but at least two records per animal are required in estimation of repeatability.

(i) Inter Class Correlation

This method is used when only two records per animal are available. Considering X and Y as the two records taken at different ages, the repeatability (r) is estimated simply as the correlation coefficient between X and Y as:

$$r_{XY} = \frac{\sum xy}{\sqrt{\sum x^2 \sum y^2}}$$

Actually the inter class correlation between repeated records on an animal is the ratio of variance attributable to permanent differences (genetic and environmental) among animals to the phenotypic variance. This ratio is repeatability. Thus the correlation between repeated records on animals is the repeatability. The inter class correlation in terms of variance components can be understood from the measurement P_{ij} taken on i^{th} animal at j^{th} time and the measurement (P_{ij}) is defined as:

$$P_{ij} = \mu + S_i + e_{ij}.$$

The measurements at two different times (j and j') on the same individual will differ because e_{ij} and $e_{ij'}$ are different representing temporary environment effects but theses two measurements will be similar to some extent because two measurements have S_i in common representing permanent effects (genetic and environmental) as:

$$P_{ij} = \mu + S_i + e_{ij} \text{ and}$$
$$P_{ij'} = \mu + S_i + e_{ij'}$$

Therefore, the covariance of two measurements taken at two times will be as:

$$\text{Cov}(P_{ij} P_{ij'}) = \text{Cov}(S_i + e_{ij})(S_i + e_{ij'})$$

$$= \sigma^2_s.$$

The correlation (r) between two records: $r = \dfrac{\text{Cov}(P_{ij} P_{ij'})}{P_{ij} P_{ij'}}$

$$= \dfrac{\sigma^2_s}{\sigma^2_{p'}}$$

(ii) Regression Method

In case of two repeated records (X and Y), the correlation between them is equal to the regression of one record on the other. This is based on the assumption that the variances of the two records (V_X or V_Y) do not differ ($\sigma^2_X = \sigma^2_Y$), so $\sigma_X = \sigma_Y$. Therefore, r $_{XY} = b_{YX}$. Thus the regression of future record (second record, Y) on the previous record (b_{YX}) = correlation between these two records (r_{XY}). This regression of future record on the previous record (b_{YX}) estimates the repeatability of the character.

$$\text{Repeatability (r)} = b_{yx} = \dfrac{\sum xy}{\sum x^2}$$

The repeatability in terms of regression can be used to predict gain in future performance of the herd by selection based on earlier record. The repeatability is the predicted deviation in future records per unit deviation in early records. This means that repeatability is the proportion of individual's deviation from population mean for one record expected to be retained in future record of the same trait. The predicted superiority in future record will be equal to b_{YX} time superiority of the individual for first record over the population mean. Thus, the repeatability is the proportion of an individual superiority for a trait expected to be retained in future record.

(iii) Intra Class Correlation

Most often more than two records per animal are available. The repeatability, based on n animals with k records each, is estimated considering the k records of each animal as the records of a family and conducting the analysis of variance similar to the estimation of intra class correlation of paternal half sibs, as done for estimation of heritability. Here, in this case of estimation of repeatability by intra class correlation based on the different records of the same animal, the expected composition of variance between animals will be different from the expected composition of variance between half sibs because in case of repeatability estimation the different records are of the same animal whereas in case of heritability estimation the different records are of the different progeny of the same sire or dam. Therefore, in this case of estimation of repeatability, the expected composition of variance between animals denoted by $\sigma^2 a$ will be:

$$\sigma^2 a = \sigma^2_G + \sigma^2_{EP}$$

$$= V_A + V_D + V_I + V_{EP}.$$

Thus, the between animal variance ($\sigma^2 a$) will estimate all the genetic variance (V_G) plus the permanent environmental variance peculiar to the animal (V_{EP}).

The $\sigma^2 e$ is the within animal variance due to temporary environmental effects and so, $\sigma^2 e = \sigma^2_{ET}$. The ANOVA is conducted as:

S.V.	D.F.	S.S.	M.S.	E.M.S.
Animals	n-1	S.S.a	M.S. a	$\sigma^2 e + K \sigma^2 a$
Within animal	n (k-1)	S.S.e	M.S. e	$\sigma^2 e = \sigma^2_{ET}$

Where, $\sigma^2 a = (MS\,a - MS\,e)/k$

$$K = \text{Av. no. of records per animal} = \frac{1}{N-1}\left[n. - \frac{\sum n^2_i}{n.}\right]$$

N = No. of animal;

$n.$ = Σn_i = Total no. of records;

n_i = no. of records of jth animal

The **repeatability is the intra class correlation** among the repeated measurements of a trait. This intra class correlation is the proportion of the variation containing genotypic variation (V_G) plus variation due to permanent environment effects (V_{EP}) to the total phenotypic variation (V_P). Therefore, repeatability (t) is:

$$t = r = \frac{\left(\sigma^2_G + \sigma^2_{EP}\right)}{\sigma^2_{P.}}$$

$$= \frac{\sigma^2_a}{\left(\sigma^2_a + \sigma^2_e\right)}$$

Thus, the repeatability indicates the proportion of total phenotypic variance attributed to the variance among individuals due to permanent differences (both genetic and environmental). This is because the repeated records are the records of the same animal and hence the same sets of genes are responsible for the expression of the character at different times.

This procedure of analysis of variance of repeated records for estimating repeatability is useful in estimating the variance due to temporary environmental effects (σ^2_{ET}).

(iv) Difference Method

The repeatability can also be approximated by regression of the difference in future performance on the difference in previous performance (Lush *et al*, 1941).

$$\text{Repeatability (r)} = \frac{\left(\overline{X}_{2H} - \overline{X}_{2L}\right)}{\left(\overline{X}_{1H} - \overline{X}_{1L}\right)}$$

$$= \frac{\text{Difference at } 2^{nd} \text{ age}}{\text{Difference at } 1^{st} \text{ age}}$$

Where, 1 and 2 subscripts indicate the first and second record

H and L subscripts indicate the high and low performing group

21.4 Repeatability of Multiple Records

The permanent environmental effects along with the genotype determine the real potential of an animal's performance during its whole life. In dairy animals, the real potential for milk yield is termed as "real Producing ability", or "most probable producing' ability" (MPPA) coined by Lush (1945).

The variance caused by temporary environmental effect (V_{Et}) is decreased by increasing the number of observations (n) by $\dfrac{1}{n}$ times the variance caused by temporary environmental effects and it becomes equal to $\dfrac{V_{ET}}{n}$. This reduction in variance is only in the V_{ET} part because only the temporary environmental factors are independent of period. Thus, only the variance caused by temporary environ mental factors is correspondingly reduced.

The variance of the mean of n measurements as a proportion of the variance of one measurement is expressed in terms of repeat ability. Thus the repeatability is,

$$\text{Repeatability} = \frac{V_{(Pn)}}{V_P} = \frac{1 + (n-1)r}{n}$$

Where, r is the repeatability, or the correlation between measurements of the same individual.

$$\frac{V_{(Pn)}}{V_P} = \frac{\left(V_G + V_{EP} + \dfrac{1}{n} V_{ET}\right)}{V_P}$$

$$= \frac{\left(V_G + V_{EP}\right)}{V_P} + \frac{\left(\dfrac{1}{n} V_{ET}\right)}{V_P}$$

$$= r + \frac{1}{n}(1-r)$$

$$= r + \frac{1}{n} - \frac{r}{n}$$

$$= \frac{(rn + 1 - r)}{n}$$

$$= \frac{[1 + r(n-1)]}{n} = \frac{1 + (n-1)r}{n}$$

Thus, $V_{(Pn)} = V_{\bar{P}} = \dfrac{\sigma^2{}_P[1 + (n-1)r]}{n}$

$$r(n) = \frac{(V_G + V_{EP})}{V_{(Pn)}}$$

$$= \frac{(V_G + V_{EP})}{V_P}$$

$$= \frac{(V_G + V_{EP})}{\left\{ \dfrac{V_P[1 + (n-1)r]}{n} \right\}}$$

$$= \left[\frac{r}{\dfrac{1 + (n-1)r}{n}} \right]$$

$$= \frac{nr}{[1 + (n-1)r]}$$

The repeatability is the intra class correlation among the repeated measurements of a trait of the same individual. The intra-class correlation between repeated measurements of the same individual is the proportion of the variation containing genotypic variation ($\sigma^2{}_G$) plus the variation due to permanent environmental effect ($\sigma^2{}_{EP}$) to the total phenotypic variation ($\sigma^2{}_P$), and it can be written as:

$$r = \frac{\left(\sigma^2{}_G + \sigma^2{}_{EP} \right)}{\sigma^2{}_P}$$

Thus the repeatability indicates the proportion of the variance among individuals due to permanent differences (both genetic and environmental). This is based on the fact that the repeated measurements are in real sense the measurements of the same character genetically. This is because same set of genes is responsible for the phenotypic expression of the character at different times.

Solved Examples and Exercises

Example 21.1

The birth weights of calves born to 10 cows are given below. Estimate the repeatability of birth weight by different methods.

Cows/Records	1	2	3	4	5	6	7	8	ΣX_i
1	22	22	22	23	24	22	–	-	137
2	21	22	21	22	22	–	-	–	108
3	24	25	25	24	26	25	23	–	172
4	23	22	23	24	24	24	–	-	140
5	21	21	21	22	22	21	22	23	173

Cows/Records	1	2	3	4	5	6	7	8	ΣX_i
6	21	22	22	23	23	23	23	–	157
7	24	25	26	25	26	27	26	28	207
8	22	23	22	24	23	23	24	–	161
9	21	22	22	23	24	21	21	23	178
10	22	22	23	24	25	22	23	24	185
Sum	221	226							1616

Solution

    (i) *Intra-class Correlation Method*

$\Sigma X = 1616;$

$\Sigma X^2 = 37436; N = 70;$

$$\text{Correction Factor} = \frac{\left(\Sigma X\right)^2}{N} = 37306.51$$

Total SS $= \Sigma X^2 - CF = 37436 - 37306.5$

                $= 129.49$

Cow SS $= \dfrac{\left(137\right)^2}{6} + \dfrac{\left(108\right)^2}{5} + \ldots + \dfrac{\left(185\right)^2}{8} - \text{C.F.}$

                $= 37423.41 - 37306.51$

                $= 116.9$

Error SS $= \text{TSS} - \text{Cow SS}$

                $= 129.49 - 116.9$

                $= 12.59$

ANOVA Table

Source of Variation	DF	SS	MS
Bet. Cows	9	116.9	12.99
Bet. Records within cow	60	12.59	0.21

$$K = \frac{1}{C-1}\left[\frac{\sum n. - \sum n_4{}^2}{\sum n.}\right]$$

$$= \frac{1}{9}\left[\frac{70 - 500}{70}\right]$$

$$= 6.98$$

$$\sigma_C{}^2 = \frac{(12.99 - 0.210)}{6.98} = 1.83$$

$$\sigma_P{}^2 = 1.831 + 0.21 = 2.041$$

$$\text{Repeatability (t)} = \frac{\sigma_C{}^2}{\sigma_P{}^2}$$

$$= \frac{1.831}{2.041}$$

$$= 0.897$$

(ii) *Regression of II record on I record*

$\sum X_1 = 221$; $\sum X_1{}^2 = 4897$; $n_1 = 10$; $CF_1 = 4884.1$; $\sum x_1{}^2 = 12.9$

$\sum X_2 = 226$; $\sum X_2{}^2 = 5124$; $n_2 = 10$ $CF_2 = 5107.6$; $\sum x_2{}^2 = 16.4$

$Cov_{12} = 5007$; $CF = 4994.6$ $Cov_{x2} = 12.4$

$$\text{Repeatability (byx)} = \frac{12.4}{12.9}$$

$$= 0.96$$

(iii) *Correlation between I and II record:*

$$\text{Repeatability } (r_{XY}) = \frac{12.4}{\sqrt{(12.9)(16.4)}}$$

$$= \frac{12.4}{14.54}$$

$$= 0.85$$

Example 21.2: Orthogonal Data

The greasy fleece weights (x 10gm) of 10 Nali ews for 7 clips recorded are given below: Calculate the repeatability of greasy fleece weight from intra-class correlation method.

Sheep	1	2	3	4	5	6	7	Sum
1	82	89	77	69	96	78	63	554
2	73	84	94	85	87	90	70	583
3	87	87	94	93	78	88	90	617
4	84	86	75	75	80	94	75	569
5	78	82	80	75	78	69	68	530
6	91	86	95	88	91	100	76	627
7	80	91	91	98	82	81	78	601
8	74	93	78	96	73	88	72	574
9	66	82	76	87	78	75	64	528
10	87	90	85	75	70	73	64	544
Sum	802	870	845	841	813	836	720	5727

Solution

(i) Intra-class correlation method:

$N = 70; \Sigma X = 5727; \Sigma X^2 = 474229$

$$C.F.' = \frac{(5727)^2}{70} = 468550.41$$

T.S.S. $= 474229 - C.F. = 5678.58$

$$\text{Sheep S.S.} = \frac{(554^2 + 583^2 + 544^2)}{7} - C.F.$$

$= 470097.29 - C.F. = 1546.88$

Year S.S. $= 802^2 + 870^2 + ... + 720^2 - C.F = 1417.1$

Error S.S. $=$ TSS $-$ Sheep SS $-$ year S.S.

$= 5678.58 - 1546.88 - 1417.1 = 2714.6$

ANOVA Table

S.V.	d.f.	S.S	M.S
Year	6	1417.10	236.18
Sheep	9	1546.88	171.87
Error	54	2714.60	50.27

$$\sigma^2_B = \frac{(171.87 - 50.27)}{7} = 17.37$$

$$\sigma^2_P = 17.37 + 50.27 = 67.64$$

$$\textbf{Repeatability} = \frac{\sigma^2_B}{\sigma^2_P} = \frac{17.37}{67.64}$$

$$= 0.256$$

(ii) The repeatability may also be worked out based on first two records (X and Y) by regression (b_{YX}) and correlation methods (r_{XY}).

Exercise 21.3

The milk productions (x 100 kg) of 10 Tharparkar cows for 6 lactations have been given as under. Estimate the repeatability of the trait.

Cows/Lact.	1	2	3	4	5	6
1	21	22′	23	23	22	20
2	24	27	28	26	24	21
3	21	27	28	27	25	25
4	23	23	29	28	27	25
5	20	25	26	27	25	23
6	21	26	27	28	28	22
7	24	29	27	28	26	24
8	21	22	25	27	26	22
9	22	23	25	26	23	21
10	27	30	29	28	25	22

Exercise 21.4

The high and low producing cows averaged 2650 and 2500 kg milk in first lactation while in second lactation their milk production averaged 2800 and 2750 kg respectively. Find out the repeatability of milk production.

Chapter 22

Correlation among Characters

It is of great interest and importance to know the variation in two character that how they vary together. This helps to understand the relationship between them. When two characters have a relationship between them, it means there is a simultaneous change (variation) in both the characters. Two characters may be related to each other in such a way that a change (variation) in one character correspond with a particular directional change in the other. If there is an increase in the value of one character, it may lead to either an increase or decrease in the value of other character. The simultaneous change (variation) in two characters is measured in terms of *co-variation* which indicates that the two characters vary together and have dependency on each other. The measurement of the co-variation is the *covariance* which is the mean product between the deviations of the two characters measured on the same individuals. The covariance indicates the direction and strength of relationship between two characters and used to estimate the degree of relationship (dependency) between two characters in terms of correlation and regression.

The degree of mutual relationship between two characters is measured by *correlation coefficient* which is a measure of simultaneous change in two characters *i.e.* how the two characters change together. It is denoted by the letter *r*. The coefficient of correlation is defined as the ratio of the variance common to the two characters (Covariance) to the geometric mean of the variances of the two characters. This is the *simple correlation*. Thus, the correlation is obtained by dividing the covariance of two characters (Cov_{XY}) by the square root of the product of the variances of two characters as:

$$r_{XY} = \frac{Cov_{XY}}{\sigma_X \, \sigma_X}$$

Thus, the correlation is the covariance between two characters when compared to their average variability and it is the covariance per unit of average change.

In general, most of the economic characters have correlation with each other to some extent. The existence of correlation among characters requires certain common causes which affect the different characters. The correlation between two characters assumes the cause and effect relationship between them and depends upon their biological relationship, but the correlation coefficient does not give the idea that which one is the cause and which is the effect.

22.1 Phenotypic Correlation – Causes and Types

The correlation directly estimated from phenotypic values of two characters is known as the *phenotypic correlation.* This measures the linear association between two traits and indicates the deviation of an individual's phenotypic value of one trait from the population mean in relation to the deviation of other trait from its population mean. Therefore, the phenotypic correlation (r_p) gives the idea of the extent to which the individuals above average in one trait are above, below or near average in the other trait.

The two characters are correlated due to certain causes. It is known that the different causes which affect the different characters are the genetic and environmental in origin. Thus, the characters showing correlation among them selves may be affected by some common genes and by some common environment. Therefore, the genetic and environmental factors are two possible causes which are responsible to create a correlation between characters. The correlations are of two types *viz.* genetic and environmental, depending upon the nature of the factors which cause correlation.

The genetic factors causing correlation are the pleiotropic effect and linkage of genes. Some genes affect more than one character. Such gene effect is called pleiotropy and it is common property of genes based on their biochemical characteristics biological functions. The linkage is the presence two genes located adjacently on the same chromosome with their tendency to inherit together.

The environmental factors causing correlation include the common environment *viz.* the sheep raised under poor nutrition are likely to have low body weight and produce low fleece weight, better nutrition regime results more milk yield and more butter fat yield, and likewise poor health of animal influence appetite, growth, reproduction and production traits simultaneously.

It is important to know the relative importance of two types of causes responsible for causing correlation between characters. The portion of phenotypic correlation caused by genetic causes is termed as *genetic correlation,* whereas the part caused by common environment shared by two characters is termed as *environmental correlation.* Therefore, on the basis of nature and cause of phenotypic correlation, it is partitioned into genetic and environmental correlation.

Genetic correlation (r_g) is arisen from pleiotropic action of genes and linkage of genes affecting the characters.

Environmental correlation (r_E) is arising from common environment shared by the two characters.

Phenotypic correlation (r_P) is the correlation between the observed phenotypic values of two characters, arising from the combined effect of genotypes and environment affecting two characters. Thus, it has both genetic and environmental components.

22.2 Causes of Genetic Correlation

The possible genetic factors causing genetic correlation among characters may thus be that the same genes or same set of genes either affect the two or more characters or they may be closely linked on the same chromosome at adjacent loci.

It has been observed that some genes affect two or more characters and such type of gene effect is known as **pleiotropy**. This pleiotropy is the property of gene and said to be the most important cause of genetic correlation. The effect of some genes may be synergetic or antagonistic. The synergetic effect means that the gene affects two or more characters in the same direction *i.e.* the gene may increase or decrease the value of two or more characters causing positive correlation whereas the antagonistic effect means that they affect the two or more characters in opposite direction i.e they may increase the value of one trait and decrease the value of other trait causing negative correlation. Therefore, the pleiotropy may not be necessarily causes an appreciable amount of correlation and the magnitude of correlation due to pleiotropy depends on the direction of their effect. The genetic correlation caused by pleiotropy is similar in magnitude and direction in any population and does not change in random mating population over generations. It is difficult to identify and measure the pleiotropy as a cause of correlation but it can be imagined *viz.* the genes responsible for growth also increase the stature or size and weight of the animal and it is interpreted that such genes cause a correlation between these traits. Likewise, the genes affecting the digestion or absorption of nutrients may affect the growth and other traits like production of milk, wool, eggs, meat or work efficiency. A mutant gene for coat colour also causes sleepiness. Male sterility and weak pulmonary function are caused by a gene in human. The sickle cell gene in homozygous condition causes abnormal shape of RBC (sickle shape) also reduces the O_2 carrying capacity of blood, causing anemia and finally become fatal to the animal.

The **linkage of genes** is another genetic cause of genetic correlation and it causes a transient correlation which is decreased in every generation due to crossing over. The rate of decrease in correlation depends on the crossing over distance between two genes affecting different characters. The genetic correlation caused by linkage of genes affecting two characters is expected to differ both in amount and direction in different populations which are of different genetic background. Moreover, the genetic correlation due to linkage is also decreased in the same population over generations of random mating due to crossing over.

Types of genetic correlation: The genetic correlation is of two types. The first is the *genotypic correlation* which is estimated based on genotypic values of two characters. It is analogous to heritability in broad sense and hence can be estimated from specialized populations which are not possible in farm animals. It is not useful to measure genotypic correlation because its causation includes the interaction effect of genes which are broken in next generation. The second type of genetic correlation is the *additive genetic correlation* (r_A) which is the correlation between breeding values of two characters and hence it is analogous to heritability in narrow sense. It is used to predict

22.3 Use and Applications of Genetic Correlation

The knowledge of genetic correlation among traits is of great interest and use to the breeders for the following purposes:

1. The knowledge of genetic correlation can be used for *counter selection measures* to prevent any harmful correlated change. The magnitude of genetic correlation indicates that how the characters are likely to be changed in the next generation as a result of selection. For example, selection for higher growth rate by selecting heavier bulls will increase the size and birth weight of calves which may result in calving difficulty.

2. The genetic correlation can be used to apply *indirect selection based on correlated response.* This is useful for traits which are difficult to improve through direct selection which may be either due to low heritability of a trait, or when it is difficult to measure the trait for want of information or the information are made available in old age or after death of the animal or it is costly to measure the trait. The correlated response will be helpful in these cases. Moreover, the indirect selection based on correlated response is helpful to reduce generation interval *e.g.* selection based on part lactation (milk production) or part year production (egg production).

3. The genetic correlation is used *to predict the breeding value* for net economic merit based on two or more traits by constructing an index using the genetic correlation. The genetic correlation can also be used to estimate the breeding value of a sex limited trait which can not be measured *viz.* ovulation rate. The ovulation rate has high genetic correlation with an easily measured trait in opposite sex *viz.* weight or diameter of male genetalia in sheep and mice. The sex limited trait can be improved by selection for a genetically correlated trait of other sex.

$$\text{B.V. for sex limited trait} = r_A h_M S_M h_F \left[\frac{\sigma_{P(M)}}{\sigma_{P(F)}} \right]$$

Where, M and F indicates males and females, respectively.

S indicates the selection differential.

4. The genetic correlation of the performance of a genotype in two environments can be used to *measure the G-E interaction,* considering the performance in two environments as two traits. If the genetic correlation is low, it indicates that the performance in two environments indeed are two different traits governed by different sets of genes (G-E interaction exists)

and hence in case of low genetic correlation the selection should be done under the environment in which the improved population has to live.

22.4 Estimation of Genetic Correlation

The genetic correlation is estimated in a manner analogous to the estimation of h^2 based on resemblance between relatives. The estimation of genetic correlation requires the estimation of observational components of covariance of two traits in addition to variances of both the traits. The components of covariance of two characters are computed from analysis of covariance similar to ANOVA. The covariance of two characters is partitioned according to the sources of variation.

1. Sib Analysis

The genetic correlation can be estimated from analysis of variance of both the traits and their analysis of covariance. The composition of variance of both the traits is similar to that for estimating heritability. The composition of the covariance, in terms of expected covariance components, corresponds to that of the variance components. The analysis of covariance on FS and HS is similar to that shown in estimating heritability except that components of covariance also occur in addition of variance components. There is similarity in the variance components and covariance components.

Expected Genetic Composition

(i) The covariance component between sires [$Cov_{S(X,Y)}$] is caused mainly by association of additive effects of genes and composed as:

$$Cov_{S(X,Y)} = \tfrac{1}{4} Cov\, A_{(XY)} + \tfrac{1}{16} Cov\, AA_{(XX)} + ...$$

Where, A_{XY} indicates additive effects of traits (X and Y)

AA_{XX} indicates the additive by additive interaction

(ii) The covariance component between dams [$Cov_{D(X,Y)}$] is expected to contain additive effects, dominance effects, interaction effects and maternal effects and hence composed of genetic components as:

$$Cov_{D(X,Y)} = \tfrac{1}{4} Cov_{A\,(X,Y)} + \tfrac{1}{4} Cov_{D\,(X,Y)} + \tfrac{1}{16} Cov_{AA\,(XY)} + \tfrac{1}{16} Cov_{AD\,(XY)}$$
$$+ \tfrac{1}{16} Cov_{DD\,(XY)} + ...$$

(iii) The covariance component combined for sires and dams is expected to have the following genetic composition –

$$Cov_{(S+D)} = \tfrac{1}{2} Cov_{A\,(X,Y)} + \tfrac{1}{4} Cov_{D\,(X,Y)} + \tfrac{1}{4} Cov_{AA\,(XY)} + 1/8\, Cov_{AD\,(XY)}$$
$$+ \tfrac{1}{16} Cov_{DD\,(XY)} + ...$$

(iv) The covariance component within progenies (Cov_w) is expected as:

$$Cov_{W(X,Y)} = \tfrac{1}{2} Cov_{A\,(X,Y)} + \tfrac{3}{4} Cov_{D\,(X,Y)} + \tfrac{3}{4} Cov_{AA\,(XY)} + 7/8\, Cov_{AD\,(XY)}$$
$$+ \tfrac{15}{16} Cov_{DD\,(XY)} + ...$$

(v) The expected composition of mean cross product [E (MCP)] for all the sources of variation is also the same as that of the expected composition of the variance components for both half sibs and full sib analysis.

(i) Half Sib Correlation

The ANOVA for estimating genetic correlation for two traits is similar to that given for estimating heritability.

The analysis of covariance is also similar and given below:

Analysis of Covariance for Half Sibs

Sources of Variation	D.F.	MCP	E (MCP)
Between sires	S – 1	MCP_S	$Cov_W + K\,Cov_S$
Within sires	N – S	MCP_W	Cov_W

$Cov_W = MCP_W = Cov_{W(XY)}$

The components of variance for $\sigma^2_{S(X)}$, $\sigma^2_{S(Y)}$, $\sigma^2_{W(X)}$, $\sigma^2_{W(Y)}$ are estimated from analysis of variance as given earlier.

The *genetic correlation* from sire component of variance and covariance as:

$$r_A = \frac{Cov_{S(XY)}}{\sqrt{\left[\sigma^2_{S(X)}\,\sigma^2_{S(Y)}\right]}}$$

The *environmental correlation* from error variance and covariance as:

$$r_E = \frac{Cov_{W(XY)}}{\sqrt{\left[\sigma^2_{W(X)}\,\sigma^2_{W(Y)}\right]}}$$

The r_E can also be estimated as under -

$$r_E = \frac{\left[Cov_{W(XY)} - 3\,Cov_{S(XY)}\right]}{\sqrt{\left[\sigma^2_{W(X)} - 3\sigma^2_{S(X)}\right]\left[\sigma^2_{W(Y)} - 3\sigma^2_{S(Y)}\right]}}$$

The *phenotypic correlation* from phenotypic variance and covariance as:

$$r_P = \frac{\left[Cov_{S(XY)} + Cov_{W(XY)}\right]}{\sqrt{\left[\sigma^2_{S(X)} + \sigma^2_{W(X)}\right]\left[\sigma^2_{S(Y)} + \sigma^2_{W(Y)}\right]}}$$

The genetic correlation can also be estimated from intra class correlation estimated from parental half sibs by portioning the phenotypic covariance in a similar way. The intra class correation (t xy) between two traits (X and Y) in paternal half sib analysis is –

$$t_{xy} = \frac{Cov_{S(XY)}}{\left[Cov_{S(XY)} + Cov_{W(XY)}\right]}$$

The genetic correlation (rg) is estimated as 4 t xy for the same reason explained for estimating heritability by paternal half sib correlation method. Therefore,

$$r_g = \frac{4\,Cov_{S(XY)}}{\left[Cov_{S(XY)} + Cov_{W(XY)}\right]}$$

(ii) Full Sib Correlation (Nested Design)

The analysis of full sib data give the information on two traits as covariance of two traits between sires, between dams within sires, and between progenies within sires, similar to the ANOVA for single trait.

The analysis of covariance is given below:

Analysis of Covariance for Full Sibs

Sources of Variation	D.F.	MCP	E (MCP)
Bet. Sires	S – 1	MCP_S	$Cov_W + K_2\,Cov_D + K_3\,Cov_S$
Bet. Dams/sire	D – S	MCP_D	$Cov_W + K_1\,Cov_D$
Bet Sibs	N – D	MCP_W	Cov_W

$$Cov_W = MCP_W \qquad\qquad\qquad = Cov_{W(XY)}$$
$$Cov_D = (MCP_D - MCP_W)/K_1 \qquad = Cov_{D(XY)}$$
$$Cov_S = (MCP_S - MCP_D)/K_3 \qquad = Cov_{S(XY)}$$

The components of variance for $\sigma^2_{S(X)}$, $\sigma^2_{S(Y)}$, $\sigma^2_{D(X)}$, $\sigma^2_{D(Y)}$, $\sigma^2_{W(X)}$, $\sigma^2_{W(Y)}$ are estimated from analysis of variance as given earlier.

(a) *Genetic correlation* (r_A) is estimated from sire component, dam component, Sire + dam component of covariance and variance.

$$r_A\,(\text{Sire component}) = \frac{Cov_{S(XY)}}{\sqrt{\sigma^2_{S(X)}\,\sigma^2_{S(Y)}}}$$

$$r_A\,(\text{Dam component}) = \frac{Cov_{D(XY)}}{\sqrt{\sigma^2_{D(X)}\,\sigma^2_{D(Y)}}}$$

$$r_A\,(\text{Sire + Dam}) = \frac{\left[Cov_{S(XY)} + Cov_{D(XY)}\right]}{\sqrt{\left[\sigma^2_{S(X)} + \sigma^2_{D(X)}\right]\left[\sigma^2_{S(Y)} + \sigma^2_{D(Y)}\right]}}$$

The r_A (Sire component) is more nearly unbiased because it contained only additive by additive epistacy (AA xy), while the $r_{A(D)}$ and $r_{A(S+D)}$ contain both dominance and epistacy. This is evident from the expected genetic composition of these components given earlier.

(b) *Environmental correlation* is estimated in 3 ways as under-

$$r_E = \frac{\left[Cov_{W(XY)} - 2\,Cov_{S(XY)}\right]}{\sqrt{\left[\sigma^2_{W(X)} - 2\sigma^2_{S(X)}\right]\left[\sigma^2_{W(Y)} - 2\sigma^2_{S(Y)}\right]}}$$

$$= \frac{\left[Cov_{W(XY)} - 2\,Cov_{D(XY)}\right]}{\sqrt{\left[\sigma^2_{W(X)} - 2\sigma^2_{D(X)}\right]\left[\sigma^2_{W(Y)} - 2\sigma^2_{D(Y)}\right]}}$$

$$= \frac{\left[Cov_{W(XY)} - Cov_{S(XY)} - Cov_{D(XY)}\right]}{\sqrt{\left[\sigma^2_{W(X)} - \sigma^2_{S(X)} - Cov_{D(X)}\right]\left[\sigma^2_{W(Y)} - \sigma^2_{S(Y)} - Cov_{D(Y)}\right]}}$$

(c) *Phenotypic correlation* is estimated as -

$$r_P = \frac{\left[Cov_{W(XY)} + Cov_{S(XY)} + Cov_{D(XY)}\right]}{\sqrt{\left[\sigma^2_{W(X)} + \sigma^2_{S(X)} + Cov_{D(X)}\right]\left[\sigma^2_{W(Y)} + \sigma^2_{S(Y)} + Cov_{D(Y)}\right]}}$$

2. Parent Offspring Regression

Similar procedure to that used to estimate heritability is applied.

(i) Paret Offspring Mean

Hazel (1943) had shown the method of estimating the genetic correlation between two traits (X and Y) from cross covariance of one trait in progeny (O) and other trait in the parent (P). The following four co-variances are estimated:

Cov_{PxOy} = Covariance of X trait of parent with Y trait of offspring

Cov_{PyOx} = Covariance of Y trait of parent with X trait of offspring

Cov_{PxOx} = Covariance of X trait of parent and offspring

Cov_{PyOy} = Covariance of Y trait of parent and offspring

The genetic correlation (r_A) may be estimated either from the geometric or arithmetic average of the covariances as:

The r_A from *geometric method* is

$$r_A = \frac{\sqrt{\left(Cov_{PxOy}\right)\left(Cov_{PyOx}\right)}}{\sqrt{\left(Cov_{PxOx}\right)\left(Cov_{PyOy}\right)}}$$

Since it is assumed that $Cov_{PxPy} = Cov_{OxOy} = \frac{1}{2}\,Cov_{A(XY)}$

$Cov_{PxOx} = \frac{1}{2}\,V_{A(X)}$ and $Cov_{PyOy} = \frac{1}{2}\,V_{A(Y)}$

Now, $r_g = \dfrac{Cov_{A(XY)}}{\sigma_{A(X)}\,\sigma_{A(Y)}}$

The r_A from *arithmetic method* is estimated as:

$$r_A = \frac{Cov_{PxOy} + Cov_{PyOx}}{2\sqrt{Cov_{PxOy}\,Cov_{PyOy}}}$$

$$\text{or } r_A = \frac{Cov_{PxOy}}{\sqrt{\left[Cov_{PxOx} \, Cov_{PyOy}\right]}}$$

$$\text{or } r_A = \frac{Cov_{PyOx}}{\sqrt{\left[Cov_{PxOx} \, Cov_{PyOy}\right]}}$$

The expected genetic compositions of these covariances are as:

$$Cov_{PxOy} = Cov_{PyOx} = \tfrac{1}{2} Cov_{A(XY)}$$

$$= \tfrac{1}{2}\sigma^2_{A(XY)} + \tfrac{1}{4}\sigma^2_{AA(XY)}$$

$$Cov_{PxOx} = \tfrac{1}{2}\sigma^2_{A(X)} + \tfrac{1}{4}\sigma^2_{AA(X)}$$

$$Cov_{PyOy} = \tfrac{1}{2}\sigma^2_{A(Y)} + \tfrac{1}{4}\sigma^2_{AA(Y)}$$

This shows that the genetic correlation obtained by parent offspring correlation has additive by additive epistacy involved in its estimation and thus has the same limitations as the heritability estimated from parent offspring regression.

Robertson (1959) used the following formula to estimate the standard error of genetic correlation:

$$S.E.(r_A) = \left[\frac{1-r^2}{\sqrt{2}}\right] \left[\sqrt{\frac{SE_{(h^2_x)} SE_{(h^2_y)}}{h^2_x h^2_y}}\right]$$

This formula is applicable to estimate the SE of r_A obtained fro sib analysis as well as parent – offspring analysis. The genetic correlations are having large sampling variance and hence not very much precise. The genetic correlation is influenced by gene frequencies and hence differs for different generations.

(ii) Intra Sire Dam mean of Offspring

The 4 covariances are computed within sire progenies, as in case of heritability and then pooled. The ANOCOVA is as given below for Cov_{PxOy}, as example:

Soureces of Variation	SCP
Sires	$\sum \left(\dfrac{P_{Xi} O_{Yi}}{n_i}\right) - C.F.$
Dam/Sire	$\sum\sum P_{Xij} O_{Yij} - \sum \left(\dfrac{P_{Xi} O_{Yi}}{n_i}\right)$

All the other covariances are obtained similarity and the genetic correlation is estimated as given in 2(i).

3. Ratio of Differences of Two Traits among Daughters

The genetic correlation can be estimated with modification of the method suggested by Lush and Strans (1942) to estimate the h^2. The herd is divided in two groups according to the two traits *i.e.* better halves and poor halves in respect of the two traits. The ratio of the difference for trait x and for trait y is estimated. The four differences are obtained *viz.*

$D_{(Y)}x$ = difference in daughters Y trait based on division of dams according to x trait.

$D_{(X)}x$ = difference in daughters X trait based on division of dams according to x trait.

$D_{(Y)}y$ = difference in daughters Y trait based on division of dams according to y trait.

$D_{(X)}y$ = difference in daughters X trait based on division of dams according to y trait.

$$\text{Ratio 1} = \frac{D_{(Y)x}}{D_{(X)x}} = r_g \sqrt{\frac{\sigma^2_{A(Y)}}{\sigma^2_{A(X)}}}$$

$$\text{Ratio 2} = \frac{D_{(X)y}}{D_{(Y)y}} = r_g \sqrt{\frac{\sigma^2_{A(X)}}{\sigma^2_{A(Y)}}}$$

The product of these two ratio estimates r^2_g. Thus r_9 can be obtained as $\sqrt{r^2_g}$.

4. Isogenic Lines

The method of estimating h^2 from isogenic lines has been discussed earlier and the same procedure is used to estimate the genetic correlation. As the h^2 estimated from isogenic lines was the h^2 in broad sense, the genetic correlation estimated is also the correlation between genotypic values instead of breeding values. Thus the genetic correlation so estimated is not free from dominance and epistatic effects. The between lines and within lines components of variances of both traits and the covariance of the two traits are obtained similarly. The form of analysis of covariance is as given here

Sources of Variation	D.F.	MCP	E (MCP)
Between lines	*l* -1	MCP *l*	$\text{Cov}_{W(X,Y)} + K \, \text{Cov}_{G(X,Y)}$
Within line	N -1	MCP w	$\text{Cov}_{W(X,Y)}$

The $\sigma^2_{G(X)}, \sigma^2_{G(Y)}, \sigma^2_{W(X)},$ and $\sigma^2_{W(Y)}$ are obtained as before.

$$r_G = \frac{\text{Cov}_{G(X,Y)}}{\sqrt{\sigma^2_{G(X)} \sigma^2_{G(Y)}}} \; ; \; r_E = \frac{\text{Cov}_{W(X,Y)}}{\sqrt{\sigma^2_{W(X)} \sigma^2_{W(Y)}}}$$

5. Correlated Response Method (realized r_g)

The genetic correlation can be estimated when the correlated response is measured by selection experiment and the heritability of the two traits are known. This requires a double selection experiment:

Selection of X character in one line and

selection of Y character in another line.

This will measure both the direct and the correlated responses of each character.

Now let us understand about the correlated response, which is the associated change in second character (Y) as a result of change due to selection in character one (X). Thus the expected response in character Y, for which there is no selection, when selection is applied for its correlated character X, is called the correlated response (of character Y). The response in character X for which selection is applied is called the directed response (DR) The resulting change in Y character is the regression of breeding value of Y on the breeding value of $X_{[bA(yx)]}$, and this can be written as

$$b_{A(YX)} = r_{A(YX)} \left[\frac{\sigma_{A(Y)}}{\sigma_{A(X)}} \right]$$

The direct response of character X denoted as DR(X) is

$$DR(x) \quad = i\sigma_{P(X)} h^2_{(X)}$$
$$= i\sigma_{A(X)} h_{(X)}$$

The correlated response of character Y, denoted as $CR_{(Y)}$ can be predicted if the genetic correlation and the heritability of both the traits are known. The $CR_{(Y)}$ is

$$CR_{(Y)} \quad = b_{A(YX)} DR_{(X)}$$

$$= r_{A(YX)} \left[\frac{\sigma_{A(Y)}}{\sigma_{A(X)}} \right] i\sigma_{A(X)} h_{(X)}$$

$$= r_A \sigma_{A(Y)} i h_{(X)}$$
$$= r_A h_{(Y)} \sigma_{P(Y)} i h_{(X)} \text{ Since } \sigma_{A(Y)} = h_{(Y)} \sigma_{P(Y)}$$

The above equation of $CR_{(Y)}$ indicates that the expected $CR_{(Y)}$ would be small if the genetic correlation is small. The correlated response will be decreased if the genetic correlation is to a great extent was due to linkage. This is because the linkage relationship of genes is diminished through recombination and there is a consequent decrease in magnitude of genetic correlation which thereby reduces the correlated response.

The equation of $CR_{(Y)}$ can also be derived as:

$$CR_{(Y)} \quad = b_{A(YX)} DR_{(X)}$$

$$= \frac{Cov_{AY AX}}{\sigma^2_{A(X)}} i\sigma_{(P)} \left[\frac{\sigma^2_{A(X)}}{\sigma^2_{P(X)}} \right] \left[\frac{\sigma_{A(Y)}}{\sigma_{A(Y)}} \right] \left[\frac{\sigma_{P(Y)}}{\sigma_{P(Y)}} \right]$$

$$= r_{A(XY)} \, i \, \sigma_{P(Y)} h_X h_Y$$

Thus r_A can be estimated as

$$r_{A(XY)} = \frac{CR(Y)}{i\sigma_{P(Y)} h_X h_Y}$$

Therefore, if $CR_{(Y)}$ is known along with the hx and hy, then the genetic correlation is the realized genetic correlation.

Similarly, the selection can be applied for both X and Y traits in two experiments. The product of the ratio of $CR_{(Y)}$ to $DR_{(X)}$ is equivalent to:

$$\frac{CR_y}{DR_x} = r_A \sqrt{\frac{\sigma^2_{G(Y)}}{\sigma^2_{G(X)}}}$$

$$\frac{CR_x}{DR_y} = r_A \sqrt{\frac{\sigma^2_{G(X)}}{\sigma^2_{G(Y)}}}$$

Thus, the product of two ratios of CR to DR gives the square of the genetic correlation as:

$$\left(\frac{CR_y}{DR_y}\right)\left(\frac{CR_x}{DR_x}\right) = r^2_A$$

22.5 Correlated Response

The genetic correlation between two characters results the change in both the characters due to selection for either of the character. The amount and direction of associated change in second character (Y) as a result of change due to direct selection in first character (X) depends upon the size and sign of genetic correlation between the two characters. This associated change in the second character (Y) due to direct selection in first character (X) is called the *correlated response to selection.* This correlated response (C.R.) is for the second character (Y) for which no selection was made where as the change in character X for which selection was applied is called the *direct response* (D.R.) to selection. Thus, the C.R. indicates the change in correlated character (Y) when selection is applied for another trait X which is genetically correlated with Y.

The associated change in character Y will be equal to the regression of BV of Y on the BV of X (b_{YX}). This regression is

$$b_{A(YX)} = \frac{Cov_{A(YX)}}{\sigma^2_{A(X)}} = r_{A(YX)} \left[\frac{\sigma_{A(Y)}}{\sigma_{A(X)}}\right]$$

Therefore, the C.R. in character Y will be obtained as:

$$CR_{(Y)} = b_{A(YX)} DR_{(X)}$$

$$= r_{A(YX)} \left[\frac{\sigma_{A(Y)}}{\sigma_{A(X)}} \right] \left[i_{(x)} h_{(x)} \sigma_{A(X)} \right]$$

$$= r_{A(YX)} \, \sigma_{P(Y)} h_{(Y)} h_{(X)} i_{(X)}$$

Thus, CR can be predicted if genetic correlation between two characters and their heritability estimates are known. The magnitude of CR also depends on the magnitude of genetic correlation. The causes of genetic correlation also influence the CR. The CR will be decreased if the genetic correlation is more due to linkage of genes. This is because the linkage between genes is diminished by crossing over and recombination. This will decrease the magnitude of genetic correlation.

Use of Correlated Response

(i) Estimation of Genetic Correlation

The CR can be measured by conducting two way selection experiments. The selection is done for character X in one line and for character Y in other line. The DR and CR for each character is measured. The realized heritability estimates are obtained for both the characters from the response to selection. The genetic correlation can be estimated as the square root of the product of the ratios of CR to DR for the two characters as-

$$\left(\frac{CR_Y}{DR_Y} \right) \left(\frac{CR_X}{DR_X} \right) = \left(\frac{i \, h_X \, r_A \, \sigma_{A(Y)}}{i h_Y \, \sigma_{A(Y)}} \right) \left(\frac{i \, h_Y \, r_A \, \sigma_{A(X)}}{i h_X \, \sigma_{A(X)}} \right) = r^2_{\ A}$$

and therefore, $r_A = \sqrt{\left(\frac{CR_Y}{DR_Y} \right) \left(\frac{CR_X}{DR_X} \right)}$

(ii) Prediction of Performance in Another Environment

The performance levels of a character in two environments are taken as two different traits. The genetic correlation between them decides the magnitude of CR in the trait under second environment where the population has to live based on selection of the trait under the first environment. When the CR is low the improvement should be carried out in the environment under which the population has to live whereas in case of high CR the improvement can be made in any environment.

(iii) Improvement through Indirect Selection

The CR is used to apply the indirect selection for making improvement in the traits for which direct selection is not possible for any reason.

22.6 Indirect Selection

The concept of *correlated response* (C.R.) is extended to indirect selection. The *indirect selection* means the direction selection applied to the character (X) other than the one (Y) that is to be improved. For example, the improvement is required in character Y but the direct selection is not possible due to some reason (low h^2 of trait, not possible or difficult to measure the character, costly to measure the trait and the traits expressed at later ages or after death of animal). In this situation (when character Y can not be selected directly), it is better to select for the character X having desired genetic correlation with character Y, so as there is C.R. in character Y. Thus, direct selection is done for character X when change is required in character Y rather than to go for direct selection for Y.

Basis of Indirect Selection

It is the high genetic correlation between the character under direct selection (X) and the character for which no direct selection can be done but requires improvement (Y) and hence the C.R. is the basis.

Applications of Indirect Selection

The indirect selection is advantageous or applicable under the following conditions-

☆ When C.R. is higher than direct response (D.R.) due to high genetic correlation and high heritability of the character under selection (h^2_x) than $h^2 y$

☆ When it is more difficult to measure character Y than character X, or when it is costly to measure the character Y (efficiency of feed conversion) than easily measured character X (growth rate). Like wise, the sex ration in offspring is a parental trait and can not be changed applying direct selection but the selection for blood pH may produce a correlated change in sex ratio.

☆ When desired character is sex limited but correlated character is measurable in both the sexes, a higher intensity of selection is possible by indirect selection.

☆ Indirect selection can be applied to reduce generation interval, *e.g.* selection based on part year production in poultry for egg production (X) will lead to a rapid genetic gain in annual egg production (Y).

Measurement of Indirect Selection

The character which is under direct selection (X) is called the secondary character because the primary character is one in which improvement is required (Y) through indirect selection. The relative efficiency of direct and indirect selection for character Y can be compared by calculating genetic gain and finding out the ratio of two gains (Q) as:

$$Q = CR_Y/DR_Y = \text{Gain by indirect selection/Gain by direct selection}$$

$$= \frac{r_A\, h_X\, h_Y\, i_X\, \sigma_{PY}}{h_Y\, i_X\, \sigma_{AY}}$$

$$= r_A \frac{h_X}{h_Y}$$

Therefore, when Q is greater than one, the indirect selection is more effective. This is possible if the secondary character (X) has higher heritability than desired trait (Y) and also r_A is high.

Examples of Indirect Selection

Some of the examples of indirect selection are:

☆ Selection of weaner fleece for increased adult fleece

☆ Selection for birth weight or weight at early age for increased adult weight

☆ Selection based on par year record

☆ Selection based on FLMY for increased lifetime or subsequent production in later lactations.

☆ It is required to improve feed efficiency in pigs but the amount of feed consumed is difficult to measure and hence selection for gain will give the idea from good $- r_A$ that as the gain is increased the feed conversion becomes better (less kg. feed per kg. gain)

☆ Selection for yearling body weight in sheep to increase fertility (lambs born) because the fertility has low heritability for which direct selection for fertility will be slow.

Solved Examples and Exercises

Example 22.1

The data on two characters were recorded on 527 progenies of 50 sires. The analysis of the data for the variances **and covariance of** two traits indicated as under. Estimate all types of correlations taking K = 10.5

S.V.	d.f.	MS (x)	MS (y)	MCP(xy)
Sires	49	899376.9	3969.6	12252.1
Progenies/Si	477	449571.2	3224.4	3870.4

Solution

$$\sigma^2_{s(X)} = \frac{(899376.9 - 449571.2)}{10.5} = 42838.64$$

$$\sigma^2_{s(Y)} = \frac{(3969.6 - 3224.4)}{10.5} = 70.97$$

$$\text{Cov}_{s(XY)} = \frac{(12252.1 - 3870.4)}{10.5} = 798.26$$

$$r_g = \frac{\text{Cov}_{s(XY)}}{\sqrt{\sigma^2_{s(x)}\sigma^2_{s(Y)}}}$$

$$= \frac{798.26}{\sqrt{(42838.64)(70.97)}}$$

$$= \frac{798.26}{1741.63} = 0.458$$

$$r_E = \frac{\text{Cov}_{W(XY)}}{\sqrt{\sigma^2_{w(x)}\sigma^2_{w(y)}}}$$

$$= \frac{3870.4}{\sqrt{(449571.2)(3224.4)}}$$

$$= \frac{3870.4}{38073.6} = 0.101$$

$$or\ r_E = \frac{(3870 - 3 \times 798.26)}{\sqrt{[(449571.2 - 3 \times 42838.64)(3224.4 - 3 \times 70.97)]}}$$

$$= \frac{1475.62}{\sqrt{(320996.06 \times 3011.49)}}$$

$$= \frac{1475.62}{31091.44} = 0.0474$$

$$r_P = \frac{(3870.4 + 798.26)}{\sqrt{[(449571.2 + 42838.64)(3224.4 + 70.97)]}}$$

$$= \frac{4668.66}{\sqrt{(492409.84 + 3295.37)}}$$

$$= \frac{4668.66}{462824.17} = 0.0116$$

$$\text{SE (rg)} = \left[\frac{1 - r^2}{\sqrt{2}}\right]\left[\sqrt{\frac{\text{SE}_{(h2X)}\text{SE}_{(h2Y)}}{h^2_X h^2_Y}}\right]$$

$$= \left[\frac{1 - 0.21}{\sqrt{2}}\right]\left[\sqrt{\frac{(0.135 \times 0.095)}{(0.348 \times 0.086)}}\right]$$

$$= \left[\frac{0.79}{1.4142}\right]\left[\sqrt{\frac{(0.135 \times 0.095)}{(0.348 \times 0.086)}}\right]$$

$$= 0.5589 \times 0.6542$$

$$= 0.3656$$

Example 22.2

Nested Design: Seventeen (17) sires were each mated to four (4) dams and each mating produced three (3) progeny. The analysis of two characters of this sample resulted as under. Estimate genetic, environmental and phenotypic correlation. $K_1 = K_2 = 3; K_3 = 12$

S.V.	d.f.	MS (x)	MS (y)	MCP(xy)
Sires	16	143114.21	8.63	501.9
Dams/Sire	51	102038.11	4.65	362.7
Progeny/dam	136	80054.1	3.65	310.5

Solution

$$\sigma^2_{S(X)} = \frac{(143114.21 - 102038.11)}{12} = 3423.0$$

$$\sigma^2_{S(Y)} = \frac{(8.63 - 4.65)}{12} = 0.33$$

$$\text{Cov}_{S(XY)} = \frac{(501.9 - 362.7)}{12} = 11.6$$

$$\sigma^2_{D(X)} = \frac{(102038.11 - 80054.1)}{3} = 7328.0$$

$$\sigma^2_{D(Y)} = \frac{(4.65 - 3.65)}{3} = 0.33$$

$$\text{Cov}_{D(XY)} = \frac{(362.7 - 310.3)}{3} = 17.4$$

The *genetic correlation* may be estimated from sire, dam and full sib components as:

$$r_{A \text{ (sire component)}} = \frac{11.6}{\sqrt{(3423 \times 0.33)}} = \frac{11.6}{33.61} = 0.345$$

$$r_{A \text{ (dam component)}} = \frac{17.4}{\sqrt{(7328 \times 0.33)}} = \frac{17.4}{49.17} = 0.354$$

$$r_{A \text{ (sire + dam component)}} = \frac{(11.6+17.4)}{\sqrt{(3423+7328)(0.33+0.33)}}$$

$$= \frac{29.0}{84.23} = 0.344$$

The *environmental correlation* may be obtained in either of 3 ways:

$$r_E = \frac{310.5 - 2 \times 11.6}{\sqrt{[80054.1 - 2 \times 3423][3.65 - 2 \times 0.33]}}$$

$$= \frac{287.3}{467.86} = 0.614$$

Or

$$= \frac{310.5 - 2 \times 17.4}{\sqrt{[80054.1 - 2 \times 7328][3.65 - 2 \times 0.33]}}$$

$$= \frac{275.75}{442.199} = 0.623$$

Or

$$= \frac{(310.5 - 11.6 - 17.4)}{\sqrt{[80054.1 - 3423 - 7328][3.65 - 0.33 - 0.33]}}$$

$$= \frac{281.5}{455.21} = 0.618$$

The *phenotypic correlation* is estimated as:

$$r_P = \frac{(310.5 + 11.6 + 17.4)}{\sqrt{(80054.1 + 3423 + 7328)(3.65 + 0.33 + 0.33)}}$$

$$= \frac{339.5}{635.59} = 0.542$$

Example 22.3 Parent-Offspring Records

The body weight (X) and age at first calving (Y) were recorded in dams (P) and daughters (0). The covariances of the two traits were found as:

$$\text{Cov}_{\text{Py Ox}} = 27.99, \; \text{Cov}_{\text{Px Oy}} = 14.99$$

$$\text{Cov}_{\text{Px Ox}} = 25.83, \; \text{Cov}_{\text{Py Oy}} = 60.55$$

Estimate the genetic correlation using the different formulae.

Solution

Arithmetic methods:

$$r_g = \frac{Cov_{PyOx}}{\sqrt{(Cov_{PxOx})(Cov_{PyOy})}}$$

$$= \frac{27.99}{\sqrt{25.83 \times 60.55}} = \frac{27.99}{39.56} = 0.71$$

or $r_g = \dfrac{Cov_{PxOy}}{\sqrt{(Cov_{PxOx})(Cov_{PyOy})}}$

$$= \frac{14.99}{39.56} = 0.379$$

or $r_g = \dfrac{Cov_{PxOy} + Cov_{PyOx}}{2\sqrt{(Cov_{PxOx})(Cov_{PyOy})}}$

$$= \frac{(27.99 + 14.99)}{2 \times 39.56} = 0.543$$

Geometric Method

$$r_A = \sqrt{\frac{Cov_{PxOy}\ Cov_{PyOx}}{(Cov_{PxOx})(Cov_{PyOy})}}$$

$$= \sqrt{\frac{29.99 \times 14.99}{25.83 \times 60.55}} = \frac{21.20}{39.56} = 0.536$$

Exercise 22.4

The milk yield and fat percentage were recorded for 10 dams and daughter pairs and given below:

Dam-daughter	Dam's Records		Daughter's Records	
Pairs	M.Y. (X)	Fat per cent (Y)	M.Y. (X)	Fat per cent (Y)
1	10.0	5.4	12.0	4.7
2	10.5	5.2	10.2	5.8
3	9.0	6.0	10.3	6.4
4	8.7	6.5	11.0	5.9
5	10.2	5.6	11.0	5.4
6	11.5	4.8	12.2	5.0

Dam-daughter	Dam's Records		Daughter's Records	
Pairs	*M.Y. (X)*	*Fat per cent (Y)*	*M.Y. (X)*	*Fat per cent (Y)*
7	10.5	5.4	12.2	5.0
8	10.2	5.6	11.5	4.6
9	11.8	5.0	10.4	5.8
10	9.1	6.2	10.1	5.6
Total	101.5	55.7	110.9	54.2

ΣP_X = 101.5 ΣP_Y = 55.7

ΣO_X = 110.9 ΣO_Y = 54.2

Cov_{PxOx} = 1128.03 – CF   = 1128.03 – 1125.63 = 2.395

Cov_{PyOx} = 616.20 – CF   = 616.20 – 617.71 = – 1.51

Cov_{PxOy} = 548.23 – CF   = 548.23 – 550.13 = – 1.90

Cov_{PyOy} = 303.01 – CF   = 303.01 – 301.89 = 1.12

Now calculate the r_g by gometric method and all the 3 arithmetic methods.

Exercise 22.5

Estimate the genetic correlation from the following data recorded on two characters on 12 progenies of 4 sires, (3 progenies of each sire):

Progeny	Sire 1		Sire 2		Sire 3		Sire 4	
	X	Y	X	Y	X	Y	X	Y
1	3	3	4	4	3	3	4	3
2	4	2	3	4	3	3	3	3
3	4	4	3	3	2	2	2	2
Total	11	11	10	11	8	8	9	8

Chapter 23
Genetics of Threshold Characters

The characters are divided into three classes on the basis of their inheritance pattern. The *qualitative traits* are governed by major genes few in number, not affected by the environment, and show discrete distribution in phenotypic values dividing the population in groups. The *quantitative traits* are governed by polygenes, affected by environment, show continuous distribution in phenotypic values, and measured in metric units. There is another class of characters which are like qualitative character on a phenotypic scale (dividing the population into discrete phenotypic classes) but they are, on the contrary, affected by polygenes as well as by the environment like quantitative characters. Such traits can be further divided in two categories *viz.* meristic traits and threshold traits.

1. Meristic Traits

The phenotypes for these traits are expressed in discrete, integral numbers. The characteristic feature of these traits is that the phenotype of an animal is a simple integer which equals the number of elements of the traits displayed by the individual. *The examples of these traits are*:

Number of offspring carried by a dam (litter size),

Number of bristles in Drosophila,

Number of ears on a stalk of corn plant,

Number of flowers on a petal, etc.

In Drosophila, the bristles occur on the sternites of ventral abdomen and these are called abdominal bristles or sternital bristles. These are usually on the fifth or sixth (or on both) sternite in females and the fourth or fifth (or both) sternite in males. Normally there are 14 to 24 bristles per sternite.

2. Threshold Traits

These types of polygenic traits are also discrete traits. These are either expressed (present) or not expressed (absent) in any one individual, in contrast to the meristic traits which are expressed in all the individuals of a population. For the description of phenotypic values of such a trait, there are two separate scales *viz.* the underlying scale (polygenic distribution) which is continuous, and the visible scale (phenotypic distribution) which is discontinuous. These two scales of distribution are connected by a point of discontinuity or 'threshold". This is a point on the continuous scale which corresponds with the discontinuity on a visible scale. The individuals whose phenotypic values on the underlying polygenic scale exceed the threshold appear in one visible class while the individuals below the threshold appear in the other visible class. Thus, the relationship between polygenes and expression of discontinuous character comes about through the establishment of "threshold".

The characters whose inheritance is polygenic but exhibit all-or-none, or one-or other kind of phenotypic expression are called "Threshold characters". The concept of the "Threshold model" for all-or-none traits was first introduced by Wright (1934) in a study on the inheritance of digit number in guinea pigs with 4 toes rather than the normal 3 toes on hind feet. Theses characters are also called quasi-continuous characters (Gruneberg 1952) for the reason that the phenotypic values are discontinuous like qualitative traits but the mode of inheritance is like quantitative characters.

The examples of such traits are:

Resistance to a disease (healthy- sick),

Survivability (survive – dead),

Fertility (pregnant – non pregnant),

Litter size (one – two offspring),

Type of birth (normal vs abnormal births),

Hatchability of eggs (hatched-not hatched),

Presence or absence of any organ or structure (present-absent) like, supernumerary teats, fur defect (normal-defective), polydactylism in guinea pigs, number of lumber vertebrae in mice etc.

These characters have been called "quisi-continuous" because the phenotypic values are discontinuous like qualitative traits but the mode of inheritance is polygenic like that of a quantitative trait.

The threshold traits are measured like that of the qualitative traits. The type of variation in these traits among the individual of a population and the distribution of individuals is also like quantitative traits. The causes of variation, both genetic and environmental, in these traits are similar to the quantitative traits. The method of analysis of these characters is different than the methods used for quantitative traits.

23.1 Cause and Effect Variables

It is known that the prevalence of a disease is the result of environment stimuli. No living being always suffers with a disease but suffers under certain environmental conditions. For example, pneumonia mostly prevailed during colder months, heavy smoking leads to coughing, sugar intake in excess amount for longer time causes diabities, etc

How a character governed by polygenes and the environment may show all or none phenotypic expression? This can be viewed from the two points of cause variable and effect variable. The cause variable is continuously distributed but the effect variable (expression of character) is discontinuous.

Cause Variable (Underlying Variable)

It is the cause variable which causes the expression of the character. The cause variable is the joint effect of the polygenes and of the environment. The cause variable is known as the underlying variable which could be the quantity of a substance from biochemical pathway or the rate of some biochemical reaction or the rate with which the development process progress in the final expression of the character as a result of the action of the polygenes and the environment.

In case of susceptibility to disease, the cause variable is the toxin substance in terms of its quantity which depends upon the level of infection and other environmental factors. The animal is affected with the disease when the quantity of toxin substance surpasses a certain limit (threshold). The level of a substance from biochemical pathway or the rate of biochemical reaction or the rate of development process are the examples of *cause variable* and called the *phenotypic potential* of the individual which is determined by the biology of the individual influenced by genes, environment and their interaction effect. Thus, this phenotypic potential is the joint genetic and environmental potential that decides the phenotype of the individual (effect variable). This phenotypic potential, which in case of disease susceptibility is the quantity of a toxin could in principle be measured and studied in metric units. When the phenotypic potential of an individual exceeds a threshold, which separate the two discrete phenotype classes, then the phenotype will be put up in a higher phenotypic class otherwise in a lower phenotypic class. The phenotypic potential (cause variable) is the underlying variable and its scale of measurement is called the underlying scale which is continuous whereas the phenotype of a character (effect variable) is discontinuous measured by a visible (phenotypic) scale. Therefore, these two scales are required to describe the phenotypic values for threshold characters. These two scales are connected by a threshold which is a point of discontinuity on the visible scale. Thus, threshold is a point of discontinuity which imposes discontinuity in phenotypic values. The threshold characters have the underlying continuity of cause variable (phenotypic potential) with a threshold for expression of the phenotype (effect variable). Therefore, the value of underlying variable (cause variable or phenotypic potential) in a particular individual could depend on both genetic and environmental factors and the expression of character (effect variable) could require that this value (underlying or cause variable) exceeds to the point of threshold.

Effect Variable

The expression of a character (phenotype) is known as the effect variable. The phenotype of a character (effect variable) is discontinuous measured by a visible (phenotypic) scale. However, the expression of some of the threshold characters shows continuous distribution in phenotypic values to certain limit, for example, susceptibility to a disease and mortality. It can be seen that these characters with all or non phenotypic expression have an underlying continuity such that the animals which died are not uniform and likewise those which survive are also not uniform. This is because some animals died quickly without any struggle, others are sick for sometime showing resistance and struggling but they will succumb, still others seem to survive but finally die. Likewise among survivors, some seems about to die, others are sick without being in a critical danger, still others seem to suffer with only a little discomfort from sickness even to be completely immune to it. In this way, the resistance can be treated itself as a continuously distributed variable or nearly so in terms of "time of survival" or degree of severity but final expression is forced to be categorized into one or the other phenotypic class *viz.* dead and survival, resistant and susceptible. The animals whose resistance levels are below a certain threshold will die and others will survive in which resistance levels are above the threshold point because of the minimum requirement for life to continue.

The phenotypic potential of different individuals of one phenotypic class differs markedly depending upon genetic and environmental factors but their phenotypes do not. The genetic merit of the individual thus can not be accurately estimated on the basis of the phenotype and hence the phenotype for these characters is a poor indicator of genetic merit of the individual. This creates a problem for genetic selection for threshold character. The direct estimation of the phenotypic potential of an individual can not be measured. The procedures to record and to code the data, the statistical and genetic analysis of the threshold traits differ from those used for quantitative traits. These have been given as under.

23.2 Data Recording

The phenotype is recorded as 1 or 0 for the individuals expressing the character (affected animals) and not expressing the character, respectively. The total numbers of individuals in the population are counted, out of which the number of affected individuals (those expressing the trait) are counted separately. The grouping of individuals is further made. These groups may be breed groups, sire-progeny groups (progenies of different sires), age groups, lactation wise groups, year wise groups, season wise groups. The total number of individuals in a groups (i^{th} group) are denoted as n_i, the number of individuals expressing the character in i^{th} group are denoted by a_i and the number of individuals not expressing the character are taken by substraction as $n_i - a_i$.

23.3 Estimation of Mean and Variance

The arithmetic mean of phenotypes of all the individual of a group is estimated to enable a person to compare the mean values of the different groups. The mean value of a group or of the whole population is expressed in terms of proportion or percentage of the total animals expressing the character. This percentage is called as the incidence or the prevalence in case of human disease. This incidence in percentage describes the mean value of the group or the whole population with respect to the character and denoted by P. Thus P is taken as mean.

Falconer (1965) has expressed the mean incidence in terms of the mean liability and made comparison in mean liability of different groups by taking the threshold as being fixed which means the same level of liability in all the groups. The threshold is treated as the origin or the zero-point on the scale of liability and the mean of any group is expressed as deviation in standard deviation units of liability from the threshold.

The variance (σ^2) for proportion data is taken as

$$\sigma^2 = \frac{pq}{n}$$

Where,   P = is the incidence in proportion

q = 1-p

n = is the number of animals exposed.

23.4 Quantification of Threshold Traits

Tests of Normal Distribution: Some statistical tests *viz.* X^2, skewness and kurtosis are conducted in order to test whether the distribution of phenotypic potentials of different individuals is normally distributed in the population which gives an indication of the multifactorial or polygenic nature of the threshold characters.

All the animals are first grouped into sire-progeny groups. The total animals (n) and the affected animals (a) with a disease are counted sire wise and the percentage susceptibility (percent or proportion of animals expressing the threshold trait) is estimated for all the sires. The arcsin transformation (angular transformations) of the proportion data is made. The total range of arcsin values of all the sire groups is divided into classes taking an appropriate class interval. Then the frequency distribution of sires falling in different class intervals is obtained and this is taken as observed frequency (o).

To test the normality of the data the expected frequency of sires in different classes is estimated with the help of normal distribution as described by Snedecor and Cockren (1967) and given as under

The Z_1 and Z_2 values corresponding for the lower and upper class limit are found out as

$$Z_1 = \frac{(X_1 - U)}{\sigma} \qquad \text{and} \qquad Z_2 = \frac{(X_2 - U)}{\sigma}$$

Where, X_1 and X_2 the lower and upper limit of class interval, respectively.

U = is the mean occurrence of a trait in the population.

σ = is the standard deviation of the trait. The area between Z_1 and Z_2 from the cumulative normal frequency distribution table is taken as Z1- Z2 and this value is multiplied by the total observed frequency (total number of sires = N). This resultant quantity is the expected frequency for that particular class. Thus, the expected frequency (E) = $N(Z_1 - Z_2)$.

23.5 Statistical Analysis

The difference in incidence among groups (breeds, sires, year, season, lactation etc.) can be tested either by chi-square test or by the technique of analysis of variance.

23.5.1 Chi-square (χ^2) Test

The χ^2 test of significance among different levels of an effect is applied as described by Chandel (1963):

(i) $\chi^2 = \left[\sum \left(\dfrac{a_i^2}{n_i} \right) - \dfrac{\left(\sum a_i \right)^2}{\sum n_i} \right]\left[\dfrac{\left(\sum n_i \right)^2}{\sum a_i \left(\sum n_i - a_i \right)} \right]$

This is tested with N- 1 degree of freedom, (N is the number of levels of an effect).

The quantity $\left(\sum \left(\dfrac{a_i^2}{n_i} \right) - \dfrac{\left(\sum a_i \right)^2}{\sum n_i} \right)$ in the formula is the sum of squares

between classes and $\left[\dfrac{\left(\sum n_i \right)^2}{\sum a_i \left(\sum n_i - a_i \right)} \right]$ is equal to $\dfrac{1}{pq}$.

Thus, the chi – square is also taken as:

$$\chi^2 = \frac{\text{S.S. between classes}}{pq} = \frac{\left[\sum \left(\dfrac{a_i^2}{n_i} \right) - \dfrac{\left(\sum a_i \right)^2}{\sum n_i} \right]}{pq}$$

(ii) $\chi^2 = \dfrac{N^2}{C_1 C_2} \sum \left[\dfrac{a_i^2}{(a_i + b_i)} \right] - \dfrac{C_1^2}{N}$

Where, a_i = no. of individuals affected in i[th] level of effect

b_i = no. of individuals not affected in i[th] level of effect

$C_1 = \Sigma a_i$ = Total no. of individuals affected in the population

$C_2 = \Sigma b_i$ = Total no. of individuals not affected in the population

$N = C_1 + C_2$ = Total no. of individuals in the population

(iii) The χ^2 for proportion data can also be computed as under:

$$\chi^2 = \frac{\left[pqN - \sum p_i \, q_i \, n_i\right]}{pq}$$

Where,

p_i = incidence of the trait in i^{th} group.

$q_i = 1 - p_i$

p = overall incidence of the trait in the population

$q = 1 - p$

n_j = no. of animals exposed in jth group (level of effect)

n = No. of levels of the effect

$N = \Sigma n_i$

23.5.2 Analysis of Variance

The significance of the different effects can be tested by partitioning the variance into the corresponding components attributable to the effects. The analysis of variance to binomial data is conducted by transformation of percent data into arcsin or angular transformation.

The angular transformation is used for binomial proportion. The angular transformation makes the variance independent of mean and hence justifies the use of analysis of variance technique. The first step is to count the number of animals affected (a_i) out of the total number of animals (n_i) under various cells developed according to the various effects under study *e.g.* under each age group, in each year under each season etc. and then converted into proportions or percentage (the proportion of affected animals in different cells). The proportion is changed to angle whose sin is $\sqrt{proportion}$.

Angle = Arcsin $\sqrt{proportion}$ = $Sin^{-1} \sqrt{p}$.

Having obtained the arcsin values, the analysis of variance of angles is conducted as usual. The transformation does not remove inequalities in variance due to different number of observations. Bartlett (1947) suggested a device which improves the equality of the variance in the angles. With n less than 50, a zero proportion is counted as ¼ n before angular transformation and 100 per cent proportion is taken as $(n - ¼)/n$. A weighted analysis in the angular scale is advisable if n vary widely.

The alternate method of transformation is used. This also involves the counting of the affected and unaffected animals in different cells developed according to the effects under study. The phenotypic values are given codes as 1 for affected and 0 for unaffected animals. The value 0 is taken as ¼ n_i. while the value 1 is taken as $\frac{(n_{i-¼})}{n_i}$.

with n_i as the total number of animals in the ith cell and denoted as P and P', respectively. The P and P' are transformed to angles Q and Q' respectively. Q = $Sin^{-1}\sqrt{p}$ and Q' = $Sin^{-1} \sqrt{p'}$. The analysis of variance is conducted on these transformed values by estimating the sum of squares as usual.

$$\text{Correction factor} = \frac{\left[\sum a_i Q_i + \sum (n_i - a_i) Q'_i\right]}{N}$$

Total S.S. $= [\Sigma a_i Q_i^2 + \Sigma (n_i - a_i) Q'^2_I] - \text{C.F.}$

$$\text{Group S.S.} = \frac{\sum \left[a_i Q_i^2 + \sum (n_i - a_i) Q'^2_i\right]}{n_i} - \text{C.F.}$$

Where, $a_i Q_i$ = total phenotypic values of affected animals in i[th] cell

$(n_i - a_i) Q'_i$ = total phenotypic values of unaffected animals in i[th] cell

$a_i Q_i^2$ = Square of phenotypic values of affected animals in i[th] cell

$(n_i - a_i) Q'^2_I$ = Square of phenotypic values of unaffected animals in i[th] cell

23.6 Estimation of Heritability

The methods of estimating genetic parameters of quantitative characters showing continuous variation are not applicable to threshold characters because the underlying continuous distribution cannot be observed. Therefore, other techniques have been used to deal with threshold characters. The methods which are in use and simple to apply have been given here.

(1) Sib Correlation Method

Lush *et al.* (1948) proposed a method of estimating heritability of viability in the fowl. The method is based on the assumption that a normal distribution of genetic and environmental effects underlies the discontinuous distribution of the phenotypes with a linear relationship between the genetic values on the two scales, *viz.* normal and binomial scales. The experimental design was that a number of sires (s_i) were each mated to several dams (d_j) and each mating produces several progenies (n_{ij}) out of which a_{ij} survives. Therefore, the kth progeny of jth dam mated to i[th] sire (Y_{ijk}) is considered a variable which takes the phenotypic value 1 if the kth progeny survive otherwise it is given the value zero. The model is as under:-

$$Y_{ijk} = U + S_i + d_{ij} + e_{ijk}$$

The total numbers of progeny surviving from dam (d_{ij}) are taken as a_{ij} and equal to total sum of n_{ij} observation. Each a_{ij} progeny is given the value 1 while those died $(n_{ij} - a_{ij})$ are given the value 0. All the effects are random and independent with expectation zero and variance

$E(S_i)^2 = \sigma^2 s$, $E(d_{ij})^2 = \sigma^2_D$ and $E(e_{ijk}) = \sigma^2 w$.

The binomial data on progeny are subjected to hierarchal ANOVA, between sires (BS), between dams with sire (BD), and between progeny within dams (W D)). The ANOVA for full sibs is carried out as for metric traits.

ANOVA Full Sib Families

Sources	D.S.	S.S.	E.M.S.
Sires	$S-1$	BS	$\sigma^2 w. + k_2 \sigma^2_D + k_3 \sigma^2_s$
Dam/Sire	$\Sigma (d_i - 1)$	BD	$\sigma^2 w. + k_1 \sigma^2_D$
Progeny/dams	$\Sigma (n_{ij} - 1)$	WD	$\sigma^2 w$

where, K_1 = Average no. of dams per sire = $\dfrac{\left[n. - \left(\Sigma \dfrac{n^2_{ij}}{n_i} \right) \right]}{(D-S)}$

K_2 = Average no. of progeny per dam = $\dfrac{\left[\left(\Sigma \dfrac{n^2_{ij}}{n_i} \right) - \left(\Sigma \dfrac{n^2_{ij}}{n.} \right) \right]}{(S-1)}$

K_3 = Average no. of progeny per sire = $\dfrac{\left[n. - \left(\Sigma \dfrac{n^2_{i.}}{n.} \right) \right]}{(S-1)}$

N = n. = Total no. of progeny;

$n_{i.}$ = No. of progeny per sire.

n_{ij} = No. of progeny per dam;

$a.$ = Total no. of progeny survive;

$a_{i.}$ = no. of progeny survive per sire

a_{ij} = no. of progeny survive per dam

S = No. of sires;

D = No. of dams

The sums of squares corresponding to different sources of variation are estimated as:

$$C.F. = \frac{(a.)^2}{n.}$$

$$\text{Total S.S.} = \frac{a. - (a.)^2}{n.}$$

$$\text{Sire S.S.} = \Sigma \left[\frac{(a_i)^2}{n_i} \right] - C.F.$$

Dam within sire S.S. $= \dfrac{\sum(a_{ij})^2}{n_{ij}} - \dfrac{\sum(a_{ij})^2}{n_i}$

Progeny within dam S.S. $= a. - \dfrac{\sum(a_{ij})^2}{n_{ij}}$

The heritability is estimated either from half sib covariance (sire component or dam component) or from full sib component as described under section 17.5.4. The estimates of standard error of heritability are also estimated as described under section 17.5.4.

This method is not strictly valid as it involves conducting analysis of variance for a binomial variable, because in such case the variance is not independent of mean. Therefore, it is desirable to use angular transformation to make the variance independent of mean so as to justify the analysis of variance technique. The values 1 and 0 are converted as outlined under section 20.5.2 above.

(2) Intra-Herd Regression of Daughter on Dam

Lush (1950) studied the inheritance of susceptibility of mastitis in dairy cattle. The method is based on the logic that the incidence of the disease should be high among the daughters of the susceptible dams than it is expected among the daughters of resistant dams in the same herd. This amounts to regression of daughters on dam. The two groups of dams are 100 per cent apart in their phenotypic susceptibility when classified in this way. Since it is assumed that the sires of the two groups of daughters would be about equal to each other in transmitting the susceptibility to mastitis and therefore, the phenotypic averages of the unselected daughters would differ by only ½ as much as the genetic average of their dams. The susceptibility of the two daughter groups which represent percent daughters susceptible out of susceptible and resistant dams are represented by X and Y. The heritability is estimated as:

$$h^2 = \dfrac{2(X-Y)}{100}$$

To estimate X and Y the information on the dam and daughters with regard to susceptibility can be collected as under

Table 23.2: Distribution of Dam – Daughters Based on their Response to Disease

No. of Susceptible Dams ($N_1 + N_2$)		No. of Resistant Dams ($N_3 + N_4$)	
No. Susceptible Daughters (N_1)	No. of Resistant Daughters (N_2)	No. Susceptible Daughters (N_3)	No. of Resistant Daughters (N_4)

X   = Per cent daughters susceptible out of susceptible dams

$$= \frac{N_1}{(N_1 + N_2)}$$

= Per cent daughters susceptible out of resistant dams.

$$= \frac{N_3}{(N_3 + N_4)}$$

The standard error of heritability obtained by this method of Lush (1950) has been given by Tomar and Verma (1981) by the formula:

$$S.E\,(h^2) = \sqrt{\left[\frac{P_1(1-P_1)}{n_1} + \frac{P_2(1-P_2)}{n_2} \right]}$$

Where, $P_1 = \dfrac{X}{100}$; $P_2 = \dfrac{Y}{100}$

n_1 and n_2 are the number of susceptible and resistant dams, respectively.

(3) Regression of Relatives on Propositi (Affected Animal)

Falconer (1965) suggested the method for estimating heritability on the underlying scale for disease liability in which the increased performance of the progeny of the selected parents is taken as the selection response and compared to selection differential. In the case of liability of disease, the increased incidence of the disease in the relatives of the propositi (affected individuals) is taken as response and the incidence in the affected individuals estimates the selection differential. The ratio of response (R) to selection differential (S) is the regression of relatives on propositi, $b_{OP} = R/S$.

From parent generation the unaffected (resistant) individuals are selected as parents and are bred to produce offspring. The response to selection is the difference in mean between the parents and progeny generation which is taken as 0.5, assuming the variances of the two generations to be equal. The selection differential is the mean liability of the affected individuals in the parent generation as a deviation from their population mean. The mean of the affected individuals in standard deviation units is equivalent to the intensity of selection, i, corresponding to the incidence as the proportion selected.

From the calculations explained above, the correlation of liability between relatives of any sort is given by

$$t = \frac{m_P - m_R}{i} = \frac{X_P - X_R}{i}$$

Where, the subscript P and R refer to the population and the relatives.

m = mean as a deviation from the threshold

x = normal deviate of the threshold from the mean

= mean deviation of affected individuals from the (parental) population mean.

The h^2 is then calculated from the correlation as $h^2 = t/r$.

Where, r is the coefficient of relationship among the relatives.

(4) Genetic Analysis of Proportion Data without Transformation

Tomar *et al* (*1991*) devised a method to estimate heritability without transformation of proportion data by conducting the analysis of variance on data of mortality of Murrah Buffaloe female calves. The sums of squares were estimated as:

	I Method	II Method
Total sum of squares	$= pN - p^2N$	$= pqN$
Sire sum of squares	$= \Sigma p_i^2 n_i - p^2N$	$= pqN - \Sigma p_i q_i n_i$
Error sum of squares	$= pN - \Sigma p_i^2 n_i$	$= \Sigma p_i q_i n_I$

Where, n_i = number of total progenies for i^{th} sire

a_i = number of affected progenies of ith sire

$N = \Sigma n_i$ = Total number of progenies

$P_i = \dfrac{a_i}{n_i}$ is the average incidence of the trait among the progenies

of ith sire

$q_i = 1 - p_i$

$\bar{p} = \Sigma a_i / \Sigma n_i$ is the average incidence of the trait in the population.

$\bar{q} = 1 - p$

The sire-wise data on progeny with regard to survivability is arranged in a tabular form.

23.7 Estimation of Repeatability

The basis of the method for estimation of repeatability depends on directly estimating the regression of performance in any one year on that of the previous year (Lush, 1950). The animals are classified in two groups. viz, susceptible and resistant to a disease in the previous lactation/age groups and the percent susceptibility of these animals is computed for the following lactation/age *i.e.* percentage animals susceptible in the following lactation which were susceptible in the previous lactation (denoted by x) as well as the percentage of animals susceptible in the following lactation which ere resistant in the previous lactation (denoted by Y). The X and Y are estimated as shown in Table 20.2 by treating the previous age corresponding to dams and the future age corresponding to daughters. The repeatability (t) is then taken as:

$$t = \frac{(X-Y)}{100}$$

23.8 Estimation of Correlation (Threshold Characters)

(i) Test of Association

The incidence of diseases is the examples of threshold characters. The association between the incidences of two diseases can be estimated by χ^2 test. To apply χ^2 test, the frequency distribution of the numbers of animals susceptible (affected) (i) to both the diseases, (ii) only to first disease, (iii) only to second disease, and (iv) to neither disease are counted and these numbers are denoted by a, b, c, and d, respectively.

The χ^2 test of association is applied as described by Chandel (1963):

$$\chi^2 = \frac{\left[(ab-bc)^2 n\right]}{R_1 R_2 C_1 C_2}$$

Where, n = Total no. of animals exposed

C_1 = a + b = total of first column

C_2 = c + d = total of second column

R_1 = a + c = total of first row

R_2 = b + d = total of second row

The calculated χ^2 value is tested at 1 degree of freedom.

(ii) Genetic Correlation

The method of estimation of genetic correlation between two threshold characters can be explained taking the example of mortality. The total mortality is divided into the death due to one disease (A) and due to second disease (B).

The data coding and grouping of data into various groups like sire groups, dam groups etc. is done as outlined under section 23.2 in this chapter.

The variances between classes and within classes are estimated as in case of heritability. The covariances between classes and within classes are estimated from cross products of two diseases. For details see solved example 23.7.

Solved Examples

Example 23.1

The following data were recorded on type of calving from 23 HF sires at NDRI, Karnal. Estimate the heritability of abnormal births from half sib method.

Sire No.	Total Births	Abnormal Births	Sire No.	Total Births	Abnormal Births
(s_i)	(n_i)	(a_i)	(S_i)	(n_i)	(a_i)
1	29	3	13	49	4
2	20	1	14	32	2
3	22	1	15	38	1
4	21	1	16	24	3
5	32	0	17	56	0
6	33	1	18	25	0
7	36	0	19	28	0
8	24	3	20	37	2
9	44	3	21	19	0
10	33	0	22	41	3
11	134	5	23	30	1
12	129	3			
			Total 23	936	37

Solution

1. Lush *etal* Method:

$$\text{T.S.S.} = \sum a_i - \frac{\left(\sum a_i\right)^2}{\sum n_i}$$

$$= 37 - \frac{(37)^2}{936} = 37 - 1.4626 = 35.5374$$

$$\text{Sire S.S.} = \sum \frac{a^2_i}{n_i} - \frac{\sum a_i^2}{\sum n_i}$$

$$= 2.5334 - 1.4626 = 1.0708$$

Error S.S. = TSS – Sire SS = 35.5374 – 1.4626 = 34.4666

Or

$$= \sum a_i - \sum \frac{a^2_i}{n_i} = 37 - 2.5334 = 34.4666$$

ANOVA Table

S.V.	D.F.	S.S.	M.S.
Sire	22	1.0708	0.04867
Error	913	34.4666	0.03775

$\sigma^2_s = (0.04867 - 0.03775)/39.725 = 0.000275$

$\sigma^2_p = \sigma^2_s + \sigma^2_e = 0.038025$

$h^2 = 4t = 4\,\sigma^2_s/\sigma^2_p = 0.0238$

2. Tomar *et al* Method:

    TSS = pqN = 0.0395 x 0.9605 x 936 = 35.5116

    Sire SS = TSS $- \Sigma p_i q_i n_i$ = 35.5116 - 34.466 = 1.045

    Error SS = $\Sigma p_i q_i n_i$ = 34.466

ANOVA Table

S.V.	D.F.	S.S.	M.S.
Sire	22	1.045	0.0475
Error	913	34.666	0.03775

$$\sigma^2_s = \frac{(0.0475 - 0.03775)}{39.725} = 0.0002454$$

$$\sigma^2_p = \sigma^2_s + \sigma^2_e = 0.03799$$

$$h^2 = 4t = 4\frac{\sigma^2_s}{\sigma^2_p} = 0.0258$$

Example 23.2

Tomar (1984) analyzed the data on disease resistance of Murrah buffaloes and recorded the following results on dam – daughter pairs. Estimate the h^2 of disease resistance for various diseases by *regression of daughters on dam* method.

Disease	Susceptible Dams Bore		Resistant Dams Bore		Difference between Two Groups (%) $= b_{OD}$
	Susceptible Daughters	Resistant Daughters	Susceptible Daughters	Resistant Daughters	
Diarrhoea	22	17	46	39	
Tympany	1	10	2	111	
Pneumonia	1	4	8	111	

Contd...

Disease	Susceptible Dams Bore		Resistant Dams Bore		Difference between Two Groups (%) = b_{OD}
	Susceptible Daughters	Resistant Daughters	Susceptible Daughters	Resistant Daughters	
Eye opacity	3	9	10	102	
TDS	3	9	10	97	
FMD	2	23	6	93	
UVD	2	6	20	96	
Udder problems	2	10	14	98	
Per cent female births	38	39	18	19	
Repeat breeding	2	8	11	42	
Anoestrus	10	19	19	31	

Solution

Heritability of Diarrhoea

Per cent daughters susceptible from susceptible dams = $\left[\dfrac{22}{(22+17)}\right](100) = 56.41$

Per cent daughters susceptible from resistant dams = $\left[\dfrac{46}{(46+39)}\right](100) = 54.11$

Difference between daughters from two groups of dams = 56.41 – 54.11 = 2.3

(Regression of daughters on dam, $b_{OD} = h^2$) = $\dfrac{2.3}{100}$ = 0.023

Similarly, the h^2 of other ailments can be estimated by finding the difference.

Example 23.3

The repeatability of various diseases in a herd of Murrah buffaloes based on first *two lactation records* were estimated by Tomar (1984). The following data were recorded, arranged and given below. Estimate the repeatability of various disorders.

Disease	I Lactation	Susceptible		Resistant	
	II Lactation	Susceptible	Resistant	Susceptible	Resistant
Vaginal prolapse		6	7	11	287
ROP		2	21	16	272
Metritis		1	12	17	281
Mastitis		4	15	20	272

Disease	I Lactation	Susceptible		Resistant	
	II Lactation	Susceptible	Resistant	Susceptible	Resistant
Teat block		1	13	11	286
Anoestrus		41	47	46	110
Conceived I service		74	60	92	107
Repeat breeding		9	32	31	150
Abnormal births		2	16	18	275
Male births		67	62	73	52

Solution

Repeatability of vaginal prolapse

Per cent susceptible buffaloes in II lactation out of those susceptible in I lactation

$$= \left[\frac{6}{(6+7)}\right](100) = 46.15$$

Per cent susceptible buffaloes in II lactation out of those resistant in I lactation

$$= \left[\frac{11}{(11+287)}\right](100) = 3.69$$

Repeatability = Difference between two groups of buffaloes

$$= \frac{(46.15 - 3.69)}{100} = 0.4246$$

Example 23.4

Based on 243 calving records of 40 Murrah buffaloes, find out the *repeatability* of sex ratio (per cent male births) *based on multiple records* from the data given below:

Cow No.	Total Births (n)	Male Births (a)	Cow No.	Total Births (n)	Male Births (a)
1	3	3	21	6	4
2	4	2	22	10	6
3	7	1	23	9	8
4	7	1	24	7	5
5	4	2	25	8	4
6	3	1	26	4	3

Contd...

Cow No.	Total Births (n)	Male Births (a)	Cow No.	Total Births (n)	Male Births (a)
7	5	2	27	8	5
8	5	2	28	7	1
9	5	3	29	6	4
10	6	4	30	5	2
11	6	3	31	3	1
12	5	3	32	4	2
13	11	5	33	5	3
14	11	7	34	9	6
15	4	2	35	4	1
16	5	3	36	4	3
17	9	4	37	7	3
18	4	1	38	9	7
19	5	3	39	7	4
20	5	2	40	7	5
			Total	243	131

Solution

$\Sigma a_i = 131$ $\qquad$ $\Sigma n_i = 243$

C.F. $\quad = \dfrac{\sum a_i^{\,2}}{\sum n_i} = \dfrac{(131)^2}{243} = 70.6214$

T.S.S. $\quad = \Sigma a_i - C.F. = 131 - 70.6214 = 60.3786$

Cow S.S. $\quad = \sum \dfrac{a_i}{n_i} - C.F. = 79.8094 - 70.6214 = 9.188$

Error S.S. $\quad = TSS - Cow\ SS = 60.3786 - 9.188 = 51.1906$

ANOVA Table

S.V.	D.F.	S.S.	M.S.
Cows	39	9.1888	0.2356
Error	203	51.1906	0.2522

$$K = \frac{1}{(C-1)}\left[\sum n_i - \left(\frac{\sum n_i^2}{\sum n_i}\right)\right]$$

$$= \frac{1}{39}\left[243 - \frac{1661}{243}\right] = 6.05$$

$$\sigma^2_c = \frac{(0.2356 - 0.2522)}{6.05} = -0.0027$$

$$\text{Repeatability (t)} \quad = \frac{\sigma^2_c}{\sigma^2_c + \sigma^2_e}$$

$$= \frac{-0.0027}{0.2495} = -0.011$$

Example 23.5

Consider the data of example 23.1 for total births and abnormal births of 23 HF sires in NDRI herd. Find out whether the incidence of abnormal births differed significantly among the progenies of different sires.

Solution

The character is threshold and hence χ^2 test can be applied. The informations required to estimate χ^2 are as under:

a_i = Number of abnormal births among the total births of ith sire

b_i = Number of normal births among the total births of ith sire

$n_i = (a_i + b_i)$ = Number of total births of ith sire

$C_1 = \Sigma a_i$ = Total abnormal births in the population = 37

$C_2 = \Sigma b_i$ = Total normal births in the population = 899

$N = C_1 + C_2$ = Total births in the population = 936

$$\sum\left(\frac{a_i^2}{n_i}\right) = 2.5334 \text{ (as calculated in example 23.1)}$$

$$\chi^2 = \frac{N^2}{C_1 C_2}\sum\frac{a_i^2}{n_i} - \frac{C_1^2}{N}$$

$$= \frac{\sum n_i}{\sum a_i \sum b_i}\sum\frac{a_i^2}{n_i} - \frac{\sum a_i^2}{\sum n_i}$$

Where, $\sum \dfrac{a_i^2}{n_i} - \dfrac{\left(\sum a_i\right)^2}{\sum n_i} = $ Corrected sire S.S.

Thus, $\chi^2 = \dfrac{\sum n_i}{\sum a_i \sum b_i}$ (Corrected sire S.S.)

$$= \dfrac{(936)^2}{37 \times 899}\left[2.5334 - \dfrac{(37)^2}{936}\right]$$

$$= \dfrac{8096}{33263}\left(2.5334 - \dfrac{1369}{936}\right)$$

$$= 26.3384\,(2.5334 - 1.4626)$$

$$= 26.3384 \times 1.0708$$

$$= 28.2031$$

Tabulated χ^2 at 22 D.F. ($P_{<0.05}$) = 33.924

Thus, the calculated χ^2 is less than tabulated and hence non-significant. Therefore, the sire effect was not significant on the incidence of abnormal births in the herd.

Example 23.6

Tomar (1984) estimated the association between the occurrence of diarrhea and respiratory ailment in a herd of 688 Murrah buffaloes. The numbers of buffaloes counted under different categories (susceptible to either diarrhea or respiratory ailments and resistant as well as susceptible to both disorders) are as given under. Apply χ^2 test of association between the occurrence of two types of ailments.

		Diarrhoea (1)	
		Susceptible	Resistant
Respiratory ailments (2)	Susceptible	14 (a)	23 (c)
	Resistant	91 (b)	560 (d)

Solution

$$\chi^2 = \dfrac{\left[(ab - bc)^2 N\right]}{R_1 R_2 C_1 C_2}$$

$$= \frac{\left[(14 \times 560 - 91 \times 23)^2 \times 688\right]}{105 \times 583 \times 37 \times 651}$$

$$= \frac{\left[(7840 - 2093)^2 \times 688\right]}{1474485705}$$

$$= \frac{\left[(5747)^2 \times 688\right]}{1474485705}$$

$$= 15.41^{**}$$

The calculated χ^2 value is highly significant. This indicated the association between the occurrence of diarrhea and respiratory disease in this herd.

Example 23.7

Data recorded on the survivability of 138 female calves sired by 6 sires and exposed to cause A and B in a herd of Tharparkar cattle have been given below. Estimate the heritability of mortality due to cause A and cause B, and the *genetic correlation* between two causes of mortality from the following data:

Sire No.	No. of Calves Exposed	No. Died Due to Cause			No. Survived from		
		A	B	Both	A	B	Both
1	25	1	2	3	24	23	22
2	20	0	3	3	20	17	17
3	18	0	4	4	18	14	14
4	23	1	0	1	22	23	22
5	25	2	2	4	23	23	21
6	27	5	3	8	22	24	19
Total	138	9	14	23	129	124	115

Solution

The variances due to two causes separately and the covariance due to both the causes are first estimated as under:

Variance due to cause A:

C.F. $\quad = \dfrac{\left(\sum a_i\right)^2}{\sum n_i} = \dfrac{(129)^2}{138} = 120.5869$

TSS $\quad = \Sigma\, a_i - \text{C.F.} = 129 - \text{C.F.} = 8.413$

$$\text{Sire SS} \quad = \sum\left(\frac{a_i^{\,2}}{n_i}\right) - \text{C.F.} = \frac{(24)^2}{25} + \frac{(20)^2}{20} + \dots + \frac{(23)^2}{25} + \frac{(22)^2}{27} - \text{C.F.}$$

$$= 121.1694 - \text{CF}$$

$$= 0.5825$$

Error SS = TSS – Sire SS

$$= 8.413 - 0.5825 = 7.8305$$

Variance due to cause B

C.F. $\quad = \dfrac{(124)^2}{138} = 111.4202$

TSS $\quad = 124 - \text{CF} = 12.5797$

$$\text{Sire SS} \quad = \frac{(23)^2}{25} + \frac{(17)^2}{20} + \dots + \frac{(23)^2}{25} + \frac{(24)^2}{25} + \frac{(24)^2}{27} - \text{C.F.}$$

$$= 111.9922 - \text{CF}$$

$$= 0.5720$$

Error SS = TSS – Sire SS

$$= 12.5797 - 0.5720 = 12.0077$$

Covariance due to two causes

C.F. $\quad = \dfrac{(129 \times 124)}{138} = 115.9130$

Total SCP $\quad = 115 - \text{CF} = -0.913$

$$\text{Sire CP} \quad = \frac{(24 \times 23)}{25} + \frac{(20 \times 17)}{20} + \dots + \frac{(22 \times 24)}{27} - \text{C.F.}$$

$$= 115.7955 - \text{CF} = -0.1174$$

Error CP = TSCP – Sire CP

$$= -0.9130 - (-0.1174) = -0.7956$$

ANOVA and ANOCOVA Table

S.V.	D.F.	Sum of Square		Mean Square		Cross Product	Mean CP
		A	B	A	B		
Sires	5	0.5825	0.5720	0.1165	0.1144	– 0.1174	– 0.0235
Error	132	7.8305	12.0077	0.0593	0.0909	– 0.7956	– 0.0060

K = 23.0

Heritability due to cause A ($h^2_{(A)}$)

$$\sigma^2_{S(A)} = \frac{(0.1165 - 0.0593)}{23}$$

$$= 0.0024$$

$$\sigma^2_{P(A)} = 0.0024 + 0.0593 = 0.0617$$

$$h^2_{(A)} = \frac{4(0.0024)}{0.0617} = \frac{0.0096}{0.0617} = 0.1556$$

Heritability due to cause B ($h^2_{(B)}$)

$$\sigma^2_{S(B)} = \frac{(0.1144 - 0.0909)}{23}$$

$$= 0.0010$$

$$\sigma^2_{P(B)} = 0.0010 + 0.0909 = 0.0919$$

$$h^2_{(B)} = \frac{4(0.001)}{0.0919} = 0.0440$$

Genetic correlation between two causes

$$Cov_{S(AB)} = \frac{[-0.0235 - (-0.0060)]}{23} = \frac{-0.0175}{23} = -0.00076$$

$$r_{A(AB)} = \frac{Cov_{S(AB)}}{\sqrt{\sigma^2_{S(A)}\sigma^2_{S(B)}}}$$

$$= \frac{-0.00076}{(0.0024 \times 0.001)}$$

$$= \frac{-0.00076}{0.00155}$$

$$= -0.490$$

Exercise 23.8

Estimate the heritability of FMD, udder problems and anoestrus from the data given in Example 23.2

Exercise 23.9

Estimate the repeatability of ROP, mastitis and male births from the data given in Example 23.3

Part III
Biometrical Techniques

Chapter 24
Univariate Analysis

The application of statistical procedures to study the biological problems is called **Biometry** or Biometrics whereas the use of the statistical procedures to deal with the genetics of quantitative characters is known as **Biometrical Genetics** or Quantitative Genetics. The different statistical procedures used in biometrical genetics are known as the biometrical techniques. This chapter has covered in brief the description of some common biometrical techniques for univeriate population and their use in Animal Breeding Programmes.

24.1 Use of Biometrical Methods

An animal breeder or a plant breeder uses the various biometrical techniques in the following ways -

1. Estimation of Mean and Variability

The variability is estimated in three ways:

(i) Simple measures of variability: These include the estimation of range, variance, standard deviation, standard error, coefficient of variation. (See Section 5.5)

(ii) Partitioning of variance into its components : The techniques used are the analysis of variance based on individual observations on groups of relatives, analysis of generation means, diallel, partial diallel, line x tester analysis and biparental matings.

(iii) Estimation of genetic diversity (distance): The genetic distance means the variability among different genotypes (strains, lines, breeds) of a species. The important biometrical technique used for this purpose is the D^2 statistic.

2. Selection of Superior Germplasm

The best germ plasm is selected on the basis of some criteria known as selection criterion which is used to estimate the genetic value (breeding value) of an individual.

The selection criteria may be the phenotypic value of an individual (individual selection) or of its relatives (pedigree, family, and progeny). The choice and use of these selection schemes depends on the availability of data, gene action, genetic variability present in a population, number of traits under selection (single or multi trait selection). These schemes are often used in a single purebred population.

Sometimes, the direct selection (*i.e.* the selection for the trait in which the improvement is required) is either not possible or not effective and hence it is desirable to go for indirect selection on the basis of correlated response based on correlation among characters. This requires the knowledge of the relative contribution of various correlated traits. The biometrical techniques applied to fulfill the objective include the correlation analysis (used to estimate simple, partial and multiple correlation as well as to partition the simple correlation into genetic and environmental correlation), the path coefficient analysis (used to detect direct, indirect and residual effects), and the discriminant function analysis to construct the selection indices.

The selection criteria may be based on the combining ability measured as the average phenotypic value of the offspring produced by crossbreeding the individuals with individuals of another population. The selection procedures for combining ability are the recurrent selection and the reciprocal recurrent selection. The selection of best germ plasm as parents of next generation for hybridization on the basis of combining ability require the diallel cross analysis, partial diallel, line x tester analysis, and the biparental cross analysis (North Carolina Designs I. II and III).

3. Assessment of Suitability of a Genotype over Environments

It is more important in plant breeding to assess the performance of improved varieties for large scale propagation in multi-environments like locations, years or both. The G-E interaction posses the problem in identify the superior variety in different environments. Thus the varietal adaptability to environmental variations is important to stabilize the crop production over regions and years. The adaptability indicates the ability of a genotype to have little variation in its performance over environments. This means that a genotype should have a buffering capacity to environmental variations which is called as the genetic homeostasis (Lerner, 1954.). In literature, the adaptability refers to the variability over the locations while the term stability refers to the variability over years at a location (location specific environments). The farmer is more interested in the stability of the improved varieties at his farm over the years and not concerned in yield response pattern in other locations (adaptability). However, in terms of G-E interactions, the term stability includes both stability and adaptability of genotypes. Therefore, the stability refers the suitability of a genotype over a wide range of environments. The phenotypic stability has been measured by different methods by different workers. The details have been given Singh and Chaudhary (1977) in their book.

24.2 Variable

The variable is the characteristic of a population whose value is represented numerically and takes different values for different individuals of the population. For example, the height of human population is such a character whose value can be represented numerically which is different for different persons. The other examples of variable are age, weight, number of fruits on a tree, number of children in a family, crop yield, milk yield etc. On the other hand, beauty is such a character which can not be represented numerically and therefore it is not a variable but such a character is called attribute.

Types of Variables

There are two types of variables namely, random variable arid non random variable.

(i) Random Variable

It is that variable which takes each of the different values according to the law of predetermined probability. It is also called as variate *e.g.* crop yield, height and weight of any organism. It is of two types

(a) Continuous : This can take any value with in the range, *e.g.* crop yield, number of accidents occur daily, height and weight of army organism, milk yield, age etc.

(b) Discrete variate: This takes only some of the values within the range *e.g.* number of fruits on a plant, number of children in a family, number of accident in a factory etc.

(ii) Non Random Variable

It is that variable whose value is not determined by probabilistic law but is according to some deterministic law *e.g.* salary of an employee which is decided under the pay scale.

Population and Sample

The population is very large including all individuals of a breed or species within a large geographical area. It is thus not possible rather difficult to examine every individual of the population. It is labourious, time consuming and costly to record measurements on every individual of a population. Therefore, small numbers of individuals are recorded (examined) and studied as a measure or indicator of the characteristics of the whole population. This smaller numbers of individuals of the population is called a *sample*. The sample having some individuals from a population is examined and studied to learn the facts in order to make the correct inference about the population. However, each sample is different from another for the reason of variation among biological individuals due to heredity and environment.

Random Sample

It is assumed that the data are a random sample from population. This means that each member of the population has an equal chance of appearing in the sample, without affecting the other members coming in to the sample.

Probability

The probability is the chance of a given variable, say X turning up when a very large number of random selection is made.

24.3 Normal Distribution

The continuous variables are distributed in many ways. The normal distribution is mostly followed by most of the quantitative traits. The other distributions are bimodal, exponential and U shaped distribution.

1. Characteristics of Normal Distribution

When individuals of a population are measured for some quantitative traits and assigned to classes delineated by equal intervals between the mid points of those classes, the resulting distribution shows the frequency of individuals in each class confirming more or less continuous distribution known as normal curve of distribution. This way the distribution of measurements on a quantitative trait can be fitted to a continuous line known as the normal distribution curve. This curve is obtained by taking the phenotypic values (intervals for the numerical measure of the trait) are taken on horizontal axis (X-axis) and the frequency of observations on the Y-axis (vertical axis). The important feature of this curve is that the curve is high in the centre (which represents the higher frequencies for the most common observation) and tapers off (thinning) equally at both the extremes for the rare observation (extreme measurements are relatively rare and intermediate measurements are common). In other words, the measurements are clustered at a mid point thinning out symmetrically towards both ends. This is because there are as many individuals in one class interval above the average of the trait as there are at the corresponding class interval below the average. The phenotypic array for the trait affected by *n* loci with two alleles, which are non interacting have additive gene action and equal frequencies of alleles at each locus show this type of distribution. Thus, *symmetry of curve is an important characteristic feature of the normal distribution curve.* A quantitative trait following this curve is said to be normally distributed. Thus, normal distribution is assumed for quantitative traits.

There is a relationship between the frequency and area occupied in the curve. The more common values representing the mean value occupy a lesser area of the curve than the rare values which appear on both tails of the curve.

The normal distribution is completely determined by two population parameters which are mean (μ) and standard deviation (σ). The mean locates the centre of the distribution while standard deviation is a measure of the spread or variation of the individual measurements. The frequency decreases more rapidly within one σ on either side of the μ and thereafter the decrease is slow and the frequency are negligibly small when the variable X, takes the value $\mu \pm 3\sigma$.

Dividing the normal curve into σ the entire area of the curve can be included within ± 3.5 σ to either side of μ. The relationship between σ and the area of the curve is that 1 σ from μ includes about 68 per cent of the observation (μ ± σ = 68 per cent), 2 σ from μ includes 95 per cent of the population (μ ± 2 σ = 95 per cent) and 3 σ from μ on either side includes 99.7 per cent of the population (μ ± 3 σ = 99.7 per cent). In this way, the values are clustered at a mid point (near the mean value of observations) and thinning out symmetrically toward both extremes. The height of the normal curve at a particular point represents the frequency of individuals with that particular value.

The ordinate or height of the normal curve is $Y = \dfrac{1}{\sigma\sqrt{2\pi}} e^{-\frac{1}{2}}$

The curve $Y = \dfrac{1}{\sigma\sqrt{2\pi}} e^{-\frac{1}{2}}$ is called the normal probability curve with respect to

mean μ and standard deviation σ. This has the following characteristics:-

It is symmetrical about the ordinate $\overline{X} = p$. and extends to infinity on either side. The ordinate decreases rapidly as X increases numerically, the maximum ordinate is

$\dfrac{1}{\sigma\sqrt{2\pi}}$ and occurs at $\overline{X} = \mu$. The ordinate at $\overline{X} = \mu$ divides the area under normal

curve into two equal parts, so the median of the curve is at $\overline{X} = \mu$ and coincides with the mode. That is to say, that in the symmetrical distribution the mean, mode, and median will coincide while in asymmetrical or skewed distribution the mean and median are different. The skewness is either + or – depending upon whether the median lies above or below the mean.

The standard deviation σ has a specific role to determine the shape of the curve. The larger value of σ makes the curve lower at the mean and the curve is more spread which indicates that population is more variable.

The normal distribution with μ = 0 and σ =1 shows that the μ represent the mid point and that the σ represents the variability equal to 1. All the standard tables of normal distribution are for the distribution with μ = 0 and σ =1. There may be different normal curves because the normal curve depends on the μ and σ. In order to use a table of the normal distribution, the rescaling of a measurement X with mean μ and standard deviation σ is required so that the mean becomes 0 and the standard deviation becomes 1. The rescaled measured is taken as

$Z = \dfrac{\left(\overline{x} - \mu\right)}{\sigma}$

The **Z** is called a standard normal deviate or variate.

2. Reasons to Use Normal Distribution

The followings are certain reasons to use the normal distribution:

(i) The distributions of most of the continuous variables are approximately normal. The standard statistical techniques are based on the assumption of normal distribution. Therefore, the normal distribution has been extensively and accurately tabulated which is used as a time saving device to analyze the data.

(*ii*) When the measurements are not distributed normally, it then requires the transformation of measurements to another scale to induce the normality. The square root, arcsin (angular) and logarithmic transformations are used to stabilize the variance.

(*iii*) The distribution may be far from normal but the distribution of sample averages tends to become normal with the increase in sample size.

3. Deviation from Normality and its Tests

The uni-model frequency distribution may deviate from normal shape. There are two types of deviations -

(a) Symmetry of Curve

The main characteristic: The feature of the normal distribution is the symmetry of the curve. In some cases the symmetry is disturbed and the spread of the curve is more towards one side (tail) of the curve, and produces asymmetry in the curve. This is then called as asymmetrical distribution or skewed distribution and the phenomenon is called skewness.

(b) Height or Flatness of the Curve

The flatness of the mode is changed in some cases. This type of departure is called Kurtosis. The kurtosis is used to study the flatness of the mode. It is of three types *viz.*

☆ *leptokurtic* which is produced when there is usually an excess of values near the mean and far from it with a corresponding depletion of the flanks of the curve,

☆ *platykurtic* which make the curve flat (flat topped curve) and

☆ *mesokurtic* which are the normal curves.

Tests of Normality

The standard statistical techniques are based on the assumption of normality. As the normal curves deviate from normality in some cases, it is, therefore, necessary to judge this departure in normal distribution. Three tests are discussed here to test the normal distribution:-

(i) Chi Square – Goodness of Fit Test

To use this test the data is grouped into different classes and a frequency distribution is made, and the sample mean (X) as well as the sample standard deviation (S) are also calculated. With the help of mean and standard deviation, the expected frequencies of each class are obtained using normal tables as:

$$Z_1 = \frac{(X_L - \mu)}{\sigma_X} \quad \text{for lower limit of the class}$$

$$Z_2 = \frac{(X_U - \mu)}{\sigma_X} \quad \text{for upper limit of the class.}$$

Cumulative normal frequency distribution table is used to find the values or area for Z_1 and Z_2. The $Z_1 - Z_2$ will indicate the area. The theoretical frequency or expected frequency in this class is taken as $N (Z_1 - Z_2)$ where N is the total number of observations. The test criteria is

$$\chi^2 = \sum \frac{(O - E)^2}{E}$$

It should follow the theoretical x^2 distribution with (n – 3) degree of freedom where n is the number of classes. If the computed x^2 is smaller than the theoretical value, it then indicates that the observed frequencies agree with the expectation on the assumption of normality but in case of lesser computed x^2 value than the theoretical a departure from normality is indicated.

However, the χ^2 test does not indicate any type of departure from normality and hence χ^2 is a non-specific test. Therefore, some other tests are used to detect the type of departure. These tests are test of skewness and kurtosis.

(ii) Test of Skewness and Kurtosis

To make the test of normality more confirmatory, the tests of skewness and kurtosis are applied. These tests indicate the variability in the shape of uni-model frequency distribution. The skewness tells about the departure from symmetry of a distribution or the degree of peak of a distribution.

The lack of symmetry in the curve indicates the skewness. The measure of the amount of skewness in a population is the average value of $(X - u)^3$ divided by σ^3. An other departure from normality is measured by kurtosis which is the average value $(X - u)^4$ divided by σ^4. The skewness and kurtosis are thus called the third and fourth movement about the mean.

The sample estimates of these coefficients are denoted by $\sqrt{b_1}$ and b_2 respectively. These are calculated as follow (Snedenor and Cochren, 1967).

$$\text{Skewness} = \sqrt{b_1} = \frac{m_3}{m_2\sqrt{m_2}}$$

Kurtosis = $b_2 = \dfrac{m_4}{(m_2)^2} - 3$

Where, $m_2 = h_2 - h_1^2$

$m_3 = h_3 - 3h_1 h_2 + 2h_1^3$

$m_4 = h_4 - 4h_1 h_3 + 6 h_1^2 h_2 - 3h_1^4$

$h_1 = \sum \dfrac{fU}{n}$

$h_2 = \sum \dfrac{fU^2}{n}$

$h_3 = \sum \dfrac{fU^3}{n}$

$h_4 = \sum \dfrac{fU^4}{n}$

n = total number of observations

U = Difference between coded values and assumed mean of coded values.

f = Observed frequency.

The skewness is measured by the third movement about the mean. The third movement will be positive if large value extend fan from the mean and low values tend to close to the mean. This is because the large positive contribution $(X - \overline{X})^3$ when X exceeds $\overline{X}$ will predominate over the small negative contribution $(X - \overline{X})^3$ of X's being less than $\overline{X}$. This will result skewness toward positive values from the $\overline{X}$. The reverse will indicate the negative skewness.

The third movement about the mean is divided by σ^3 to make it independent of the scale on which the measurements were recorded. The sample estimate of skewness coefficient is denoted by $\sqrt{b_1}$.

Skewness is the measure of the shape of curve rather than its size and indicates the asymmetry. The skewness is measured with the objective to estimate the direction and extent to which the curve has deviated from normal curve. The skewness is positive if the curve is more elongated to the right side and it yields the mean greater than mode or median. In the reverse case, the skewness is called negative.

The peaked distribution (Leptokutic) having the value of b_2 greater than 3 shows positive kurtosis while the flat topes distribution (platy kurtic) having the value of b_2 lesser than 3 shows negative kurtosis. The b_2 is normally distributed with mean 0 and

$\sigma = \sqrt{\dfrac{\sigma}{n}}$ in large samples.

It is now clear that the conditions for normal distribution which is symmetrical about the mean and is mesokurtic (with medium height)are:

$\sqrt{b_1} = 0$ and $b_2 = 3$.

It can be proved that all the movements of odd order about the mean vanished for the symmetrical distribution and in particular $U_3 = 0$ and so $b_1 = 0$. When the sample size increases the measures of skewness and kurtosis both go to zero, in the distribution of $\overline{X}$. But the kurtosis is reduced much faster than skewness. The kurtosis has an effect on the distribution of $\$^2$ (sample variance). Or, say that the distribution of s^2 is sensitive to amounts of kurtosis. Any amount of kurtosis increases the sample variance (S^2) than it is in normal distribution.

4. Non-normality and Transformation of Data

The skewness in the distribution tends to give too many significant results in F-test and t-test, besides a loss of efficiency in the analysis. This is because when errors are non-normal, the mean of the observed values for a treatment does not provide most accurate estimate of the corresponding mean for that treatment. The variance is often related to the mean is one feature of non-normal distribution. The variance equals to mean in Poisson distribution and the variance is $p(1-p)/n$ with mean p for a binomial distribution. The measurements are transformed before analysis to induce normality.

(i) Square Root Transformation

This is applied for counts of rare events like number of defects or of accidental events. Such events show poisson distribution. The transformed value is taken as $\sqrt{X}$ on the transformed scale instead of X on the original scale to stabilize the variance effectively. When variance of x (σ^2) is proportional to its mean $\left(\overline{X}\right)$ *i.e.* $\sigma^2 = K\overline{X}$ the squre root transformation is used. This is mostly observed with counts, when the numbers or counts are large in some cases but low in others like the effects of treatments on the numbers of plants or tillers in crop experiments with the result of wide range leading to heterogeneous variance. Analysis of data on original scale yields the error mean square to be too large for testing differences among certain treatments but too small for other treatments.

The K value is used to test the poisson distribution. If K is near 1, it indicates the poisson distribution. The K is estimated from error variance from the analysis in the square root scale as: $K = 4(\sigma^2_e)$.

(ii) Logarithmic Transformation

This scale is used when the standard deviation on the original scale varies directly with mean or to put it in other words when the coefficient of variation is constant. This type of relation between mean and standard deviation is produced when the effects are proportional instead of being additive, *e.g.* when an effect is giving consistently higher or lower results compared to another effect. The log transformation of data stabilizes the variance (equality of variance) and the effects additive. When the data is highly variable, the log transformation has been found effective.

(iii) Arcsin or Angular Transformation

This type of transformation is used for binomial proportions, when the percent values range beyond 30 to 70. The percent values are transformed into angles = Arcsin $\sqrt{p}$, where p = proportion. For example a $_{ij}$ is the percentage of calves died or survived which were born in ith year of jth season and n is the total number of calves,

then $p = \dfrac{a_{ij}}{n}$. It has variance $p_{ij} = \dfrac{(1 - p_{ij})}{n}$. When the proportions are near 0 or 1, these

are spread out in the angular scale and it increases their variance. However, if n vary widely, the inequalities in variance is not removed by the transformation.

In order to improve the equality of variance in angles, Bartlett (1947) suggested that with n < 50, the zero proportion should be taken as ¼ n before transforming into

angles and 1 (or 100 per cent proportion) as $\dfrac{\left(n - \frac{1}{4}\right)}{n}$.

5. Genetic Interpretation of Normal Curve

The normal distribution curve of the values of quantitative trait indicates that the appearance of such characters is not determined by major gene effects but by polygenes or minor genes with small quantitative effects. Secondly, this type of distribution also indicates that the gene action is additive and independent of each other and no interaction among loci. In a perfectly symmetrical distribution, the mean, mode, and median coincide. The frequencies of particular classes are related to the number of polygenes carried. The class with the intermediate phenotype carrying the intermediate number of polygenes is with the highest frequency and the other classes are symmetrically distributed in frequency around the mean value depending upon the number of polygenes carried by them.

6. Genetic Causes of Skewness

Frequency curves for the distribution of quantitative measurements do not always follow the normal symmetrical curve. The curve become asymmetric or skewed at either tail due to greater frequency of phenotypes at that end of the curve compared at the other end. One of the reasons may be less number of observations, small sample size, which result chance fluctuations in some classes. There are certain genetic causes of skewness in the curve which are discussed below:-

(i) Non-Additive Effects of Genes

The interaction effect of genes *e.g.* dominance between alleles is one type of the effect that cause skewness. The effect of dominance on the shape of the curve further depends upon the number of gene pairs affecting a trait. The segregation of one gene pair produces F_2 distribution with a ratio of 3:1. More number of gene pairs affecting a trait makes the distribution curve less skewed and it is difficult to distinguish the type of gene action, (dominance and additive) as the numbers of gene pairs are 10 or more. The distribution is continuous and normal due to the effects of additive genes and environmental effects but skewed towards the dominant parents.

(ii) Multiplicative Gene Action

The presence of certain genes which have multiplicative effects cause the distribution of phenotypes to depart considerably than expectation of their additive effects. The additive genes only increase the value of a trait by a constant arithmetic amount and show no greater variability when their number is high or low. The presence of genes with multiplicative effects when their number is high has a much greater phenotypic effect than when their number is low. The multiplicative gene action produces a geometric series of phenotypic values like 2, 4, 8, 16. for the contribution of 1,2,3,4 active alleles respectively producing skewness in curve while the additive gene action forms an arithmetic series like 2, 4, 6, 8 for the contribution of 1, 2, 3, 4 active alleles respectively giving a normal phenotypic distribution with F_1 mean intermediate of parental populations. The evidence of the multiplicative gene action is indicated:

(a) If a skewed distribution becomes normal distribution by changing the scale to logarithmic. The geometric series 1, 10, 100, and 1000 with a multiplicative increment of 10 on being converting to logarithms becomes an arithmetic series of 0, 1, 2, 3 with an additive increment of one unit. That is to say that the effect of multiplicative gene may be eliminated by changing the scale of measurement which converts observed measurements into units which are multiples of arithmetic numbers. This will lead to the effect of each multiplicative gene to appear to be additive and will provide a normal distribution similar to that of genes whose effects are additive and measured on arithmetic scale. Logarithms, which are the exponents of a particular base number, are useful for this purpose.

(b) When the variation is proportional to the mean. That is to say the variance is dependent upon the mean so that as the mean increases the variance is increased proportionately. The co-efficient of variation thereby remains constant in segregating population. On the other hand, in a normally distributed population the mean and variance are independent and thus the extent of increase in variance cannot be predicted if the population mean is increased.

(c) When the variability differs between strains that have high and low mean values, the multiplicative gene action is assumed to be an alternative. For example, the two strains differ in their mean plant height being 40 inches and 10 inches respectively. The absence of multiplicative allele of a gene produce the height of 40 inches but the presence of multiplicative allele that double the height will produce the plants of 80 inches in height. In other stock of 10 inches height, the presence or absence will only produce a difference of only 10 inches, against a difference of 40 inches in the first strain. Further, suppose each gene increasing the value of a trait may act by doubling the value of the trait and by adding two such genes would quadruple the value. Thus if an inbred strain has a large number of multiplicative alleles, the variability of the strain will be much higher than the same strain having few such alleles.

(iii) Bimodal Distribution

The segregation of a single major gene affecting a quantitative trait produces bimodality in the curve. A bimodal curve consists of two separate overlapping populations which are considered as one group showing continuous variation. Hutt (1959) reported the effect of dwarf gene with major effect in fowl affecting body size which is a metric trait. The dwarf gene, *dw*, is a sex linked gene which is completely recessive and reduces the adults size in homozygous females by 26 to 32 per cent and in homozygous males by about 43 per cent. All female progeny of one sire showed biomodal distribution for adult body size. The distribution within each of the two groups showed continuous variation from smallest to largest. When the *dw* gene is not present the size of body conforms in crosses to expectation. A similar dwarfing caused by deficiency in pituitaryhormone is known in the mouse but those affected are sterite.

Bimodal distribution of human height (men and women) is expected, the men and women differ in their mean height but the two groups will overlap to make one bimodal distribution. A bimodal distribution indicates the effect of genes with major effect on metric traits. A similar bimodal distribution is formed for the concentration of potassium in the blood *viz.* one group is having high potassium (HK group) and the other as low potassium (LK group).

(iv) Transgressive Inheritance

Sometimes in the F_2 generation a few exceptional individuals are observed which exceed the range of variation of both parental types. For example, following crosses between parents that differ in size, some of the descendants will be even small than the smaller parent or larger than the larger parent. This is called the transgressive inheritance when it is not caused by the environmental influences. A small animal could contribute to a cross genes for size different from those of its larger mate and from this cross some of the individuals in second generation will be larger than the larger parent. This can be made clear citing an example of colours of kernels in wheat. In addition to A-a and B-b inducing red colour, there is a third gene pair C-c with similar effect. The cross between dark red and light red wheat will produce some individuals more dark than the dark red parent.

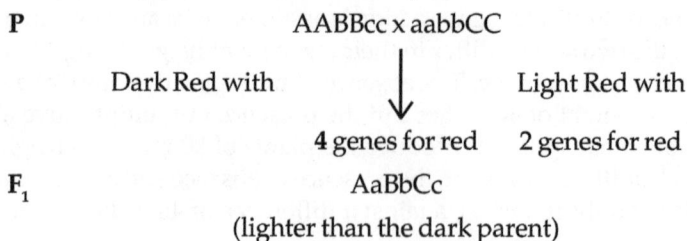

P   AABBcc x aabbCC

   Dark Red with   ↓   Light Red with

                              4 genes for red   2 genes for red

F_1 AaBbCc

                          (lighter than the dark parent)

F_2 There will be 27 different genotypes – including AABBCC and AABBCc genotypes which will have darker colour than the dark red parent due to more number of genes (5 or 6) for red.

A similar example of the behaviour of a metric character in crosses between parents of different types was cited by Punnett (1923). Sun bright hens weigh about 600 gm while males 750 gm but the Hamburg hens are about 500 gm heavier (1100 gm) than Senbright hens while cocks are about 1350 gm in weight. Progeny of this cross were intermediate in weight between the two parents but closer to the larger one. Among F_2 males a wide range in size was noted with several individuals larger than Hamburg male and some ones smaller than the Senbright.

The various environmental factors also cause skewness. Sickness, low nutrition and low management factors affecting some of the individuals of a population force this portion of the population to take extreme values. For example, the curve for slaughter weight may be skewed if certain animals remain sick or have slow growth due to some reason.

24.4 Concept of Model

A number of genetic and environmental factors are responsible for creating and maintaining the variability in economic characters. It is virtually difficult or rather impossible to consider at a time all the factors of variability. Therefore, attention is focused on the most relevant and important aspects, excluding those factors which seems to be of little concern, to simplify the more complicated situation. The simplification of complex situation is known as the model. The concept of model can he understood by considering that a person tries many possibilities before reaching any conclusion about any fact or partial truth. He makes mental images in an effort to generalize his experience or observations. The observations are related to mental images to achieve the organized observation. The use of mental images is important in abstraction of observations and no observation can be abstracted without the use of mental images. *The designing of mental image to simplify the complex real situation to meet the objective of abstracting some important aspect is called the model building or model.*

A model can not reflect all the aspects of the true situation because all the complexities of the true situation cannot be taken into the model and hence it is always unsatisfactory in some respects. Mathematically, a model becomes unmanageable in a try to make the model more close to the nature (true situation). A complex model lost its modality. It is not a model if made as complex as the true situation. A model assumes a set of hypothesis that specifies the mathematical relations between the measurable quantities (parameters) in a process or system. An ideal model includes all the essential aspects of the system and excludes the unimportant ones. The usefulness of the model depends on the close approximation of ideal situation. Inclusion of every aspect of the system makes the model complex and hence some aspects of the actual system are intentionally excluded from the model. Therefore, a compromise is made between reality and manageability in constructing a model because mathematical handling of the complete real model become complex. However, a model should not be such simple that it becomes unrealistic and useless. Thus, a model is valid within certain limits beyond which it becomes misleading. A model is however, simpler than the real situation. In testing the validity of a model it is determined whether the hypotheses in formulating a model and the results of the model are consistent with observations.

The mathematical models are of great use:

(_i_) The hypothesized mathematical relationship between parameters arc concisely expressed.

(_ii_) The most important parameters in a system are revealed and critical experiments or observations are therefore, suggested.

(_iii_) Guidelines are obtained in collection, organization and interpretation of observed data.

(_iv_) The quantitative predictions can be made with confirmation or proved as false about the behaviour of a system.

Models of Population Genetics

Theoretical population genetics is concerned with models that are mathematical in nature. The population genetics, like any other science, is a set of organized observations and not merely the collection of observations and facts. The subject matter of population genetics lies not in catalogues of the changes known to have occurred in the genetic composition of population but it covers the generalization in an abstract form regarding the likely genetic composition at a given time in future. The generalization can be based on probability statements with reference to the existing situation at a given locus (loci) in relation to distribution pattern of expectations or describing the events which may encounter the locus over a long period of time. Thus abstraction or abstract generalization is important in the study of population genetics rather than simple description of actual events.

The genetic variation is organized into genotypes. The mating system (assortative), though does not change the allele frequencies, determines the organization of genes into genotypes. The assortative mating system that occurs in a population has its effect on the relative frequencies of genotypes. The genotype frequencies are also affected by small population size, and by the evolutionàry forces (mutation, migration, and selection). Therefore, in population genetics, the effects of all these factors on the relative frequencies of genotypes are essential to study. All these factors interact in such a complex way that it is not easy to study their combined effects at a time. Therefore, some simplification is made by taking only one factor at a time or to include only the important factors and neglecting others. Therefore, an attempt is made to simplify the complex situation of the effects of all the factors to focus attention on the essential aspects of the situation by eliminating extraneous details.

The population geneticist is concerned with the overall effects of births, deaths, choice of mates. The total population may be increasing, or decreasing or may remain constant and the different genotypes may differ in intrinsic birth rates and death rats, depending on their response to the environment. This leads the interest with changes in proportion of different types rather than in total numbers.

The mathematical models of population growth and structure can be divided as deterministic model and stochastic model. *For deterministic model* the population is assumed to be large enough (infinite population) with constant birth and death rates leaving no scope of random fluctuations. The *stochastic model* is used to take account of the effects of the finite population and other random effects.

24.5 Statistical Inference

A population is called *univariate population* on which the information (data) for one trait is considered for study whereas the population having the data on two traits under study is known as the *bivariate population* and likewise is known as the *multivariate population* which has the data under study for three or more traits.

The phenotypic values for a quantitative trait show continuous distribution for which it is unmanageable and difficult to describe a population with respect to a metric trait. This needs the use of some statistical methods to summarize the whole data on any metric trait. The statistics deals with techniques of collecting, analyzing and drawing conclusions (inferences) from data.

An investigator faces twin problems of taking the correct sample which may truly represent the population and of making correct inference. The inference means to make quantitative statements about any character of a population from the results obtained on a sample. The statistical inference is based on two parts of statistical analysis of data *viz.* estimation and testing of hypotheses.

24.5.1 Estimation Theory

In a series of papers around 1930, R.A. Fisher founded the theory of estimation which is divided in two parts *viz.* Point estimation and interval estimation.

A single numerical value (statistic) is obtained as an estimate of the population parameter and called as point estimation. The interval estimation specifies the probable range (of an estimate) within which the true value of the population parameter is expected to lie.

(i) Point Estimation

Estimator and Estimate: The estimation is concerned with the method of assessing the magnitude of an estimate of the sample. The *estimate* or point estimate is a numerical value of character (s) obtained after making some calculations. The rule of calculation (computation) is called *estimator*. For example, in obtaining the arithmetic mean certain calculations have to be done. The procedure of calculation of arithmetic average (to obtain the estimate) is the estimator and the mean value (numerical value) of arithmetic average of data is the estimate. Thus, the procedure used for estimation of arithmetic mean, geometric mean, mode, median, harmonic mean, weighted average are the estimator and the numerical value obtained by calculating them is the estimate. Therefore, the rule(s) of calculating the estimate is known as estimator whereas the estimate is the numerical value obtained with the help of an estimator. The estimate is a constant value, has no distribution and thus static. An estimate is obtained by a number of methods and these methods are called estimator. The estimator is a procedure of preparing a function of a variable.

The numerical value obtained from an estimator in a population is called the parameter but when obtained on a sample it is called an estimate.

The examples of population parameters are as under and can be divided in two groups:

(a) *Phenotypic Parameters*: Mean, variance, standard deviation, standard error, correlation, regression etc.

(b) *Genetic Parameters*: Gene frequency, no of alleles at a locus, no of loci affecting a trait, additive and non additive gene action and the variance caused by them in terms of heritability and repeatability, heterosis and inbreeding depression, genetic correlation, inbreeding coefficient, coefficient of relationship, genetic gain, penetrance of a trait, recombination fraction in linkage studies, etc.

The various measures of central tendency are also called as the *first degree statistics* where as the various measures of dispersion are called the *second degree statistics* and all these are estimated for any character under study to characterize the population.

Properties of Good Estimator

A good and satisfactory estimator has the following criteria or properties

1. *Consistency* (Sample Size): With the increase in sample size the estimated value (estimate) obtained from an estimator (rule of calculation) approaches the parameteric value more and more closely. Such as estimator is said to be consistent,

2. *Unbiased* (Repeated Samples): An estimator whose expectation in repeated samples of the same size equals the parametric value is said to be unbiased. The estimator (Q of Q) is said to be unbiased if Q = Q which means that the mean value of the sampling distribution of the statistic is equal to the parameter *e.g.* the sample mean X is an unbiased estimate of the population mean (μ) and the sample proportion p is an unbiased estimate of the population proportion p.

3. *Efficiency* (Low Variability): The estimator with low variability is efficient. The efficiency of Q is inversely proportional to its variance. The efficiency of two estimators is compared as the ratio for their sampling variance and the efficiency of army estimator should not exceed unity. An unbiased estimator with the least variance is said to be the best unbiased estimator.

4. *Sufficiency* (All Information): This is a remarkable property possessed by some estimators. A sufficient estimator utilizes all the information that a given sample can furnish about the parameter and it contained as well as extracts all the information in the sample about the parameter. A sufficient estimator is also the most efficiency estimator, is always consistent but it may or way not be unbiased. If there exists a sufficient estimator for a parameter, it is a minimum variance unbiased estimator (M.V. U.E). The arithmetic mean is a sufficient estimator for population mean μ in the normal distribution. The median provides no more information on μ if the arithmetic

mean of a sample is available. On the contrary, if the median is estimated first, the estimation of arithmetic mean is still worth while or valuable.

Methods of Point Estimation

The estimation is concerned with the methods of assessing the magnitude of the important parameters characterizing the population. The commonly used methods to obtain the point estimates are:

Least squares method, maximum likelihood method.

The other methods are:

Method of moments; method of minimum variance; method of minimum chi-square; and method of inverse Probability theory.

(ii) Interval Estimation

An estimate obtained from a sample is likely to be subjected to an error particularly when the sample size is small. Thus an estimate is likely to differ from population parameter. Therefore, it is essential to determine with reasonable degree of confidence the range of values within which the parameter may lie. The limits of this range are called *confidence limits* (Neyman) or feducial limits (R.A. Fisher) and the range between these limits as *confidence interval* whereas the associated probability is called confidence coefficient.

The interval estimate is a statement that the parameter has a value between two specific limits. For example, instead of saying that there are 33 per cent sheep having black wool, it may be said that sheep population has black wool between 24 to 42 per cent. The limits are obtained on the basis of the standered error of the estimate which is the reliability of the estimate. The probability that the parameter has exactly the value as the estimate is extremely low. A confidence interval is one type of interval estimate. It has a feature that in repeated sampling a known proportion of the interval (say 66, 95 per cent) includes the parameter.

The true mean must lie with confidence limits so that the difference between sample mean X and population mean μ is not significantly different at a given probability level. The upper and lower limits of mean are:

$$\overline{X} \pm t_{0.05}\left(\frac{s}{\sqrt{n}}\right)$$

or $\quad \overline{X} \pm 1.96\left(\dfrac{s}{\sqrt{n}}\right)$

or $\quad \overline{X} \pm 1.96$ (S.E. of mean)

Where, $s = \sigma$

The 95 per cent confidence internal for µ is wider for small n and decreases to

$\overline{X} \pm 1.96 \left(\dfrac{s}{\sqrt{n}} \right)$ as n is increased. The 99 per cent confidence limits for µ are

$\overline{X} \pm 2.58 \left(\dfrac{s}{\sqrt{n}} \right)$. The true mean must lie within theses limits in 95 or 99 per cent of the

cases.

24.5.2 Hypothesis Testing

The Hypothesis is a statement or assumption about a population parameter. A sample estimate is found to be different from population parameter for the reason of fluctuations in sampling etc. The branch of statistics which help in taking a decision about the validity of hypothesis is known as the hypothesis testing. The theory of hypothesis testing was initiated by J. Neyman and E.S. Pearson.

Fundamentals of hypothesis testing are:

Types of hypothesis, Test of significance, Errors in hypothesis testing,

Level of significance, Critical region, and Degrees of freedom, etc.

(i) Types of Hypothesis

Null hypothesis: When it is assumed (hypothesized) that the sample result (estimate) does not differ from population parameter it is called as the hypothesis of no difference or the null hypothesis coined by R.A. Fisher. Thus, the neutral or null attitude is adopted about the sample result (estimate). Therefore, the basis of null hypothesis is the no difference. The null hypothesis is denoted by the letter H_0 which indicates that the difference between estimate and parameter or the difference between two sample estimates is not significant but the difference is just by chance. In order to test any statement about the population, it is necessary to set up the null hypothesis that it is true. For example, if it is of interest to find whether the population mean (µ) has specified value (μ_0), then proceed to set up null hypothesis H_0: $\mu = \mu_0$

Alternative hypothesis: It is complementary to null hypothesis denoted by H_A or H_I. The H_A could be as:

H_A: $\mu \neq \mu$

The *null hypothesis* is usually simple consists only a single parameter while the alternative hypothesis is usually composite. The hypothesis which completely specifies the population is called *simple hypothesis* otherwise it is called the *composite hypothesis*. The hypothesis H: $\mu = \mu_0$ and $\sigma^2 = \sigma^2_0$ is a simple hypothesis for a normal population N (μ, σ^2) because it completely specifies the distribution.

On the contrary, the *composite hypothesis* are:

$\mu = \mu_0$ (σ^2 is not known)

$\sigma^2 = \sigma^2_0$ (μ is not specified)

$\mu < \mu_0, \sigma^2 = \sigma^2_0$ and $\mu > \mu_0, \sigma^2 = \sigma^2_0$

$\mu = \mu_0, \sigma^2 > \sigma^2_0$ and so on.

(ii) Test of Significance – Test of Null Hypothesis

The null hypothesis is tested through sample results. The testing of null hypothesis involves a procedure to know the significance of difference between estimates of two samples or of the difference between estimate and parameter. This is called the test of significance. Thus a test of significance is a calculation by which the sample results are used to throw light on the truth or falsity of a null hypothesis In other words, the statistical procedure to decide whether H_0 should be rejected or accepted is called the test of significance.

A quantity called a **test criteria** is computed which measures the extent to which the sample departs from null hypothesis. The different test criteria are:

χ^2 test – used for qualitative traits

F and t test – used for quantitative traits

The sample size affects the test of significance. Based on small sample the null hypothesis is rejected where there is really large difference between sample estimate and population parameter or between two independent estimates. With a large sample, small difference from null hypothesis may be significant.

(iii) Errors in Hypothesis Testing

A decision is taken to accept or reject a null hypothesis (H_0). This involves a risk to take the wrong decision as there are four possible decisions which can be shown as:

		For the Population	
		H_0 *is True* *(Accepted)*	H_0 *is not True* *(Rejected)*
On the Basis of sample	Reject H_0	Wrong decision Error I = α	Correct decision
	Accept H_0	Correct decision	Wrong decision Error II = β

Thus, in taking one of the four possible decisions one may take two wrong decisions and hence may commit two types of errors. The sample result rejects the null hypothesis when it is true for the population and hence an error is committed. This is called type I error denoted by α. Secondly, the sample result accept H_0 when it is false for population and this is type II error denoted by β. Thus

Type I error = Probability of rejecting H_0 when it is true

$\qquad\qquad$ = Rejecting the correct result

$\qquad\qquad$ = α = Level of significance

Type II error   = Probability of accepting H_0 when it is false

                         = Accepting the wrong result

                         = β

Therefore, the probability of rejecting H_0 when it is true is the probability of error of first kind represented by α which is also called *"level of significance"*. The level of significance is the maximum size of the type I error which is put to risk. In simple words, the level of probability which is considered small for rejecting the H_0 is called the *level of significance* and this is to be necessarily fixed arbitrarily. To accept or reject the null hypothesis the most commonly used levels of significance are 5 per cent (0.05) and 1 per cent (0.01). In case 5 per cent level is used it implies that in 5 out of 100 samples, a correct H_0 is rejected and hence the decision to reject H_0 is correct to the extent of 95 per cent confidence. In rejecting a null hypothesis there is certain confidence in taking the decision which depends on the level of significance used. Therefore, the degree of confidence at 'α' level of significance in taking the decision is $1 - \alpha$ which is also called as the confidence coefficient. The H_0 is rejected when the probability of test criteria having a value as extreme as or more extreme than that observed (calculated) value is less than the level of significance (α). It is therefore possible that H_0 is rejected by test criteria when H_0 is true. This is the error of first kind and the probability of committing error is less than or equal to α, level of significance. Thus this first kind of error may be controlled by choosing the level of significance.

Secondly, it is equally possible that when H_0 is not true (but false), the test of significance does not reject H (but accept). This is the error of second type. The type II error is more serious because it is more risky to accept a wrong hypothesis than to reject a correct hypothesis.

It is ideal to reduce both types of error but it is not possible because an attempt to decrease α will lead to an increase in β or vice versa. However, if the sample size is large there are chances to reduce both α and β. Therefore, it is better to minimize more serious error after fixing the less serious one. Thus α (size of type I error) is fixed and try to obtain a criterion which minimize β (the size of type II error).

There are two parts of accepting H_0 on the basis of sample result *viz.* accepting H_0 when H_0 is true (correct decision) or false (wrong decision). Thus

Prob (accepting H_0 when it is true + accepting H_0 when it is wrong) =1

or correct decision + wrong decision = 1

Now, Prob (accepting H_0 when it is true) = $1 - \beta$

                                         = Correct decision

                                         = $1 -$ Probability to accept H_0 when it is wrong.

Therefore, the H_0 should be accepted when H_0 is true and so reducing β will increase the $1 - \beta$ which is called as the *power of test*. The whole procedure is thus to fix α and minimize β or maximize the power of test $(1 - \beta)$. Minimizing β increases power of test.

Power of test $(1-\beta)$ = Prob (rejecting H_0 when H_0 is true)

= Prob (accepting H_0 when H_0 is true)

The test which gives maximum power at a given α and given sample size is called most powerful test. The statistical test is a procedure by which it is decided either to accept or reject a given statistical hypothesis.

(iv) Critical or Rejection Region

When a number of samples of equal size are drawn from a population and compute some of the statistics for all the samples and the values of these statistics are used to test null hypotheses, it will then be observed that some values may lead to the rejection of H_0 whereas others will lead to accept H_0. Thus these values may be divided into two groups and the values which lead to rejection of H_0 are covered in a region called critical or rejection region while rest comes under acceptance region.

(v) Degrees of Freedom

This concept is of great importance. The degree of freedom is defined as the number of items or no. of cell frequencies whose values can be determined at will. The number of degree of freedom depends on the number of restrictions or constraints imposed.

24.6 Measures of Central Tendency

The central tendency of the given statistical data is represented by an average value, as some of the values are above the average while others are below or near the average. An ideal average has the following characteristics -

    (i) It should be well defined, based on all observations, easily obtained, and easily understandable.

    (ii) Its value should not fluctuate based on different samples.

    (iii) It should be explained in algebraic terms.

The arithmetic mean, median, mode, geometric mean, harmonic mean and weighted average are the measures of average.

1. Mean or Arithmetic Average

The population mean which is simply the arithmetic average of all the values is represented by the Greece letter μ. The sample mean is represented by $\overline{X}$, whereas the individual measurements in the sample are symbolized by X_1, X_2, X_3 X_n. The sample mean is simply the sum of all measurements divided by the number of measurements.

2. Geometric Mean

This is n^{th} root of the product of n values. Thus taking $X_1, X_2 X$ as the values of variates, the geometric mean (G) is taken as

$$G_x = (X_1 X_2 X_3 \ldots\ldots Xn)^{1/n}$$

The Gx is the antilog of the arithmetic mean (X) of the logarithms of the values. The geometric mean is used with the average rate of change or ratios, a quantity whose changes are directly proportional to the quantity itself like change in human population where the changes in the population is proportional to the population itself. The population increases in geometric nature. It is used for the data which are not symmetrically distributed.

3. Harmonic Mean

It is defined as the reciprocals of the mean of reciprocals of the values of the variate and symbolized by H_x. Thus, $\overline{H}_x = \dfrac{n}{\sum R_i}$

    where,   n = number of observations,

                   R_i = reciprocal of ith value

It is used in averaging the time rates and price data like if the price is given in terms of quantities *i.e.* 3 kg per rupee, instead of rupees 3 per kg which is in terms of money. Harmonic mean is computed when price is given in terms of quantities. This can he illustrated with an example. A man walks 4 miles in first hour and 3 miles in second hour. The average speed of the man will be $\dfrac{(4+3)}{2} = 3.5$ miles per hour in terms of arithmetic mean but it will be = $\dfrac{2}{\left(\frac{1}{4}+\frac{1}{3}\right)} = 3.43$ miles as harmonic mean.

4. Weighted Average

It is computed under certain special conditions when all the items are not of equal importance. The examples to estimate the weightage average are yield of a crop in two fields which vary in size, milk yield of a herd having two or more breeds with varying number, average salary of staff of different cadres etc.

5. Median

This is the middle value when all the measurements are arranged in ascending order. Median is useful when the extreme classes are not well defined like "less than" or "more than".

6. Mode

The mode is taken as the value of the class with highest frequency. The mode is more useful in industrial data *i.e.* the quality (size etc.) of the commodity with greatest market demand *e.g.* model size of shoe, ready made garments etc.

Relation between different Averages

In the symmetrical distribution, the mean, mode and median coincide, while in the skewed distribution the mean and median are different; skewness is either positive or negative according to whether the median is above or below the mean and the relationship is:

mean – mode = 3 (mean – median)

or median = 1/3 (mode + 2 mean)

Secondly, $\overline{X} > G_x > H_x$

Uses of Mean

(i) This is used to describe the sample or the population.

(ii) Use to compare the different samples or populations *viz.* herd/lines/breeds etc.

(iii) All the values are expressed as deviation from mean.

(iv) Used to calculate the variance and covariance.

(v) Used to indicate the center of the distribution of normally distributed variable.

24.7 Measures of Dispersion (Variability)

The measures of central tendency give no idea about any population whether all observations are fairly similar or variable. Any two population of equal size may have similar mean but be radically different. The mean value of a population for a quantitative trait is the average of all the observations on different individuals whose phenotypic value differ from the population mean. Thus, the individual observations vary about the mean. The measure of variability among individuals of a population is required to know the variability among the individuals of a population and to test the means of two or more populations.

The following statistics or parameters are used to estimate the degree of dispersion (variation) exhibited by a set of measurements -

Range, mean deviation, variance including standard deviation and standard error, and coefficient of variation.

1. Range

The range is the simplest measure estimated by tracing the two extreme values of observations of a sample or population (largest minus smallest observation). The range is affected by fluctuations of sampling and not related to any type of frequency distribution. The range provides some indication of variability, though it is a rough estimate. It is because the range does not give any idea whether the extremes or other middle classes away from the mean contain one or several observations.

2. Mean Deviation

The simplest measure of spread is the mean deviation which is the arithmetic mean of the deviations of all the observations from the mean ignoring signs.

3. Variance

The variation of the individual observation about the mean can be quantified in another way by overcoming the difficulty of sign by making squares of all the deviations from the mean before summing and then dividing by N. The quantified value is termed the variance. The variance is a measure of the amount of variation in a population.

The variance is defined as the mean of the squares of all the individual values expressed as deviation from their arithmetic mean. The sample variance is denoted as s^2 and the population variance as σ^2. The variance is computed by taking the deviation of each observation from the mean, squaring these deviations, taking their sum and dividing this total by the degree of freedom (one less than the. total number of observation (N-1).

The variance is always a positive quantity as the square value can not be negative. The magnitudes of observations affect the variance. An observation with more extreme value will contribute proportionately more than an observation having value close to mean. This is because in computing the variance, the deviations are squared.

To handle large number of measurements, it will be time consuming, labourious and erroneous to compute the variance by taking the deviation of each value from the mean and also to work out the mean.

Properties of Variance

The variance is described in square units. This makes it a more useful statistics than others. It is because of two main reasons: The variance has the property of additivity and subdivisibility which are not applicable with standard deviation.

(i) Additivity of Variance

The Variance is additive in the sense that the variance of two independent (uncorrelated) quantities or distributions is the sum of the variances of both when each value in one distribution is summed in all possible ways with each value in the other distribution.

Further, this additivity is not affected by either the addition of the means of the two distributions or the substraction of one from the other. This is because that both positive and negative deviation from the mean produce the variance, and they are only inter changed but not altered when the means are substracted.

(ii) Partitioning of Variance

The second property of variance is that it can be subdivided/separated/partitioned into its various components by a special analysis by which the proportion of variation in a population due to different causes (which may be genetic and environment) can be determined. The partition of variance is done, by the technique known as analysis of variance, in order to know the effect of different factors to cause variation in the variable and to estimate the per cent contribution of different causes to the total variance.

The reliability of estimate depends upon the sample drawn. When the sample is not drawn properly, there is a difference between the value expected from such a faulty sample and the population parameter. This is called the bias. Such estimates are called biased estimates and the samples which yield biased estimates are called biased samples. Thus the population parameters are subject to bias or error. The bias or error is of two types based on the sample drawn. If the sample size is small (data is not sufficient for proper estimation) this causes one type of error. The small samples cause the chance deviation or chance error. This can be corrected by increasing the sample size. Secondly, the sample drawn may not be true representative of the population. This type of error arises when the feeding and management practices differ at different farms raising the daughters of the same sires. This results in the deviation of daughter's average by the amount caused by these environmental differences inspite of the fact that the sample size is large.

Uses of Variance

(i) Use to compare the variability of different traits as well as to compare the variability of different values (P, A, etc.) for a trait.

(ii) Use to calculate the genetic parameters by its partitioning.

4. Standard Deviation

The standard deviation is a measure of the average deviation of observations from the mean. Thus it measures the variation about the mean and is computed as the square root of the variance. The standard deviation is more commonly used than variance. The unit of standard deviation is same as of the mean. The population standard deviation is denoted as σ and of the sample as S.

However, by taking the square root of the variance, the additivity property of the variance is lost which means that standard deviations are not additives.

Uses of Standard Deviation

(i) Similar to that of the variance.

(ii) Easy to conceptualize than variance for the reason of being measured in the units of the traits.

(iii) Use to correlate the distribution of observations. The standard deviation along with mean is used to describe the variation in a trait of any population. There is a consistent relationship between the mean and standard deviation for a normal distribution in a way that about 2/3 of the observations fall between one standard deviation on either side of the mean, 95 per cent between two standard deviation, and 99 per cent within 3 standard deviation. Thus, the mean ± two standard deviations include 95 per cent of the individuals in a population and only about 5 per cent of the individuals fall outside this range. The deviation is practically useful along with the mean in order to compare different samples or populations for any trait.

5. Coefficient of Variation

It is another way to express the amount of variability present in a trait. The coefficient of variation (C.V.) is the ratio of the standard deviation of the mean. Thus $C.V. = \frac{\sigma}{\overline{X}}$. The coefficient of variation (C.V.) expresses the standard deviation as a percentage of the arithmetic mean and computed as:

$$C.V. = \frac{(S.D. \times 100)}{Mean}$$

Uses of Co-efficient of Variation

The important use of this statistics is to compare two different quantitative traits measured in different units, and also to compare the variations of two unrelated groups for the same trait *viz.* growth rate in different species. In general the character with large value has more variability than those with small values *e.g.* body weight of elephant and mouse. The body weight of elephant is more than that of mouse and has more variability in terms of standard deviation. But the coefficient of variation may be nearly equal, showing that the greater variability in body weight of elephant was proportionally to their larger size. Likewise, the bull calves may be heavier than heifers at weaning age and also more variable having high standard deviations, but having nearly equal coefficient of variation. The range and standard deviation would tell us nothing because their mean differ widely. The C.V. relates the variation to the mean and measures the variation in percent. Thus, to make such comparisons, the standard deviation is expressed as a percentage of the mean and this is called the coefficient of variation.

The standard deviation divided by the mean makes the C.V. independent of the units of measurements. The knowledge of C.V. is valuable for planning and evaluating the breeding programme or any experiment. The trait with high C.V. indicates a greater scope of improvement. The improvement can either be made genetically or by providing better environment depending upon the relative magnitude of variation due to the cause *e.g.* if the genetic component of variation is high, which is expressed in terms of heritability of the trait, there is then a scope of improvement by manipulating genetic variation through selection but if the genetic variation is comparatively low the improvement can be made by providing better environment.

6. Standard Error

This is also called as standard deviation of the mean or standard error of the mean. The standard error (SE) together with mean $\left(\overline{X}\pm S.E.\right)$ describes the true mean of the population *viz.* the true mean of an infinite number of means drawn from a population. Thus it tells about the reliability of the mean of that sample from which it is estimated. In other words, if another sample is drawn from the same population and its mean is estimated, how much then the mean of the second sample come close to that of the mean of the first sample. Thus, the S.E. of the mean is a measure of the spread of the mean estimated from a number of samples from the whole population.

It is logical to think of the closeness (reliability) of the sample mean as a representative of the true mean of the entire population. The reliability of the mean depends upon the amount of variation in the population and the number of observations. The sample mean has a certain error depending upon the number of individuals measured in the sample and the sampling procedure. If the entire population is divided into many samples each with N variates with a standard deviation, then a population of means is obtained with its standard deviation as

$\dfrac{\sigma}{\sqrt{n}}$. This expression is a measure of the error with which a sample mean estimates the population mean, U. This is called the standard error of the mean or simply standard error, and it is given with the mean value, *e.g.* $\bar{X} \pm$ S.E. The standard error is thus estimated by dividing the σ of the distribution by the square root of the number of observation in the sample.

The standard error of one mean is equivalent to the standard deviation of a whole series of means that might be determined from corresponding samples of the same population.

Uses of Standard Error

(i) The mean of the distribution ± one SE includes about 68 percent of the means, the mean ± two S.E. should include about 95 per cent of the means. Thus there are five chances out of hundred that the true mean of an infinite number of means drawn from a population will not be covered by the sample mean ± two SE. In other words, if we draw a number of samples from a population, about 95 per cent of them will have a value in the range between the sample mean ± two S.E. Thus the S.E. indicates the reliability of mean. However, the reliability of the mean depends to a greater extent of the sample size. The.S.E. is greater with small sample size and therefore the mean will be less reliable.

(ii) *Comparison of two sample means:* The standard errors of two sample means can be used to determine significance of the difference between two sample means. In other words, if the means of two samples have been estimated, then it can be tested whether the means are truelly different or whether they are different due to sampling error. If the difference between the two means is about twice than the standard error of difference, it is then taken as a true difference at the 5 per cent level of probability.

24.8 Statistical Analysis

The amount of variation in a set of data is expressed as deviations from mean and measured as variance. The sum of a set of observations from mean is zero for a normal distribution because these deviations are positive, negative and zero. Therefore, the deviations are squared, added and divided by the degree of freedom to get the mean of squared values which is called the variance.

The square root of the variance is taken to express the variation in original unit of measurements of data. The square root of variance is called the standard deviation and used to measure the spread (variation) of the individual measurements.

The variations in individual measurements from the mean are due to a number of factors which may be genetic and environmental as well as the error of measurements. The variance measured is the total variance or phenotypic variance. It is most important to know the magnitude of the different factors causing the total variance. The factors causing the variation in a variable are known as *sources of variation* and the part of the variation caused by different sources are called as *components of variation*.

Data Classification

The data show two types of classifications *viz.* hierarchal classification and cross classification.

In *hierarchal classification,* each sample is composed of sub-samples which are in turn again subdivided into further samples. This repeated sub sampling results in to nested or hierarchal classification of data. For example, a number of sires are each mated to several dams and each dam produce a number of progenies. The ANOVA for hierarchal data takes the form as that for FS analysis.

In *cross classification,* an observation is affected by two or more factors like years ($r = 1, 2, …, i…$), and seasons ($c = 1, 2, …, j.$) when the sample of n observations is classified in r x c contingency table with frequencies n_{ij} (number of observations in j^{th} season of ith year).

Analysis of Non-orthogonal Data

The data having unequal numbers among sub-classes are called non-orthogonal data. In such case, the simple analysis of variance is not appropriate. Therefore some other statistical methods are used.

The data are subjected to least squares analysis to study the effect of different factors in causing the variation in a metric trait. The least squares procedure is a method of fitting constants. In this method some arbitrary restrictions are imposed. Another statistical procedure of analysis of non-orthogonal data is the maximum likelihood method.

The significance of the variation due to different levels of the effect is tested by t – test, χ^2 – test and F – test depending on the nature of data.

24.8.1 Comparison of Two Samples Means (Fisher's t- test)

It is of great interest to know whether means of two sample populations are really different or the differences are just by chance. The difference in two sample means is tested by using Fisher's t test. The standard error of difference between two sample means is given as:

$$S_d = \sqrt{\sigma^2_c \left(\frac{1}{n_1} + \frac{1}{n_2} \right)}$$

Where, σ^2_c = Combined variance of two samples (X and Y)

$$= \frac{(C.S.S._X + C.S.S._Y)}{(n_X + n_Y - 2)}$$

n_X and n_Y are number of observations of two samples

t   = Difference between two means/standard error of difference

$$= \frac{(\overline{X} - \overline{Y})}{S_d}$$

This calculated t value is tested at $(n_X + n_Y - 2)$ degree of freedom.

When there are only two levels of an effect, the F- test is equal to t – test. The F = t^2 with single D.F.

24.8.2 χ^2 Test

The χ^2-test is applied when it is of interest to test whether a particular distribution is in agreement to normal distribution or two distributions are in agreement with one another or whether two observed values are in any particular ratio or whether two sets of classification are independent of each other and so on. The χ^2 test indicates how closely the theoretical (hypothetical or expected) frequencies agree with the observed ones. Thus, the χ^2 test afford a measure of the correspondence between the fact and the theory.

(A) Testing the Independence of Attributes

The attribute is a quality characteric present in the individual like shape, colour, education, deafness, mortality, disease incidence, etc. The attribute may be present in two or more forms like illiterate, education up to high school, graduation or above. The χ^2 is applied to test the independence between two attributes in 2 x 2, 2 x n, m x n contingency table and tested with 1, n – 1 and (m – 1)(n – 1) degree of freedom, respectively.

$$\chi^2 = \sum \frac{(O-E)^2}{E}$$

Where,   O = Observed frequencies,

            E = Expected frequencies

The expected frequencies (E_{ij}) of ith row and j^{th} column are estimated as:

        $E_{ij} = (R_i \times C_j)/N$

Where, R_i = Row total for i^{th} row

            C_j = Column total for j^{th} column

            $N = \Sigma R_i = \Sigma C_j$

The χ^2 test can also be applied without calculating the expected frequencies of different cells of contingency table by the formulae given below:

(i) **2 x 2 contingency table**: This takes the form as:

		Yes	*No*	*Total*
Character A	Yes	a	b	R_1
Character B	No	c	d	R_2
	Total	C_1	C_2	N

$$\chi^2 = \frac{(ab - bc)^2 N}{R_1 R_2 C_1 C_2}$$

Where, a, b, c and d are the observed numbers in four classes

(ii) **2 x n contingency table**: This takes the form as:

Classes (levels of effect)	1	2	3	i	n	Total
No. affected	a_1	a_2	a_3	a_i	a_n	R_1
No. not affected	b_1	b_2	b_3	b_i	b_n	R_2
Total numbers	C_1	C_2	C_3	C_i	C_n	N

$$\chi^2 = \frac{N^2}{R_1 R_2}\left(\sum \frac{a_i^2}{C_i} - \frac{R_1^2}{N}\right)$$

Where, $\quad R_1 = \Sigma a_i$

$\qquad\qquad R_2 = \Sigma b_i$

$\qquad\qquad C_i = a_i + b_i$

(B) Testing the Significance of Proportions

Examples – (Sex ratio which is 1:1) or any ratio like 3:1.

$$\chi^2 = \frac{(m_2 a_1 - m_1 a_2)^2}{m_1 m_2 N}$$

Where, a_1 and a_2 = Observed numbers or ratios,

$\qquad\qquad N = a_1 + a_2$

$\qquad\qquad m_1$ and m_2 = Expected ratios

(C) χ^2 and Genetic Problems

The χ^2 is also used in testing the agreement of observed ratio of segregation with the hypothetical one like 1:2:1; 3:1; 9:3:3:1, etc. The expected numbers are calculated based on the expected ratios.

Further, the total χ^2 can also be partitioned into different components due to different factors for testing the homogeneity among the different levels of the effect like sex ratio in different breeds as well as the pooled sex ratio for all the breeds. The χ^2 is estimated for different breeds separately (χ^2_i) and their total is done to get total χ^2 as: $(\chi^2_T = \Sigma\chi^2_i)$. The χ^2 is also estimated based on pooled data of all the breeds which is χ^2 due to deviation (χ^2_D). The difference between χ^2_T and χ^2_D is the χ^2 due to heterogeneity (χ^2_H). Thus, $\chi^2_H = \chi^2_T - \chi^2_D$. The χ^2_H indicates the heterogeneity between groups like breeds.

The linkage between two attributes based on 9:3:3:1 ratio of F_2 data can also be detected by χ^2 test. The χ^2 for each of two loci affecting two characters (A and B) is calculated with a 3:1 ratio as:

$$\chi^2_{(A)} = \frac{(m_2a_1 - m_1a_2)^2}{m_1m_2N}$$

$$= \frac{(a_1 - 3a_2)^2}{3N}$$

$\chi^2_{(B)}$ = as $\chi^2_{(A)}$ is estimated.

Each of two χ^2 for two characters is tested at 1 D.F.

The $\chi^2_{(Linkage)}$ is calculated as:

$$\chi^2_{(Linkage)} = \frac{(a_1 - 3a_2 - 3a_3 - 9a_4)^2}{9N}$$

Where, $N = a_1 + a_2 + a_3 + a_4$.

The $a_{i's}$ are observed numbers in different cells.

The $\chi^2_{(Linkage)}$ is tested at 1 D.F.

$\chi^2_{(Total)} = \chi^2_{(A)} + \chi^2_{(B)} + \chi^2_{(Linkage)}$ and tested at 3 D.F.

24.8.3 F-test (Analysis of Variance)

More often it is required to compare more than two samples. The ratio of these two sources of variation (Between and within samples) is called as *F ratio* after Fisher, R.A. The variation among samples is due to the differences among the means. Therefore more is the difference among sample means, the more will be the variation among samples and the F raio will be more. Thus, the F ratio compares the variances but it is used to determine the significance of differences between two means or among more means.

Fisher in 1920's developed a method to separate out the effects of different factors in causing the total variation and provided a test called the Fisher's test or simply as F test to test the significance of the different factors in causing the variation and producing the differences in means of different levels of the effects. This method is called the analysis of variance (ANOVA). This is based on the subdivisible property of variance.

The aim of analysis of variance is to know the total variation present in a variable and assigning this total variation among the various factors responsible for the variation. The analysis of variance is thus a process to know the components of variation in a variable. However, the analysis of variance has two important roles. One is that it estimates the variance components and secondly it provides a means of testing the significance of differences among the levels of an effect.

The analysis of variance (ANOVA) is applied by calculating the total sum of squares (T.S.S.), the sum of squares due to different effects (Years, seasons, parity order, nutrition levels, sires, breeds, etc.), and the sum of squares due to remainder factors not taken in the model known as residual sum of squares or error sum of squares. The erros S.S. are obtained by taking the difference between T.S.S. and sum of sum of squares due to all the factors. The variance is taken as the sum of squares divided by degree of freedom of the respective effect (factor, like season, year). This variance is called the mean square (M. S.). The M.S. is estimated for different factors causing the variation.

Chapter 25
Bivariate Analysis

It is also of great interest and importance to know the variation in two traits together *i.e.* how two random variables vary together. This helps to understand the relationship between the two traits. Any two characters may be related to each other in such a way that a change or variation in one character correspond with a particular directional change (in the same or opposite direction) in the other. For example, if there is an increase in the value of one character it may lead to either an increase or decrease in the other character. The second situation may be that the two characters may be independent of each other. If the two characters have a relationship between them, it then means that there is a simultaneous change (variation) in both the characters. This simultaneous change or variation in two characters is measured in terms of covariation which indicates that the two characters vary together and have dependency on each other. Mathematically, the dependent variable Y is called the function of independent variable X, but in statistical terms the degree of this dependency (relationship or covariation) is measured by two statistical measures (statistics) known as coefficient of correlation and regression.

25.1 Covariance

The measurement of the covariation is the covariance which is the mean product between the deviations of the two traits measured on the same individual.

Uses of Co-variance

(i) Indicates the direction (sign) and strength of relationship between two variables.

(ii) Used to estimate the correlation and regression:

The covariance and its measures *viz.* Correlation and regression which measures the association between two or more characters are also the second degree statistics estimated for a bivariate population. The covariance is the variance common to the two traits and gives a quantitative description of the bivariate population in the manner and extent to which the two traits vary together.

25.2 Correlation Coefficient

This is a measure of the degree of mutual linear relationship between two variables (characters) indicating the manner the two characters tend to change together. The correlation coefficient between two variables is symbolized by r_{XY}.

25.2.1. Concept of Correlation

The product of chain of events:

The concept that the correlation is the result of chain of events (steps) was first conceived by Fisher (1918) and later developed by Wright (1921) in path coefficient analysis. This concept is very useful because it follows from the product rule of independent probabilities. This can be better illustrated with an example of the correlation between phenotypes of parent (x) and offspring (y) which is the resultant quantity of chain of three following events:

(i) Correlation between breeding value (A) and phenotypic value (P) of the parent (X) denoted by $r_{AP(X)}$. The $r_{AP(X)} = \sigma_{A(X)}/\sigma_{Px} = h_X$.

(ii) Genetic correlation between parent and offspring: This is the genetic effect between haploid gamete set in parent and offspring [$r_{A(XY)}$] and is equal to ½. This is because each parent transmits half of its total genes to its each offspring.

(iii) Correlation between breeding value (A) and phenotypic value (P) of the offspring (Y) denoted by $r_{AP(Y)}$. The $r_{AP(Y)} = \sigma_{A(Y)}/\sigma_{P(Y)} = h_Y$.

Therefore, total correlations between parent and offspring phenotypes ($r_{XY} = r_{OP}$) has three components and equal to:

$$r_{XY} = r_{OP} = r_{AP(X)}\, r_{A(XY)}\, r_{AP(Y)}$$
$$= h\tfrac{1}{2}h = \tfrac{1}{2}h^2.$$

This relationship can be shown diagrammatically as under:

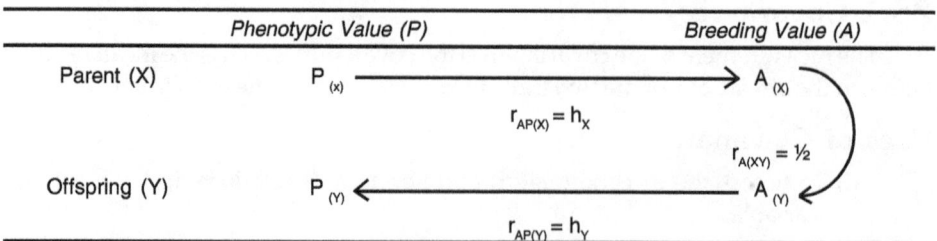

	Phenotypic Value (P)	Breeding Value (A)
Parent (X)	$P_{(x)}$ ————————————→	$A_{(x)}$
	$r_{AP(X)} = h_X$	$r_{A(XY)} = ½$
Offspring (Y)	$P_{(Y)}$ ←————————————	$A_{(Y)}$ ←
	$r_{AP(Y)} = h_Y$	

Figure 25.1: Showing Correlation as the Product of Chain of Events

25.2.2 Definition and Interpretation

Correlation Coefficient

The correlation between two variables is measured by a coefficient known as correlation coefficient. The correlation is defined as a ratio between the variance common to the two characters (covariance) to the geometric mean of the variances of the two characters. Suppose X and Y are two variables, the correlation coefficient between them denoted by r_{XY} is obtained by dividing the covariance of the two characters (Cov $_{XY}$) by the square root of the product of the variances of the two characters as:

$$r_{XY} = \sum \frac{(X - \bar{X})(Y - \bar{Y})}{\sqrt{(X - \bar{X})^2 (Y - \bar{Y})^2}}$$

$$= \frac{Cov_{XY}}{\sigma_X \sigma_Y}$$

$$= \frac{\sum XY}{\sigma_X \sigma_Y}$$

This expression of correlation coefficient gives a numerical measurement of the degree of linear association between the deviations of the two variables. This indicates that variation in either variable will cause variation in other variable. This implies that if one variable is held constant the other variable will also remain constant.

Coefficient of Determination

The squares of the correlation coefficient between two variables (r^2_{XY}) indicate the amount of variability in one variable caused by the variability in other variable (or vice versa). This is the fraction of the variance of one variable (X) determined by the variance in other variable (Y) or vice versa. This means that the variability will disappear in one variable (X) if the variability in other variable (Y) is kept constant (or vice versa). The r^2_{XY} is known as the coefficient of determination because this determines the variability in a variable due to the variability in other variable. However, it does not indicate any directional or casual relationship between two variables but it is symmetrical to both variables. This symmetry is one of the main properties of correlation coefficient.

The coefficient of determination of the dependent variable (effect) by the cause variable (X) is defined as the portion of complete determination of effect variable (Z) for which the particular cause (X) is directly responsible in the system of related variables considering all causes into account. This coefficient of determination is denoted as d_{ZX}. The sum of all the coefficients of determination of effects by the different causing factors (causes *viz.* x, y) must equal to unity. Therefore,

$$d_{ZX} + d_{ZY} + \ldots = 1.0$$

The coefficient of determination is the degree (amount) of determination of one variable by the other. This coefficient measures the portion of the variance caused by any one of the causing factors (X or Y) to the total variability in the effect (Z). Thus, r^2_{ZX} = $d_{ZX} = \sigma^2_X/\sigma^2_Z$. Therefore, the coefficient of determination is obtained in two ways as:

(i) Coefficient of determination as square of correlation coefficient:

$$d_{ZX} = r^2_{ZX}$$

(ii) Coefficient of determination as ratio of variance of cause (X) to the variance of effect (Y): $d_{ZX} = \sigma^2_X/\sigma^2_Z$.

When the two variables, say X and Y are not correlated to each other, they are said to be independent and $r_{xy} = 0$ because the sum of products of their corresponding deviations is vanished yielding $\sum(X-\overline{X})(Y-\overline{Y})=0$.

25.2.3 Variation in Dependent Variable due to its Causes

Now suppose, any variable, say Z, is linear combination of two other variables (say X and Z) which may be correlated to each other or may be independent such that

$$Z = X + Y$$

In this equation Z is the effect and X, Y are the causes responsible for causing variation in Z. Thus the variation in Z will be affected by the variation in X and Y. Therefore,

$$(Z-\overline{Z})^2 = \sum(X-\overline{X})^2 + \sum(Y-\overline{Y})^2 + 2\sum(X-\overline{X})(Y-\overline{Y})$$

$$\sigma_Z = \sigma^2_X + \sigma^2_Y + 2\sigma_{XY}$$

$$\quad = \sigma^2_X + \sigma^2_Y + 2r_{XY}\sigma_X\sigma_Y \qquad \text{when X and Y are correlated}$$

$$\quad = \sigma^2_X + \sigma^2_Y \qquad\qquad\qquad \text{when X and Y are not correlated}$$

The equation of variance of the sum of two variables indicates that the amount of variance of the causing factors (X and Y) influence the variance of the dependent variable (effect Z). The variance of dependent variable (σ^2_Z) is completely determined by the sum of the variances of the independent variables ($\sigma^2_Z = \sigma^2_X + \sigma^2_Y$) if the independent variables (X and Y) are not correlated to each other but if X and Y are correlated their covariance also contributes to the variance of the dependent variable.

Now dividing both sides with σ^2_Z amounts to:

$$\frac{\sigma^2_Z}{\sigma^2_Z} = \frac{\sigma^2_X}{\sigma^2_Z} + \frac{\sigma^2_Y}{\sigma^2_Z} + 2r_{XY}\frac{\sigma_X\sigma_Y}{\sigma^2_Z}$$

$$1.0 = \frac{\sigma^2_X}{\sigma^2_Z} + \frac{\sigma^2_Y}{\sigma^2_Z} + 2r_{XY}\left(\frac{\sigma_X}{\sigma_Z}\right)\left(\frac{\sigma_Y}{\sigma_Z}\right)$$

$$\quad = x^2 + y^2 + 2r_{XY}(x.y.) \qquad \text{if X and Y are correlated}$$

$$\quad = x^2 + y^2 \qquad\qquad\qquad \text{if X and Y are independent}$$

The x^2 and y^2 are the coefficient of determination of Z by the two causes (X and Y), respectively. This is the ratio of variance of cause to the variance of the effect and equal to the square of the corresponding correlation coefficients.

The ratio of variance of an independent factor (cause, X) to the dependent variable (effect, Z) is also equal to the coefficient of determination.

$$\frac{\sigma^2_x}{\sigma^2_z} = d_{ZX} = X^2$$

When the Causes are Uncorrelated (Z = X + Y)

Cov. $_{XY} = 0$, Cov. $_{XZ} = \sigma^2_x$ and Cov. $_{YZ} = \sigma^2_Y$. This can be shown as under:

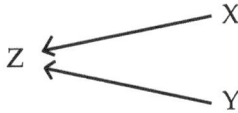

$$Z \longleftarrow \begin{array}{c} X \\ Y \end{array}$$

$$
\begin{aligned}
\sum(Z-\bar{Z})(X-\bar{X}) &= \sum\left[(X+Y)-(\bar{X}+\bar{Y})\right](X-\bar{X}) \quad \text{since } Z = X + Y \\
&= \sum(X-\bar{X})(Y-\bar{Y})(X-\bar{X}) \\
&= \sum(X-\bar{X})^2 + \sum(Y-\bar{Y})(X-\bar{X}) \\
&= \sum(X-\bar{X})^2 \qquad \text{since X and Y are not correlated} \\
&= \sigma^2_X
\end{aligned}
$$

Similarly, $\sum(Z-\bar{Z})(Y-\bar{Y}) = \sum(Y-\bar{Y})^2 = \sigma^2_Y$

From this the r_{ZX} and r_{ZY} can be obtained as:

$$r_{ZX} = \frac{\sigma_{ZX}}{\sigma_z \sigma_x} = \frac{\sigma^2_x}{\sigma_z \sigma_x} = \frac{\sigma_x}{\sigma_z}$$

$$r_{ZY} = \frac{\sigma_{ZY}}{\sigma_z \sigma_Y} = \frac{\sigma^2_Y}{\sigma_z \sigma_Y} = \frac{\sigma_Y}{\sigma_z}$$

Thus, $r^2_{ZX} = \dfrac{\sigma^2_x}{\sigma^2_z}$

$$= x^2 = \text{coefficient of deter. of Z by X}$$

$$= d_{ZX}$$

$$r^2_{ZY} = \frac{\sigma^2_Y}{\sigma^2_z}$$

$$= y^2 = \text{coefficient of deter, of } Z \text{ by } Y$$

$$= d_{ZY}$$

The important conclusion is that the sum of the coefficients of determination equal unity as:

$$r^2_{ZX} + r^2_{ZY} = 1.0$$

(*See numerical example 25.1*)

25.2.4 Characteristics and Properties of Correlation Coefficient

The r is a ratio and has the following characteristics:

☆ The r is a pure number without any unit or dimensions.

☆ The r has limits between − 1 to +1

☆ The chief property of correlation coefficient is that it is symmetrical to both traits (X and Y) yielding a numerical measurement of the degree of linear association between the deviations of X and Y.

☆ The correlation coefficient is related to the variance. The square of correlation coefficient (r^2) indicates the proportion of the total variation which can be explained by linear regression. The r^2 measures the proportion of the variance in one variable (character) that can be accounted for by variation in a related variable (character). The r^2 is therefore called the coefficient of determination. Thus, r^2 indicates that fraction of the variance of X which is determined by Y or vice versa, in the sense that this fraction disappears if Y in kept constant.

☆ The correlation between two characters assumes the cause and effect relationship between them and depends upon their biological relationship. However, r gives no idea that which variable is the cause and which is effect. Thus it does not indicate the cause and effect relationship between the characters. Thus r does not tell that which character is dependent and which one is independent.

☆ The r is a valid measure of linear relationship only and not for other type of relationship viz, curvilinear.

☆ The r is a bidirectional regression coefficient in standard measure.

Uses of Correlation

1. The *r* is of value when the relationship is linear. It measures the degree of relationship which conveys valuable information about the population. The *r* measures the intensity of the relationship of the two characters.

2. It has close relation to the slope of the linear estimate of one variable in terms of the other variable by the method of least squares as:

$$byx = rxy \left(\frac{\sigma_Y}{\sigma_x} \right) \text{ and}$$

$$bxy = rxy \left(\frac{\sigma_x}{\sigma_y} \right)$$

Where, byx and bxy represents the slop of the regression line.

3. The r is related to the covariance as:

$$Cov\, xy = rxy\, \sigma_x \sigma_Y$$

4. The correlation is easy to interpret because it is unitless and ranges from -1 to +1.

5. The square of correlation coefficient (r^2) is a useful measure of the part of variance of either of the. two variables (character) due to the other *i.e.*

$$r^2_{XY} = \frac{\sigma^2_{Y(X)}}{\sigma^2_Y}$$

$$= \frac{\sigma^2_{X(Y)}}{\sigma^2_X}$$

Where, $\sigma^2_{Y(X)}$ is the portion of variance of y due to x

$\sigma^2_{X(Y)}$ is the portion of variance of x due to y

Therefore, $\sigma^2_{Y(X)} = r^2_{XY} \sigma^2_Y$

$\sigma^2_{X(Y)} = r^2_{XY} \sigma^2_X$

The r^2 indicates the proportion of the total variation in one character that can be accounted for by the variation in a related character. Thus, r^2_{XY} shows the fraction of the variance if x is determined by y or vice versa.

25.2.5 Types of Correlations

The correlation coefficients are of three type *viz.* Simple or total, partial and multiple correlations.

(a) Estimation of Simple Correlation

The simple correlation coefficient is estimated between two variables depending upon the nature of data available and purpose of its estimation. It is estimated in the following ways:

(I) Inter Class Correlation

The inter-class correlation is estimated for the paired values on each individual. These paired values may be for two different traits of the individual or may be on one trait measured at two different times on the same set of individuals like estimation of correlation between body weight at two ages, correlation between milk yield recorded in two lactations etc. or may be for one trait of two individuals paired for some reason like the correlation between milk yield of dam and daughter. It is estimated as:

$$r_{XY} = \frac{Cov_{XY}}{\sigma_x \sigma_Y}$$

Test of Significance of r: It has been mentioned that the two independent variables has the value of r equal to zero or near zero. It is therefore important to decide the significance of association (correlation) between two variables. This depends on the magnitude of correlation (r) and the number of observations used to estimate r. A quantity with same distribution as student's t is calculated as:

$$t \quad = \frac{r}{S.E.(r)}$$

$$= \frac{r}{\sqrt{\frac{(1-r^2)}{(n-2)}}}$$

$$= \frac{r}{\sqrt{\frac{(n-2)}{(1-r^2)}}}$$

If the t value is greater than the tabulated t value for n-2 degree of freedom, the r is taken as significantly different from zero and it is then considered that the two variables are correlated to each other.

(II) Intra Class Correlation

There may be more than two observations per individual for each character. This requires finding out the correlation between the multiple measurements (observations) of the same individual or the correlation between different members of each group or family. The correlation between multiple observations is called the intra-class correlation and denoted by r' or t.

When each group or family has a large number of individuals, or each individual has multiple measurements, the intra-class correlation (r') is estimated by analysis of variance. Suppose there are n groups each with k individuals, or n individuals each with k observations (*e.g.* there are. n sires each with k daughters), it is the problem now to estimate the correlation between K observations of a group or individual. The total variability of the *nk* observations can be calculated and then it can be partitioned into between groups and within group.

$$r' \quad = \frac{(MS_B - MS_W)}{[MS_B + (k-1)MS_W]}$$

$$= \frac{\sigma^2_B}{(\sigma^2_B + \sigma^2_W)}$$

If r' is zero, it means that the variation between groups and within group is of the same order. When variation between groups is greater than the variation within group, the r' will be positive and will show that group means have a tendency to differ, while negative value of r′ will mean reverse, *i.e.* group means have got a tendency to be alike and variation between groups is less than the variation within group. For complete intra-class correlation the variance within group ($\sigma^2_w = 0$) is zero and therefore the intra class correlation is defined in terms of variance.

The r′ is used to obtain correlation between family member *viz.* half sibs and full sibs, and to estimate the correlation between repeated or multiple measurements of the individual *viz.* repeatability.

The simple correlation is of three types *viz.* phenotypic, genetic and environmental. In other words, the phenotypic correlation which is the observable correlation between two variables can be partitioned into genetic and environmental correlations which are due to the genetic and environmental effects, respectively.

(III) Rank Correlation

When the bivariate population is far from normal the computation of r is not valid. For example, when it is needed to estimate the correlation between two characters on the basis of the rank of the individual, another method of estimating correlation was given by C. Spearman (1904) and is known as rank correlation, denoted by r_s. The r_s is the simple correlation coefficient *r* between the ranked values of Individuals based on two characters. It thus can be estimated in usual way between two rankings of the same individual for two traits.

But spearman devised the following formula:

$$r_S = 1 - \frac{6\sum d^2}{n(n^2 - 1)}$$

where,   d = difference between the two ranks of an individual

n = number of individuals.

The rank correlation is used in animal breeding to estimate the correlation between the rankings of bulls for certain character (*e.g.* breeding value) by different methods etc.

(IV) Biserial Correlation

Sometimes it is important to know the correlation between a qualitative and quantitative trait of the individuals of the population *viz.* physiological status of animal (pregnancy, lactation, and dry condition of sheep) and their wool production. Such correlation is known as biserial correlation, r_B, given as (Tate, 1955):

$$r_B = \left[\frac{(\overline{X}_1 - \overline{X}_0)}{S_{\overline{X}}} \right] \sqrt{pq}$$

Where, $\overline{X}_1$ = average of X values (continuous variable) for the Z′s which are 1.

$\overline{X}_0$ = average of X values (continuous variable) for the Z′s which are 0.

$$p = N_1/n$$

$$q = N_0/n = 1 - p$$

$N_1 = Z_1$, the number of Z observations with value 1.

$N_0 = n - Z_1$, the number of Z observations with value 0

$N = N_1 + N_0$, the number of total observations

$$S_{\overline{X}} = \sqrt{\left[\frac{1}{n}\right]\left[\sum(X_{0i} - \overline{X})^2 + \sum(X_{ij} - \overline{X}_1)^2 + npq(X_1 + \overline{X}_0)^2\right]}$$

(b) Estimation of Partial and Multiple Correlation

See point 26.2 of Chapter 26.

25.3 Regression

The correlation coefficient signifies the relationship between two variables. However, it can not be used to predict the value of one variable (dependent variable, Y) from a given value of the other variable, X. Another measure of relationship is estimated to measure the expected amount of change in one variable (Y) associated with per unit change in the second variable (X). This measure is called the regression coefficient. Galton (1889) gave the idea of regression.

For example, the correlation (r_{XY}) between heart girth (X) and birth weight (Y) is found significant. Now it is of interest to know that how many Kg of birth weight on the average is associated with each cm. change in heart girth. In order to obtain this information, the regression of birth weight on heart girth (b_{YX}) is estimated. The regression coefficient is denoted by b_{YX}. Thus, the dependence of one character on the other is measured as coefficient of regression which is a measure of the covariance expressed as a proportion of the total variation of an independent variable. The regression coefficient measures this form of relationship and is estimated with the following objectives:

☆ To know whether Y is dependent on X

☆ To predict Y from X

☆ To determine the shape of regression curve

☆ To know the error in Y after adjustment has been made for the effect of a related variable (to test the best of fit).

25.3.1 Estimation of Regression Coefficient

The regression coefficient (b) may be estimated both ways *viz.* regression of Y on X (denoted as b_{YX}) and regression of X on Y (denoted as b_{XY}). The regression is defined and computed as

$$b_{YX} = \frac{\sum xy}{\sum x^2} \quad \text{and} \quad b_{XY} = \frac{\sum xy}{\sum y^2}$$

The regression of Y on X (b_{YX}) equals the covariance of X and Y (Cov $_{XY}$) divided by the variance of X (V_X), and likewise the regression of X on Y (b_{XY}) equals the Cov $_{XY}$ divided by the variance of Y. The b_{YX} indicates the expected change (predicted change) in variable Y per one unit change in variable X, the unit of measurement are taken actual. This can further be elaborated in a way that if an individual value for X variable is one unit above the mean (X), the value of Y variable for that individual is predicted to deviate b_{YX} units from the mean of Y variable. The direction of deviation will depend on the positive or negative sign of b_{YX}. In other words, it can be stated that if the values of variable X differ for two individuals by K units, then their predicted difference for Y variable is Kb_{YX} units. Thus the value of b_{YX} is a coefficient by which a unit variation in X, the independent variable will cause a variation in Y, the dependent variable.

Test of Significance

The significance of regression is tested by 't' test and 'F' test:

(a) *t–Test:* $t = b/S.E. (b)$

$$\text{Where,} \quad S.E. (b_{YX}) = \sqrt{\frac{\sum y^2 - \frac{\left(\sum xy\right)^2}{\sum x^2}}{\sum x^2(n-2)}}$$

$$S.E. (b_{XY}) = \sqrt{\frac{\sum x^2 - \frac{\left(\sum xy\right)^2}{\sum y^2}}{\sum y^2(n-2)}}$$

The significance is tested by comparing calculated t value with tabulated t value at N-2 degrees of freedom.

(b) *F-test:* F = Regression variance/Residual variance

$$\text{Where, Regression S.S.} \quad = \frac{\left(\sum xy\right)^2}{\sum x^2} \text{ for } b_{YX}$$

$$= \frac{\left(\sum xy\right)^2}{\sum y^2} \text{ for } b_{XY}$$

Residual S.S. = Total S.S. – regression S.S.

Total S.S. $= \Sigma x^2$ for b_{YX}

                        $= \Sigma y^2$ for b_{XY}

The F is tested for 1 and N-2 degree of freedom.

The regression sum of squares divided by Σy^2 or Σx^2 measures the fraction of variation in Y or X variable due to X or Y variable. For example, the fraction of variation in Y due to variation in X is 0.1896/0.27 = 0.7022. This indicates that 70.2 per cent variation in Y is explained due to variation in X. This value is exactly the same as obtained by r^2.

(i) Prediction of Y from given X

Two prediction equations are determined by the method of least squares and expressed as:

$$Y - \overline{Y} = b_{YX}\left(X - \overline{X}\right)$$

and $\qquad \hat{Y} = \overline{Y} + b_{YX}\left(X - \overline{X}\right)$

Similarly, $\qquad X - \overline{X} = b_{XY}\left(Y - \overline{Y}\right)$

and $\qquad \hat{X} = X + b_{XY}\left(Y - \overline{Y}\right)$

Where, $\hat{Y}$ and $\hat{X}$ are the estimated value of Y and X, respectively.

After having obtained such a prediction equation the value of dependent variable (Y) can be predicted by substituting the value of independent variable (X).

(ii) Fitting Regression Line

The X and Y values are plotted on graph paper and the resulting diagram is called *scatter diagram*. A line is drawn among the plotted points, the line represents the best relationship between pairs of X and Y values and called the *regression line*. This line shows the relationship between two variables. If the line is a straight one, it is then a case of linear regression. The two regression lines are obtained based on b_{YX} and b_{XY}. The slope of the line is called the *regression coefficient*. The regression line is drawn to provide the best fit to the paired observations in such a way that the squared distance between this line and all points on the graph is minimized.

The prediction equation for a straight line takes the following form:

Y = a + bX

Where, $\qquad$ Y is the predicted value,

$\qquad$ a is the Y intercept

$\qquad$ b is regression coefficient (slope of the line),

$\qquad$ X is the value of independent variable

The Y intercept is the point where the regression line crosses the Y axis when the value of X variable is zero. This is also the estimated height of the line, when X = 0.

The value of *a* is determined as

a = y – b x

Where, x and y are the mean values

(iii) Goodness of Fit of the Line

The sample points (Y) can be compared with the corresponding estimated values $\left(\hat{Y}\right)$ in order to get the measure of the goodness of fit of the line. This is done by substituting each X in the regression equation and to obtain $\hat{Y}$. The deviation from regression, $Y - \hat{Y} = d_{yx}$ measures the failure of the line to fit the data.

The sum of squares due to difference in observed Y and that expected from regression function ($\Sigma d^2_{y.x}$) gives an idea of the variance not accounted for by regression.

The mean square deviation from regression is $d^2 y.x/n - 2$ which is sample standard deviation from regression. This provides a sample standard deviation of the regression coefficient as:

$$S_b = \frac{\sqrt{\Sigma \dfrac{d^2_{y.x}}{n-2}}}{\sqrt{x^2}}$$

This is used to test the significance of b as -

$t = b/S_b$

The $\Sigma d^2_{y.x}$ may also be directly estimated as:

$$\Sigma d^2_{y.x} = \Sigma y^2 - \frac{\Sigma xy^2}{\Sigma x^2}$$

and used to estimate the SE (b).

25.4 Relation between Correlation and Regression

25.4.1 Similarities

The r is closely related to the regression coefficients in the following manner -

(1) The r measures the spread about the regression line (the intensity of the relationship of the two variables), whereas the regression coefficient measures the slope of the regression line. Taking the linear relationship between two variables, the regression coefficient is the slope of the line drawn by plotting the measurements of individuals taking the independent variable (X) on X-axis and dependent variable (Y) on the Y-axis. A line can be drawn extending from low values of two variables to their high values. Such a line will show three types of slopes *viz.* positive slope, if two variables are positively correlated; negative slop, if they are negatively correlated; and zero slope in the absence of correlation between them (r = 0).

(2) The r equals the linear regression coefficient (b) when the variances of the two variables are equal:

If $\sigma^2_X = \sigma^2_Y$, and then $r = b$

And hence $r_{XY} = \dfrac{\text{Cov}_{XY}}{\sigma^2_X} = \dfrac{\text{Cov}_{XY}}{\sigma^2_Y}$

$$= b_{YX} = b_{XY}$$

(3) Another way of showing the relation between r and b

$$b_{YX} = r_{xy}\frac{\sigma_Y}{\sigma_X} \qquad \text{Since, } b_{YX} = \frac{\text{Cov}_{XY}}{\sigma_X \sigma_X}\frac{\sigma_Y}{\sigma_Y}$$

$$= \frac{\text{Cov}_{XY}}{\sigma_X \sigma_Y}\frac{\sigma_Y}{\sigma_X}$$

Likewise, $\qquad b_{XY} = r_{xy}\dfrac{\sigma_X}{\sigma_Y} \qquad \text{Since, } b_{XY} = \dfrac{\text{Cov}_{XY}}{\sigma_Y \sigma_Y}\dfrac{\sigma_X}{\sigma_X}$

$$= \frac{\text{Cov}_{XY}}{\sigma_X \sigma_Y}\frac{\sigma_X}{\sigma_Y}$$

This again shows that the regression and correlation coefficient will be equal if and only if the standard deviation of the two traits is equal.

$$r_{XY} = b_{YX}\frac{\sigma_X}{\sigma_Y} \qquad \text{Since, } r_{XY} = \frac{\text{Cov}_{XY}}{\sigma_X \sigma_Y}\frac{\sigma_X}{\sigma_X}$$

$$= \frac{\text{Cov}_{XY}}{\sigma^2_X}\frac{\sigma_X}{\sigma_Y}$$

$$r_{XY} = b_{XY}\frac{\sigma_Y}{\sigma_X} \qquad \text{Since, } r_{XY} = \frac{\text{Cov}_{XY}}{\sigma_X \sigma_Y}\frac{\sigma_X}{\sigma_X}$$

$$= \frac{\text{Cov}_{XY}}{\sigma^2_Y}\frac{\sigma_Y}{\sigma_X}$$

$$r^2 = b_{XY}\frac{\sigma_Y}{\sigma_X} b_{YX}\frac{\sigma_X}{\sigma_Y}$$

$$= b_{XY}b_{YX}$$

And hence, $\quad r \quad = \sqrt{b_{XY}b_{YX}}$

Therefore, the geometric mean of the two regression coefficients is the correlation between X and Y.

(4) The numerator of both correlation coefficient and the regression coefficients is the covariance of X and Y.

Both the correlation and the regression coefficients take the sign of the covariance. As the correlation coefficient was standardized, the regression is also standardized in a way to divide the covariance by the variance of one character and this makes it more readily interpretable.

25.4.2 Differences

The correlation and regression coefficient differ in a number of the following ways

(1) The correlation has no unit of measurement but it is a pure number. On the other hand, the regression coefficients have actual units of measurements *viz.* the unit of measurement for byx is actual units of measurement for Y per one unit of measurement for X. For example, the variation in body weight due to the variance in heart girth can be described as the regression of body weight on heart girth in the form of kg per cm (*e.g.* byx = 0.469 kg/cm)

(2) The correlation has limits between —1 to +1, whereas the regression coefficient has no limit but may take any value depending upon the magnitude of cause and effect relationship between two variables.

(3) The correlation is bidirectional and assumes no cause and effect relationship between variables. This means that it only describes the relationship between two variables (relationship of X to Y and Y to X) and will have the same numerical value ($r_{xy} = r_{yx}$)

On the contrary, the regression coefficient is unidirectional and specifies the direction of cause and effect from one variable to the other. For example, for byx the interpretation is that the X is cause or independent variable and Y is the effect or dependent variable. Taking an example of milk yield in dairy cattle, it can be said that the milk yield of dam affects the milk yield of daughters and not the opposite. Therefore, the proper way is the regression of daughter's milk yield on dam's yield. Likewise, the changes in atmospheric temperature will affect the respiration rate and not the vice versa and it will be taken as regression of breaths per minute.

(4) The correlation and regression coefficients are used in a different way. The correlation is used to quantify and to describe the linear association between the two variables whose cause and effect relationship is not known. On the other hand, the regression coefficient is used for two purposes mainly which are

   (i) Quantification of the effect of one variable on the other variable, *e.g.* gain in body weight due to some feed additive. If the regression of gain on the amount of feed additive is estimated, it will then quantify as well as describe the cause and effect relationship between weight gain and amount of feed additive, *i.e.* average association between these two variables will be explained by the regression coefficient.

   (ii) Prediction of the value of dependent variable from the measured value of the independent variable. This is more important situation when it is of great interest to know (predict) well in time the value of dependent variable whose actual measurement is expensive and time taking (*e.g.* carcass traits and life time traits) based on the measured value of the independent (cause) variable whose value is obtained earlier. The prediction equation is

$$Y_i = a + b_{YX} X_i$$

with the symbols as described earlier.

Solved Examples

Example 25.1

The calving interval (C) is completely determined by the service period (S) and gestation period (G) such that C = S + G.

Verify the relations based on the following data of 5 cows:

Variables	Value for 5 Cows					Sum	S.S.	σ^2	σ
S	61	81	72	66	80	360	302	75.5	8.6891
G	283	285	288	286	283	1425	18	4.5	2.1213
C	344	366	360	352	363	1785	320	80.0	8.9443

Solution

The service period is more variable while the variation in gestation period is very low and these two traits are uncorrelated. Therefore, most of the variation in calving interval must be due to the variation in service period while the contribution of gestation period in causing variation in calving interval should be very less. This can be shown by estimating the coefficient of determination as under:

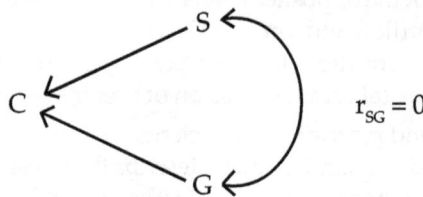

$$C = S + G$$

$$\sigma^2_C = \sigma^2_S + \sigma^2_G + 2\,Cov_{SG}$$

$$= \sigma^2_S + \sigma^2_G \text{ since } Cov_{SG} = 0$$

$$r^2_{CS} = \frac{\sigma^2_S}{\sigma^2_C} \quad ; r_{CS} = \frac{\sigma_S}{\sigma_C}$$

$$r^2_{CG} = \frac{\sigma^2_G}{\sigma^2_C} \quad ; r_{CG} = \frac{\sigma_G}{\sigma_C}$$

$r^2_{CS} + r^2_{CG} = 1.0$

$\Sigma CS = 12822$, $\Sigma SG = 102600$, $\Sigma CG = 508743$

$\text{Cov}_{CS} = 75.5$; $\text{Cov}_{CG} = 4.5$; $\text{Cov}_{SG} = 0$,

The coefficient of determination which is the square of the correlation coefficient (r^2_{CS} and r^2_{CG}) can be verified in terms of the ratio of the variance of cause to the variance of the effect

$$r^2_{CS} = \frac{\sigma^2_s}{\sigma^2_c} \; ; r^2_{CG} = \frac{\sigma^2_G}{\sigma^2_c}$$

Coefficient of determination as square of correlation efficient:

$$r_{CS} = \frac{\text{Cov}_{CS}}{\sigma_s \sigma_c} = \frac{75.5}{8.6891 \times 8.9443} = \frac{75.5}{77.7179} = 0.9717$$

$$r^2_{CS} = (0.9717)^2 = 0.9444 = d_{CS}$$

$$r_{CG} = \frac{\text{Cov}_{CG}}{\sigma_s \sigma_G} = \frac{45.5}{2.1213 \times 8.9443} = \frac{45.5}{18.9735} = 0.2372$$

$$r^2_{CG} = (0.2372)^2 = 0.0563 = d_{CG}$$

$$r^2_{CS} + r^2_{CG} = 0.9444 + 0.0563 = 1.007$$

Coefficient of determination as ratio of variance of cause to the variance of effect:

$$\frac{\sigma^2_s}{\sigma^2_c} = \frac{75.5}{80.0} = 0.9438 = s^2 = d_{CS}$$

$$\frac{\sigma^2_G}{\sigma^2_c} = \frac{4.5}{80.0} = 0.0563 = s^2 = d_{CG}$$

$$s^2 + g^2 = 0.9438 + 0.0563 = 1.0001$$

The following conclusions can be easily drawn from the results-

(i) The service period (S) and gestation period (G) are uncorrelated.

(ii) The service period is more variable with a difference of 20 days ranging from 61 to 81 days with a variance of 75.5 while the gestation period is less variable with a difference of only 5 days ranging from 283 to 288 days with a variance of 4.5.

(iii) The variance of calving interval is 80.0 which is equal to the variance of service period plus the variance of gestation period.

$$\sigma^2_c = \sigma^2_c + \sigma^2_G$$

$$80.0 = 75.5 + 4.5$$

(iv) The service period being more variable has contributed more variability (94.38 per cent) to the total variability in the calving interval while the gestation period being less variable has contributed lesser variability (5.63 per cent) to the total variability in calving interval. Thus more variable cause contributes more to the total variability in the effect. This means that more variable cause has greater effect on the dependent variable compared to the less variable cause. This is the basis of estimating the path coefficient that the total variability in dependent 'variable (effect) is proportional to the variability of the different causing factors (causes).

Chapter 26
Multivariate Analysis

The multi trait selection rather than single trait selection is more effective in bringing the genetic improvement in the overall genetic merit. Secondly, the characters of farm animals are correlated among themselves. Therefore, it is better to make use of more traits in animal improvement programme. The analysis of more than two characters in a model is known as *multivariate analysis*. The multivariate analysis may involve the data of a single population or of more populations located at the same farm or at other location. The multivariate analysis has become easy with the use of computers.

The multivariate analysis taking more than two variables of one or more populations can be conducted. In the present volume of the book it is not possible to give all the details of different methods of multivariate analysis and hence only the basic principles and use of these techniques have been given here. The readers may consult the statistical books to learn the techniques of various multivariate analyses.

26.1 Multiple Regression Analysis

The technique of regression was given by Galton (1886) taking two variables. The regression coefficients may be simple, partial and multiple depending on the number of variables.

26.1.1 Partial Regression

The characters of farm animals are inter-related to each other and hence the total correlation between two variables may be misleading. Therefore, it is better to estimate the correlation between two variables after eliminating the effects of other interrelated factors (keeping their effect constant). The association between two variables in this way (keeping constant the effect of other correlated variables) is measured by partial correlation and partial regression. The partial correlation between two variables measures the degree of covariation for two variables with third variable being constant and hence the effect of third variable is eliminated.

The partial regression coefficients are estimated with the help of regression equations as:

$$X_1 = b_{12.3} \, x_2 + b_{13.2} \, x_3 \qquad\qquad\qquad \text{................ Eq. 1}$$

Where, $b_{12.3}$ is the partial regression coeffient of 1 and 2 keeping 3 as constant,

$b_{13.2}$ is the partial regression coeffient of 1 and 3 keeping 2 as constant,

x_1 are the variables (1, 2 and 3).

The above equation 1 is multiplied by x_2 and x_3 and summing to get the following equations –

$$\Sigma x_1 \, x_2 = b_{12.3} \, \Sigma x_2^2 + b_{13.2} \, \Sigma x_2 x_3 \qquad\qquad \text{................ Eq. 2}$$

$$\Sigma x_1 \, x_3 = b_{12.3} \, \Sigma x_2 x_3 + b_{13.2} \, \Sigma x_3^2 \qquad\qquad \text{................ Eq. 3}$$

The solution of equation 2 and 3 yields the values of $b_{12.3}$ and $b_{13.2}$

Similarly, the regression equation for x_2 is obtained as:

$$x_2 = b_{21.3} \, x_1 + b_{23.1} \, x_3 \qquad\qquad\qquad \text{................ Eq. 4}$$

The eq. 4 is multiplied by x_1 and x_3, and summing to get the following equations:

$$\Sigma x_2 \, x_1 = b_{21.3} \, \Sigma x_1^2 + b_{23.1} \, \Sigma x_3 x_1 \qquad\qquad \text{................ Eq. 5}$$

$$\Sigma x_2 \, x_3 = b_{21.3} \, \Sigma x_1 x_3 + b_{23.1} \, \Sigma x_3^2 \qquad\qquad \text{................ Eq. 6}$$

Solving equation 5 and 6 give the values of $b_{21.3}$ and $b_{23.1}$

Likewise, the regression equation of third variable (x_3) is set, multiplied by x_1 and x_2, taking the summation and solve them to get the values of $b_{31.2}$ and $b_{32.1}$

26.1.2 Multiple Regressions

The technique of multiple regression involving more than two variables is used in a single population by conducting the least square analysis based on the principle of minimizing the sum of square of deviation between observed and expected variable or to minimize the sum of squares of error. The regression analysis estimates the regression coefficients which indicate the amount of change in dependent variable.

The regression analysis is conducted assuming the continuous distribution and linear relationship between the dependent and independent variables. It is also assumed that the error is normally and independently distributed with mean zero and variance one. This is because the normal curve depends on the mean and standard deviation. The normal distribution with mean zero and unit standard deviation showed that the mean represents the mid point and the standard deviation represents the variability equal to unity. Thus, the rescaling of a measurement X with mean and standard deviation is required so that the mean becomes zero and standard deviation becomes 1.

The multiple regression analysis is used to correct the data and to predict the average value of dependent variable for a particular value of independent variables.

The *relative importance of different independent variables* to cause variation in dependent variable can be estimated from regression analysis. The regression equation for n values of dependent variable (Y) and independent variables (X_1 and X_2) is:

$Y = \alpha + b_1 X_1 + b_2 X_2 + \ldots + b_K X_K + e$

$\sigma^2 y = b_1{}^2 \sigma^2{}_{x1} + b_2{}^2 \sigma^2 x_2 + \ldots + b_k{}^2 \sigma^2 x_k + \sigma^2{}_e$

The quantity $(b_1{}^2 \sigma^2 x_1)/\sigma^2 y$ is a measure of the fraction of the variation in dependent variable due to its linear regression on X_1. This portion indicates the relative importance of X_1. The square root of this quantity $[(b_1{}^2 \sigma^2 x_1)/\sigma^2 y]$ is called the *standard partial regression coefficient* which is a measure of relative importance.

Quadric Regression

The regression model may however be non-linear. In non-linear case, the models are different which may be polynomial, multiplicative, exponential or reciprocal. The second degree polynomial,

$y = a + bX + c X^2$

The best model is evaluated by some criteria like R^2, mean sum of squares due to error, etc.

26.2 Multiple Correlations

The correlation between two variables can also be estimated when the data on more than two variables is available. This is done to remove or eliminate the effect of third and or fourth variable.

26.2.1 Partial Correlation

It is the correlation between two variables (X_1 and X_2) when estimated by eliminating the effect of a third variable (X_3). The effect of third variable is eliminated by keeping it constant. This measures the true relationship between two variables for which it is also called as *net correlation*.

The partial correlations may be of first order or second order depending up on whether the effect of only one variable is held constant or of two variables.

(i) First Order Partial Correlation

It is estimated from the values of simple correlations as under:

$$r_{12.3} = \frac{(r_{12} - r_{13} r_{23})}{\sqrt{(1 - r^2{}_{13})(1 - r^2{}_{23})}}$$

The partial correlation can be estimated from partial regression coefficients as:

$$r_{12.3} = \sqrt{b_{12.3} b_{21.3}}$$

(ii) Second Order Partial Correlation

It is the correlation between two variables (1 and 2) estimated by eliminating the effects of other two variables (3 and 4) as -

$$r_{12.34} = \frac{\left(r_{12.3} - r_{14.3} \, r_{24.3}\right)}{\sqrt{\left[\left(1 - r^2_{14.3}\right)\left(1 - r^2_{24.3}\right)\right]}}$$

$$\text{or} \quad = \frac{\left(r_{12.4} - r_{13.4} \, r_{23.4}\right)}{\sqrt{\left[\left(1 - r^2_{13.4}\right)\left(1 - r^2_{23.4}\right)\right]}}$$

26.2.2 Multiple Correlations

The multiple correlation coefficient measures the joint effect of two or more independent variables $(X_2, X_3 \ldots \ldots$ etc.) on a dependent variable (X_1) and indicates the combined relation between a dependent and a series of independent variables. It is also estimated from simple correlations as:

$$R_{1.23} = \sqrt{\frac{\left(r^2_{12} + r^2_{13} - 2r_{13} \, r_{12} - r_{23}\right)}{\left(1 - r^2_{23}\right)}}$$

Where, $R_{1.23}$ is the multiple correlations

This can also be estimated from first order partial correlations as –

$$R_{1.23} = r^2_{12} + r^2_{13.2}\left(1 - r^2_{12}\right)$$

The R^2 is the coefficient of determination.

The multiple correlations can also be explained as the correlation between the observed values of dependent variable (X_1) and its estimated values(X) for the independent variables estimated from multiple regression equation. Thus, the multiple correlation between Y and X_1, X_2 X, is defined as the simple correlation between Y and its linear regression on $X_1 \ldots Xn$, *i.e.* $b_1X_1 + \ldots\ldots + b_nX_n$. The R is thus the simple correlation between Y and its estimated value, $y = b_1X_1 + \ldots\ldots + b_nX_{n.}$ This gives

$$R = \frac{\left(\sum Y\hat{y}\right)}{\left(\sum y^2\right)\left(\sum \hat{y}^2\right)}$$

Where, y is the estimated value.

The R lies between 0 and 1 and is also numerically not less than any value of r_{12}, $r_{13.2}$, $r_{14.23} \ldots$ etc. R is not less than zero. The R is also given as:

$$R = \frac{\left[b_1 \sum x_1 y + b_2 \sum x_2 y + b_3 \sum x_3 y\right]}{\sum y^2}$$

Where, $\quad x_i = \left(x_i - \overline{x}_i\right)$

$$y = \left(y - \overline{y}\right)$$

26.3 Canonical Variate Analysis

This technique was developed by Hotelling (1935). It is mainly used in one population. The traits are divided in to two sets to evaluate the relationship between these sets. One set is called the predictor characters (X set) and other set is of the criteria or response characters(Y set). The linear combination of criteria characters is obtained that maximally correlated with linear combination of predictor characters. The objective is to know the set of canonical coefficients so that the correlation between two sets is maximum. Such correlation is called *Canonical Correlation*. This technique is used when it is required to predict simultaneously more than one correlated variables.

26.4 Principle Comonent Analysis

This technique was given by Hotelling (1933) using derived variables. This is mainly conducted in single population. This technique was developed keeping in view the correlation among various characters and make these correlated variables as uncorrelated. Thus the principal objective of this technique was to transform the original set of correlated variables in to a new set of uncorrelated variable, called as the *principal components*. The newly derived variables are uncorrelated and are linear combinations of original variables. These principal components are artificial variables and have no physical meaning. It is worth while to mention here that PCA (principal component analysis) is not required if there is no correlation among the original variables.

The principal components are derived in decreasing order of importance in terms of accounting the portion of the variation in the original data. The first variable explain maximum possible variation, the second variable accounts the portion of variation next to the first variable, and so on. These derived variables are formed by specific linear combinations of original variables. A small set of derived variables is constructed from eigen values and eigen vectors of sample correlation or sample covariance matrix. The sample correlation matrix is used to estimate the principal components if the variables have large variation. Second way is to standardize the variables before computing the principal components so that new variables are created which are equally important. The sample covariance matrix is used to compute the principal components from standardized variables. This small set of derived variables summarizes the original data and hence reduces the dimensionality of original data.

The PCA is more useful when the independent variables are highly correlated. The multiple regression analysis is of little use or misleading in case of high correlation. In such case the regression analysis can be conducted after deriving the principal components. This is then called as the principal component regression.

26.5 Discriminant Analysis

Fisher, R.A. (1936) originally developed this technique and used by Smith (1936) to discriminate some of the desirable genotypes from undesirable ones based on their phenotypic performance. This can be used in single population having distinct groups or more populations. Hazel (1943) applied this technique in animal improvement discussing the genetic basis of constructing the selection index, as described in this volume of the book.

This technique is used when there are more numbers of distinct groups or populations and each individual has more than two characters. The different groups of animals are classified as best or poor animals in production performance based on two or more characters, like construction of selection index.

26.6 Genetic Divergent Analysis

This is known as genetic distance analysis given by Mahalanobis, P.C. (1928) and generally known as D^2 analysis. The D^2 is a measure of group distance based on many characters. This technique is used for more populations for classifying different groups in different clusters like the different genetic groups of crossbreds with varying inheritance and putting two or more groups in different clusters based on different characters. The significant differences among groups estimate the genetic distance values (D^2 – values). This is done to know the genetic similarity or dissimilarities among different groups. The detail procedure along with cluster formation (grouping of genotypes in to clusters) with worked example has been described by Singh and Chaudhary (1985) in their book "Biometrical Methods".

26.7 Path Analysis

See next chapter 27.

Chapter 27
Path Analysis

The method of Path coefficient was invented by Sewall Wright (1921). This method subdivides the correlation in a casual scheme and analyses the relative contribution of different causing factors interacting among themselves and ultimately influencing a character. Thus, it is used when the interacting factors are causing variation in the determination of a measured effect. This method is simple and flexible to work out the correlation between relatives and to solve a variety of complex inbreeding problems under various mating systems through a general scheme connecting zygotes and gametes. This method has practical applications in genetics and animal breeding and it gained popularity as a statistical method for cause and effect analysis of correlated variables.

Before discussing the theory of path coefficient, it is better to have the idea of cause-effect relationship, their diagrammatical representation (path diagram) and concept of path coefficient.

27.1 Cause-Effect Relationship

In a biological system, there is a complex relationship among various characters (variables) which are affected by each other directly or indirectly through variation in other characters. For example, milk yield in dairy animals is affected by age and body weight at calving, lactation length, service period etc. While age and body weight at calving are affected by birth weight and gain in weight from birth to maturity. The gain in weight is affected by birth weight, sex of animals etc., whereas the birth weight is affected by early embryonic growth, gestation period etc. The relationship is such that certain characters are causes of variation in others like the variation in early embryonic growth, foetal growth, gestation period etc. causes variation in birth weight while certain pairs of variables are correlated as effects of a certain common causes like milk yield and age at first calving are commonly affected by weight at calving; milk yield and lactation length are commonly affected by age at first calving, body weight at calving, service period etc.

27.1.1. Path Diagram

The cause and effect relationship of related variables can be represented diagrammatically by putting the arrows indicating the direction of effect of the causing factor (s). The arrows connecting the causes and effect in a net work of related variables are called "paths" and the resulting diagram is called "path diagram". The path diagram is used to represent the whole system of related variables showing the cause-effect relationship by single arrows indicating the direction of effect while the correlation is indicated by double sided arrows. Thus, a path diagram is one in which a dependent variable is shown to be represented as completely determined by a number of independent factors (causes) all of which except unknown cause (called residual factor) are represented as inter-correlated. Suppose, a variable (Y) is affected by three factors (X_1, X_2, X_3). These three causing factors are also correlated among themselves. The cause-effect relationship can be shown by a path diagram as under:

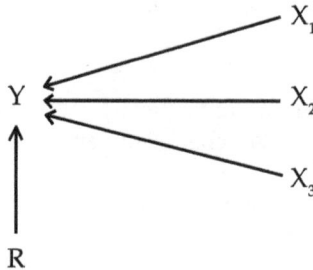

Figure 27.1: Path Diagram Showing Cause-Effect Relationship in a System of Correlated Variables

27.1.2. Assumptions in Path Analysis

The method of path analysis has certain assumptions.

(i) All the relations are linear.

(ii) The path diagram is constructed representing the every variable by arrows as either completely determined by certain factors (causes) which may in turn he represented as similarly determined or as an ultimate factor. Each ultimate factor is shown by double head arrows at both sides to be connected with other ultimate factors to indicate the correlation among them.

(iii) An unknown residual factor denoted by R is taken unless there is a reason to assume that the dependent variable (Y) is completely determined by specified independent variables (X1s)

(iv) The direct effect along a given path is measured by the standard deviation in the dependent variable after all other paths are eliminated (if the variation of other causes are kept constant) while the variation in the dependent variable is kept as great as ever irrespective of its relation with other causes which have been made constant.

27.2 Concept and Definition of Path Coefficient

It is well known that the variation in a causing factor (independent variable) causes the variation in the dependent variable. The amount of the variation in causing factor is reflected in the variation of the dependent variable. For example, body weight in humans is affected by body height. If the variation in body height is more, the variation in body weight will also be more. The variation in the dependent variable (Y) due to one of its causing factor (A) to the extent that A is affecting the dependent variable (Y) directly in a system of related variables when the dependent variable is a linear combination of a number of causing factors (A, B,.) is measured by the path coefficient. Thus path coefficient is a measure of the direct effect (along a given path) of a causing factor in causing the variation in the dependent variable (effect). This is measured by the standard deviation present in the dependent variable after eliminating other paths of effects but the variation in the causing factor (whose effect is measured) is kept as great as ever irrespective of the variation in the causing factor to the other causes which have been made constant.

Mathematically, the path coefficient is defined as the ratio of standard deviation of the effect (dependent variable) due to a given cause (σ_A) to the total standard deviation of the effect (σ_X). The standard deviation of the effect due to a given cause is taken as the standard deviation of that cause and represented as $\sigma_{X:A} = \sigma_A$ if A is the causing factor and X is the effect. Thus path coefficient is (σ_A/σ_X). The concept of path coefficient can be better clear from the following path diagram:

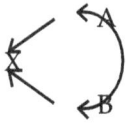

In this system X = A + B and both the causing factors (A and B) are also correlated to each other. The path coefficient for the path from cause A to the effect X is represented as:

$p\,(X \leftarrow A)$ and measured as $\left(\dfrac{\sigma_A}{\sigma_X}\right)$. This can be shown as under-

$$p\,(X \leftarrow A) = p_{X.A}$$

$$= \frac{\sigma_{X:A}}{\sigma_X} = \frac{\sigma_A}{\sigma_X}$$

Similarly, the path coefficient for the second path from second causing factor B to this effect (X) is taken as:

$$p\,(X \leftarrow B) = p_{X.B}$$

$$= \frac{\sigma_{X:B}}{\sigma_X} = \frac{\sigma_B}{\sigma_X}$$

The two path coefficients are further represented by separate small letters correspond-ing to the letters used to denote the causing factors. For example:

$$P_{X.A} = \frac{\sigma_{X.A}}{\sigma_X} = \frac{\sigma_A}{\sigma_X}$$

$$= a$$

$$= \text{path coefficient from A to X}$$

$$P_{X.B} = \frac{\sigma_{X.B}}{\sigma_X} = \frac{\sigma_B}{\sigma_X}$$

$$= b$$

$$= \text{path coefficient from B to X.}$$

In this example, each cause has direct and indirect effect on dependent variable (effect). The cause A affects the dependent variable X directly and indirectly by affecting the second cause B because both causes (A and B) are correlated to each other through some other common cause. Likewise, the cause B affects the dependent variable X directly as well as indirectly through causing variation in A because of their (A and B) relationship. The direct effect of a cause (A, B,.) on the dependent variable measured as the ratio of the standard deviation of the cause to the standard deviation of the effect (*viz.* σ_A/σ_X or σ_A/σ_X, etc.) is called the **path coefficient** for the path connecting cause and effect. There may be any number of path coefficients in a system of correlated variables, their number being equal to the number of causing factors which affect the dependent variable directly.

27.3 Characteristics of Path Coefficient

1. Path Coefficient and Correlation Coefficient

The path coefficient is an absolute number without any physical unit, irrespective of the units of measurement to measure the variables, and thus it is similar to the correlation coefficient. However, the path coefficient differs from correlation coefficient in following respects:

(i) The path coefficient may be greater than unity and may take negative values while the correlation coefficient ranges from -1 to + 1. The path coefficient may be greater than unity because no restriction is imposed on the relative magnitudes of the variance of an effect and a cause. The variance of a cause may be greater than that of the effect and hence some other path coefficient will have to be negative.

(ii) The correlation coefficient is an absolute measure of association between two variables and does not indicate the direction of effect while the path coefficient measures the effect of one variable on the other indicating the direction of the effect depending upon the cause effect relationship.

(iii) The path coefficient may be equal or less than the correlation coefficient. They are equal if the causing factors are uncorrelated but in case there is a relationship among the causing factors the path coefficient, being a measure of the direct effect of the cause on the effect, will be lesser than correlation coefficient because the correlation coefficient constitutes both direct effect and indirect effect of a cause through other correlated causes.

(iv) The path coefficient possess the chain property while the correlation coefficient has the chain property only for the chains of independent causes and not for the chains of common correlated causes. Please refer point (ii) of 27.4 (2) under the title "Tracing connecting paths".

(v) The path coefficient has a direction *viz.* $p_{X.A}$ which means that A is the cause and X is the effect. Thus, it differs from correlation coefficient which has no direction.

(vi) The correlation coefficients may be zero between two variables and yet the path coefficient from one variable to the other is not zero. This can be proved by changing the interrelationship between the variables involved. This change in interrelationship leads to a change in the direction of a path and its value but the correlation coefficient between two variables remains the same irrespective of the direction of the paths.

This principle along with its findings can be illustrated considering the causal scheme X = A + B in which A and B are uncorrelated ($r_{AB} = 0$), have equal standard deviations ($\sigma_A = \sigma_B$) and determine the X completely. Therefore,

$$X = A + B$$

$$\sigma^2_X = \sigma^2_X + \sigma^2_X$$

$$= 2\sigma^2_A = 2\sigma^2_B \text{ since } \sigma_A = \sigma_B$$

$$d_{X.A} = d_{X.B} = \frac{\sigma^2_A}{\sigma^2_X} = \frac{\sigma^2_B}{\sigma^2_X} = \frac{1}{2} \quad \text{because } d_{X.A} + d_{X.B} = 1.0$$

and hence $p_{X.A} = p_{X.B} = \sqrt{a^2} = \sqrt{b^2} = \sqrt{\tfrac{1}{2}} = r_{XA} = r_{XB}$

Now if the interrelationship is changed. This means that if the path diagram is turned around in a way that the cause A is taken as the "effect" being determined by the causes X and B it will be a different view point of the same earlier relationship, as shown in the figure below:

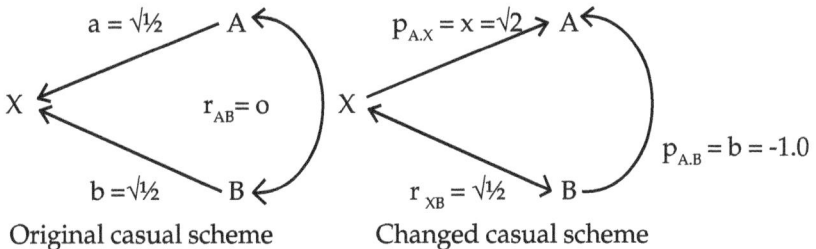

Original casual scheme　　　　　Changed casual scheme

This changed relationship can be mathematically written as:

A = X – B　　with　　$r_{XB} = \sqrt{\tfrac{1}{2}}$

As $\sigma^2_X = \sigma^2_A$, therefore in the new changed casual scheme

$$p_{A.X} = \sqrt{\frac{\sigma^2_x}{\sigma^2_A}} = \sqrt{\frac{2\sigma^2_x}{\sigma^2_A}} = \sqrt{2}$$

Further since $\sigma^2_A = \sigma^2_B$ and $A = X - B$, the value of the path from B to A will he -1 because A and B have negative relation. Therefore, $p_{A.B} = -1$. To verify the above relationship of $\sigma^2_A = \sigma^2_B$ and $A = X - B$ and the negative relationship between A and B.

$$\sigma^2_A = \sigma^2_x - \sigma^2_B$$

$$\frac{\sigma^2_x}{\sigma^2_A} = \frac{\sigma^2_x}{\sigma^2_A} - \frac{\sigma^2_B}{\sigma^2_A}$$

$$1 = d_{A.X} - d_{A.B}$$

Therefore, $\frac{\sigma^2_B}{\sigma^2_A} = d_{A.B} = d_{AX} - 1 = 2 - 1 = 1$. The path coefficient for the path B to A

$(p_{A.B})$ is negative as it takes the negative root of σ^2_B because of negative relation between A and B. Thus, $p_{A.B} = -1.0$

The new values of path coefficients can be verified from the complete determination of dependent variable by its causing factors as:

$$d_{Ax} + d_{AB} + 2 \times b \, r_{XB} = 1.0$$

$$x^2 + b^2 + 2 \times b \, r_{XB} = 1.0$$

$$2 + (-1)^2 + 2(\sqrt{2})(-1)(\sqrt{\frac{1}{2}}) = 1.0$$

$$3 + 2(\sqrt{2\frac{1}{2}})(-1) = 1.0$$

$$3 - 2 = 1.0$$

Therefore, it is proved that the correlation coefficient between two variables may be zero ($r_{AB} = 0$) and yet the path coefficient from one variables (B) to the other (A) is not zero ($p_{A.B} \neq 0$). It was also clear that the values of the reverse paths due to a change in causal scheme ($P_{X.A}$ and $P_{A.X}$) are not equal (in general) but the correlation coefficient between two variables remains the same irrespective of the direction of paths. This emphasize the importance of the formulation of casual scheme which must be adequate, complete and consistent to get valid results otherwise the values of path coefficients will be erroneous and misleading.

(*See numerical example 27.1*)

2. Path Coefficient and Regression Coefficient

The path coefficient is similar to regression coefficient which is also directional. However, they differ in the sense that physical units are attached with regression coefficient while path coefficient is without physical units.

3. Path Coefficient Equals the Standardized Regression Coefficient

The path coefficient is equivalent to the standardized regression coefficient

$\left(b_{YX}\dfrac{\sigma_X}{\sigma_Y}\right)$ which is obtained by standardizing the variables rather than to variables in original physical units. The example of regression of breeding value (A) on phenotypic value (P) can be taken here

$$b_{AP} = \frac{\text{Cov}_{AP}}{\sigma^2_P}$$

$$= \frac{\text{Cov}_{AP}}{\sigma^2_P}\frac{\sigma_P}{\sigma_A} \quad \text{(after standardizing the variables)}$$

This is because the best estimate of an individuals breeding value (A) is equal to the product of its phenotypic value and h^2 as:

$A = h^2.P$

$= b_{AP}P \quad (\text{Since } h^2 = b_{AP})$

Now, reckoning the A and P as deviation from population mean, the regression equation becomes as:

$$\left(A-\overline{A}\right)= b_{AP}\left(P-\overline{P}\right)$$

and standardizing both the variables it becomes

$$\frac{\left(A-\overline{A}\right)}{\sigma_A} = b_{AP}\frac{P-\overline{P}}{\sigma_P}\frac{\sigma_P}{\sigma_A}$$

The standardization means to divide the variable by its standard deviation. Thus both the variables taken as deviation from population mean were divided by their respective standard deviation and to balance the equation the right hand side was multiplied by the factor σ_P/σ_A. The quantity $b_{AP}(\sigma_P/\sigma_A)$ is called the standardized regression coefficient which on further solving is equal to r_{AP} and $p_{P.A}$ (path coefficient). This has been shown below:

$$\frac{\text{Cov}_{AP}}{\sigma^2_P}\frac{\sigma_P}{\sigma_A} \qquad = \frac{\sigma_{AP}}{\sigma_P\sigma_P}\frac{\sigma_B}{\sigma_A}$$

$$= \frac{\sigma_{AP}}{\sigma_A\sigma_P} = r_{AP}$$

$$\text{Now, } \frac{\sigma_{AP}}{\sigma_A\sigma_P} \qquad = \frac{\sigma^2_A}{\sigma_A\sigma_P} \qquad \text{since } \sigma_{AP} = \sigma^2_A$$

$$= \frac{\sigma_A}{\sigma_P} = \sigma_{P.A}$$

Therefore, the *standardized regression coefficient* $b_{AP} \dfrac{\sigma_P}{\sigma_A}$ is equal to the path coefficient ($p_{P.A}$) for independent causes. The path coefficient in this sense is called a standardized linear regression coefficient. The linear regression coefficient worked out with standardized variables (*standardized regression coefficient*) is equal to the correlation coefficient between two variables.

It should be emphasized that the standardized partial regression coefficients are used as measures of relative importance of independent causes (x) in causing variation in the dependent variable (Y). The estimate $[b_{YX}\, \sigma_X/\sigma_Y]$ is the standardized regression coefficient which estimates the change in Y as a fraction of σ_Y produced by one standard deviation change in X. This is in confirmation of the definition of path coefficient.

The quantity $b_{YX}\, \sigma_X$ is taken as the standard deviation of Y due to the influence of X. Thus $b_{YX}\, \sigma_X = \sigma_{Y.X} = \sigma_X$. This is also because the standardized regression coefficient

$$\left(b_{YX} \frac{\sigma_X}{\sigma_Y}\right) = P_{Y.X} = \frac{\sigma_X}{\sigma_Y}$$ and hence $b_{YX}\, \sigma_X$ is regarded as the standard deviation of Y due

to the influence of X.

27.4 Precautions to Use Path Coefficient Analysis

1. *Formulation of causal scheme*: The importance of the formulation of a causal scheme to be adequate, complete and consistent has been discussed under point (vi) of 1 of section 27.3

2. *Tracing connecting paths*: This is an important aspect of practical use of path coefficient being governed by certain rules. This is preliminary process required to calculate the total correlation between two variables. This is because the total correlation is the sum of all the paths connecting the two variables in a causal scheme.

   (i) The correct method of tracing a connecting path is the first backward and then forward motion. First forward and then backward motion in tracing any connecting path is not allowed. This is shown diagrammatically with correct connecting paths below:

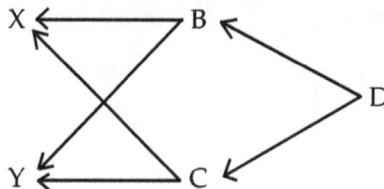

Correct paths are:

X-B-Y, and X-C-Y, these are two connecting paths if B and C are independent

X-B-C-Y is a connecting path between X and Y when B and C are correlated.

X-C-D-B-Y is a connecting path in a chain of variables.

(ii) The correlation between two causing factors is a two way path being used in either direction and shown by a line with arrow on both sides. A precaution is required to use such a line when there are a number of causing factors which are correlated in a chain fashion. The path coefficient has a chain property in the sense that in a system such as A —— B —— C in which A and C are connected by a path whose coefficient is equal to the product of the two single step path coefficient *viz.* $p_{C.A} = p_{C.B} \, p_{B.A}$. On the other hand, the correlation does not possess the chain property of path coefficient in a system such as A—— B —— C in which A and B are correlated, B and C are correlated, it is not necessary that A and C will also be correlated. This is shown below in which A is correlated with B and B with C but A and C may be independent or correlated and their correlation (r_{AC}) may not be equal to $r_{AB} \cdot r_{BC}$ It is important here to indicate the correlation between A and C by a separate correlation line like A —— C and indicating the value of r_{AC} which may not be equal to $r_{AB} \cdot r_{BC}$.

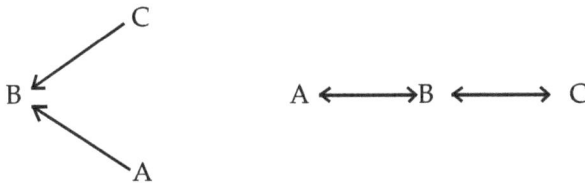

27.5 Practical Applications of Path Coefficient

The theory of path coefficient is useful particularly when correlations take negative values due to difficulties in the probability concept. Wright (1922) extended this theory to elaborate the concepts of inbreeding coefficients and coefficients of relationship. The theory of path coefficient is entirely different technique which has proved extremely effective for a number of problems in theoretical genetics and for practical applications in animal breeding as well as in the statistical analysis of cause and effect relationship in a system of correlated variables to estimate the direct effect of a cause, its indirect effect via other variables, and residual effect due to the remaining unknown cause contributing to the total variation of dependable variable. It is useful in finding out the correlation between relatives and in solving a wide variety of inbreeding problems of more complex nature.

The economic traits of farm animals are related to each other through a number of ways known as causal schemes. The aim of animal breeder is to know the relative contribution of different causing factors in the determination of a variable and to study the relative importance of different factors (in respect of their direct and indirect effect via other causing factors) responsible to cause association between two effects through analysis of variance or regression analysis, one could know the relative importance of different causing factors in the variation of an effect. However, partitioning of the direct and indirect effect of different causing factors can only be analyzed with the help of the theory of path coefficient.

The theory of path coefficient is useful for the analysis of quantitative traits in the following two ways:

(1) Complete determination of a variables determined by independent or correlated causes,

(2) Total correlation between two variables with two or more common independent or correlated causes:

27.5.1 Theory of Complete Determination of a Variable

A dependent variable (effect) is determined by a number of causing factors (causes). These causing factors may be independent to each other (uncorrelated/ independent causes) or correlated (correlated causes). Further each causing factor may be affected by a number of other factors which are not correlated to each other forming a chain of independent causes.

Certain common independent causes may also cause correlation between two effects (common causes and correlation). Secondly, there may be a situation in which the causes themselves are correlated and causing the variation in the effect, referred to as correlated causes.

(i) Complete Determination of a Variable (Effect) by Independent Causes

Correlation between breeding value and phenotypic value:

Such a relationship exists when a dependent variable is completely deter-mined by two or more uncorrelated causes *viz.* the phenotypic value (P) is determined by the breeding value (A) and the remainder part (R). The R includes the non additive effects of genes as well as the environmental effects. The two component parts (A and R) of the phenotypic value are uncorrelated such that

$$P = A+R$$

$$\sigma^2_P = \sigma^2_A + \sigma^2_R + 2 \text{ Cov}_{AR}$$

$$= \sigma^2_A + \sigma^2_R + 2 \text{ r}_{AR} \sigma_A \sigma_R$$

$$= \sigma^2_A + \sigma^2_R \qquad \text{Since A and R are uncorrelated.}$$

The path diagram will take the form as:

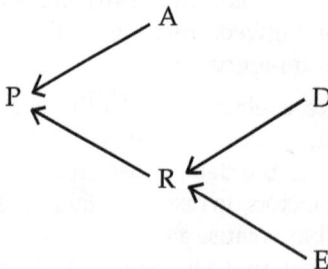

In this case, $\text{Cov}_{AR} = 0$, $\text{Cov}_{PA} = \sigma^2_A$, and $\text{Cov}_{PR} = \sigma^2_R$

Therefore,
$$r_{PA} = \frac{Cov_{PA}}{\sigma_A \sigma_P} = \frac{\sigma^2_A}{\sigma_A \sigma_P} = \frac{\sigma_A}{\sigma_P} = P_{P.A}$$

and
$$r_{PR} = \frac{Cov_{PR}}{\sigma_A \sigma_R} = \frac{\sigma^2_A}{\sigma_A \sigma_R} = \frac{\sigma_A}{\sigma_R} = P_{P.R}$$

It is thus obvious to see that the correlation coefficient between breeding value and phenotypic value (r_{AP}) is equal to the path coefficient for the path from

A to P: $P_{P.A} = \dfrac{\sigma_A}{\sigma_P}$.

Therefore, in case of independent causes the correlation coefficient and path coefficient are equal.

$$P_{P.A} = r_{PA} \text{ and } r^2_{PA} = \frac{\sigma^2_A}{\sigma^2_P} = d_{PA}$$

$$P_{P.R} = r_{PR} \text{ and } r^2_{PR} = \frac{\sigma^2_A}{\sigma^2_R} = d_{PR}$$

The degree to which the variation of phenotypic value (p) is determined by breeding value (A) is $d_{PA} = \sigma^2_A/\sigma^2_P$ and therefore it is confirming the complete determination of a variable as:

$$d_{PA} + d_{PR} = \frac{\sigma^2_A}{\sigma^2_P} + \frac{\sigma^2_A}{\sigma^2_R} = 1.0$$

The above expressions can thus be written as:

$$\sqrt{d_{P.A}} = P_{P.A} = r_{PA} = \frac{\sigma_A}{\sigma_P}$$

$$\sqrt{d_{P.R}} = P_{P.R} = r_{PR} = \frac{\sigma_A}{\sigma_R}$$

(See numerical example 27.2)

The relationship between path coefficient, correlation coefficient and coef-ficient of determination holds true if the dependent variable (effect) is a linear combination of more than two causing factors which are independent to each other. In this situation the deviations of dependent variable are additive indicating that a given amount of change in one causing factor is reflected in the effect (dependent variable), irrespective of its own value of other causes.

Chains of Independent Causing Factors

P = G + E and G = A + D

The path coefficient has a chain property in a chain system of cause- effect relationship of independent causes. In such a relationship the effect is caused by all the ultimate independent variables. This can be understood by taking the components of phenotypic value (P) as genotypic value (CI) and environmental deviation (E) and in turn G is determined by breeding value (A) and dominance deviation (D). Thus the relationship is equivalent to have 3 independent causes of the effect, P. Therefore,

$$P = G + E$$
$$= A + D + E \text{ Since } G = A + D$$

Thus $\quad \sigma^2_P \quad = \sigma^2_G + \sigma^2_E$

$$= \sigma^2_A + \sigma^2_D + \sigma^2_E$$

The chain of independent causes satisfying the above relations can be shown by the following figure:

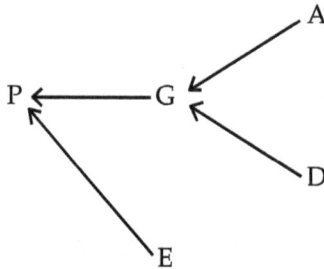

Figure 27.2: Chain of Independent Causes.

The phenotypic value (P) will be completely determined by:

$$P = d_{P.G} + d_{P.E}$$
$$= d_{P.A} + d_{P.D} + d_{P.E}$$

The genotypic value (G) will be completely determined by:

$$G = d_{G.A} + d_{G.D}$$

Now, based on the theorem of complete determination of a variable by two or more independent causes, the following relations will be used to get $d_{P.A}$ and $d_{P.D}$

$$d_{P.G} = \sigma^2_G / \sigma^2_P;$$
$$d_{G.A} = \sigma^2_A / \sigma^2_G; \text{ and}$$
$$d_{P.A} = \sigma^2_A / \sigma^2_P;$$

Therefore, $d_{P.A} = \sigma^2_A / \sigma^2_P$ can be obtained by multiplying $d_{P.G}$ with d_{GA} as:

$$d_{P.A} \quad = d_{P.G} \, d_{G.A}$$

$$= \frac{\sigma^2_G \, \sigma^2_A}{\sigma^2_P \, \sigma^2_G}$$

$$= \frac{\sigma^2_A}{\sigma^2_P}$$

Likewise, $d_{P.D}$ can also be obtained by multiplying $d_{P.G}$ with $d_{G.D}$ as:

$$d_{P.D} = d_{P.G}\, d_{G.D}$$

$$= \frac{\sigma^2_G\; \sigma^2_D}{\sigma^2_P\; \sigma^2_G}$$

$$= \frac{\sigma^2_D}{\sigma^2_P}$$

From the above relation of coefficients of determination, the combined path coefficients for a path connecting an effect with a remote cause through intermediate cause (s) along the connecting path can be obtained as:

$$P_{P.A} = P_{P.G}\, P_{G.A} = \frac{\sigma_G\, \sigma_A}{\sigma_P\, \sigma_G}$$

$$= \frac{\sigma_A}{\sigma_P}$$

$$P_{P.D} = P_{P.G}\, P_{G.D} = \frac{\sigma_G\, \sigma_D}{\sigma_P\, \sigma_G}$$

$$= \frac{\sigma_D}{\sigma_P}$$

Further, in case of independent causes affecting a dependent variable, the correlation coefficient is equal to path coefficient. Therefore

$$r_{PA} = P_{P.A} = P_{P.G}\, P_{G.A}$$

$$= r_{PG}\, r_{GA}$$

$$r_{PD} = P_{P.G} = P_{P.G}\, P_{G.D}$$

$$= r_{PG}\, r_{GD}$$

Therefore, the combined path coefficient for the path connecting an effect with a remote cause (through intermediate causes) equals the products of the individual path coefficient along the connecting path. Similar are the combined correlation coefficient and the combined coefficient of determination.

(*See numerical example 27.3*)

(ii) Complete Determination of a Variable by Correlated Cause

The correlated causing factors may be two or more to cause the variation in a dependent variable (effect).

(a) Two Correlated Causing Factors

The dependent variable (effect) may be affected by two causing factors which may be correlated to each other. Let Y be a dependent variable being affected by two correlated variables (A and B). The causal scheme and the path diagram will be as given below:

Causal scheme: X = A + B, where the causing factors (A and B) are correlated.

Path diagram:

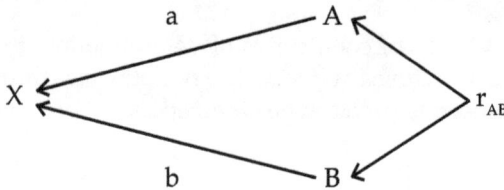

Figure 27.3: Two Correlated Causes.

In this situation of correlated causes (A and B) influencing the dependent variable (X), the path coefficient ($P_{X.A}$) and correlation coefficient between X and A (r_{XA}) will not be equal but the r_{XA} will be greater/lesser than $p_{X.A}$. The reason is that the causing factor A affects the dependent variable (X) directly through the path A to X plus indirectly (by affecting the second cause, B) through the path A $\leftrightarrow$ B $\rightarrow$ X. The correlation between A and B will reduce the σ^2_A equal to $\sigma^2_A r^2_{AB}$ when the variable B is kept constant. Thus, σ^2_A will be reduced to $\sigma^2_A (1 - r^2_{AB})$. Thus the total correlation between X and A can be partitioned into *direct effect* and *indirect effect* through other variable (B) as explained here:

The complete determination of X affected by causes (A and B) can be obtained by partitioning the correlation between A and X (r_{XA}) as:

$$r_{XA} = \frac{Cov_{AX}}{\sigma_A \sigma_X}$$

$$= \frac{\left|Cov_{A(A+B)}\right|}{\sigma_A \sigma_X} \qquad \text{Since } X=A+B$$

$$= \frac{Cov_{AA}}{\sigma_A \sigma_X} + \frac{Cov_{AB}}{\sigma_A \sigma_X}$$

$$= \frac{\sigma^2_A}{\sigma_A \sigma_X} + \frac{r_{AB} \sigma_A \sigma_B}{\sigma_A \sigma_X} \qquad \text{Since } Cov_{AB} = \gamma_{AB} \sigma_A \sigma_B$$

$$= \frac{\sigma_A}{\sigma_X} + r_{AB}\left(\frac{\sigma_B}{\sigma_X}\right)$$

$$= a + r_{AB} b$$

Where, $a = \dfrac{\sigma_A}{\sigma_X}$ = path coefficient from A to X

$b = \dfrac{\sigma_B}{\sigma_X}$ = path coefficient from B to X

The above equation of correlation (r_{XA}) has thus two parts *viz.*

(a) *Direct effect:* It is equal to "a" which is the path coefficient from A to X and

(b) *Indirect effect:* This is equal to $r_{AB}\, b$ which is the correlation between two variables (r_{AB}) times the path coefficient (b) via other variable (B).

Similarly, the correlation between X and B (r_{XB}) can also be partitioned as:

$r_{XB} = b + r_{AB}\, a$

Thus, the general relationship between a dependent and an independent variable can be written as:

$r_{iX} = P_{X.i} + P_{X.j}\, r_{ij}$

$\qquad = a + b\, r_{ij}$

Total correlation = Direct effect + indirect effect

The following two simultaneous equations are obtained

$r_{XA} = a + r_{AB}\, b$

$r_{XB} = b + r_{AB}\, a$

These simultaneous equations are solved to get the values of different path coefficient either directly, or by elimination method or by matrix method.

(II) More than Two Correlated Causing Factors

The dependent variable (effect) may be affected by more than two causing factors which may be correlated to each other. Let Y be a dependent variable (effect-say milk yield) being affected by three correlated variables (X_1, X_2, X_3) plus unknown cause denoted by R. The causal scheme and the path diagram will be as given below:

Causal Scheme

$Y = X_1 + X_2 + X_3 + R$

Path Diagram

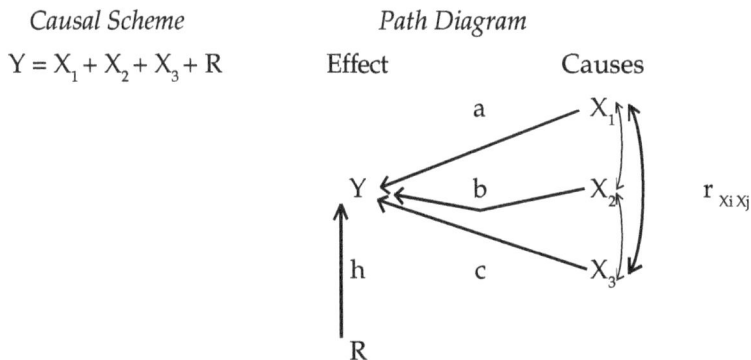

Figure 27.4: More than two Correlated Causes.

The **first step** is to estimate the correlation coefficients of dependent variable with all the cause variables (A vector), and correlation coefficients (taking two cause variables at a time) among all the cause variables which form the B matrix.

The correlation coefficient between cause variable (X_1) and effect variable (Y) is estimated as:

$$r_{X1Y} = \frac{Cov_{(X1,Y)}}{\sigma_{X1}\sigma_Y}$$

$$= \frac{Cov[X_1(X_1 + X_2 + X_3 + R)]}{\sigma_{X1}\sigma_Y}$$

$$= \frac{Cov_{X1X1}}{\sigma_{X1}\sigma_Y} + \frac{Cov_{X1X2}}{\sigma_{X1}\sigma_Y} + \frac{Cov_{X1X3}}{\sigma_{X1}\sigma_Y} + \frac{Cov_{X1R}}{\sigma_{X1}\sigma_Y}$$

Now, $Cov_{X1X1} = V_{(X1)};$ $\quad Cov_{X1R} = 0;$ $\quad Cov_{X1X2} = r_{(X1X2)}\sigma_{X1}\sigma_{X2}$

Thus, the equation becomes:

$$r_{X1Y} = \frac{\sigma^2_{X1}}{\sigma_{X1}\sigma_Y} + \frac{\left[r_{(X1X2)}\sigma_{X1}\sigma_{X2}\right]}{\sigma_{X1}\sigma_Y} + \frac{\left[r_{(X1X3)}\sigma_{X1}\sigma_{X3}\right]}{\sigma_{X1}\sigma_Y}$$

$$= \frac{\sigma_{X1}}{\sigma_Y} + \frac{r_{(X1X2)}\sigma_{X2}}{\sigma_Y} + \frac{r_{(X1X3)}\sigma_{X3}}{\sigma_Y}$$

$$= a + r_{(X1X2)}b + r_{(X1X3)}c$$

Where, $\quad a = \dfrac{\sigma_{X1}}{\sigma_Y}$, path coefficient from X_1 to $Y = p_{Y.X1}$

$$b = \frac{\sigma_{X2}}{\sigma_Y}, \text{ path coefficient from } X_2 \text{ to } Y = p_{Y.X2}$$

$$c = \frac{\sigma_{X3}}{\sigma_Y}, \text{ path coefficient from } X_3 \text{ to } Y = p_{Y.X3}$$

The total effect is partitioned into:

(i) Direct effect of $X_1 = \sigma_{X1}/\sigma_Y = a$

(ii) Indirect effect of X_1 via other causes:

Indirect effect of X_1 via $X_2 = r_{(X1X2)}b$

Indirect effect of X_1 via $X_3 = r_{(X1X3)}c$

Similarly, the correlation coefficients of effect variable (Y) with other cause variables $(X_2$ and $X_3)$ are also estimated. The subset of equations become as:

$$r_{X1Y} = a + r_{(X1X2)}b + r_{(X1X3)}c$$

$$r_{X2Y} = r_{(X1X2)}a + b + r_{(X2X3)}c$$

$$r_{X3Y} = r_{(X1X3)}a + r_{(X2X3)}b + c$$

$$r_{RY} = h$$

The **second step** is to get the solution of C vector (path coefficients) by matrix method after setting the simultaneous equations equal to the number of causing factors as:

$$
\begin{matrix} A & B & C \end{matrix}
$$

$$
\begin{bmatrix} r_{X1Y} \\ r_{X2Y} \\ r_{X3Y} \end{bmatrix} = \begin{bmatrix} r_{X1X1} & r_{X2X1} & r_{X3X1} \\ r_{X1X2} & r_{X2X2} & r_{X3X2} \\ r_{X1X3} & r_{X2X3} & r_{X3X3} \end{bmatrix} \begin{bmatrix} a \\ b \\ c \end{bmatrix}
$$

In matrix form, the equations can be written as:

A = B.C

Where,   A = Vector of correlation coefficients of dependent (effect) variable with all independent (cause) variables,

B = Matrix of correlation coefficients among all the cause variables

C = Vector of path coefficients equal to the number of cause variables.

$$C = AB^{-1}$$

The **third step** is to determine the residual effect (R) after obtaining the values of C vector. The effect of residual factor (R) is obtained as:

$$\sigma^2_X = \sigma^2_A + \sigma^2_B + 2\,r_{AB}\,\sigma_A\sigma_B$$

$$\frac{\sigma^2_X}{\sigma^2_X} = \frac{\sigma^2_A}{\sigma^2_X} + \frac{\sigma^2_B}{\sigma^2_X} + \frac{2r_{AB}\,\sigma_A\,\sigma_B}{\sigma^2_X}$$

$$1.0 = a^2 + b^2 + 2\,r_{AB}\,a\,b$$

$$1.0 = a^2 + b^2 + c^2 + h^2 + 2\,r_{X1X2}\,ab + 2\,r_{X1X3}\,ac + 2\,r_{X2X3}\,bc$$

$$h^2 = 1.0 - [a^2 + b^2 + c^2 + 2\,r_{X1X2}\,ab + 2\,r_{X1X3}\,ac + 2\,r_{X2X3}\,bc]$$

Thus, the value of h^2 is derived which equals to residual effect of all those factors which were not included in the model.

The direct and indirect effects of different causes can be obtained by estimating the values of path coefficients and their correlations times the path coefficient through other cause as obtained for two causes above. Thus,

$$Y = X_1 + X_2 + X_3 + R$$

$$\sigma^2_Y = \sigma^2_{X1} + \sigma^2_{X2} + \sigma^2_{X3} + \sigma^2_R + 2\,r_{X1X2}\,\sigma_{X1}\sigma_{X2} + 2\,r_{X1X3}\,\sigma_{X1}\sigma_{X3} + 2\,r_{X2X3}\,\sigma_{X2}\sigma_{X3}$$

Now dividing both sides of above equation with σ^2_Y will yield as under -

$$1 = a^2 + b^2 + c^2 + h^2 + 2\,r_{X1X2}\,ab + 2\,r_{X1X3}\,ac + 2\,r_{X2X3}\,bc$$

The values of a, b, and c are the path coefficients due to respective variables and whose values may be obtained directly from the ratio of their standard deviation or by setting the simultaneous equations to get the values of path coefficients which can be obtained either by elimination procedure or by matrix method.

Extension of the Theorem

The theorem of complete determination of a variable by correlated causes can be extended in two ways:

   (i) taking the effect of a common cause of correlated variables

  (ii) taking some more remote causes other than the correlated causes and assuming that the remote causes are independent of each other omitting the intermediate causes.

The first and the second type of relationship of the extension of theorem can be diagramed into the following path diagram.

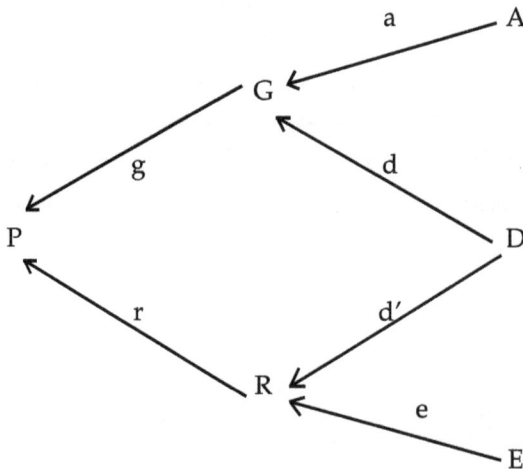

Figure 27.5: Correlated Causes.

In the first scheme, the D is the common cause of correlated variables (causes) G and R. Thus two common causes, G and R, are correlated to each other through common cause D. Therefore, the coefficient of determination of P by G and R taking the effect of D will be estimated as under

$$P = G + R$$

$$\sigma^2_P = \sigma^2_G + \sigma^2_R + 2\,\text{Cov}_{GR}$$

$$= \sigma^2_G + \sigma^2_R + 2\,r_{GR}\sigma_G\sigma_R$$

$$1.0 = g^2 + r^2 + 2\,r_{GR}\,g\,r$$

$$= d_{P.G} + d_{P.R} + d_{P.GR}$$

It will be seen in subsequent section on the theory of total correlation that r_{GR} = $P_{G.D} P_{R.D}$ = dd'. Therefore, the complete determination of an effect by correlated causes will be as under -

$$P = d_{P.G} + d_{P.R} + d_{P.GR}$$
$$= g^2 + r^2 + 2\,g\,r\,d\,d'$$

Thus, the variation in common cause of correlated variables is known, the correlation between the correlated causes can be obtained in terms of the path coefficients by the cross product of the two path coefficients for the paths connecting the two correlated variables to their common cause.

In the second scheme, the effect P is considered as a linear combination of independent causes A, D, E, if omit the intermediate variables (G and R) from the causal scheme. However, the cause D is connected with P through two paths (G and R). Thus it is important to find the value of the path from D to P considering intermediate individual steps.

Since, A, D, E are independent of each other, so

$$d_{P.D} + d_{P.A} + d_{P.E} = 1.0$$
$$d_{G.A} + d_{G.D} = 1.0$$
$$d_{R.E} + d_{R.D} = 1.0$$

According to the theorem of chains of independent cause

$$d_{P.G} = d_{P.G} (d_{G.A} + d_{G.D})$$
$$= d_{P.A} + d_{P.G} d_{G.D}$$
$$d_{P.R} = d_{P.R} (d_{R.E} + d_{R.D})$$
$$= d_{P.E} + d_{P.R} d_{R.D}$$

The coefficient of determination of P by D ($d_{P.D}$) may be obtained from $P_{P.D}$ = gd + rd' as:

$$d_{P.G} = d_{P.R} + d_{P.GR} \quad = (d_{P.D} + d_{P.A}) + d_{P.E} = 1$$

Therefore, $d_{P.D}$
$$= (d_{P.G} + d_{P.R} + d_{P.GR}) - d_{P.A} - d_{P.E}$$
$$= d_{P.G} d_{G.D} + d_{P.R} d_{R.D} + d_{P.GR}$$
$$= g^2 d^2 + r^2 d'^2 + 2\,gdd'$$

It can further be seen that D is independent of A and E, hence

$$P_{P.D} = r_{PD} = gd + rd'$$
$$= d_{P.G} d_{G.D} + d_{P.R} d_{R.D}$$

The value of $d_{P.D}$ (coefficient of determination of P by D) can also be obtained as:

$$d_{P.D} = (d_{P.D})^2$$
$$= (gd + rd')^2 = g^2 d^2 + r^2 d'^2 + 2\,gd\,rd'$$
$$= d_{P.G} d_{G.D} + d_{P.R} d_{R.D} + d_{P.GR}$$

27.5.2 Theory of Total Correlation of Two Variables

The two effects (dependent variables) may be affected either by a single common cause or by two common causes which in turn may be independent or correlated among them. Thus there are a number of causal schemes and some of them have been given here. It is of interest and useful in animal breeding to find the correlation between two variables *e.g.* computing the correlation between relatives which are related through their common ancestors. The correlation between two variables can be estimated in terms of path coefficients from their common causes.

(i) Single Common Cause Affecting Two Variables

Consider two effects (dependent variables) designated as X and Y which are commonly affected by the variable B, plus affected separately by A and D respectively. The path diagram of this causal scheme will take the following form similar to the pedigree of half sibs (X and Y) with common parent B.

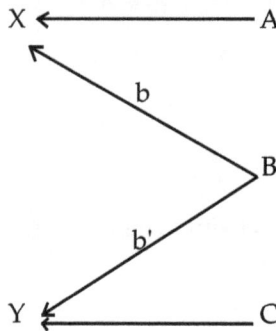

Figure 27.6: Single common cause affecting two variables.

Thus, all the three causes (A, B, C) are independent to each other. The effect X is influenced by A and B while other effect Y is influenced by B and C. Therefore, both X and Y variables are affected by B in common.

This path diagram showing the relationship between X and Y through one common cause (B) is identical to the pedigree of half sibs (X and Y) having B as their common parent and their second parents as A and C respectively which do not contribute common genes to X and Y. Therefore, A and C do not contribute to the correlation between X and Y (r_{XY}).

The path coefficients are denoted by the small letters corresponding to the causes. Thus in this cause-effect relationship, the path coefficient for the path from A to X is: $p(X \leftarrow A) = p_{X.A} = a$. The path coefficient for the other effect is designated by primed small letter and thus $p(Y \leftarrow B) = P_{Y.B} = b'$.

The path coefficient is a measure of the direct effect along a given path of a causing factor (cause) in causing variation in the dependent variable (effect). In this scheme the common cause (B) is affecting both dependent variables (X and Y) and hence causing similarity between them. The extent to which B is influencing two effects (X and Y) are two independent event and hence the combined effect of B, responsible for causing relationship between X and Y, will be obtained by multiplying the separate effect of B to influence X and Y. Therefore, r_{XY} will be obtained as:

$$r_{XY} = b\,b' = P_{X.B}\,P_{Y.B}$$

$$= \frac{\sigma_B}{\sigma_X}\,\frac{\sigma_B}{\sigma_Y}$$

$$= r_{XB}\,r'_{YB}$$

Therefore, the total correlation between two effects is equal to the product of the path coefficients connecting the two effects with the common cause:

(ii) Two Common Independent Causes

The two effects (Say X and Y) may be affected by two common causes which are not correlated.

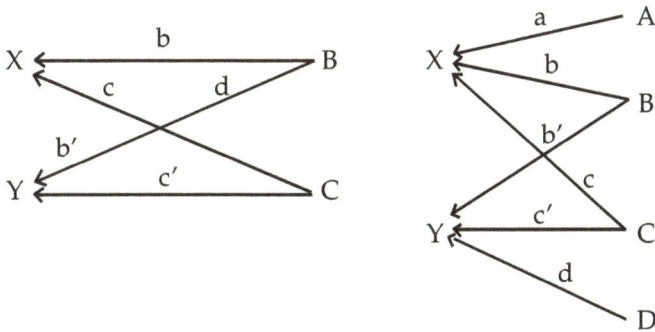

Figure 27.7: Two Common Independent Causes Affecting Two Variables.

This is identical to the pedigree of two full sibs (X and Y) with both parents (B and C) as common. Thus r_{xy} will represent the correlation between two full sibs. The two effects (X and Y) are commonly affected by B and C. Besides this, the two effects may also be affected by some other variables which do not affect the two effects commonly:

In this case, obviously A and D do not contribute to r_{xy} at all. Therefore, a and d' need not to compute. Two effects (X and Y) are correlated through two common causes (B and C). The correlation between X and Y (r_{xy}) due to B is equal to bb' and due to C is equal to cc'. Therefore, the total correlation through two common causes will be

$$r_{XY} = bb' + cc'$$

Therefore, the total correlation between two effects is equal to the sum of the products of the pairs of path coefficients connecting the two effects with each common cause when the causes are uncorrelated.

(iii) Two Common Correlated Causes

When two common causes are correlated and affecting the two effects, the path diagram can be drawn as under:

This path diagram is identical to the pedigree of two full sibs (X and Y) whose parents (B and C) are relatives.

In a biological system two variables (characters) besides being affected by common causes may be affected by some other causes which are not common to the two effects. The path diagrams then can be drawn as: A

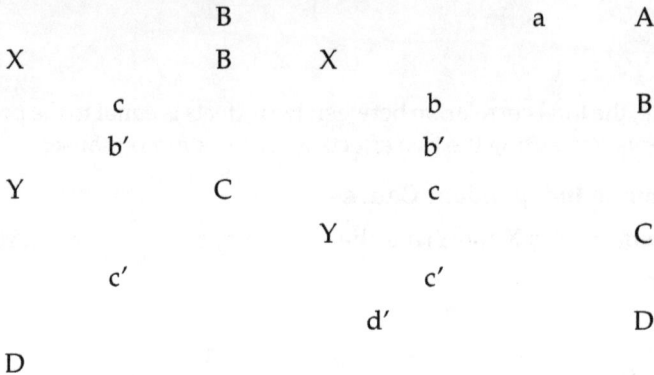

Figure 27.8: Two Common Correlated Causes Affecting Two Variables.

However, A and D are not contributing to r_{XY}.

The $r_{XY} = bb' + cc'$ when B and C are not correlated. But when B and C are correlated, the r_{XY} will be increased and will be higher than bb' + cc'. This is because the common causes (B and C) are more similar being correlated and hence they will increase r_{XY}. The r_{XY} can then be computed as under -

$$r_{XY} = bb' + cc' + bc'\, r_{BC} + b'c\, r_{BC}$$

Thus the correlation between two variables is the sum of the products of the chains of individual path coefficients along all the paths by which they are related.

Solved Examples and Exercises

Example 27.1

The principle of the difference between correlation coefficient and path coefficient can be numerically illustrated from the values of the example No. 25.1 for calving interval which is the sum of service period and gestation period. Which of the two causal scheme is adequate?:

Original Scheme	Changed scheme
CI = S.P. + G.P.	SP = C.I. – G.P.

P_{CS} · SP P_{SC} · SP

CI $r_{SG} = 0$ CI $P_{SG} = -0.2441$

$\quad$ GP $\quad$ GP

P_{CG} r_{CS}

Solution

Original scheme: (C.I.=S.P.+G.P.)

$$1.0 = d_{C.S} + d_{C.G} + 2 \, c \, g \, r_{CG}$$
$$= 0.9438 + 0.0563 = 1.0001 \qquad \text{since } r_{SG} = 0.0$$

Revised scheme: (S.P.=C.I.–G.P.)

$$1.0 = d_{S.C} + d_{S.G} + 2 \, c \, g \, r_{CG}$$
$$= 1.0596 + 0.0596 - 2 \,(1.0294)\,(- 0.2441)\,(0.2372)$$
$$= 1.1192 - 0.1192 = 1.00$$

In this example the revised causal scheme is not adequate and consistent. Thus, it will lead to misleading values of path coefficients. Therefore, the causal scheme must be adequate and complete.

Example 27.2

Verify that the correlation coefficient and path coefficients are equal in case of independent causes from the following example assuming

$$P = A + R \text{ and } Cov_{AR} = 0$$

	Values								Total	Mean	C.S.S.
A	43	34	28	31	28	37	17	6	224	28.0	956
R	7	16	19	9	15	4	12	6	88	11.0	200
P	50	50	47	40	43	41	39	12	312	39.0	1156

Solution

$$Cov_{PA} = \frac{\sum PA - \dfrac{\sum A \sum P}{N}}{N} = \frac{(9692 - 8736)}{8} = 119.5$$

$$Cov_{AR} = \frac{\sum AR - \dfrac{\sum A \sum R}{N}}{N} = \frac{(2464 - 2466)}{8} = 0.0$$

$$\sigma^2_A = \frac{956}{8} = 119.5 \text{ and } \sigma_A = 10.9$$

$$\sigma^2_R = \frac{200}{8} = 25 \text{ and } \sigma_A = 5$$

$$\sigma^2_P = \frac{1156}{8} = 144.5 \text{ and } \sigma_A = 12.02$$

$$r_{PA} = \frac{Cov_{AP}}{\sigma_A \sigma_P} = \frac{\sigma^2_A}{\sigma_P \sigma_A} = \frac{\sigma_A}{\sigma_P} = P_{PA}$$

$$r^2_{PA} = d_{P.A} = \frac{\sigma^2_A}{\sigma^2_P} = \frac{119.5}{144.5} = 0.8276$$

$$r_{PR} = \frac{Cov_{PR}}{\sigma_P \sigma_R} = \frac{\sigma^2_R}{\sigma_P \sigma_R} = \frac{\sigma_R}{\sigma_P} = P_{P.R}$$

$$r^2_{PR} = d_{P.R} = \frac{\sigma^2_R}{\sigma^2_P} = \frac{25}{144.5} = 0.1733$$

$$r^2_{PA} + r^2_{PR} = 1$$

or $d_{P.A} + d_{P.R} = 1$

$0.8276 + 0.1733 = 1.0009$

The squared correlation co-efficient is known as co-efficient of determination. In case of independent causing factors, the following relationship holds true:

$$r^2_{PA} \quad = p^2_{P.A} = d_{P.A}$$

and $\qquad r^2_{PR} \quad = p^2_{P.R} = d_{P.R}$

The $r^2_{PA} = p^2_{P.A} = d_{P.A}$ measures the portion of variance in phenotypic value (P) which is determined by that of breeding value (A) and in this example $r^2_{PA} = h^2$, while $r^2_{PR} = P^2_{P.R} = d_{P.R}$ measures the portion to which the variance of P value is determined by that of R and in this example r^2_{PR} is equal to $1-h^2$. Therefore, 82.76 per cent of the variation in phenotypic value is due to the variation in breeding value while 17.33 per cent is due to combined effect of non-additive gene effects and environmental effects.

The relationship among path coefficient, correlation coefficient and coefficient of determination holds true if the dependent variable (effect) is a linear combination of more than two causing factors which are independent to each other. In this situation the deviations of dependent variable are additive indicating that a given amount of change in one causing factor is reflected in the dependent variable, irrespective of its own value of other causes.

Example 27.3

The values of following variables are given below.

Variables		Values				Total	Mean	C.S.S.
A	29	20	28	14	9	100	20.0	302
D	13	16	11	14	11	65	13.0	18
G	42	36	39	28	20	165	33.0	320
E	9	47	42	9	33	140	28.0	1304
P	51	83	81	37	53	305	61.0	1624

Verify the following relations:

(i) $d_{P.A} = d_{P.G} d_{G.A}$ and $p_{P.A} = p_{P.G} p_{G.A}$

(ii) $d_{P.D} = d_{P.G} d_{G.D}$ and $p_{P.D} = p_{P.G} p_{G.D}$

(iii) Complete determination of $G = d_{G.A} + d_{G.D} = 1.0$

(iv) Complete determination of $P = d_{P.G} + d_{P.E} = d_{P.A} + d_{P.D} + d_{P.E} = 1.0$

Solution

The variation based on numerical values is as under -

(i) $d_{P.A}$ $= d_{P.G} d_{G.A}$

$$\frac{302}{1624} = \frac{320}{1624} \times \frac{302}{320}$$

$$= \frac{320}{1624} = 0.1860$$

$p_{P.A}$ $= p_{P.G} p_{G.A}$

$$\sqrt{\frac{302}{1624}} = \sqrt{\frac{320}{1624}} \times \sqrt{\frac{302}{320}}$$

$$= \sqrt{\frac{320}{1624}} = \sqrt{0.1860} = 0.4312$$

(ii) $d_{P.D}$ $= d_{P.G} d_{G.D}$

$$\frac{18}{1624} = \frac{320}{1624} \times \frac{18}{320}$$

$$= \frac{18}{1624} = 0.0111$$

$p_{P.D}$ $= p_{P.G} p_{G.D}$
$= \sqrt{0.0111} = 0.1053$

(iii) Complete determination of $G = d_{G.A} + d_{G.D} = 1.0$

$$d_{G.A} \quad = \frac{302}{320} = 0.9437$$

$$d_{G.D} \quad = \frac{18}{320} = 0.0563$$

Thus,

$d_{G.A} + d_{G.D} = 0.9437 + 0.0563 = 1.0$

(iv) Complete determination of $P = d_{P.G} + d_{P.E} = 1.0$

$$= d_{P.A} + d_{P.D} + d_{P.E} = 1.0$$

$$d_{P.G} = \frac{320}{1624} = 0.1970;$$

Also $d_{P.G} = d_{P.A} + d_{P.D}$
$$= 0.1860 + 0.011 = 0.197$$

$$d_{P.E} = \frac{1304}{1624} = 0.8030$$

Thus, $P = d_{P.G} + d_{P.E}$
$$= 0.197 + 0.803 = 1.0$$

Example 27.4

The correlated causes as per casual scheme given in figure 27.5 (X=G+R) where G=A+D and R=D+E, the intermediate causes G and R are correlated by their common cause D.

The standard deviation of A=8.69, $\sigma_D = 2.12$, $\sigma_E = 24.92$, $\sigma_G = 8.94$, $\sigma_R = 25.02$,

$$Cov_{GR} = 18$$

(i) Find out the values of path coefficients g, r, d, d'

(ii) Verify that $r_{GR} = d\,d'$

(iii) Find out the values of dP.A., dP.D and dP.E taking P=A+2D+E and see whether they are equal to unity.

Example 27.5

The casual scheme of uncorrelated causes (B and C) given in figure 27.7 is that X=B+C and Y=B+3C whereas the $\sigma_B = 8.94$; $\sigma_C = 4.63$; $\sigma_X = 10.07$; $\sigma_Y = 16.53$; $Cov_{XB} = Cov_{YB} = 80.0$; $Cov_{XC} = 86$; $Cov_{YC} = 3 \times 86 = 258$; $Cov_{XY} = 144.5$; $Cov_{BC} = 0$. Find out the values of 4 path coefficients b, b', c, c' and verify that $r_{XY} = bb' + cc'$

Example 27.6

Consider the casual scheme of given in figure 27.8 for correlated common causes (B and C) and that X=A+B+C and Y=10C+3C+D. The $\sigma_A = 11.68$; $\sigma_B = 5.34$; $\sigma_C = 21.38$; $\sigma_D = 82.72$; $\sigma_X = 28.53$; $\sigma_Y = 139.90$; $Cov_{XB} = 109$; $Cov_{XC} = 484$; $Cov_{BC} = 84$

(i) Find out the values of 6 path coefficients.

(ii) Verify that $a^2 + b^2 + c^2 + 2bcr_{BC} = 1.0$

(iii) Show that $r_{XY} = bb' + cc' + (bc' + cb')r_{BC}$

9 789351 306634